T0271932

CONCISE BIOCHEMISTRY

ANATOLY BEZKOROVAINY

MAX E. RAFELSON, JR.

**Rush Medical College
Rush-Presbyterian–St. Luke's Medical Center
Rush University
Chicago, Illinois**

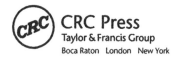

CRC Press
Taylor & Francis Group
Boca Raton   London   New York

CRC Press is an imprint of the
Taylor & Francis Group, an informa business

Library of Congress Cataloging-in-Publication Data

Bezkorovainy, Anatoly.
    Concise biochemistry / Anatoly Bezkorovainy, Max E. Rafelson. Jr.
      p.   cm.
    Includes bibliographical references and index.
    1. Biochemistry. I. Rafelson, Max E. II. Title.
    QP514.2.844 1995   95-25212
    574.19′2—dc20   CIP
    cloth: ISBN 0-8247-9659-4 (alk. paper)
    paper: ISBN 0-8247-9736-1 (alk. paper)

The publisher offers discounts on this book when ordered in bulk quantities. For more information, write to Special Sales/Professional Marketing at the address below.

Marcel Dekker, Inc.
270 Madison Avenue, New York, New York 10016

Current printing (last digit):
10 9 8 7 6 5 4 3 2 1

To the memory of
PROFESSOR RICHARD J. WINZLER
mentor, colleague, and friend

Preface

Biochemical educators are forever on the lookout for the text most suitable for their biochemistry courses, be they in the undergraduate, graduate, medical, nursing, medical technology, or veterinary school environments. Some medical school biochemistry teachers feel that the "major leap forward [in designing a suitable text] came with the publication of the first edition of Stryer's *Biochemistry* in 1975," and it is now expected that every new text should conform to this standard of "excellent illustrations and a bright style" (K. R. F. Elliott, History, trivia and TIBS defined, but little else. *TIBS* 15(1):35–36, 1990). However, as such books become more and more voluminous and more and more lavishly and elaborately illustrated, one wonders if there isn't a place in the biochemical world for a textbook of the nuts and bolts type, which would present the basic material in a concise, cost-effective, and rational manner. This need for a comprehensive yet concise text is especially obvious when one looks at the demands placed upon first-year medical students. The explosion in knowledge of the past decades, and the rapid pace at which this knowledge, rightly or wrongly, is being communicated during the preclinical years, allows for only a limited number of daily hours that can be devoted to reading. Thus, although a 1200-page biochemistry text may be "required" by a professor, few, if any, students may in fact read it carefully, and they may depend heavily on handouts instead.

Years ago, Rafelson and Binkley recognized this need and published *Basic Biochemistry* (Macmillan), which went through four editions after it first appeared in 1965. The book was limited to less than 400 pages, and the authors stated that their intent was to introduce "to the student in life sciences and allied disciplines the principles and viewpoints of biochemistry and a core of essential facts, without presenting an overwhelming amount of factual material." The current text continues the tradition set by *Basic Biochemistry*, although it is no longer possible to achieve its goals within only 400 pages.

This text is designed to meet the needs of students in those health care–oriented professions that require biochemistry in their curricula. Judging from our personal experience, this text would meet the needs of students in medical, podiatric medicine, optometry, and medical technology programs. Its health sciences orientation may make it suitable for undergraduate premedical biochemistry courses as well. As an aide to learning, behavioral objectives are stated at the beginning of each chapter, and multiple-choice questions are posed at the end of each chapter. Answers with the appropriate explanations are also provided. The questions are designed solely for a review process and not necessarily to prepare students for their licensure exams. In addition to these questions, each chapter contains open-ended queries that require more than rote learning. Many of these have been taken from published case reports, with the citations provided in the instructor's manual. Successful handling of these questions may require some outside reading.

Many illustrations in this volume have been taken from previous editions of *Basic Biochemistry*, many others are reproduced with permission from the primary biochemical literature, review articles, and specialized monographs, and still others have been drawn for this text. Those reproduced from the primary or secondary research literature should provide a link between the students in the classroom and the world of research scientists.

Special care has been taken to present the material in a rational order or sequence. Part I of the book is concerned with properties of biologically important materials. Part II is concerned with the properties of nucleic acids, their metabolism, and their function as carriers of genetic information. The last part, Part III, discusses intermediary metabolism and its regulation. This order of presentation and structures of individual chapters may not be very conventional and not to everyone's liking. But this approach makes sense to us, and we have used it successfully in various teaching situations.

Several individuals and organizations have been extremely helpful in our quest to produce this text. We are appreciative of those colleagues and publishers who gave us permission to reproduce their tables and figures. We thank Dr. Klaus Kuettner, Chairman of the Department of Biochemistry at Rush, who gave his enthusiastic and unequivocal support for this project. Ms. Shirley Moore was our principal typist, and Theresa Snarski was our expert illustrator.

Finally, we would like to pay homage to our predecessors and thank them for the leadership and inspiration they have provided to the biochemical profession. We fondly remember the late Dr. Stephen B. Binkley, a colleague and an author of the first three editions of *Basic Biochemistry*. One of us also had the unforgettable experience as a student of using the first edition of A. White et al., *Principles of Biochemistry* (McGraw-Hill) in the mid-1950s. It is therefore with a great degree of admiration and gratitude that we endeavor to join our forebears and hope that our contribution will complement theirs in our common goal to provide the most effective and efficient education possible to future biomedical professionals.

Anatoly Bezkorovainy
Max E. Rafelson, Jr.

Contents

Appendixes

I

COMPONENTS OF CELLS

1

Characteristics of Cells

After completing this chapter, the student should

1. Know the differences in cellular architecture between prokaryotic and eukaryotic cells.
2. Be able to describe the structures and general functions of cell walls, plasma membranes, nucleus and nucleoid region, mitochondria, lysosomes, peroxisomes, endoplasmic reticulum, cytoskeleton, and extracellular matrix.

1.1 INTRODUCTION

We know that all living organisms are composed of cells and cell products, that all cells arise from other cells, and that all organisms have arisen from a common primordial ancestor by evolutionary diversification. Several different evolutionary scenarios have been proposed, and each has its proponents. Although it is not possible to make an absolute choice on the bases of current biochemical and morphologic data, we have arbitrarily selected the scheme shown in Figure 1.1. In this scheme, the putative and undefined common ancestor is believed to be far less complex than any known *prokaryotic organism* (cells without a membrane-bound nucleus). This common ancestor is presumed to have diverged to yield three different prokaryotic lines. The archaebacteria and eubacteria (true bacteria) kept the prokaryotic pattern of cellular organization, whereas *eukaryotic* organisms (cells with a membrane-bound nucleus) evolved from a third prokaryotic ancestor and developed a compartmentalized cellular structure. Archaebacteria are amazing organisms: they thrive in the most hostile of environments, for example under extreme salt conditions (halophilous), hot acid conditions (sulfur bacteria), bogs, where they reduce CO_2 to methane (methanogens), and at extreme ocean depths.

Compared with eukaryotes, prokaryotes have a much simpler internal structure, but are nevertheless biochemically diverse and complex. Table 1.1 compares some general properties of prokaryotic and eukaryotic cells. The gram-negative bacterium *Escherichia coli* is the best understood prokaryote both bio-

Table 1.1 General Comparison of Prokaryotic and Eukaryotic Cells

	Prokaryotes	Eukaryotes
Cell size	1–10 μm[a] in linear length	10–1000 μm in linear length
Cell division	Binary fission, budding, spore formation by a few	Mitosis (or meiosis)
Nuclear membrane	Absent	Present
Nucleolus	Absent	Present
Number of chromosomes	One	More than one
DNA	Single, circular, double-helical molecule densely coiled, not bound to histones; not membrane bound	Very long linear molecules with extensive noncoding regions; complexed histones and other proteins; organized into chromosomes in membrane-bounded nucleus
Cell structures		
Nucleus	Absent	Present
Endoplasmic reticulum	Absent	Present
Mitochondria	Absent	Present
Golgi apparatus	Absent	Present
Lysosomes	Absent	Present
Peroxisomes	Absent	Present
Chloroplasts	Absent	Present in plants
Ribosome size	70S	80S
Microtubules	Absent	Present
Microfilaments	Absent	Present
Intermediate filaments	Absent	Present
Cell wall with peptidoglycans[b]	Present, except in archaebacteria and mycoplasms	Absent
Functional characteristics		
Endocytosis[c]	Absent	Present
Exocytosis[d]	Absent	Present
Site of electron transport	Cell membrane	Organelle membranes
RNA and protein synthesis	Together in same compartment	RNA synthesized in nucleus; protein synthesized in cytoplasm

[a]Micrometer = 10^{-6} m.

[b]Complex of covalently linked carbohydrates and amino acids; can be thin, as in *E. coli* (a gram-negative bacterium), or thick with several layers, as in *Bacillus* (gram-positive organisms: those stained by the dyes crystal violet and iodine).

[c]Uptake of extracellular solutes or particles by infolding of the plasma membrane, followed by budding of a membrane-bound vesicle and its movement into the cell.

[d]Fission of vesicular membranes with plasma membrane with the subsequent expulsion of the vesicular contents to the extracellular environment.

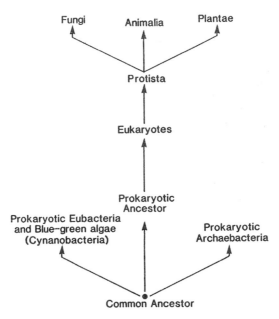

Figure 1.1 Evolutionary scheme proposed by C. R. Woese and G. E. Fox. Protista are defined as any eukaryotic organism not included in Animalia, Fungi, or Plantae.

chemically and genetically, and we use it in our discussion here as well as in subsequent chapters.

Eukaryotic cells are much larger and much more complex in structure than prokaryotic cells. They include fungi, most algae, protozoa, plants, and animals. Such cells contain several membrane-bound organelles specialized to carry out specific cellular processes (Figure 1.2 and see Table 5.1). These components include the nucleus, mitochondrion, lysosome, Golgi apparatus, peroxisomes, and the smooth and rough (with ribosomes) endoplasmic reticulum. Everything other than these compartments is referred to as cytosol.

1.2 CELL MEMBRANES, CELL WALLS, AND CELL COATS

Escherichia coli (gram negative) is surrounded by an outer membrane characterized by unique lipopolysaccharides, whose highly specific polysaccharide side chains extend outward. Also present are matrix proteins (*porins*), which are specific pores through which extracellular molecules must pass to enter the cell. In addition, there is a lipoprotein that anchors the outer membrane to a thin cell wall consisting of peptidoglycan and associated protein. Beneath this is the cytoplasmic membrane. The area between the outer and inner membrane is the *periplasmic space* and is filled with peptidoglycan that is dense near the outer membrane and fluid near the cytoplasmic membrane (Figure 1.3). Also present are specific binding proteins that facilitate the transport of specific nutrient molecules across the inner cytoplasmic membrane, specific chemoreceptors that sense the concentration of substances in the environment and enable cells to move toward or away from them,

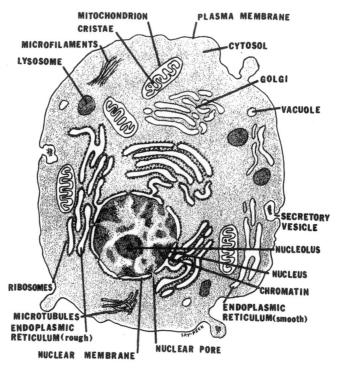

Figure 1.2 Typical eukaryotic cell. (Courtesy of Dr. Howard H. Sky-Peck, Rush Medical College.)

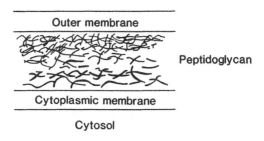

Figure 1.3 Arrangement of peptidoglycan in gram-negative bacteria.

and hydrolytic enzymes that degrade nutrient molecules. Inserted within the inner phospholipid-containing cytoplasmic membrane are the components of the oxidative phosphorylation system (flavoproteins, quinones, iron sulfur proteins, and cytochromes). Two-dimensional gel electrophoresis has shown that more than 200 proteins are localized in this membrane. In the cytosol are the enzymes for the synthesis and degradation of soluble substrates and for DNA replication, transcription (mRNA synthesis), and translation (protein synthesis).

Gram-positive cells are composed of a thick porous cell wall composed of a sugar–amino acid heteropolymer (peptidoglycan), polyolphosphate polymers (teichoic acids), and generally little lipid. It is generally believed that gram-positive cells do not have an outer lipopolysaccharide membrane, although it is possible that there are some proteins on the outer surface of these cells and that the difference between gram-negative and gram-positive cells is caused primarily by the difference in the amount of peptidoglycan in each. A cytoplasmic membrane lies beneath the cell wall with properties similar to that in gram-negative organisms.

Cell walls in bacteria are porous structures that provide structural integrity and physically protect the cell from swelling and bursting in a hypotonic environment. If the cell wall is removed, the bacteria assume a spherical shape. Cell walls contain specific antigens useful for the diagnosis of some infectious diseases. Inhibitions of the biosynthesis of the bacterial cell wall is the basis for the bactericidal action of penicillin and some other antibiotics.

Eukaryotic cells are also characterized by one or more structures exterior to the cytoplasmic membrane. Plant cells have a rigid cellulose-containing cell wall, and animal cells have a cell coat composed of *glycoproteins* (contain carbohydrate) and other components that do not confine the cell but are important in cell–cell recognition.

Membrane structure and function are discussed in some detail in Chapter 9 and in the discussion of the intracellular organelles that follows. It is worthwhile to note here that biologic membranes, whether the cytoplasmic membrane or those of intracellular organelles, play active and unique roles in the integrated metabolism and function of cells.

1.3 NUCLEOID REGION AND NUCLEUS

In *E. coli* and other prokaryotes, DNA is localized in a nucleoid region with no surrounding membrane. All genes are contained on a single, double-stranded, supercoiled, circular DNA molecule. The extended length of the "circle" is about 1300 μm, with a diameter of 2×10^{-3} μm. Because *E. coli* has a diameter and a length of about 1 and 2–3 μm, respectively, it is obvious that its DNA must be highly coiled and folded to reside in the cell.

A highly compact structure can be isolated that contains a single, supercoiled DNA molecule and protein. This is the bacterial chromosome or *nucleoid*. Because removal of protein decreases the compactness of this structure, it is concluded that the protein acts as a scaffold to keep the nucleoid in a compact state by binding to specific regions of the DNA molecule. The nucleoid DNA is also attached to the cytoplasmic membrane.

In addition to the nucleoid DNA, small circular molecules of double-stranded DNA occur in bacteria and replicate autonomously as the host cell proliferates. These are *plasmids*, and they carry the genes required for replication of themselves as well as for other functions, such as resistance to antibiotics. They can be readily separated from the nucleoid DNA, modified by splicing a piece of "foreign" DNA into it, and used as a vehicle for the cloning of the "foreign" DNA (Chapter 15).

The nucleus of the eukaryotic cell is separated from the cytoplasm by the double-membrane nuclear envelope, which provides a continuous boundary between the nucleoplasm and the cytoplasm, except where it is penetrated by nuclear pores, each of which is surrounded by a disklike structure, the nuclear pore complex. These pores serve an export–import function for an exchange of materials between the nucleus and the cytosol. This is necessary in eukaryotic cells in which *transcription* (RNA synthesis) and *translation* (protein synthesis) are separated both spatially and temporally. In prokaryotic cells, transcription and translation take place concurrently.

Eukaryotic DNA is organized into distinct units, *chromosomes*, each containing a single enormous DNA molecule. Such a DNA molecule may have a molecular weight greater than 10^{10} and an extended length of $1.2 \times 10^4\ \mu m$. The ratio of length to width ($2 \times 10^{-3}\ \mu m$) is 6×10^6! Because a chromosome is more compact than the DNA molecule, the DNA is compacted by a series of foldings, each of which is mediated by one or more protein molecules.

Basic proteins, *histones* (Chapter 10), are bound in roughly equal amount to the DNA to form the complex *chromatin*. Chromatin has repeating beadlike structures, *nucleosomes*, that consist of various histones and 150–240 base pairs of DNA. Chromatin and chromosome structures change as the cell proceeds through its growth cycle (Chapter 13). The nucleus contains a distinct intranuclear organelle, the *nucleolus*, which contains both granular and fibrillar components and functions in ribosomal RNA synthesis and ribosome assembly. The appearance of the nucleolus also changes during the cell cycle.

1.4 OTHER EUKARYOTIC ORGANELLES

1.4.1 Mitochondria

These organelles are the sites of energy production of aerobic cells and contain the enzymes of the tricarboxylic acid cycle, the respiratory chain, and the fatty acid oxidation system. The mitochondrion is bounded by a pair of specialized membranes that define the separate mitochondrial compartments, the internal matrix space and an intermembrane space. Molecules of 10,000 daltons or less can penetrate the outer membrane, but most of these molecules cannot pass the selectively permeable inner membrane. By a series of infoldings, the internal membrane forms *cristae* in the matrix space. The components of the respiratory chain and the enzyme complex that makes ATP are embedded in the inner membrane as well as a number of transport proteins that make it selectively permeable to small molecules that are metabolized by the enzymes in the matrix space. Matrix enzymes include those of the tricarboxylic acid cycle, the fatty acid oxidation system, and others.

In mammalian cells, some 1% of the total cellular DNA is found in the mitochondria. This DNA is double stranded, circular, and small, with a molecular weight of about 10 million, which is in the same range as that of viral DNAs. Some four to ten molecules of DNA per mitochondrion, along with some ribosomes, are found in the matrix space. DNA replication, transcription, and synthesis of *some* mitochondrial proteins take place in the matrix space. This protein synthesis very much resembles that of bacteria. The mitochondrial genetic code differs from the "universal" genetic code (Chapter 12) used for nuclearly encoded proteins and bacteria. The reasons for this are unknown.

1.4.2 Lysosomes

Most animal cells contain *lysosomes*, which have a single limiting membrane and contain a variety of hydrolases (some 40 enzymes) used for the controlled intracellular digestion of macromolecules. The enzymes are all acid hydrolases optimally active near the pH of 5 maintained within this organelle. Proteins, nucleic acids, and unneeded intracellular organelles, as well as foreign substances, are internalized by *pinocytosis*, which involves the ingestion of fluids and their solutes, or by *phagocytosis*, which involves the ingestion of large particles, such as microorganisms or cell debris. These are two types of *endocytosis*, in which the material to be ingested is enclosed by a portion of the plasma membrane, which invaginates and then is pinched off to form an intracellular vesicle containing the ingested material. Normal lysosomal digestive products can diffuse across the lysosomal membrane and be reutilized by the cell. Accumulated indigestible material can be removed by *exocytosis*.

There are numerous inherited disorders of lysosomal metabolism in humans. These disorders result from the lack of a specific acid hydrolase and have several clinical manifestations. A variety of substances may accumulate that interfere with normal cell functions, as is the case with the lipidoses (Chapter 9) or mucopolysaccharides (glycosaminoglycans) in the Hurler's disease (gargoylism).

1.4.3 Peroxisomes

These are single membrane-bounded organelles, present in almost all eukaryotic cells and specialized for carrying out oxidative reactions with molecular oxygen. Peroxisomes contain D-amino acid oxidase, urate oxidase, and most of the cell's catalase, which uses H_2O_2 generated by these and other enzymes to oxidize substrates, such as alcohol, formaldehyde, formic acid, and phenols. Half of ingested alcohol is oxidized to acetaldehyde by this reaction. Because H_2O_2 is highly toxic, the cell is protected by having the peroxide-producing and utilizing enzymes in the same cellular compartment.

In addition, most peroxisomes catalyze the oxidation of long-chain fatty acids to acetyl CoA (coenzyme A), which can be transported through the cytosol to mitochondria for use in the tricarboxylic acid cycle.

1.4.4 Endoplasmic Reticulum

The endoplasmic reticulum (ER) is characterized by several membrane complexes that are interconnected by separate organelles. These membranes and the aqueous channels they enclose are *cisternae*. The ER merges with the outer membrane of the nuclear envelope and is closely associated with the Golgi apparatus. Near the nucleus, the ER is coated on the cytoplasmic side with ribosomes and is called rough endoplasmic reticulum. Microsomes, which do *not* occur in cells, are formed during cell fractionation from the rough ER. These are vesicles studded with ribosomes on the outside surface. The interior corresponds to the luminal space of the ER. The·smooth endoplasmic reticulum has no attached ribosomes and forms smooth microsomes that can be separated from rough microsomes by sedimenting the mixture to equilibrium in sucrose density gradients. Rough ER synthesizes membrane lipids and proteins for export via the lumen of the cisternae. Smooth ER is not involved in protein snythesis but is involved in the modification and transport of proteins synthesized in the rough ER and in lipid production.

1.4.5   Golgi Apparatus

The *Golgi apparatus* is a network of flattened smooth membranes and vesicles and is closely associated with the ER. It apparently receives proteins from the ER on one side and releases via secretory vesicle modified proteins on the other side. Carbohydrates and lipids are added to proteins to form glyco- and lipoproteins.

1.4.6   Eukaryotic Cytoskeleton

Eukaryotic cells have an internal scaffolding called the cytoskeleton or cytomatrix that maintains their cellular morphology and enables them to migrate, undergo shape changes, and transport vesicles. *Microfilaments*, made of actin, *intermediate filaments*, which are composed of laminin and other proteins, and *microtubules*, formed from the protein tubulin, along with many different accessory proteins, comprise the cytoskeleton. Both the microfilaments and the microtubules can assemble and disassemble rapidly in the cell, whereas disassembly of intermediate filaments may require their destruction. Although much is known about the molecular composition of the cytoskeleton, the molecular events involved in most cell movements are still unknown.

1.4.7   Extracellular Matrix

Cells in tissues are in contact with a complex network of extracellular macromolecules (the *extracellular matrix*). Besides holding cells and tissues together, this matrix provides a lattice within which cells can migrate and interact with each other. This matrix contains three major fiber-forming proteins, collagen, elastin, and fibronectin, enmeshed in a network of glycosaminoglycan chains. Collagen can assemble in highly ordered arrays (Chapter 8). Elastin fibers impart elasticity to the network, and fibronectin forms fibers that promote cell adhesion. All these macromolecules are secreted locally by cells in contact with the matrix.

1.4.8   Cytosol

Most intermediary metabolism takes place in the cytosol, which represents about 55% of the total cell volume. It is here that the biosynthesis of sugars, amino acids, fatty acids, nucleotides, and the reactions of glycolysis and gluconeogenesis take place. It is unlikely that the sequential enzymes in glycolysis, for example, are running around looking for their substrates, or vice versa. It is more likely that the variety of cytoskeletal proteins impart some organization to the cytosol so that nonrandom encounters are maximized. It is known that the cytosol immediately surrounding the Golgi apparatus is not identical to that surrounding the nucleus. When cells are disrupted, however, this type of organization cannot be preserved for study. Little if anything is known about the mechanisms by which such organization could be achieved.

1.5   VIRUSES

Because viruses are not cellular, they are neither prokaryotes nor eukaryotes. All known viruses contain a core of either DNA or RNA (but never both) surrounded by a protective protein coat (*capsid*). Some capsids are complex and

Table 1.2 Virus Types

Nucleic acid	Virus example	Long dimension (nm)	No. of genes
Single-stranded DNA	ϕx174	18	5
Double-stranded DNA	Adeno	70	30
	T_4-phage	200	150
Single-stranded RNA	Tobacco mosaic	300	6
	Polio	30	8
	Influenza	50	12
Double-stranded RNA	Reovirus	100	22

contain many proteins, as well as carbohydrate and lipid molecules, whereas in the small RNA bacterial viruses the capsid contains only one type of protein and no lipid or carbohydrate. Their size can range from about 18 to 300 nm (nm = 10^{-9} m), and each virus has its own characteristic shape. Their genome (nucleic acid) may be single-stranded or double-stranded RNA or DNA and can contain as few as 4 genes or as many as 250 genes. Some representative virus types and their properties are shown in Table 1.2.

Are viruses alive? The answer is no: no known virus can give rise directly to any other virus by any self-duplication process. Instead, they must subvert the metabolic and genetic machinery of a host cell for the synthesis of capsid protein(s) required for the packaging of the RNA or DNA that arises by copying the genetic information of the parent virus. Some viruses specify proteins that alter host cellular metabolism to enhance selective expression of the viral genome. For example, they may encode a virus-specific RNA polymerase or a nuclease that destroys the host DNA. Viruses may be regarded as small pieces of itinerant genetic material enclosed in a protective protein coat that facilitates their transport from one cell to another. Like a cellular chromosome, a viral chromosome can replicate only in the complex environment of a living cell. Genetic mechanisms are very similar in viruses and cells; for example, virus genes are also subject to mutations and recombinations. Because viruses have no protein-synthesizing systems of their own, they must appropriate that of the host cell. As a result, it is perhaps not surprising that the virtually universal genetic code (Chapter 12) encoded for viral proteins as well as those of prokaryotic and eukaryotic cells.

QUESTIONS

In Questions 1.1–1.4, indicate the occurrence as follows:
    a. Prokaryotes   c. Both
    b. Eukaryotes   d. Neither

1.1.   Cell wall
1.2.   Plasma membrane
1.3.   Nuclear membrane
1.4.   Microsomes

In Questions 1.5–1.10 choose answers from the following:
  a. Mitochondria   d. Cytosol
  b. Nucleus   e. Extracellular space
  c. Lysosomes

1.5.   Repository of hydrolytic enzymes
1.6.   Contains circular DNA
1.7.   Collagen and proteoglycans located in ____
1.8.   Glycolytic pathway enzymes located in ____
1.9.   Contains a double membrane, one relatively porous the other nonporous
1.10. Contains a single chromosome

Answers

1.1.   (c)   Cell wall is present in both the bacterial cells and some eukaryotic systems, such as plants.
1.2.   (c)   Both eukaryotes and prokaryotes have cell membranes that enclose the cell contents and act as barriers to the entry of a number of substances.
1.3.   (b)   Eukaryotes have only subcellular particles, including the nucleus.
1.4.   (d)   Microsomes are not present in either cell type. They are artifacts of endoplasmic reticulum preparation.
1.5.   (c)   Lysosomes contain proteolytic and other hydrolytic enzymes.
1.6.   (a)   Circular DNA is present in prokaryotes and in the mitochondria of eukaryotes.
1.7.   (e)   Collagen, a fibrous protein, and proteoglycans constitute the matrix in which cells are located.
1.8.   (d)   The glycolysis pathway is an intermediate metabolism pathway for glucose oxidation located in the cytosol.
1.9.   (a)   Mitochondria are encased in outer (porous) and an inner (nonporous) membrane.
1.10. (a)   The only eukaryotic structures that contain DNA are the nucleus and the mitochondria. In mitochondria there is one chromosome; in the nucleus, many chromosomes.

PROBLEM

It has been hypothesized that mitochondria arose from bacteria during the course of evolution. List some similarities between the bacteria on the one hand and mitochondria on the other. To make this hypothesis stronger, what other evidence should be obtained?

BIBLIOGRAPHY

Alberts B, Bray D, Lewis J, Raff M, Roberts K, Watson J. Molecular Biology of the Cell, 3rd ed. New York: Garland, 1994.
Hopkins CH. Structure and Function of Cells. Philadelphia: WB Saunders, 1978.
Piez KA., Reddi AH. Extracellular Matrix Biochemistry. New York: Elsevier, 1984.
Watson J, Hopkins N, Roberts J, Steitz J, Werner A. Molecular Biology of the Gene, Vol. 1, 4th ed. Menlo Park: Benjamin-Cummings, 1987.
Woese CR. Bacterial evolution. Microbiol Rev 51:221–271 (1987).

2

Bioenergetics

After completing this chapter, the student should

1. Be familiar with the concepts of the first and second laws of thermodynamics.
2. Be able to calculate free energies from equilibrium constants and redox potentials and do so under nonstandard conditions using the appropriate equations involving reactant and product concentrations at the beginning of the reaction.
3. From free energy and redox potential calculations, be able to predict in which direction chemical reactions will proceed.
4. Know the effect of temperature on equilibrium constants, free energy, and entropy and enthalpy changes.
5. Be familiar with the concept of a high-energy phosphate bond, and be able to calculate the overall free energy change for reactions coupled to ATP hydrolysis.
6. Understand why anhydride bonds are unstable from a chemical point of view.
7. Be able to calculate the energy charge and phosphorylation potential for a cell.
8. Be able to calculate the ATP yield for any organic substance.

2.1 INTRODUCTION

Tissues carry out an enormous number of chemical reactions. Collectively these are referred to as *metabolism*. Some reactions or reaction sequences (often referred to as metabolic pathways) create complex molecules from simpler molecules, and these processes are then called *anabolism*. Many reactions, however, serve to break down complex molecules into simple molecules, and these processes are called *catabolism*. Among the latter is the degradation of foodstuffs, such as proteins, carbohydrates, and fats. Often these are degraded to CO_2 and H_2O, which are excreted by the organism. The purpose of doing this is to acquire useful energy, which is in turn required for the various life processes, including muscle contraction, maintenance of gradients across membranes, cell replication, and intestinal motility.

Every chemical reaction, including those in the living organism, is accompanied by an energy change. Whereas a high percentage of anabolic processes require an energy input, the reverse is true for catabolic processes. The degradation of foodstuffs results in the release of energy that the organism can harness for its needs. Energy may be expressed in calories or joules. One calorie is that amount of energy required to raise the temperature of 1 g water from 14.5 to 15.5°C; 1000 cal is a kilocalorie (kcal). Food package labeling often includes nutritional information, including the energy content of one "serving." This is usually given in "calories," which in reality are kilocalories. For various reasons, recent trends in the bioenergetics field have utilized joules rather than calories. Each calorie is equal to 4.18 J, and 1000 J is a kilojoule (kJ).

2.2 FIRST LAW OF THERMODYNAMICS

The first law of thermodynamics is the law of conservation of energy. Energy can be neither created or destroyed. Thus,

$$Q = W + \Delta U \tag{2.1}$$

where Q is the energy added or subtracted to or from a system, W is work done, and ΔU is an internal energy change. When Q is negative, heat is lost from the system to its surroundings, and when Q is positive, energy is absorbed. Work is done by the system on its surroundings when W is negative. If it is of the $p\Delta V$ type, where p is pressure and V is volume, then

$$Q_p = p\Delta V + \Delta U \tag{2.2}$$

Here, Q is at constant pressure. All in vivo biologic reactions are considered to take place at a constant pressure.

When the only work performed is of the $p\Delta V$ type, Q_p is termed the *enthalpy change* (ΔH). It can be measured in a constant-pressure calorimeter. If heat is given off in such a calorimeter experiment, the reaction is exothermic and ΔH is negative. If heat is absorbed, the reaction is endothermic and ΔH is positive. In chemical compounds, enthalpies of formation are related to the sum of their bond energies.

The first law of thermodynamics allows us to rate foods in terms of their energy contents. These are really ΔH of combustion values. Thus, carbohydrates, fats, proteins, and ethanol yield approximately 4, 9, 4, and 7 kcal/g, respectively when combusted. A normally active person requires between 2000 and 2500 kcal/day in foodstuffs to function normally. Persons doing heavy work may require as much as 5000 kcal/day or more.

2.3 SECOND LAW OF THERMODYNAMICS

2.3.1 Definition of Free Energy

The second law of thermodynamics is of major importance in the biomedical sciences, because it can be used to predict the direction of chemical reactions. It states that all systems tend to reach an equilibrium, that is, the thermodynamically most stable state. This is the state of maximum randomness or disorder. A measure of randomness is the *entropy S*. It increases as randomness increases, so that at equilibrium it is maximum. Changes in entropy are designated ΔS.

A reaction occurs spontaneously if the entropy of the system and its surroundings increases. Thus, the entropy of the universe is always on the increase: it never decreases. Unfortunately, changes in entropy cannot be measured directly. Instead, another thermodynamic parameter, the free energy change ΔG, is used. ΔG is that amount of energy generated by a chemical reaction that can do useful work. ΔS and ΔG are related by Equation (2.3):

$$\Delta G = \Delta H - T\Delta S \tag{2.3}$$

This relationship indicates that useful work ΔG is equal to the overall energy (heat) change ΔH minus that amount of energy not available to do useful work and in some sense is dependent on a change in the internal randomness of molecules $T\Delta S$. T is the temperature in degrees Kelvin, ΔG and ΔH are in calories, and ΔS is in cal/degree (entropy units). Equation (2.3) may be derived from the concepts of the first law of thermodynamics as follows: From Equation (2.2), we can write $\Delta U = \Delta H - p\Delta V$. Substituting the expression for ΔU in Equation (2.1), we obtain $Q = W + \Delta H - p\Delta V$. If we define W as $p\Delta V + W'$, where W' is useful work of the non-$p\Delta V$ type, then $Q = \Delta H + W'$. If no work is done, then $Q = \Delta H$. Rearranging this equation, we obtain

$$-W' = \Delta H - Q \tag{2.4}$$

Considerations from the classic Carnot cycle define ΔS as Q/T and $Q = T\Delta S$. Substituting this relationship into Equation (2.4) and substituting ΔG for W', we obtain Equation (2.3), $\Delta G = \Delta H - T\Delta S$.

The term ΔG is extremely useful, because, unlike ΔS, it can be determined, and it predicts the direction of chemical reactions. If ΔG is negative, the reaction proceeds as written, that is, it is spontaneous in the direction in which it is written. If ΔG is positive, the reaction proceeds in a direction opposite to that in which it is written. When ΔG is 0, the reaction is in equilibrium. However, ΔG provides no information on how fast a reaction will go or what path it will take. Its magnitude will be the same no matter what path is taken, as long as the starting and the finishing points are the same. A negative ΔH and a positive ΔS certainly contribute to the spontaneity of a chemical reaction (negative ΔG); however, a negative ΔH and a positive ΔS need not coexist to result in a negative ΔG. For example, a large negative ΔH can overcome a small negative ΔS to give a high negative ΔG, as in the combustion of alcohols.

2.3.2 Determination of Free Energy Changes

Free energy change cannot be determined directly: it may be calculated from other data. The standard free energy ΔG_0 can be calculated from the equilibrium constant of a chemical reaction. It represents that amount of useful work that can be done when the concentrations of all reactants and products are initially 1 M each. If this is done at pH 7, it is termed $\Delta G_0'$. The pertinent expression is

$$\Delta G_0' = -RT \ln K \tag{2.5}$$

Here R is the gas constant (1.987 cal/degree-M or 8.314 J/degree-M), $\Delta G_0'$ is in cal/M (in many cases, the M is ignored, and $\Delta G_0'$ is expressed as calories only), T is temperature (K); K is the equilibrium constant, and ln is natural logarithm, or 2.303 log. Note that when $K = 1$, $\Delta G_0' = 0$; when K is larger than 1, $\Delta G_0'$ is negative; and when K is smaller than 1, $\Delta G_0'$ is positive.

Both K and $\Delta G_0'$ depend on temperature. The relationship between the equilibrium constant K and temperature is given by the *Gibbs-Helmholtz* equation, the integrated version of which is

$$\ln K = \frac{\Delta H_0}{RT} + C \tag{2.6}$$

where C is an integration constant. It is clear that C and ΔH_0 can be determined by plotting ln K versus $1/T$, where C is the y intercept and the slope is $-\Delta H_0/R$, as shown in Figure 2.1. This equation also indicates that C and ΔH_0 are temperature independent. In Figure 2.1, representing $N_2 + O_2 \rightarrow 2NO$, the slope is about -9600, and $\Delta H_0 = -(-9600)(2.303)(1.987) = 43,900$ cal. The y intercept C is equal to $\Delta S/2.303R$. The y intercept is 1.365, and ΔS is therefore 6.2 entropy units. Thus the entropy change is also temperature independent under these conditions.

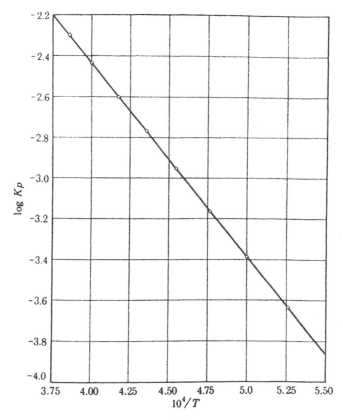

Figure 2.1 Relationship between the equilibrium constant and temperature. Reproduced with permission from Daniels F, Alberty RA. Physical Chemistry. New York: John Wiley & Sons, 1955. p. 257.

There are situations in which the concentrations of reactants and products are initially not 1 M each, and a $\Delta G'$ must be calculated to predict in which direction the reaction may proceed. For this purpose, Equation (2.7) may be used. The $\Delta G_0'$ must be known to use this equation.

$$\Delta G' = \Delta G_0' + 2.303RT \log \frac{[C][D]}{[A][B]} \tag{2.7}$$

where $[A]$, $[B]$, and so on, are the initial concentrations of reactants and products for the reaction $A + B \rightleftharpoons C + D$, not those at equilibrium.

Example 2.1

The equilibrium constant K for $A + B \rightleftharpoons C + D$ is 100. Determine the direction of the reaction at 27°C (300 K) when $[A] = [C]$, $[D] = 10^{-3}\ M$, and $[B] = 10^{-7}\ M$.

Solution: First, $\Delta G_0' = -2.303 \times 1.987 \times 300 \times \log 100 = -2746$ cal. Now, $\Delta G' = -2746 + 2.303 \times 1.987 \times 300 \times \log 10^{-3}/10^{-7} = -2746 + 5491 = 2745$ cal/M.

Thus, under "standard" conditions, $\Delta G_0'$ is a negative number; should $[A] = [B] = [C] = [D] = 1\ M$, the reaction goes to the right. However, in this specific situation, $[D] \gg [B]$ with $[A] = [C]$. This shifts the reaction in the other direction (law of mass action), so that the resulting $\Delta G'$ becomes a positive number and C and D are converted to A and B. Were $[B] = 10^{-4}\ M$ with $[D] = 10^{-3}\ M$, the $\Delta G'$ would be -1373 cal and the reaction would proceed as written.

2.3.3 Free Energy of Multistep Reactions

Metabolic pathways consist of several individual enzymatic reaction steps, each with its own $\Delta G_0'$. The overall $\Delta G_0'$ of the pathway is the sum of the individual step $\Delta G_0'$ values, and whether a pathway proceeds as written under a set of conditions depends on the overall $\Delta G_0'$. In addition, if there are two series of reactions leading to the same product from a common set of reactants, the two overall free energy changes is the same, because ΔG depends only on the initial reactants and final products, not the path taken. Thus, for

$$A \underset{(\Delta G_0')_1}{\rightarrow} B \underset{(\Delta G_0')_2}{\rightarrow} C \underset{(\Delta G_0')_3}{\rightarrow} D$$

and for

$$A \underset{(\Delta G_0')_4}{\rightarrow} E \underset{(\Delta G_0')_5}{\rightarrow} F \underset{(\Delta G_0')_6}{\rightarrow} D \tag{2.8}$$

The overall $\Delta G_0'$ for the conversion of A to D is then

$$\text{Overall } \Delta G_0' = (\Delta G_0')_1 + (\Delta G_0')_2 + (\Delta G_0')_3 = (\Delta G_0')_4 + (\Delta G_0')_5 + (\Delta G_0')_6 \tag{2.9}$$

2.4 REDOX REACTIONS

2.4.1 Redox Potential and Free Energy

A special type of a chemical reaction that is of great importance in intermediary metabolism results in an exchange of electrons between two compounds. These are termed *redox reactions*. The compound losing electrons is called a *reducing* agent and that gaining electrons is called *oxidizing* agent. The propensity of a compound to gain electrons is expressed by its *redox potential ΔE*, in volts or millivolts. Those substances that have a high capacity to gain electrons, that is, are good oxidizing agents, have the most positive redox potentials. Those substances that do not gain electrons easily but are instead good reducing agents have the more negative redox potentials.

Redox potentials for some compounds of biochemical interest are given in Table 2.1. Notice that oxygen occupies the uppermost position, with the most positive ΔE. In the living organism, oxygen is the ultimate oxidizing agent, to which all electrons flow from the oxidation (catabolism) of foodstuffs. Note that in Table 2.1 the redox potentials are given for various compounds *accepting* electrons, that is, in the direction of reduction. Table 2.1 could just as well be written in the oxidation direction, but then the signs of all redox potentials would have to be reversed. Further, the redox potentials are given as $\Delta E_0'$ values. This again means that we are dealing with conditions at pH 7 and that the concentrations of reactants and products at the beginning of the redox reaction are 1 M each. Last, note that most biochemical redox reactions involve the exchange of two electrons (a pair of electrons), which usually goes hand in hand with the exchange of protons.

The half-reactions shown in Table 2.1 do not occur naturally. If electrons and protons are to be gained, they must come from some other compound. Thus, to conduct a redox reaction, one must combine two half-reactions, making sure that both sides of the overall reaction have a reducing agent and an oxidizing agent. Suppose we choose two half-reactions from Table 2.1:

$$\text{Oxaloacetate} + 2H^+ + 2e^- \rightarrow \text{malate} \quad \Delta E_0' = -0.10 \text{ V}$$
$$NAD^+ + 2H^+ + 2e^- \rightarrow NADH + H^+ \quad \Delta E_0' = -0.32 \text{ V}$$

Table 2.1 Reduction-Oxidation Potentials of Some Biologically Important Half-reactions

Half-reaction	$\Delta E_0'$
$\frac{1}{2}O_2 + 2H^+ + 2e^- \rightarrow H_2O$	0.82
$2 \text{ cyt a-Fe}^{3+} + 2e^- \rightarrow 2 \text{ cyt a-Fe}^{2+}$	0.29
$2 \text{ cyt c-Fe}^{3+} + 2e^- \rightarrow 2 \text{ cyt c-Fe}^{2+}$	0.25
Ubiquinone $+ 2H^+ + 2e^- \rightarrow$ ubiquinone-H_2	0.10
Fumarate $+ 2H^+ + 2e^- \rightarrow$ succinate	0.03
$FAD + 2H^+2e^- \rightarrow FADH_2$	−0.06
Oxaloacetate $+ 2H^+ + 2e^- \rightarrow$ malate	−0.10
Pyruvate $+ 2H^+ + 2e^- \rightarrow$ lactate	−0.19
$NAD^+ + 2H^+ + 2e^- \rightarrow NADH + H^+$	−0.32

We can write two potentially naturally occurring reactions as

1. Oxaloacetate + NADH + H^+ → malate + NAD^+
2. Malate + NAD^+ → oxaloacetate + NADH + H^+

So, which reaction will proceed as written? To determine this, we must calculate the overall $\Delta E_0'$. If it is positive, the reaction will go as written, and if it is negative, the reaction will go in the opposite direction. For reaction 1, overall $\Delta E_0' = -0.10 + 0.32 = 0.22$ V, whereas for reaction 2, $\Delta E_0' = 0.10 - 0.32 = -0.22$ V. Thus, reaction 1 but not reaction 2 will go as written. Note that in reaction 1, oxaloacetate is converted to malate, and hence we retain the $\Delta E_0'$ of -0.10 V. However, the NADH + H^+ is converted to NAD^+; that is, it is written in a direction opposite to that seen in Table 2.1. Hence we change its sign to 0.32 V. The algebraic sum of -0.10 and 0.32 gives a positive $\Delta E_0'$ of 0.22 V. At this point it should be obvious that when two half-reactions are considered, the one with the more positive $\Delta E_0'$ oxidizes the one with the less positive $\Delta E_0'$.

$\Delta E_0'$ may be used to calculate the $\Delta G_0'$, for either a half-reaction or an overall reaction constructed from two half-reactions. The following equation is used:

$$\Delta G_0' = -nF\,\Delta E_0' \qquad (2.10)$$

where n is the number of electrons changing hands (usually 2) and F is the *Faraday constant* (23,000 cal/V-mol, or 96,400 J/V-mol). For the overall reaction 1, $\Delta G_0'$ is $-10,120$ cal. The negative sign indicates that the reaction will go as written. Thus a positive $\Delta E_0'$ gives a negative $\Delta G_0'$, and vice versa.

Example 2.2

Consider the following two half-reactions and their redox potentials:

Fumarate + $2H^+$ + $2e^-$ → succinate $\Delta E_0' = 0.030$ V
Pyruvate + $2H^+$ + $2e^-$ → lactate $\Delta E_0' = -0.19$ V

Write the overall redox reaction that will take place spontaneously at reactant and product concentration of 1 M each, and determine the $\Delta G_0'$.

Solution: The fumarate-succinate system has a more positive $\Delta E_0'$ than the pyruvate-lactate system, and hence the fumarate will oxidize lactate:

Fumarate + lactate → succinate + pyruvate

To calculate the overall $\Delta E_0'$, we leave the redox potential of the fumarate-succinate system at 0.030 V, but the sign of the pyruvate-lactate system must be reversed, because in the overall reaction lactate is being oxidized. Therefore, the overall $\Delta E_0' = 0.030$ V + 0.19 V = 0.22 V. The $\Delta G_0'$ is calculated as $\Delta G_0' = -2 \times 23,000$ cal/V $\times 0.22$ V = $-10,120$ cal.

2.4.2 Nernst Equation

The foregoing discussion was applicable to redox potentials, and the concentrations of reactants and products were assumed to be 1 M each. If it is not so, a correction must be made as was the case with $\Delta G_0'$. Such a correction may be made via the *Nernst equation*, which for the reaction $A + B \rightarrow C + D$ can be written as

$$\Delta E' = \Delta E_0' - \frac{RT}{nF} \ln \frac{[C][D]}{[A][B]} \qquad (2.11)$$

Note again that the concentrations of reactants and products are the initial concentrations, not those at equilibrium.

2.5 HIGH-ENERGY PHOSPHATE BOND

2.5.1 Nature of ATP and Its Hydrolysis

By *high-energy bond*, one understands a covalent linkage whose hydrolysis yields a high number of energy units. Thus, the energy generated by oxidizing foodstuffs in the organism can be partially recovered in the form of high-energy compounds, which are then capable of providing energy for the operation of essential life processes, such as muscle contraction. The most abundant and versatile high-energy compound is ATP (adenosine triphosphate). Its structure is given in Figure 2.2. The high-energy bonds of ATP are the two anhydride-type bonds joining the phosphate residues. Such high-energy phosphate bonds are universal throughout the plant and animal kingdoms. The bond joining the ribose moiety to the phosphate residue is of the ester type, not of the high-energy variety. The two anhydride bonds are unstable at neutral pH, and they

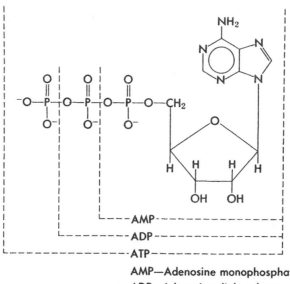

AMP—Adenosine monophosphate
ADP—Adenosine diphosphate
ATP—Adenosine triphosphate

Figure 2.2 Structure of ATP and its hydrolysis products ADP and AMP.

Example 2.3

Suppose for the reaction oxaloacetate + NADH + H$^+$ → malate + NAD$^+$ ($\Delta E_0'$ = 0.22 V), [NAD$^+$] = 10^{-3} M, [NADH] = 10^{-4} M, and [oxaloacetate] = [malate] = 10^{-5} M. Temperature is 300 K. What is the $\Delta G'$ of the reaction? Calculate the $\Delta G'$ if [malate] = [NAD$^+$] = 0.1 M, [NADH] = 10^{-4} M, and [oxaloacetate] = 10^{-6} M.

Solution: First, calculate $\Delta E'$ from the Nernst equation as follows: $\Delta E'$ = 0.22 − (1.987 × 300)/(2 × 23,000) × 2.3 log $(10^{-5})(10^{-3})/(10^{-5})(10^{-4})$ = 0.19 V $\Delta G'$ = −2 × 23,000 × 0.19 = −8749 cal. This reaction has a negative $\Delta G'$ and will go as written.

Now taking the second scenario, we have $\Delta E'$ = 0.22 − (1.987 × 300)/ (2 × 23,000) × 2.3 log $(10^{-1})(10^{-1})/(10^{-6})(10^{-4})$ = −0.02 V $\Delta G'$ = −2 × 23,000 × (−0.02) = 920 cal. The $\Delta G'$ is now positive, and the reaction will now go in the opposite direction until it reaches equilibrium.

Example 2.4

Will the reaction fumarate + NADH + H$^+$ → succinate + NAD$^+$go as written if fumarate, succinate, NAD$^+$, and NADH are present in 10^{-2}, 10^{-5}, 10^{-7}, and 10^{-3} M amounts? Temperature is 300 K.

Solution: We write the two half-reactions:

Fumarate + 2H$^+$ + 2e$^-$ → succinate $\Delta E_0'$ = 0.030 V
NAD$^+$ + 2H$^+$ + 2e$^-$ → NADH + H$^+$ $\Delta E_0'$ = −0.32 V

For this reaction, the fumarate-succinate system has a more positive redox potential than the NAD$^+$/NADH system, and hence fumarate will oxidize NADH under standard conditions ($\Delta E_0'$ = 0.35 V). Using the Nernst equation, we obtain $\Delta e'$ = 0.35 − (1.987 × 300)/(2 × 23,000) × 2.3 log $(10^{-7})(10^{-5})/(10^{-2})(10^{-3})$ = 0.56 V. Because $\Delta E'$ is positive, the reaction will go as written.

---

release some 8400 cal energy when hydrolyzed. Thus, the hydrolysis of 1 M equivalent of one high-energy phosphate bond has a $\Delta G_0'$ of −8400 cal, and through appropriate enzyme reactions, this energy of hydrolysis can be utilized to operate processes with positive $\Delta G_0'$ values.

The reasons the anhydride phosphate bonds in ATP are unstable and contain so much energy are at least threefold. First, there are contiguous negative charges on the phosphate residues. Second, the hydrolysis products have a greater number of resonance forms than ATP, and hence the hydrolysis products are more stable. Thus for inorganic phosphate, a product of ATP hydrolysis, we can write four resonating structures:

$$
\begin{array}{cccc}
\text{O} & \text{O}^- & \text{O}^- & \text{O}^- \\
\parallel & | & | & | \\
{}^-\text{O–P–O}^- & \text{O=P–O}^- & {}^-\text{O–P=O} & {}^-\text{O–P–O}^- \\
| & | & | & \parallel \\
\text{OH} & \text{OH} & \text{OH} & \text{+OH}
\end{array}
\qquad (2.12)
$$

Finally, when ATP is hydrolyzed, one of the products is a proton (H^+). In a living system, cellular buffers at pH 7 immediately buffer the protons thus produced and shift the reaction toward hydrolysis.

The hydrolysis of ATP and related compounds can proceed as follows:

$$ATP + H_2O \rightarrow ADP + P_i + H^+ \qquad \Delta G'_0 = -8400 \text{ cal}$$
$$ATP + H_2O \rightarrow AMP + PP_i + H^+ \qquad \Delta G'_0 = -9900 \text{ cal}$$
$$ADP + H_2O \rightarrow AMP + P_i + H^+ \qquad \Delta G'_0 = -8500 \text{ cal}$$
$$PP_i + H_2O \rightarrow 2P_i + H^+ \qquad \Delta G'_0 = -7000 \text{ cal}$$

In this series of reactions, P_i designates inorganic phosphate ($H_2PO_4^-$ and HPO_4^{2-}) and PP_i designates *pyrophosphate*,

$$\overset{\displaystyle O \quad\; O}{\underset{\displaystyle OH \quad OH}{{}^-O-\overset{\parallel}{P}-O-\overset{\parallel}{P}-O^-}}$$

For the hydrolysis of ATP to AMP and $2P_i$, we can write two pathways, both producing the same number of calories:

$$ATP \underset{P_i}{\overset{}{\rightarrow}} ADP \underset{P_i}{\overset{}{\rightarrow}} AMP \qquad \Delta G'_0 = -8400 + (-8500) = -16,900 \text{ cal}$$

$$ATP \underset{AMP}{\overset{}{\rightarrow}} PP_i \rightarrow 2P_i \qquad \Delta G'_0 = -9900 + (-7000) = -16,900 \text{ cal}$$

Other di- and trinucleotides (compounds in which the adenine moiety is replaced by another purine or pyrimidine base, such as guanine in GTP, cytosine in CTP, or uracil in UTP; Chapter 10) are also of the high-energy type and perform certain biologic functions requiring high-energy phosphate bonds.

In addition to the di- and trinucleotides, certain other compounds contain high-energy phosphate bonds; these are metabolic pathway intermediates, such as phosphoenolpyruvate ($\Delta G'_0 = -12,800$ cal), 1,3-diphosphoglycerate ($\Delta G'_0 = -11,800$ cal), creatine phosphate ($\Delta G'_0 = -10,500$ cal), and acetyl phosphate ($\Delta G'_0 = -10,000$ cal), which is found in bacteria. These compounds contain phosphoanhydride bonds with a greater $\Delta G'_0$ of hydrolysis than that of ATP, and it is therefore possible for these compounds to transfer their high-energy bonds to ADP to form ATP, as shown in Equation (2.13). Phosphoenolpyruvate and 1,3-diphosphoglycerate are components of the glycolysis pathway, which gives rise to ATP through the so-called substrate-level phosphorylation reactions (see Chapter 18).

$$\underset{\substack{\displaystyle CH_2 \quad\; O^- \\ \text{Phosphoenolpyruvate}}}{\overset{\substack{\displaystyle COOH \quad O \\ \displaystyle | \qquad \parallel}}{C-O-\overset{|}{P}-O^-}} + ADP \rightarrow \underset{\substack{\displaystyle CH_3 \\ \text{pyruvate}}}{\overset{\substack{\displaystyle COOH \\ \displaystyle |}}{C{=}O}} + ATP \qquad (2.13)$$

In Equation (2.13), the overall $\Delta G_0' = -12,800 - (-8400) = -4400$ cal.

Many other organic phosphates exist in nature, but their bonding is not of the anhydride type and their hydrolysis does not result in the release of large amounts of energy. Many such compounds are phosphate esters, whose formation may be envisioned to involve a reaction of phosphate with an alcohol:

$$
\begin{array}{ccc}
\overset{\displaystyle O}{\underset{\displaystyle O^-}{\overset{\|}{\underset{|}{^-O-P-OH}}}} & + & \overset{\displaystyle H}{\underset{\displaystyle H}{\overset{|}{\underset{|}{HO-C-R}}}} \rightarrow \overset{\displaystyle O}{\underset{\displaystyle O^-}{\overset{\|}{\underset{|}{^-O-P-}}}} O \overset{\displaystyle H}{\underset{\displaystyle H}{\overset{|}{\underset{|}{-C-R}}}}
\end{array}
\qquad (2.14)
$$

Phosphate   alcohol   phosphate ester

For example, the hydrolysis of glucose-6-phosphate has a $\Delta G_0'$ of -3300 cal and that of glycerol phosphate, -2300 cal.

2.5.2 Energy Charge and Phosphorylation Potential

As pointed out earlier, the $\Delta G'$ of a chemical reaction depends not only on the $\Delta G_0'$ but also on the initial concentrations of reactants and products. Thus, in rat muscle, whereas $[ATP] = [ADP] = 8 \times 10^{-3} M$, $[P_i] = 0.9 \times 10^{-3} M$. At 37°C, $\Delta G'$ of this system is potentially $-13,310$ cal/mol, and it is evident that under the in vivo conditions of the rat muscle, ATP can deliver quite a bit more energy than would be predicted from its $\Delta G_0'$.

There are several ways of expressing the energy states of tissues. One is to calculate the so-called energy charge, as shown in Equation (2.15):

$$
\text{Energy charge} = \frac{[ATP] + \frac{1}{2}[ADP]}{[ATP] + [ADP] + [AMP]}
\qquad (2.15)
$$

In most healthy tissues, the energy charge is around 0.96, indicating a relatively high ATP concentration.

Another way of expressing the availability of energy, that is, ATP, is to calculate the so-called phosphorylation potential:

$$
\text{Phosphorylation potential} = \frac{[ATP]}{[ADP][P_i]}
\qquad (2.16)
$$

There are numerous enzyme systems in the human organism, which respond to changes in the energy status of cells. A high-energy charge (or phosphorylation potential) tends to shut down those systems that produce ATP directly or indirectly. On the other hand, a low-energy status of cells turns on such pathways and turns off those that utilize ATP.

2.5.3 Coupled Reactions

Energy contained in a high-energy phosphate bond can be utilized to run *endergonic* reactions, that is, reactions with a positive $\Delta G'$. Such reactions are said to be *coupled* to ATP hydrolysis. Most such reactions result in the hydrolysis of ATP to ADP or ATP to AMP and PP_i. ADP rarely participates in biologic reactions to utilize its phosphate bond energy. One such reaction is catalyzed by adenylate kinase (myokinase), where $2ADP \rightarrow ATP + AMP$.

Normally, the formation of an ester from an alcohol and a fatty acid is difficult; the $\Delta G_0'$ is about 4000 cal/M or more. However, in the presence of an appropriate enzyme system, this can be coupled to ATP hydrolysis:

$$R - COOH + ATP \rightarrow R - \overset{\overset{\displaystyle O}{\|}}{C} - O - AMP + PP_i \qquad\qquad \Delta G_0' = 2500 \text{ cal}$$

$$R - \underset{\underset{\displaystyle O}{\|}}{C} - O - AMP + HO - R' \rightarrow R - \underset{\underset{\displaystyle O}{\|}}{C} - O - R' + AMP \qquad \Delta G_0' = -6000 \text{ cal}$$

$$R - COOH + HO - R' + ATP \rightarrow R - \underset{\underset{\displaystyle O}{\|}}{C} - O - R' + AMP + PP_i \quad \Delta G_0' = -3500 \text{ cal net}$$

The pyrophosphate thus produced is often degraded by a ubiquitous enzyme, *pyrophosphatase*, to inorganic phosphate, thus pushing the reaction ever further toward completion. Another process that requires energy input is the formation of peptide bonds, which hold amino acids together in proteins. Peptide bonds cannot form spontaneously, and their biosynthesis requires at least four ATP equivalents, amounting to some 33,600 cal. The whole point of ATP hydrolysis in biologic systems is thus to drive forward those reactions that would otherwise not occur because of unfavorable $\Delta G'$.

2.5.4   Calculation of ATP Yields

The number of ATP molecules one can generate by combusting any substance can be calculated, assuming that appropriate enzyme mechanisms are in place in the organism. Consider the combustion (oxidation) of a hypothetical substance $C_xH_yO_z$:

$$C_xH_yO_z + nO_2 \rightarrow xCO_2 + \frac{y}{2}H_2O \tag{2.17}$$

We may calculate n by

$$n = x + \frac{y}{4} - \frac{z}{2} \tag{2.18}$$

ATP yield is then $6n$, and $\Delta G_0' = -6 \times 18n = -108n$ kcal. Consider the oxidation of glucose:

$$C_6H_{12}O_6 + 6O_2 \rightarrow 6CO_2 + 6H_2O \tag{2.19}$$

Here $n = 6$, and ATP yield per mole glucose is $6 \times 6 = 36$. $\Delta G_0' = -108 \times 6 = -648$ kcal. In reality, because each mole of ATP (hydrolyzed to ADP) is worth only 8.4 kcal/M, the oxidation of glucose yields only 302 kcal. The other 346 kcal is wasted as heat. The metabolic engine is therefore only about 47% efficient, which for engines is excellent.

QUESTIONS

For Questions 2.1 through 2.3, use the following half-reactions:

$$NAD^+ + 2e^- + 2H^+ \rightarrow NADH + H^+ \qquad \Delta E_0' = -0.32 \text{ V}$$

$$Pyruvate + 2e^- + 2H^+ \rightarrow lactate \qquad \Delta E_0' = -0.19 \text{ V}$$

$$Ubiquinone + 2e^- + 2H^+ \rightarrow hydroubiquinone \qquad \Delta E_0' = 0.10 \text{ V}$$

2.1 Which reaction will go as written, given a 1 M concentration of reactants and products?
   a. $NADH + pyruvate + H^+ \rightarrow NAD^+ + lactate$
   b. $Lactate + NADH + H^+ \rightarrow NAD^+ + pyruvate$
   c. $Hydroubiquinone + pyruvate \rightarrow ubiquinone + lactate$
   d. $Hydroubiquinone + NAD^+ \rightarrow NADH + ubiquinone + H^+$
   e. $NAD^+ + ubiquinone \rightarrow NADH + hydroubiquinone + H^+$

2.2. What is $\Delta G_0'$ in kcal/mol if a pair of electrons is transferred from 1 mol lactate to 1 mol ubiquinone ($F = 23,000$ cal/V-mol, $R = 1.987$ cal/degree-mol, and $T = 310$ K).
   a. -4.14 c. 4.14 e. 5.98
   b. -13.3 d. -12.4

3. If in Question 2.2 [ubiquinone] = [hydroubiquinone] and pyruvate and lactate are 10^{-4} and 10^{-2} M, respectively, what would be the $\Delta G_0'$ in kcal/mol?
   a. -6.9 c. -13.3 e. -16.1
   b. 10.5 d. 16.1

For Questions 2.4–2.6, use the following information:

$$ATP + H_2O \rightarrow ADP + P_i + H^+ \qquad \Delta G_0' = -8400 \text{ cal}$$

$$B + C \rightleftharpoons D \qquad K_{eq} = 0.1$$

$$R = 1.987 \text{ cal/degree-M} \qquad T = 310 \text{ K} \qquad \ln X = 2.3 \log X.$$

2.4. If the reaction $B + C \rightleftharpoons D$ were coupled with the hydrolysis of ATP to ADP, the overall $\Delta G_0'$ would be near (cal/mol)
   a. -9800 c. 9800
   b. -7000 d. 3600
   e. Not necessarily to couple; the reaction will go as written.

2.5. To achieve a $\Delta G' = 0$ for $B + C \rightleftharpoons D$, what should be the initial concentration of B if initially $D = C = 1$ M?
   a. $0.1 M$ c. $10 M$ e. $B = C$
   b. $1 M$ d. $2 M$

2.6. Hydrolysis of ATP as just indicated was assigned a $\Delta G_0'$ of -8400 cal/mol. This means that
   a. One obtains 8400 cal useful work when 1 mol ATP is hydrolyzed to 1 mol ADP and phosphate.
   b. This is the amount of energy one obtains from 1 mol ATP in the cell at pH 7.
   c. It is necessary to add 8400 cal to hydrolyze 1 mol ATP.
   d. At equlibrium, when there are 1 mol each of ATP, ADP, and phosphate, the $\Delta G' = \Delta G_0' = -8400$ cal/mol.
   e. One obtains 8400 cal useful work when at the beginning of the reaction ATP, ADP, and phosphate concentrations are 1 M each.

2.7. How many ATP equivalents can one obtain from lactic acid?

```
      COOH
       |
   H–C–OH
       |
      CH₃
```

a. 3 c. 18 e. 36
b. 6 d. 24

For Questions 2.8–2.12, use the following code:
 a. 1, 2, and 3 are correct.
 b. 1 and 3 are correct.
 c. 2 and 4 are correct
 d. 4 only is correct.
 e. All are correct.

2.8. Entropy
  1. Maximum at equilibrium
  2. Change can be measured in a calorimeter
  3. Related to degree of randomness
  4. Temperature dependent

2.9. ATP
  1. Can be produced only by oxidation of carbohydrates and fats
  2. Yields energy only if hydrolyzed to ADP and P_i
  3. Has approximately the same amount of energy per phosphate bond as glycerol-3-phosphate
  4. Complete hydrolysis yields $3P_i$ + ribose + adenine

2.10. The high-energy phosphate bond
  1. Is present only in ATP
  2. Carries an ester character
  3. Has more resonance forms than its hydrolysis products
  4. Would be more stable in an acidic solution than in an alkaline solution

2.11. The equilibrium constant(s)
  1. Is 1 when $\Delta G_0' = 0$
  2. Is dependent on temperature
  3. Can be used to calculate entropy change at a set of temperatures
  4. Cannot be changed by adding a catalyst

2.12. The Nernst equation
  1. Can be used in the calculation of a tissue's phosphorylation potential
  2. Can be used for the calculation of a $\Delta G'$
  3. Requires the knowledge of the equilibrium constant
  4. Can be used to predict the direction of a chemical reaction

Answers

2.1. (a) Equations in b and e are nonsensical, whereas c and d will have negative $\Delta E_0'$ (−0.29 and −0.42 V, respectively).

2.2. (b) Lactate + ubiquinone → pyruvate + hydroubiquinone, $\Delta E_0' = 0.29$; $\Delta G_0' = -2 \times 23{,}000 \times 0.29 = -13.3$ kcal/mol.

2.3. (e) $\Delta G' = -13{,}300 + 1.987 \times 310 \times 2.3 \times \log 10^{-4}/10^{-2} = -16{,}100$ cal/mol.

2.4. (b) For $B + C \rightleftharpoons D$, $\Delta G_0' = -2.3RT \log 0.1 = 1417$ cal/M. Overall $\Delta G_0' = -8400 + 1417 = -6983$ cal.

2.5. (c) $0 = 1417 + 2.3 \times 1.987 \times 310 \times \log 1/B = 1417 - 1417 \log B$. Log B must be 1, and $B = 10\ M$.

2.6. (e) The definition of $\Delta G_0'$ is the amount of useful work that can be obtained when at the beginning of the reaction the concentrations of all reactants and products are $1\ M$ each.

2.7. (c) For lactic acid, $C_x H_y O_z + nO_2 \rightarrow xCO_2 + (y/2)H_2O$, $x = 3$, $y = 6$, $z = 3$, and $n = x + (y/4) - (z/2) = 3 + 6/4 - 3/2 = 3$; moles ATP $6n = 18$.

2.8. (b) Entropy increases to a maximum as equilibrium is attained. It cannot be measured directly, nor is it temperature dependent as for the Gibbs-Helmholtz equation.

2.9. (d) ATP can be generated by the oxidation of many compounds and yields energy if hydrolyzed to ADP + P_i or to AMP + PP_i. Glycerol-3-phosphate is not a high-energy compound.

2.10. (d) There are many high-energy phosphate compounds, and they carry an anhydride character. One reason they provide a lot of energy by hydrolysis is because the products have a greater number of resonance forms than the high-energy compound.

2.11. (e) When $\Delta G_0' = 0$, $K_{eq} = 1$. K_{eq} values can be used to calculate ΔS by the Gibbs-Helmholtz equation. K_{eq} is dependent on temperature and is not altered by a catalyst.

2.12. (c) The Nernst equation is useful only when a redox reaction is involved and provides us with an overall $\Delta E'$ when the concentrations of reactants and products at the beginning of a reaction are known. The $\Delta E'$ can then be used to calculate the $\Delta G'$ and predict the direction of the reaction.

PROBLEMS

2.1. For the biochemical reaction $A \rightarrow B + C$, the $\Delta G_0'$ is 6000 cal. If one starts with $10^{-4}\ M$ of A, how much B and C will be found at equilibrium? In a living cell, explain how this reaction could be shifted toward the production of B and C. Use $T = 310$ K and $R = 1.987$ cal/deg/mol.

2.2. In $A \rightarrow B + C$, the equilibrium constant is 0.2. Using $T = 310$ K and $R = 1.987$ cal/deg/mol, what must be the initial concentration of A when $[B] = 10^+\ M$ and $[C] = 10^{-3}\ M$ for the reaction to move as written?

2.3. The following quantities of FAD, FADH$_2$, pyruvate, and lactate are mixed in the presence of an enzyme that catalyzes their interconversion: 10^{-4}, 10^{-3}, 0.1, and 0.01 M, respectively. Write the reaction that would take place, and calculate its $\Delta G'$.

2.4. In Prob. 2.3, calculate the amounts of FAD, FADH$_2$, pyruvate, and lactate when equilibrium has been established.

BIBLIOGRAPHY

Harold FM. A Study of Bioenergetics. San Francisco: WH Freeman, 1987.
Klotz IM. Introduction to Biomolecular Energetics. Orlando: Academic Press, 1986.
Lehninger A. Bioenergetics. New York: WA Benjamin, 1965.
Mitchell RA. Yields from biological oxidations—ideas new and not so new. Biochem Educ 11:64–65, 1983.

3

Concepts of Acid and Base Chemistry

After completing this chapter, the student should

1. Be able to derive the pH expression and the Henderson-Hasselbalch equation.
2. Know the difference between strong and weak acids and the meaning of the pK.
3. Be able to manipulate the Henderson-Hasselbalch equation to calculate parameters important for buffer preparations.
4. Be able to interpret titration curves of weak mono- and polyprotic acids.
5. Be familiar with and be able to perform calculations on the bicarbonate–CO_2 buffer system.
6. Recognize the various acidotic and alkalotic conditions from the acid–base status of an individual.

3.1 PROPERTIES OF WATER AND pH EXPRESSION

Between 60 and 70% of the human organism's weight is water. It is present both outside the cells (extracellularly), such as in the bloodstream, and inside the cells (intracellularly). Water is a unique substance serving as a solvent for many biologically important substances, as a means of controlling body temperature, as a means of removing waste products, and in many other capacities. Under normal circumstances, a substance with a molecular weight (MW) of 18 should be a gas (e.g., NH_3, MW 17, or even propane, MW 44). Yet water remains a liquid up to 100°C because it forms intermolecular *hydrogen bonds*. These are physical interactions in which a hydrogen atom with a partial positive charge forms a bond with an atom carrying an unshared pair of electrons, such as =O or −O. H atoms attached to O or N, but not to C, form hydrogen bonds. There is a partial positive charge (δ^+) on such atoms because the bonding electrons in −OH, for example, are closer to the O atom (because of its larger nucleus) than they are to the H atom. Subsequently, O atoms may carry a partial negative charge (δ^-). In liquid water, we therefore have the following, where the dotted lines represent hydrogen bonds:

$$\cdots O-H\cdots O \left\{ \begin{array}{l} H\cdots\cdot O \left\{ \begin{array}{l} H\cdots \\ H\cdots \end{array} \right. \\ H\cdots\cdot O \left\{ \begin{array}{l} H\cdots \\ H\cdots \end{array} \right. \end{array} \right. \tag{3.1}$$

Water has other unique properties as well. It is a permanent dipole, and it has a rather high dielectric constant. These properties of water and other substances are amply described in general chemistry textbooks. The formation of hydrogen bonds, the dipolar nature of water, and its other properties allow water to act as a solvent for a number of ionic and nonionic substances. Such water-soluble substances are termed *hydrophilic*. Those substances that do not interact with water (e.g., the hydrocarbons) are termed *hydrophobic*. Among substances that are hydrophilic because of hydrogen bond formation are amines, ketones, aldehydes, mercaptans, and alcohols. Ionic compounds, both organic and inorganic, are generally water soluble because of the dipolar nature of water: positive ions (e.g., Na^+) interact with the negatively charged portions of the water dipole (the O atom), whereas negatively charged ions (e.g., Cl^-) interact with the positively charged H atoms of the water dipole:

$$\text{(3.2)}$$

Body water itself is poorly ionized, but it contains numerous solutes that maintain the organism in a stable environment, *homeostasis*. Water is dissociated as follows: $2H_2O \rightleftharpoons H_3O^+ + OH^-$. H_3O^+ is the *hydronium ion*. However, for the sake of simplicity, it is customary in the biomedical sciences to refer to H_3O^+ as simply H^+ or a proton, so that the dissociation of water can also be expressed as $H_2O \rightleftharpoons H^+ + OH^-$. Writing a dissociation constant for this as $K_d = [H^+][OH^-]/[H_2O]$, we obtain $[H_2O]K_d = [H^+][OH^-] = K_w$. Because K_d and $[H_2O]$ are constants ($[H_2O] = 55.5\ M$), K_w is also a constant and is equal to 10^{-14} at 25°C, so that

$$[H^+][OH^-] = 10^{-14} \tag{3.3}$$

If logs are taken on both sides of Equation (3.3), we obtain $-14 = -\log [H^+] + \log [OH^-]$; changing signs, we obtain $14 = \log [H^+] - \log [OH^-]$. The term $-\log [H^+]$ is the pH, whereas $-\log [OH^-]$ is pOH. Thus, pH + pOH = 14. When $[H^+] = [OH^-] = 10^{-7}$, the pH and pOH are both 7 and the aqueous solution is said to be at neutrality. If pH < pOH, we have an acidic solution, and when pOH < pH, we have an alkaline or basic solution. The pH of blood plasma is close to 7.4, whereas that of other extra- and intracellular fluids may deviate quite drastically from neutrality: the pH of gastric juice is between 1 and 2, that of pancreatic juice is between 7.5 and 8, and that of urine, depending on diet, may vary between 4.5 and 7.5.

Example 3.1

Determine the pH of a blood sample that has $[H^+] = 5 \times 10^{-8} M$.

Solution: Because pH $= -\log [H^+]$, then pH $= -\log 5 \times 10^{-8} = -(\log 5 + \log 10^{-8}) = -(0.7 - 8) = 7.3$. The blood sample pH is slightly below the normal value of 7.4.

3.2 WEAK AND STRONG ACIDS

Many substances in solution have the capability of releasing or absorbing protons. According to the classic *Brønsted* definition, *acids* are those substances that release protons and *bases* (alkalis) are those that accept protons. Thus, acetic acid is an acid, but acetate is a base. Ammonium ion (NH_4^+) is an acid, whereas ammonia (NH_3) is a base. When an acid loses its proton, its *conjugate base* is formed, whereas when a base gains protons, its conjugate acid is generated.

Certain acids dissociate in water completely: all their protons are released into solution. Such acids are termed *strong acids*. Thus, 1 M HCl, a strong acid, will dissociate into 1 M H^+ ions and 1 M Cl^- ions. Similar strong acids are HI, HF, HBr, and HNO_3. Other acids when dissolved in water release only a small portion of their component protons. These are termed *weak acids*. They include carboxylic acids (e.g., acetic and citric acids) and such inorganic acids as H_3PO_4 and H_2SO_4.

The tendency of a compound to release protons into solution is quantitatively expressed in terms of its dissociation constant K_d, defined for acetic acid,

$$CH_3-COOH \rightleftharpoons CH_3-COO^- + H^+ \tag{3.4}$$

as

$$K_d = \frac{[H^+][CH_3-COO^-]}{[CH_3-COOH]} \tag{3.5}$$

Because the use of dissociation constants is somewhat cumbersome, a new parameter, analogous to the pH, has been developed. This is the pK, defined as

$$pK = -\log K_d \tag{3.6}$$

Thus, for acetic acid, $K_d = 1.8 \times 10^{-5}$, and its p$K = -\log 1.8 \times 10^{-5} = (\log 1.8) + \log 10^{-5}) = 4.70$. Ammonium ion is a weaker acid ($NH_4^+ \rightleftharpoons NH_3 + H^+$). Its p$K$ is 9.25. Thus, the lower the pK of an acid, the stronger (more dissociated) the acid. One might also say that the pK is a measure of the propensity of an acid to give up protons. For a strong acid, such as HCl, K_d is almost infinity, because it is completely dissociated under normal conditions in water solutions. The pH of a strong acid is therefore calculated directly from its molarity: the pH of a 0.1 M HCl is 1 ($-\log 0.1$), and that of 1 M HCl is 0. Negative pH values are also possible. K_d values, like all equilibrium constants, depend on temperature (see Chapter 2).

Example 3.2

What is the pH of 0.15 M acetic acid? Its K_d is 1.8×10^{-5}.

$Solution:$ First, let x be the amount of acetic acid dissociated. Then, for

$$CH_3-COOH \rightarrow CH_3-COO^- + H^+$$
$$0.15 - x \qquad\qquad x \quad\ x$$

and we can write

$$K_d = 1.8 \times 10^{-5} = \frac{[x][x]}{0.15 - x} = \frac{x^2}{0.15 - x}$$

Because x is very small compared with 0.15, we can ignore it, and

$$K_d = 1.8 \times 10^{-5} = \frac{x^2}{0.15}$$

$$x^2 = (1.8 \times 10^{-5})(0.15)$$

and

$$x = [H^+] = \sqrt{(1.8 \times 10^{-5})(0.15)} = 1.64 \times 10^{-3}\ M$$
$$pH = -\log(1.64 \times 10^{-3}) = -(\log 1.64 + \log 10^{-3}) = 2.79$$

3.3   BUFFERS

Suppose we have a weak acid solution, and to this we add its sodium salt, such as acetic acid and sodium acetate. The pH of the acetic acid solution will increase because a common ion, acetate, shifts the equilibrium of acetic acid dissociation toward its undissociated form, thus removing protons from solution and making it more alkaline. We now have a mixture of a weak acid and its conjugate base.

If to a mixture of a weak acid and its conjugate base one adds protons (e.g., HCl), the conjugate base (the acetate ion) will combine with the protons to form undissociated acetic acid to maintain the K_d at the appropriate level [Equation (3.5)]. The proton concentration and the pH will remain relatively stable. Likewise, if to the mixture of a weak acid and its conjugate base one added OH^- ions (e.g., NaOH), the OH^- will combine with the protons present to form the inert H_2O. To maintain the K_d [Equation (3.5)], acetic acid will dissociate to replenish the protons removed, again resulting in reestablishment of nearly the original pH.

Solutions that consist of a weak acid and its conjugate base, which resist changes in pH, are $buffers$. Buffers may also consist of weak bases and their conjugate acids, such as NH_3 and NH_4^+. A buffer solution best resists change in pH in both the alkaline and acidic directions when its pH = pK. A buffer solution is considered effective about 1 pH unit above and below the pK. Note, however, that even if a buffer pH is at the right level, its capacity to buffer H^+ and OH^- is not limitless. Such capacity to buffer depends on the concentration of the buffer as well as its pH. Thus, a 0.1 M acetate buffer at pH 5 may have a higher capacity to buffer OH^- ions than a 0.01 M acetate buffer at pH 4.7 (pK of acetic acid).

Although this qualitative view of buffering action is quite informative, both clinical and research activities involving buffered solutions, biologic fluids or laboratory made, require a quantitative approach. This can be achieved via the *Henderson-Hasselbalch* equation derived from Equation (3.5) as follows: taking logs on both sides of Equation (3.5), we have

$$\log K_d = \log [H^+] + \log [CH_3COO^-] - \log [CH_3COOH] \tag{3.7}$$

Rearranging Equation (3.7), we obtain

$$-\log H^+ = -\log K_d + \log \frac{[CH_3COO^-]}{[CH_3COOH]} \tag{3.8}$$

Because $-\log H^+ = $ pH and $-\log K_d = $ pK, Equation (3.8) simplifies to the Henderson-Hasselbalch equation,

$$pH = pK + \log \frac{[CH_3COO^-]}{[CH_3COOH]} \tag{3.9}$$

where CH_3COO^- is the conjugate base or unprotonated species of the buffer, whereas CH_3COOH is the acid or the protonated species of the buffer. For acetic acid, the pK = 4.7. In the NH_3/NH_4^+ system, Equation (3.9) would be

$$pH = pK + \log \frac{[NH_3]}{[NH_4^+]} \tag{3.10}$$

where the pK = 9.25.

Looking at Equation (3.9), it becomes clear that the pH = pK when $[CH_3COO^-] = [CH_3COOH]$, or in Equation (3.10), $[NH_3] = [NH_4^+]$. One can therefore define the pK in another way, as that pH at which the protonated and unprotonated forms of a buffer system are present at equal concentrations.

There are numerous weak acids and bases that, with their conjugate partners, can serve as buffers at pH values near their pK values. Some weak acids, such as citric acid, can release more than one proton and can thus be used as buffers in several pH ranges. Each proton has its own typical pK value. Thus, phosphate buffers can be used in the following pH ranges: 1–3 (pK = 2.0), 5.7–7.7 (pK = 6.7), and 11–13 (pK = 12). Table 3.1 lists some weak acids with their pK values.

Example 3.3

An acetate buffer is made by mixing 500 mL of 1 M acetic acid and 500 mL of 2 M sodium acetate. What will be the pH? The pK of acetic acid is 4.70.

Total volume will be 1 L, and this will now be 0.5 M acetic acid (acid) and 1 M sodium acetate (conjugate base). Using the Henderson-Hasselbalch equation, we have

$$pH = 4.70 + \log \frac{1}{0.5} = 4.70 + \log 2 = 4.70 + 0.3 = 5.0$$

Table 3.1 pK Values for Some Common Weak Acids

Acid	Structure	Protons released	pK_a[a]
Acetic	CH_3COOH	1	4.70
Boric	H_3BO_3	1	9.23
Citric	$C_3H_5(COOH)_3$	3	3.09, 4.25, 5.41
Formic	HCOOH	1	3.77
Oxalic	$(COOH)_2$	2	1.25, 4.14
Phenol	C_6H_5OH	1	9.95
Phosphoric	H_3PO_4	3	2.0, 6.7, 12.0
O-Phthalic	$C_6H_4(COOH)_2$	2	2.98, 5.28
Propionic	CH_3CH_2COOH	1	4.87
Sulfuric	H_2SO_4	2	0.40, 1.92
Methylamine	$CH_3NH_4^+$	1	10.62
Ammonium	NH_4^+	1	9.25
Tris (tris-hydroxymethyl-aminomethane)	$(CH_2OH)_3CNH_3^+$	1	9.25

Source: From Fasman GD, Handbook of Biochemistry and Molecular Biology, 3rd ed., Vol. 1, Boca Raton, FL: CRC Press, pp. 307–351, 1976.
[a]All are thermodynamic constants.

Note that Table 3.1 provides dissociation constants K_d for weak acids, that is, the pK values listed indicate the propensity to release protons. These are often termed pK_a values, where a means acid. The propensity of the corresponding conjugate bases to accept protons can be expressed numerically by pK_b, where b means base. pK_b values can be calculated from pK_a + pK_b = 14, which in turn comes from

$$K_b = \frac{K_w}{K_a} = \frac{10^{-14}}{K_a} \tag{3.11}$$

One often needs to calculate the pH of a salt solution that comes from a weak acid and a strong base, such as sodium acetate. For this salt, $K_b = 10^{-14}/(2 \times 10^{-5}) = 5 \times 10^{-10}$, where 2×10^{-5} is the K_a of acetic acid. Because sodium acetate solutions are alkaline because of the hydrolysis phenomenon,

$$CH_3COO^- + H_2O \rightarrow CH_3COOH + OH^- \tag{3.12}$$

we can calculate the $[OH^-]$ and hence the pH. Thus, from

$$K_b = \frac{[CH_3COOH][OH^-]}{[CH_3COO^-]} = 5 \times 10^{-10} \tag{3.13}$$

We have $[CH_3COOH] = [OH^-]$. For 0.05 M sodium acetate solution, $5 \times 10^{-10} = [OH^-]^2/0.05$ and $[OH^-] = 5 \times 10^{-6}$ mol. This translates to pOH 5.3 and pH 8.7.

3.4 TITRATION CURVES

Suppose one has 10 ml of 0.1 M acetic acid (1 mmol). To this one adds 1 ml increments of 0.1 M NaOH (0.1 mmol), and the pH is determined at each step.

The addition of NaOH causes a decrease in CH_3COOH and an increase in CH_3COO^-:

$$CH_3COOH + NaOH \rightarrow Na^+ + CH_3COO^- + H_2O \qquad (3.14)$$

The pH can in fact be calculated via the Henderson-Hasselbalch equation after the addition of each NaOH increment. For instance, after the addition of 3 ml of 0.1 M NaOH (0.3 mmol) to 10 ml of the 0.1 M acetic acid, there will be 0.3 mmol CH_3COO^- and 0.7 mmol CH_3COOH. The pH will be

$$pH = 4.7 + \log \frac{0.3}{0.7} = 4.4 \qquad (3.15)$$

The results following the addition of each NaOH increment are listed in Table 3.2. Note that the pH first increases rather rapidly as the NaOH is added, but then it slows as the acetate–acetic acid ratio approaches 1. At this point, the pH is 4.7, the pK of acetic acid. As this ratio goes beyond 1, the pH again shows a higher rate of change.

Data in Table 3.2 can be represented in graph form, the *titration curve*. This is shown in Figure 3.1, and it is generated by plotting NaOH added versus pH. It shows a plateau approximately between pH 3.7 and 5.7 and an inflection point at pH 4.7, the pK of acetic acid. pH 3.7–5.7 is considered the acetic acid buffer buffering range.

Note also that as we add NaOH to the acetic acid, the total volume of the buffer solution increases. At the end of the titration, this volume is 20 mL. Will the volume change have an effect on the pH? Only minimally so! The pH of a

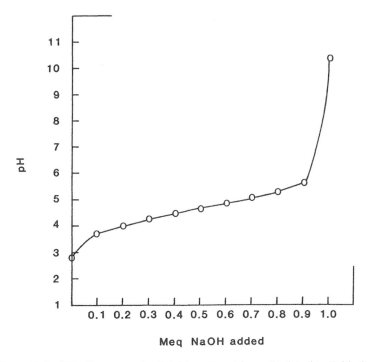

Figure 3.1 Titration curve for 0.1 M acetic acid as calculated in Table 3.1.

Table 3.2 Addition of 1 mL Portions of 0.1 M NaOH to 10 mL of 0.1 M Acetic Acid

mL NaOH added	mmol acetic acid remaining	mmol acetate present	Acetate/ acetic acid	pH (calculated)	ΔpH
0	1.0	Very small	Very small	2.85	—
1	0.9	0.1	1:9	3.81	0.92
2	0.8	0.2	1:4	4.16	0.35
3	0.7	0.3	3:7	4.39	0.23
4	0.6	0.4	2:3	4.58	0.19
5	0.5	0.5	1	4.70 (pK)	0.18
6	0.4	0.6	3:2	4.84	0.18
7	0.3	0.7	7:3	5.13	0.19
8	0.2	0.8	4	5.36	0.23
9	0.1	0.9	9	5.71	0.35
10	Very small	1.0	Very high	8.70	3.0

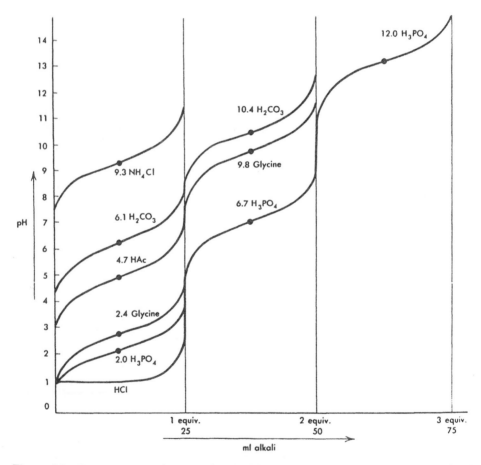

Figure 3.2 Titration curves for several acids. We are titrating 25 ml of 0.1 M acid with 0.1 M NaOH. Note that H_3PO_4 has three plateau regions, and therefore, phosphoric acid may serve as a buffer at three pH ranges, 1–3, 5.7–7.7, and 11–13; for example, an amino acid, glycine, has two plateau (buffering regions). The numbers at the inflection points of each plateau region indicate the pK values.

buffer solution depends largely on its unprotonated and protonated species ratio. As a buffer is diluted, however, its total buffering capacity per unit volume will change: 10 mL of 0.1 M acetate buffer at pH 4.7 can easily handle the addition of 1 ml 0.1 M NaOH; its pH will increase to 4.84. The addition of 1 mL of 0.1 M NaOH to 10 ml of 0.01 M acetate buffer at pH 4.7, however, results in a pH of about 8.4.

3.5 PHOSPHATE BUFFER SYSTEM

Numerous acids have several functional groups capable of releasing protons (Table 3.1). Taking phosphoric acid (H_3PO_4) as an example, we see that three protons can be released. Each proton has its own typical pK, as shown in the titration curve in Figure 3.2. Other titration curves are also shown for comparison purposes. The dissociation of phosphoric acid can be represented as

$$H_3PO_4 \rightarrow H_2PO_4^- \rightarrow HPO_4^{2-} \rightarrow PO_4^{3-} \qquad (3.16)$$

$$\begin{array}{ccc} H^+ & H^+ & H^+ \\ pK = 2.0 & pK = 6.7 & pK = 12 \end{array}$$

Phosphate buffers are the principal intracellular buffering systems in living organisms, because the second pK of 6.7 is near neutrality. The protonated and unprotonated buffer species are $H_2PO_4^-$ and HPO_4^{2-}, respectively. Their ratio depends on the pH of the cell.

Example 3.4

What quantity of 1 M NaOH must be added to 100 ml of a solution of 0.1 M phosphoric acid to give a buffer solution at pH 7.5? What will be the total phosphate concentration?

Solution: First, we must choose the correct pK. This is 6.7, because the desired buffer pH of 7.0 is nearest to that figure. At this pH, the acid is $H_2PO_4^-$ and the conjugate base is HPO_4^{2-}, as per Equation (3.16). Their total amount is 0.1 M × 100 mL = 10 mmol (i.e., [HPO_4^{2-}] + [$H_2PO_4^-$] = 10 mmol). Using the Henderson-Hasselbalch equation, we then have 7.0 = 6.7 + log [HPO_4^{2-}]/[$H_2PO_4^-$], and [HPO_4^{2-}]/[$H_2PO_4^-$] = 2.

Because total phosphate is 10 mmol, the absolute quantity of HPO_4^{2-} at pH 7.0 must be 6.7 mmol (two-thirds of 10), and that of $H_2PO_4^-$ must be 3.3 mmol (one-third of 10). Now, because we started with H_3PO_4, one must add 10 mmol NaOH (10 ml of 1 M NaOH) to convert all the H_3PO_4 to $H_2PO_4^-$. On the titration curve (Figure 3.2), we have moved from the 0 point to where the X axis is labeled "1 equiv." Then an additional 6.7 mmol NaOH (6.7 ml of 1 M NaOH) must be added to convert 6.7 mmol $H_2PO_4^-$ to HPO_4^{2-}, leaving 3.3 mmol $H_2PO_4^-$ behind. On the titration curve, we end up on the second plateau region beyond the inflection point labeled 6.7. Thus a total of 16.7 ml of 1 M NaOH must be added to the original 100 ml of 0.1 M H_3PO_4 to generate a buffer with pH = 7.0. The total volume of the buffer is 116.7 mL, and the phosphate concentration is 10 mmol/116.7 = 0.086 M.

3.6 BICARBONATE–CARBON DIOXIDE SYSTEM

Human plasma under normal circumstances has a pH of 7.4, which is maintained by a HCO_3^-/H_2CO_3 buffering system. H_2CO_3 in actuality is a combination of true H_2CO_3 and dissolved CO_2. Their relationship to HCO_3^- and to each other is shown in Equation (3.17):

$$CO_2 + H_2O \rightleftharpoons H_2CO_3 \rightleftharpoons HCO_3^- + H^+ \tag{3.17}$$

For each reaction, an equilibrium constant can be written as

$$K_1 = \frac{[HCO_3^-][H^+]}{[H_2CO_3]} \quad \text{and} \quad K_2 = \frac{[H_2CO_3]}{[CO_2][H_2O]} \tag{3.18}$$

A combined pK derived from both K_1 and K_2 is 6.1 and is used in the Henderson-Hasselbalch equation involving blood bicarbonate buffer system. The conjugate base is HCO_3^-, and the acid is designated H_2CO_3. Both are expressed in terms of meq/L. The HCO_3^- is also termed the *metabolic* component of the buffer system, whereas H_2CO_3 is referred to as the *respiratory* component. The latter depends on the partial pressure of CO_2, or pCO_2. Under normal conditions, we can write the Henderson-Hasselbalch expression for the bicarbonate system as shown in Equation (3.19):

$$7.4 = 6.1 + \log \frac{[HCO_3^-]}{[H_2CO_3]} \quad \text{and} \quad \frac{[HCO_3^-]}{[H_2CO_3]} = 20 \tag{3.19}$$

In red blood cells, the enzyme that catalyzes the conversion of CO_2 and H_2O to HCO_3^- and H^+ is *carbonic anhydrase*, and it plays a crucial role in maintaining the pH of the organism at a constant level.

   In the clinical biochemistry laboratory, measurements of "total CO_2" and pCO_2 can be performed. Blood pH is also determined routinely. pCO_2 is often expressed in mm Hg, and the normal value for an adult male is 35–48 mm Hg. Total CO_2 is the sum of $[H_2CO_3]$ and $[HCO_3^-]$ and is measured in terms of meq/L. Normal values in adults are in the range 22–29 meq/L. To convert pCO_2 in mm Hg to $[H_2CO_3]$ in meq/L, the pCO_2 value is multiplied by 0.0301, a factor derived from the solubility of CO_2 in water, as well as standard temperature and pressure parameters (STP). Notice that CO_2 occupies 22.26 L/mol at STP. We therefore have the following relationship:

$$H_2CO_3 \text{ in meq/L} = \frac{pCO_2 \text{ (mm Hg)} \times 1000 \times 0.510}{760 \text{ (mm Hg)} \times 22.26 \text{ L/mol}} = pCO_2 \times 0.301 \tag{3.20}$$

0.510 is the CO_2 solubility coefficient. pCO_2 is, of course, equal to $P \times (\% \ CO_2)/100$, where P is atmospheric pressure and % CO_2 is the percentage of CO_2 in the atmosphere or environment. Thus, for a pCO_2 of 40 mm Hg, the normal pCO_2 of arterial blood, $[CO_2]$ is 1.2 meq/L.

   Example 3.5 indicates that the blood of the patient is abnormally acidic. We also note that pCO_2 is normal, whereas the bicarbonate is severely depressed. Because the pH is less than 7.4, the patient is said to be acidotic, and because the bicarbonate is largely responsible for this and the bicarbonate part of the Henderson-Hasselbalch equation has been termed the metabolic component, the patient is suffering from pure *metabolic acidosis*. This is often seen in untreated

---

Example 3.5

A patient has a blood "total CO_2" of 16.27 meq/L and a pCO_2 of 41 mm Hg. What is his blood pH?

Solution: Converting pCO_2 from mm Hg to meq/L, we have 41 × 0.0301 = 1.23. $[HCO_3^-]$ is now 16.27 − 1.23 = 15.04. Setting up the Henderson-Hasselbalch equation, we have pH = 6.1 + log 15.04/1.23 = 6.1 + 1.87 = 7.19.

---

diabetics or persons with lactic acidosis. Other "pure" acid–base disturbances observed in clinical medicine are *metabolic alkalosis* (normal pCO_2 and high HCO_3^-), *respiratory acidosis* (high pCO_2, normal HCO_3^-, and low pH), and *respiratory alkalosis* (low pCO_2, normal HCO_3^-, and high pH).

The organism can "compensate" for such pure acid–base disturbances, either partially or almost fully, by adjusting the plasma pH back toward the normal value of 7.4. In patients with disturbances of the metabolic component (HCO_3^-), compensation involves an adjustment of pCO_2. In metabolic acidosis, pCO_2 is lowered by increasing the rate of respiration, the result of which is a faster removal of CO_2 from the organism. In metabolic alkalosis, pCO_2 is increased by lowering the respiration rate to retain CO_2 in the organism. If there is a primary disturbance in the respiratory component, that is, pCO_2, compensation involves adjustment of bicarbonate by the kidney. In respiratory alkalosis (low pCO_2), bicarbonate is excreted in greater quantities in the urine, which also carries away Na^+ and K^+ ions. In respiratory acidosis (high pCO_2), blood HCO_3^- is increased as follows: CO_2 combines with H_2O as a result of the carbonic anhydrase action to generate H_2CO_3. This dissociates into H^+ and HCO_3^- in the usual manner. The protons produced are excreted in the urine (the urine becomes acidic), whereas the bicarbonate is reabsorbed into the bloodstream. Associated with these disturbances in acid–base status are alterations in other blood electrolytes, such as Na^+, K^+, and Cl^-. These are discussed more fully in Chapter 16.

The acid–base status of a patient can also be determined from a plot of $[HCO_3^-]$ against pH containing pCO_2 isobars, as shown in Figure 3.3. Metabolic acidosis and alkalosis situations are seen in quadrants I and IV, respectively. Compensatory events can also be followed on this graph: suppose a patient is suffering from pure metabolic alkalosis, represented by point B. His pCO_2 = 40 mm, but $[HCO_3^-]$ = 35 meq/L. He compensates by breathing more slowly, that is, retaining CO_2, and moves from point B toward pH 7.4 via a line drawn toward point C. when and if fully compensated, his pCO_2 should be 65 mm Hg and $[HCO_3^-]$ = 38 meq/L. In a patient with pure respiratory alkalosis (point F), the pCO_2 is 20 mm Hg and $[HCO_3^-]$ = 20 meq/L. Renal compensation involves excretion of HCO_3^- in the urine. The patient's blood then approaches point E, and when fully compensated, the pCO_2 is still 20 mm Hg, but $[HCO_3^-]$ = 12 meq/L at pH 7.4.

Treatment of acid–base disturbances requires a determination of how much "acid" (NH_4Cl) or "alkali" ($NaHCO_3$) to add to the patient's system. For this

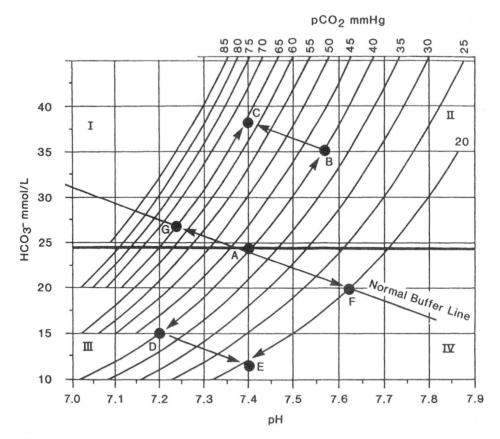

Figure 3.3 Relationships among pCO_2, pH, and $[HCO_3{}^-]$ for the extracellular bicarbonate–CO_2 buffer system. "True plasma" means that the plasma was separated from blood cells under anaerobic conditions to preserve its CO_2 content. The normal buffer line provides a standard reference for the relationship among pCO_2, $[HCO_3{}^-]$, and pH. Its slope depends on blood hemoglobin content.

reason, *base excess* in metabolic alkalosis or *base deficit* in metabolic acidosis may be calculated. In Figure 3.3, base excess is represented by the distance between points A and C along the y axis, amounting to some 14 meq/L. The base deficit between points A and E amounts to about 13 meq/L.

In practical terms, it is often difficult to establish exactly which form of acid–base disorder is present in a patient, especially in view of the existence of compound (mixed) disorders. A nomogram presented in Figure 3.4 provides a rapid method for assessing uncomplicated disorders of this sort within a 95% confidence limit. Anything falling outside the shaded areas can be viewed as an acid–base disorder of compound nature.

A very important blood buffer is hemoglobin, a red blood cell protein carrying oxygen to various tissues of the human organism. Red blood cells also contain carbonic anhydrase, which converts the CO_2 generated by peripheral tissue metabolism to H_2CO_3 [Equation (3.17)], and this in turn ionizes to $HCO_3{}^-$ and H^+. The protons thus generated are buffered largely by hemoglobin, and

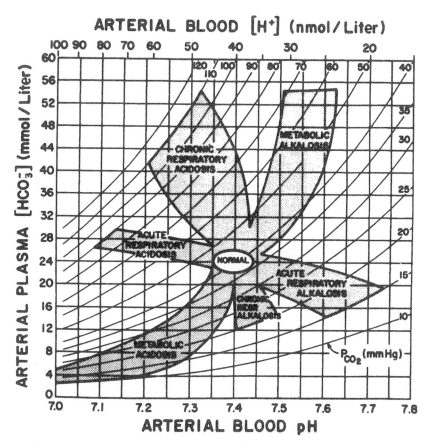

Figure 3.4 Identification of various acid–base disturbances. Acute disorders are synonymous with uncompensated disturbances, whereas chronic conditions are synonymous with partially compensated or compensated disturbances. If a specific case falls outside the shaded areas, a compound acid–base disturbance may be suspected, such as the coexistence of respiratory acidosis (partially compensated) and metabolic alkalosis. Unshaded areas may also indicate a transient state between an acute (uncompensated) state and a chronic (partially compensated) condition. (From Cogan MG, Rector FC Jr., Seldin DW. In Brenner BM, and Rector FC Jr, eds. The Kidney, 2nd ed., Vol. 1, Philadelphia: WB Saunders, 1986, p. 860.)

Example 3.6

A patient with slow and shallow breathing had a pCO_2 of 58 mm Hg and a total CO_2 of 33.8 meq/L. What is the acid–base status?

Solution: The $[H_2CO_3]$ is $0.0301 \times 58 = 1.75$ meq/L, hence $[HCO_3^-] = 33.8 - 1.75 = 32.05$ meq/L pH $= 6.1 + \log 32.05/1.75 = 7.36$. The patient is slightly acidotic, with both the pCO_2 and the $[HCO_3^-]$ above normal. The patient therefore has a partly compensated respiratory acidosis. If the patient had a metabolic alkalosis with partial respiratory compensation, his or her blood pH would have been above 7.4.

this serves to induce hemoglobin to release oxygen. This phenomenon, known as the *Bohr effect*, is discussed in greater detail in Chapter 7.

QUESTIONS

3.1 Which statement about the pK is *incorrect*?
    a. pK is a constant independent of temperature.
    b. pK reflects the capacity to donate protons.
    c. The higher the pK, the less acid the substance.
    d. Buffer capacity with respect to both H^+ and OH^- is highest at the pK.
    e. pK is a pH at which the protonated and unprotonated form concentrations of an acid are equal.

3.2. Which of the following has the highest *capacity* to buffer both the H^+ and OH^- ions?
    a. 0.5 M acetic acid.
    b. 0.1 M acetate buffer at pH 3.76.
    c. 0.1 M acetate buffer at pH 4.70.
    d. 1.0 M acetate buffer at pH 4.60.
    e. 0.5 M sodium acetate.

3.3. What is the approximate pH of 10^{-8} M HCl?
    a. 5   b. 6   e. −8
    c. 7   d. 8

3.4. Which expression is *incorrect*?
    a. $[OH^-][H^+] = 10^{-14}$.
    b. $pCO_2(mm) \times 0.0301 = CO_2(mEq/L)$.
    c. $pH = \log 1/[H^+]$.
    d. $pH = pK$ for Na^+ acetate-acetic acid buffer when $[Na^+] = [acetate]$.
    e. Normal plasma $[HCO_3^-]/[H_2CO_3] = 20$.

3.5. What is the pH of an acetate buffer ($pK = 4.76$) prepared by adding 20 ml of 1 M HCl to 100 ml of a solution of 0.3 M sodium acetate (MW 82)?
    a. 4.25   b. 4.46   e. 5.26
    c. 4.76   d. 5.06

For Questions 3.6–3.8, consider the following facts: a patient comes in with a blood pCO_2 of 25 mm Hg and a "total CO_2" of 25 meq/L.

3.6. What is the patient's blood bicarbonate in mEq/L?
    a. 0.75   b. 24.25   e. 37.5
    c. 25.8   d. 50.0

3.7. What is the patient's plasma pH (use $pK = 6.1$)?
    a. 7.51   b. 7.40   e. 7.61
    c. 7.35   d. 7.47

3.8. The patient is most likely suffering from
    a. Compensated respiratory alkalosis.
    b. Uncompensated respiratory alkalosis.
    c. Uncompensated metabolic alkalosis.
    d. Overcompensated metabolic acidosis.
    e. The patient is normal.

3.9. The pH of 0.1 M formic acid solution will be
    a. 1.70   b. 2.39
    c. 4.08   d. 3.77   e. 1.88

3.10. Suppose a patient's plasma has a pH of 7.2 and a bicarbonate concentration of 18.5 mEq/L. What is the base deficit? Use Figure 3.2.
    a. 15   b. 5.5   c. 18.5
    d. 24   e. 9.0

3.11. What is the base excess in meq/L in a patient with fully compensated respiratory acidosis having an initial pH of 7.2 and $[HCO_3^-] = 28$ meq/L?
    a. 20   b. 28   e. 15
    c. 44   d. 4

For Questions 3.12–3.15, use the following answers:
    a. Organic and inorganic phosphates   d. Citric acid (protonated)
    b. "Total CO_2"   e. Methylamine (protonated)
    c. H_2SO_4 (protonated)

3.12. Find the weakest acid in Table 2.
3.13. What is the principal intracellular buffer system?
3.14. Which is a diprotic acid?
3.15. Which conjugate base is uncharged?

Answers

3.1. (a) pK is derived from K_d, which is temperature dependent, as are all equilibrium constants.
3.2. (d)   Although pH 4.60 is not the pK, the buffering capacity of this buffer will exceed that in c because of its 10-fold higher concentration.
3.3. (c)   pH will approach 7, because the $[H^+]$ contributed by water (10^{-7} M) is higher than that contributed by HCl (10^{-8} M).
3.4. (d) $pK = pH$ only when [acetate] = [acetic acid].
3.5. (b)   100 ml of 0.3 M NaAc represents 30 mmol, and the addition of 20 mmol HCl will convert 20 mmol NaAc to HAc, leaving 10 mmol NaAc. Then pH = 4.76 + log 10/20 = 4.76 − log 2 = 4.76 − 0.30 = 4.46.
3.6. (b) $[H_2CO_3] = 0.0301 \times 25 = 0.75$ meq/L. $[HCO_3^-] = 25 − 0.75 = 24.25$ meq/L.
3.7. (e)   pH = 6.1 + log 24.25/0.75 = 6.1 + log 32.3 = 7.61.
3.8. (b)   High pH, normal $[HCO_3^-]$, and low pCO_2 are consistent with uncompensated (pure) respiratory alkalosis (see Figure 3.3).
3.9. (b) $K_d = \dfrac{[H^+]\,[formate]}{[formic\ acid]} = 1.7 \times 10^{-4}$; because [formate] = $[H^+]$ and [formic acid] = $0.1 − [H^+]$, $1.7 \times 10^{-4} = \dfrac{[H^+]^2}{0.1 − [H^+]}$; ignoring $[H^+]$ in the denominator, we have $[H^+]^2 = 1.7 \times 10^{-5}$ and $[H^+] = 4.12 \times 10^{-3}$ M; pH = $-\log 4.12 \times 10^{-3} =$ 2.39.
3.10. (e)   Mark the point at which pH 7.2 corresponds to $[HCO_3^-] = 18.5$ (at the $pCO_2 =$ 50 mm isobar). Now draw a line parallel to the normal buffer line through this point. It intersects the pH 7.4 line at the 15 meq/L point. Base deficit is 24 (normal) − 15 = 9 meq/L.
3.11. (a)   Find the point corresponding to pH = 7.2 and $[HCO_3^-] = 28$ meq/L (at the $pCO_2 = 75$ mm isobar). Now move along the isobar to the pH 7.4 line, which intersects it at 44 meq/L. Base excess = 44 − 24 (normal) = 20 meq/L.
3.12. (e)   The weakest acid has the highest pK; it is protonated methylamine ($CH_3NH_3^+$).
3.13. (a)   Phosphates are intracellular, whereas bicarbonate and H_2CO_3 are extracellular buffers.
3.14. (c) H_2SO_4 is a diprotic acid because it releases two protons in solution.

3.15. (e) The conjugate base in the Henderson-Hasselbalch equation is the unprotonated form of the weak acid. In methylamine, it is CH_3-NH_2.

PROBLEMS

3.1. The pK_a for hydroxylamine, NH_2OH, is 8.0. What is the pH of a 0.1 M hydroxylamine solution? How would you prepare 1 L of 0.1 M hydroxylamine buffer at pH 7.5?

3.2. Calculate the pH and acetate ion concentration when a buffer solution is prepared by mixing 400 ml of 0.1 M formic acid and 200 ml of 0.1 M sodium acetate. The pK_a values of formic and acetic acid are 3.75 and 4.76, respectively. Is there an advantage to preparing buffers of this sort as opposed to simple acetate and formate buffers?

3.3. Explain the following phenomenon: If one added 5 mmol HCl to 1 L of a closed solution containing 24 mmol bicarbonate and 1.2 mmol H_2CO_3, the pH would change from 7.4 to 6.58. However, if this is done in vivo in the bloodstream, the pH change is much smaller, from 7.4 to 7.3. Why?

BIBLIOGRAPHY

Davenport HA. The ABC of Acid–Base Chemistry, 5th ed. Chicago: University of Chicago Press, 1971.

Lowenstein J. Acid and Basics. New York: Oxford University Press, 1993.

Tarr RS, Norwell DY. A unifying clinical basis for teaching acid–base balance in biochemistry. Biochem Educ 12:14–17, 1985.

4

Amino Acids and Proteins

After reading this chapter, the student should

1. Know the names, structures, and classification of all amino acids and their side chains present in proteins, and be familiar with their physical and chemical properties, such as conformation, absorption of ultraviolet light, and reactions with ninhydrin.
2. Be able to solve acid–base problems involving amino acids, draw structures at various pH values, estimate isoelectric points and net charges, and construct and interpret their titration curves.
3. Be familiar with the general structure of peptides and their synthesis and the properties of the peptide bond; be familiar with methods of end-group analysis; and be able to apply the concepts of acid–base chemistry to peptides, including estimation of net charges and isoelectric points.
4. Know basic language to describe and/or classify proteins: primary, secondary, tertiary, and quaternary structures, the different types of conjugated proteins, and acidic and basic proteins.
5. Be familiar with methods for protein molecular weight determination and the limitations of such methods: gel filtration, gel electrophoresis, and hydrodynamic methods.
6. Be familiar with the principles governing primary structure determinations in proteins: hydrolysis for amino acid composition, fragmentation with CNBr, trypsin and chymotrypsin and their application to the discovery of hemoglobin S; relation among proteins (homologies) on the basis of primary structures, including the serine proteinase group, the cytochrome c group, the lysozome group, the β-lactoglobulin group, and the hemoglobin group; explain the principle of amino sequence determination of proteins directly and from their mRNAs and cDNAs.
7. Be familiar with the various secondary structures of proteins and their dimensions: the α helix, β turns, pleated sheet structures, and collagen and what dictates the assumption of such

shapes; know the general principles of the x-ray diffraction method.

8. Be familiar with why proteins assume the three-dimensional shapes that they do, including physical and covalent bonding, the relationship between polarity and shape and Chothia's classification of proteins; the mechanism and agents for denaturation, and what parameters change when a protein is denatured.

9. Understand how proteins act as polyelectrolytes; discuss separation methodologies based on ionic properties of proteins: electrophoresis, ion-exchange chromatography, and isoelectric focusing.

4.1   INTRODUCTION

Proteins are large molecules that play a vital role in the organization and function of living organisms. They are polymers of amino acids, and their sizes range from a few thousand to the tens of millions of daltons. Among the more important functions performed by proteins are the following. (1) They provide the structural framework of cells and tissues. Examples are collagen and elastin. (2) They act as antibodies in the bloodstream to immobilize foreign materials, such as viruses and bacteria. (3) They act as biologic catalysts, called enzymes. (4) They perform mechanical work, such as skeletal muscle contraction and the pumping action of the heart. (5) They act as transport media in the bloodstream for a variety of substances, such as lipids and oxygen.

A mammalian cell may contain as few as 2000 different proteins and as many as 50,000 at any given time. Each of these is uniquely suited to the function it performs, and this in turn depends on its size, shape, solubility in aqueous media, acid–base properties, propensity to form fibers, and numerous other physical and chemical properties. The component amino acids are largely responsible for the ability of proteins to perform their biologic roles. The properties of amino acids are therefore of paramount importance in determining how proteins work.

4.2   PROPERTIES OF AMINO ACIDS

4.2.1   Structures of Amino Acids

An *amino acid* may be defined as a compound possessing an amino and an acid group, which is almost always a carboxyl group. The most important amino acids from the biomedical point of view are the α-amino acids, which with the exception of glycine possess a *chiral* (asymmetric) carbon in the α (number 2) position. We thus have α-D- and α-L-amino acids:

$$
\begin{array}{llll}
\text{COO}^- & 1 & & \text{COO}^- & 1 & & \text{CHO} \\
\text{}^+\text{NH}_3-\overset{|}{\underset{|}{\text{C}}}-\text{H} & 2 & \alpha & \text{H}-\overset{|}{\underset{|}{\text{C}}}-^+\text{NH}_3 & 2 & \alpha & \text{HO}-\overset{|}{\underset{|}{\text{C}}}-\text{H} \\
\overset{|}{\underset{|}{\text{C}}} & 3 & \beta & \overset{|}{\underset{|}{\text{C}}} & 3 & \beta & \text{H}_2\overset{|}{\text{C}}-\text{OH} \\
\overset{|}{\underset{|}{\text{C}}} & 4 & \gamma & \overset{|}{\underset{|}{\text{C}}} & 4 & \gamma & \text{L-glyceraldehyde} \\
\overset{|}{\underset{|}{\text{C}}} & 5 & \delta & \overset{|}{\underset{|}{\text{C}}} & 5 & \delta & \text{CHO} \\
\overset{|}{\text{C}} & 6 & \epsilon & \overset{|}{\text{C}} & 6 & \epsilon & \text{H }\overset{|}{\underset{|}{\text{C}}}-\text{OH} \\
& & & & & & \text{H}_2\overset{|}{\text{C}}-\text{OH}
\end{array}
\tag{4.1}
$$

L–amino acid   D–amino acid   D-glyceraldehyde

The configurations of amino acids have been related to the two optical isomers of glyceraldehyde, whose absolute configurations are known and used as reference compound; the L-amino acids are of the same configuration as L-glyceraldehyde, and D-amino acids are related in this context to D-glyceraldehyde. The D and L forms of an amino acid rotate plane-polarized light in opposite directions, and they are termed *enantiomers*. A 1:1 mixture of the two forms is a *racemic mixture*, and it does not rotate plane-polarized light. The carbon atoms in Structure (4.1) are also labeled 1–6 and α through ϵ. Carbon 2 is referred to as the α carbon, and the carboxyl (carbon 1) and amino groups attached to it are termed α-carboxyl and α-amino groups, respectively. An ϵ-amino group would be located on carbon 6, as in lysine. Most naturally occurring α-amino acids have the L configuration. Some amino acids have additional chiral carbon atoms (threonine and isoleucine). Only about 20 different α-amino acids are found in proteins, all present in the L configuration. D-Amino acids are rarely found in nature.

Hydroxylysine and hydroxyproline are normally found in collagen-like proteins, and γ-carboxyglutamic acid is found only in prothrombin and other calcium binding proteins. All amino acids other than glycine contain *side chains*, that is, chemical groupings attached to their α-carbon atoms. These side chains are extremely important in imparting various properties to proteins. Amino acids may be classified on the basis of their side chain properties. Thus, the acidic amino acids have acidic side chains, the aromatic amino acids have benzene rings in their side chains, and so on. The various α-amino acids with their structures and names of side chains are given in Table 4.1.

In addition to those listed in Table 4.1, other amino acids are present in small amounts in specialized proteins, including several types of methylhistidines in muscle proteins, phosphoserine in casein and certain enzymes, and pyroglutamic acid as N-terminal amino acid in several proteins.

The most abundant amino acid in the human organism does not occur in proteins and does not have a carboxyl group. Its acidic residue is the sulfonate group, and its name is *taurine* ($\text{N}^+\text{H}_3-\text{CH}_2-\text{CH}_2-\text{SO}_3^-$). It occurs in the free state (exact function often unknown) and in bile salts, in which it plays an important role in fat digestion and absorption (see Chapters 9 and 19). Other amino acids that do not occur in proteins are *ornithine* and *citrulline*. They are important intermediates in the urea cycle described in Chapter 20.

Table 4.1 Amino Acids Encountered in Proteins[a]

Amino acid	Abbreviation	Structure	Common name of side chain	$[\alpha]_d$	pI
		Neutral aliphatic amino acids			
Glycine	Gly G		None	0	6.1
L-Alanine	Ala A		Methyl	13.7[b] 2.42[c]	6.0
L-Valine	Val V			28.8[b] 6.42[c]	6.0
L-Leucine	Leu L			15.2[b] −10.6[c]	6.0
L-Isoleucine	Ile I			40.6[b] 11.3[c]	6.0
L-Serine	Ser S			15.0[d] −6.83[c]	5.7
L-Threonine	Thr T			−28.3[c]	5.6
		Sulfur amino acids			
L-Cysteine	Cys C		Sulfhydryl group	7.6[d]	5.1
L-Cystine	Cys-Cys		Disulfide group	−214[d]	n.a.

Table 4.1 Continued

Amino acid	Abbreviation	Structure	Common name of side chain	$[\alpha]_d$	pI
L-Methionine	Met M	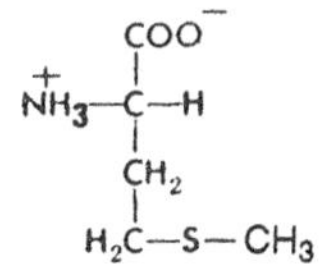	Mercaptomethyl group	-8.11^c 23.4^d	5.7

Acid amino acids

Amino acid	Abbreviation	Structure	Common name of side chain	$[\alpha]_d$	pI
L-Aspartic acid	Asp D	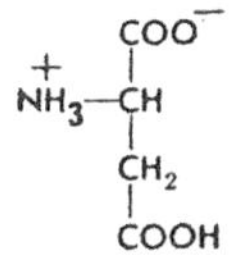	β-Carboxyl group	24.6^b 4.7^c	2.8
L-Glutamic acid	Glu E	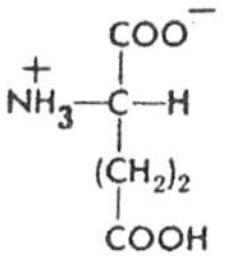	γ-Carboxyl group	31.2^b 11.5^c	3.2
L-Carboxylglutamic acid		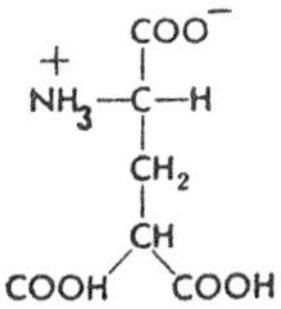	γ-Carboxyl group	NA	n.a.

Aminidinated amino acids

Amino acid	Abbreviation	Structure	Common name of side chain	$[\alpha]_d$	pI
L-Asparagine	Asn N	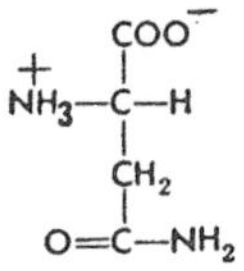		34.3^d -5.3^c	5.4
L-Glutamine	Gln Q	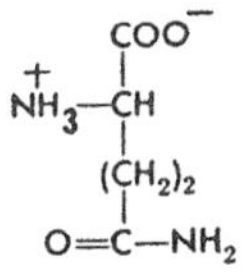		5.0^c	5.7

Basic amino acids

Amino acid	Abbreviation	Structure	Common name of side chain	$[\alpha]_d$	pI
L-Lysine	Lys K	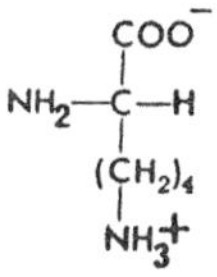	ϵ-Amino groups	25.9^b 14.6^c	9.7
L-Arginine	Arg R	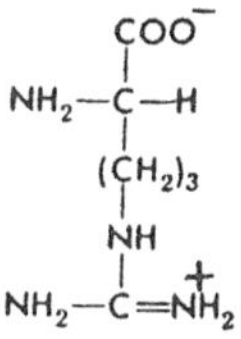	Guanido groups	27.6^b 12.5^c	10.8

Table 4.1 Continued

Amino acid	Abbreviation	Structure	Common name of side chain	$[\alpha]_d$	pI
L-Hydroxylysine	OH-Lys	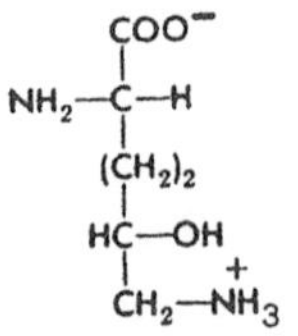	ϵ-Amino group δ-Hydroxyl group	14.5[b]	9.1

Heterocyclic amino acids

L-Tryptophan	Trp W	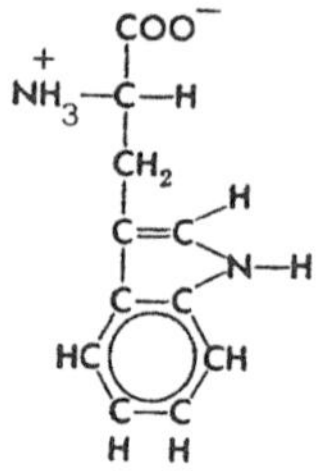	Indole group	−31.5[c] 2.4[d]	5.9
L-Proline	Pro P	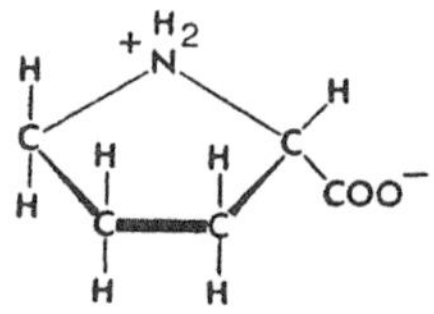	Imino group	−52.6[d] −85.0[c]	6.3
L-Hydroxyproline[e]	OH-Pro	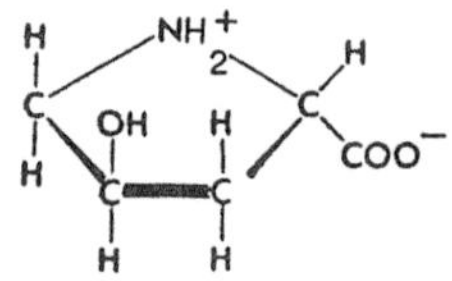	Hydroxyimino group	−47.3[d] −75.2[c]	5.7
L-Histidine	His H	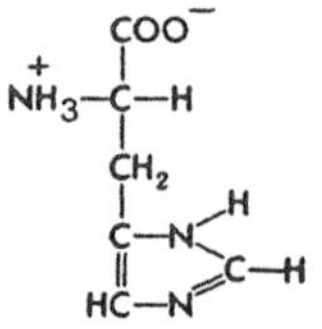	Imidazole group	13.3[b] −39.0[c]	7.6

Aromatic amino acids

L-Phenylalanine	Phe F	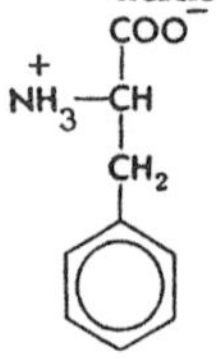	Phenyl group	−35.1[c]	5.5
L-Tyrosine	Tyr Y	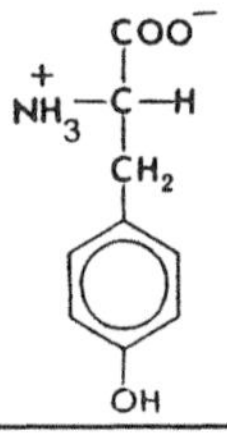	Phenolic group	−8.6[b]	5.7

4.2.2 Physical and Chemical Properties of Amino Acids

Among the properties of amino acids that are most pertinent to the biomedical scientist are their optical rotations, already discussed, which are listed for each amino acid in Table 4.1. Note the dramatic differences between optical rotations in the *zwitterionic* (water) and fully protonated (HCl) forms. Further, all amino acids absorb ultraviolet light in the range 190–220 nm. The C=O bond in carboxyl residues is largely responsible. Moreover, aromatic amino acids, especially tryptophan, absorb in the 260–285 nm range. Protein concentrations in solutions are often determined via absorption at 210 or 280 nm.

Amino acids are chemically reactive at their α-amino groups and their side chains. The carboxyl groups are relatively unreactive unless activated. A very useful reaction is the oxidative deamination of amino acids with *ninhydrin*. The reaction produces a blue pigment, which can be used for the detection of amino acids both qualitatively and quantitatively. The series of reactions producing the blue complex is given in Equation (4.2).

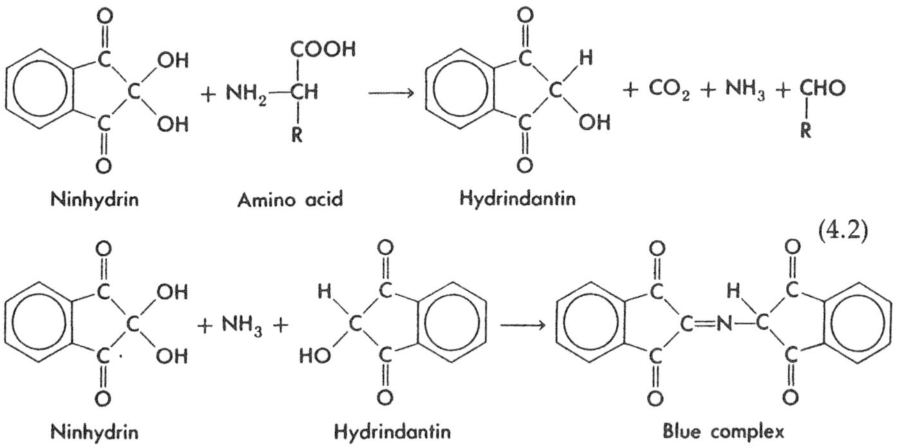

(4.2)

A very important property of amino acids is their ability to accept and donate protons, that is, to act as acids and bases. A compound that can act as both an acid and a base is said to be *amphoteric* or an *ampholyte*. Both the α-amino and carboxyl groups, as well as several side chains, can participate in proton exchange reactions. This means that amino acids can be titrated and can be used as buffers. When carboxyl, the phenolic, or the sulfhydryl groups lose protons, they become negatively charged; on the other hand, when an amino, imidazole, or guanido group gains a proton, it becomes positively charged. When the number of positive charges is exactly equal to the number of negative

Notes to Table 4.1

[a]The structures are drawn in their zwitterionic forms with a net charge of 0. [α], optical rotation, Na D line; NA, not available; pI, isoelectric point.
[b]In 6 N HCl.
[c]In water.
[d]In 0.5–3 N HCl.
[e]Structure shown is that of 4-hydroxyproline, which occurs largely in collagen. A less commonly occurring 3-hydroxyproline is also present in collagen.

charges, the structure is then called a *zwitterion*. For glycine, this form may be represented by

$$
\begin{array}{c}
\text{COO}^- \\
\;\;\;\; | \\
\overset{+}{\text{NH}_3}\text{- C-H} \\
| \\
\text{H}
\end{array}
\qquad\qquad (4.3)
$$

Amino acid forms shown in Table 4.1 are given in their zwitterionic (uncharged) states.

Each titrable group of an amino acid has a characteristic pK value, that is, a pH at which 50% of a specific group present is protonated and the other half is nonprotonated. Table 4.2 lists the pK values of various titrable groups of amino acids. Each amino acid also has a characteristic pH at which it exists in the zwitterionic form; that is, it has a net charge of 0. Such pH values, termed *isoelectric points* (pI), are listed for each amino acid in Table 4.1. For each individual amino acid, the pI can be calculated by averaging two pK values. Thus, for glycine, the pK values for the α-carboxyl and amino groups are 2.4 and 9.8, respectively. The pI is therefore 6.1. For acidic amino acids (aspartic and glutamic), the pK values of the two acidic groups are averaged: for aspartic acid, pI = (2.0 + 3.9)/2 = 3.0. For basic amino acids, such as lysine, the two higher pK values are averaged: pI = (9.2 + 10.8)/2 = 10. Acidic amino acids thus have low pI values, basic amino acids have high pI values, and neutral amino acids have pI values near 6. Further, at pH below the pI, an amino acid is positively charged, whereas at pH above the pI, the amino acid is negatively charged.

The acid–base behavior of amino acids may also be illustrated via titration curves. If one started with aspartic acid hydrochloride, that is, aspartic acid crystallized from solution in hydrochloric acid, one would require 3 mol base to remove completely the protons from 1 mol aspartic acid. The titration curve obtained with structures at each step of the reaction series is shown in Figure 4.1. Note that the *isoelectric point* is attained after one proton equivalent has been removed from the molecule. At this point, aspartic acid contains one positive and one negative charge: it is zwitterionic.

Table 4.2   pK Values of Titrable Amino Acid Groups

Group name	pK range for most amino acids
α-Carboxyl group	1.8–2.4
α-Amino group	9.0–10.0
ϵ-Amino group	10.8
Guanido group	12.5
Imidazole group	6.0
Sulfhydryl group	10.5
Phenolic group	10.1
β-Carboxyl group	3.9
τ-Carboxyl group	4.1

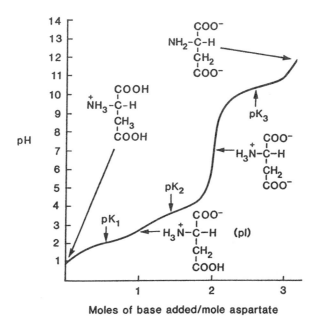

Figure 4.1 Titration curve of aspartic acid. pK_1, pK_2, and pK_3 are pK values of the α-carboxyl, γ-carboxyl and α-amino groups, respectively. The fully protonated form is present at a very low pH (e.g., pH 1); the fully deprotonated form is present at a very high pH (e.g., pH 12). The zwitterionic form (net charge 0) is present at pH $\simeq$ 3, which is also the pI.

All amino acids can be used as buffers. The buffering regions are pH values near the pK values of each titrable group. For aspartic acid, buffering regions most likely are around pH 2, 3.9, and 9.9 (pK of the α-amino group). These can be identified as plateau regions in Figure 4.1.

Example 4.1

To 100 ml of a solution containing 0.1 M monosodium glutamate is added 17 ml of 1 M HCl. What is the final pH, and which molecular forms are present?

Solution: Monosodium glutamate has the following ionic structure and undergoes the following conversion to more protonated states:

$$
\begin{array}{ccc}
\text{COO}^- & \text{COO}^- & \text{COOH} \\
| & | & | \\
\overset{+}{\text{NH}_3}-\text{CH} & \overset{+}{\text{NH}_3}-\text{CH} & \overset{+}{\text{NH}_3}-\text{CH} \\
| & | & | \\
\text{CH}_2 \xrightarrow[\text{HCl}]{\text{10 m moles}} & \text{CH}_2 \xrightarrow[\text{HCl}]{\text{7 m moles}} & \text{CH}_2 \\
| & | & | \\
\overset{+}{\text{Na}} \quad \text{CH}_2 & \text{CH}_2 & \text{CH}_2 \\
| & | & | \\
\text{COO}^- & \text{COOH} & \text{COOH} \\
\text{Monosodium} & \text{Zwitterionic} & \text{Fully protonated} \\
\text{glutamate,} & \text{form} & \text{form} \\
\text{10 m moles}
\end{array}
\tag{4.4}
$$

There are a total of 10 mmol glutamate; 10 mmol HCl (of a total of 17 mmol added) converts the singly negatively charged glutamate ion to its zwitterionic form. The additional 7 mmol HCl converts 7 mmol zwitterionic glutamate to 7 mmol fully protonated glutamate, leaving 3 mmol zwitterionic glutamate behind. The pH is then calculated using the Henderson-Hasselbalch equation as follows (pK values of glutamate are 2.1, 4.1, and 9.5): pH = 2.1 + log 3/7 = 1.73. There will be 3.0 mmol of the zwitterionic form and 7 mmol of the fully protonated form in solution [see Equation (4.4)]. Note that pK 2.1, rather than 4.1 or 9.5, was used in the Henderson-Hasselbalch equation. This was chosen because pH 2.1 represents the interconversion of the fully protonated and the zwitterionic forms of glutamate, the forms present in the buffer.

4.3 PEPTIDES

4.3.1 Structures and Properties of Peptides

The most important reaction of amino acids from a biologic point of view is their ability to form *peptide linkages*, that is, the reaction of the amino group of one amino acid with the carboxyl group of another:

$$
\begin{array}{ccc}
\text{COOH} & \text{COOH} & \text{O} \quad \text{H} \quad \text{COOH} \\
| & | & \| \quad | \quad | \\
\text{NH}_2-\text{C}-\text{H} + \text{NH}_2-\text{C}-\text{H} \longrightarrow \text{NH}_2-\text{CH} & \text{C}-\text{N}-\text{CH} & + \text{H}_2\text{O} \\
| & | & | \quad\quad\quad R_2 \\
R_1 & R_2 & R_1
\end{array}
\qquad (4.5)
$$

Amino acid$_1$ Amino acid$_2$ Dipeptide

The peptide formed has retained a carboxyl and an amino group, which are free to form peptide linkages with other amino acids. In this fashion, *peptides* of various lengths may be formed. Very long peptides are called polypeptides and proteins. Shorter peptides are termed di-, tri-, tetrapeptides, and so on, on the basis of the number of amino acids they contain. Specific peptides are named in accordance with the amino acids they contain (in addition to, of course, any trivial name they may possess). The name begins with the N-terminal amino acid (amino acid residue possessing a free α-amino group), and the suffix *yl* is added to it. One proceeds in this fashion until the C-terminal amino acid is reached, for which the original name is retained. Thus, Ala-Pro-Glu-Lys is named alanylprolylglutamyllysine.

The physical and chemical properties of peptides are similar to those of amino acids except that the peptide bonds add another dimension to these compounds. Amino and carboxyl groups involved in the peptide linkage can no longer accept or donate protons. The peptide bond itself carries a partially planar (double-bonded) character because of the resonance effects that are possible:

$$
\begin{array}{ccc}
\text{O} & & \text{O}^- \\
\| & & | \\
\text{C}-\text{C}-\overset{..}{\text{N}}-\text{C} & \rightleftharpoons & \text{C}-\text{C}=\overset{+}{\text{N}}-\text{C} \\
| & & | \\
\text{H} & & \text{H}
\end{array}
\qquad (4.6)
$$

where the $-O^-$ and the $-H$ of N^+-H are positioned trans to each other.

Structure Proofing of Peptides

All peptides and proteins, unless they are cyclic, contain the so-called N- and C-terminal residues: a free α-amino group at one end and a free α-carboxyl group at the other. The identity of such groups may be determined by various chemical and enzymatic means. One of the first such methodologies utilized *fluorodinitrobenzene* (FDNB) for N-terminal group analysis:

$$\text{(4.7)}$$

| Amino group | Fluorodinitrobenzene | Dinitrophenylated amino acid |

FDNB reacts with all free $-NH_2$ groups, including ϵ-amino groups. Following acid hydrolysis of the dinitrophenylated protein, a separation of the dinitrophenylated N-terminal amino acid from the rest of the hydrolysis products can be achieved by organic solvent extraction of the hydrolysate. A more modern procedure utilizes dansyl chloride instead of FDNB. This method requires less protein, because dansylated amino acids can be identified via fluorescence measurements.

$$\text{(4.8)}$$

| Amino group | Dansyl chloride | Dansylated amino acid |

Another N-terminal amino group identification procedure is *Edman degradation* using phenylisothiocyanate as the reagent. This procedure has the advantage of not requiring the hydrolysis of the protein into its component parts following modification with the reagent. The phenylthiohydantoin of the N-terminal amino acid comes off under mildly acidic conditions, leaving the protein minus its N-terminal amino acid intact. In fact, the latter can then be used to determine the next few amino acids at the N terminus of the peptide or protein. The Edman procedure has been automated to provide sequence data for peptides and proteins.

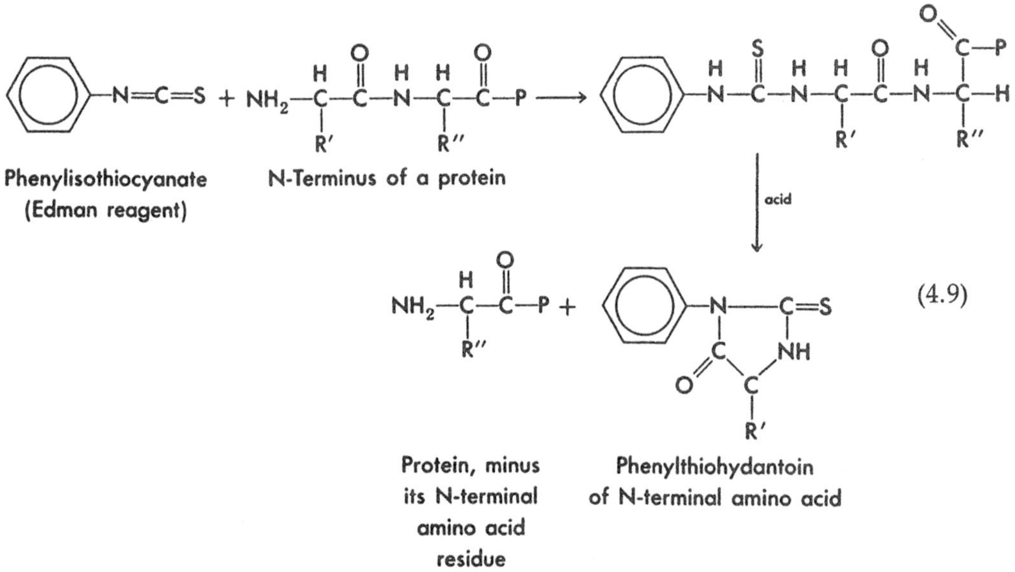

Phenylisothiocyanate
(Edman reagent)

N-Terminus of a protein

(4.9)

Protein, minus
its N-terminal
amino acid
residue

Phenylthiohydantoin
of N-terminal amino acid

Carboxyl-terminal amino acid residues can be identified using exopeptidases called carboxypeptidase A and B. These are enzymes normally found in mammalian small intestine. Carboxypeptidase A causes the removal of amino acids, other than proline and basic amino acids, from the C terminus of peptides and proteins. The C-terminal amino acid appears first, followed by the next in line, and so forth. Carboxypeptidase B removes basic amino acids from the C termini of peptides and proteins.

4.3.2 Naturally Occurring Peptides

Numerous biologically active peptides are known, some having hormone function, others being antibiotics, and so on. *Glutathione* is a ubiquitous peptide that plays a role as an antioxidant and possibly an amino acid transporter. It is a rare example of a peptide linkage involving the γ-carboxyl group of glutamate:

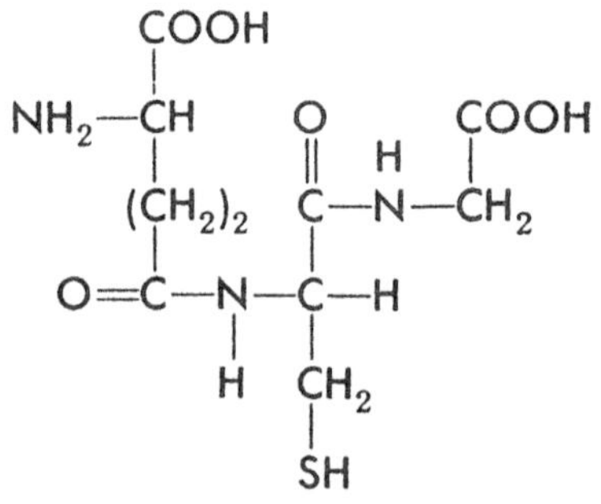

(4.10)

Glutathione
(γ-glutamylcysteinylglycine)

Other examples include the pituitary hormones vasopressin (antidiuretic hormone, ADH), oxytocin, and adrenocorticotrophic (stimulating) hormone (ACTH):

$$(4.11)$$

NH$_2$-Ser-tyr-ser-met-glu-his-phe-arg-trp-gly-lys-pro-val-gly-lys-lys-arg-arg-pro-val-lys-val-tyr-pro-asp-ala-gly-glu-asp-glu-ser-ala-glu-ala-phe-pro-leu-glu-phe-COOH

Human ACTH

Among the peptide antibiotics are gramicidin S (from *Bacillus brevis*) and bacitracin A (from *Bacillus subtilis*), which contain D-amino acids in addition to L-amino acids:

$$(4.12)$$

4.3.3 Chemical Synthesis of Peptides

In biologic systems, elaborate mechanisms exist for the joining of amino acids to form peptides and proteins with the expenditure of energy in the form of ATP or by genetic engineering techniques described in Chapter 15. Small proteins and peptides may also be synthesized in the laboratory by strictly chemical means, however. Steps must be taken to assure that the reactions proceed as desired: carboxyl and amino groups that are not to participate in peptide bond formation must be blocked, and the carboxyl group that *is* to participate must be activated with, for example, PCl$_5$. The latter step may be omitted if a carbodiimide compound is used as a condensing agent. The synthetic procedure is presented in Equation (4.13):

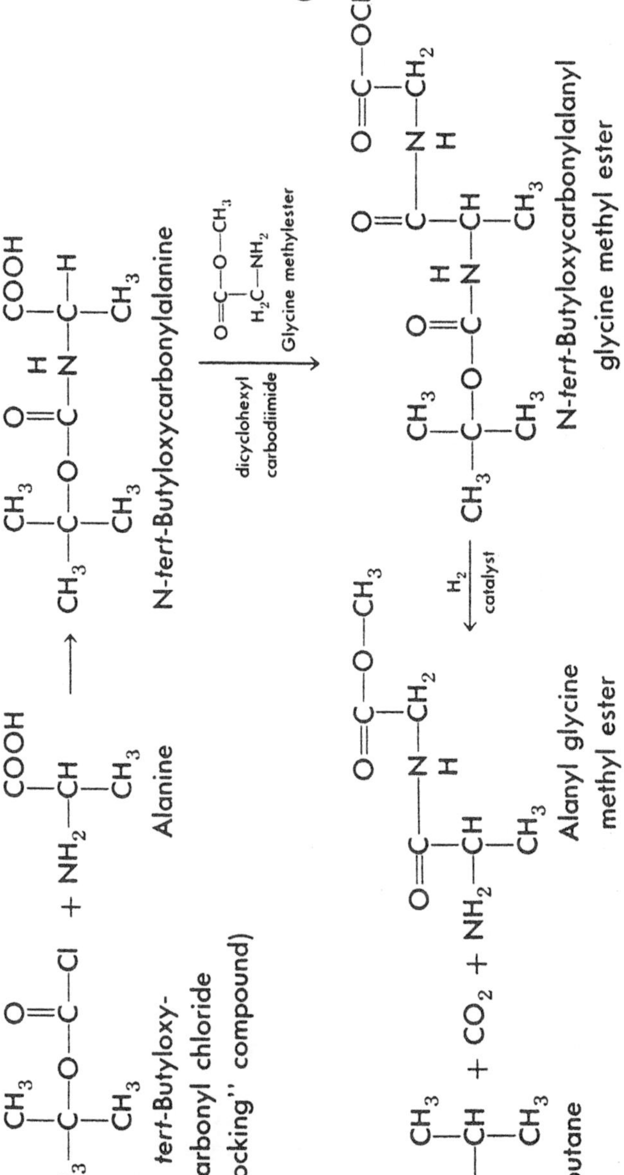

$$
\begin{array}{c}
\text{CH}_3 \\
\text{CH}_3\!-\!\overset{\displaystyle \text{CH}_3}{\underset{\displaystyle \text{CH}_3}{\text{C}}}\!-\!\text{O}\!-\!\overset{\displaystyle \text{O}}{\overset{\|}{\text{C}}}\!-\!\text{Cl} \;+\; \overset{\displaystyle \text{COOH}}{\text{NH}_2\!-\!\text{CH}}\!-\!\text{CH}_3
\end{array}
$$

tert-Butyloxy-carbonyl chloride ("blocking" compound)   Alanine

$\longrightarrow$

$$
\text{CH}_3\!-\!\overset{\text{CH}_3}{\underset{\text{CH}_3}{\text{C}}}\!-\!\text{O}\!-\!\overset{\text{O}}{\overset{\|}{\text{C}}}\!-\!\overset{\text{H}}{\underset{}{\text{N}}}\!-\!\overset{\text{COOH}}{\text{C}}\!-\!\text{H} \quad (\text{CH}_3)
$$

N-*tert*-Butyloxycarbonylalanine

dicyclohexyl carbodiimide │ $\text{O}=\text{C}-\text{O}-\text{CH}_3$, $\text{H}_2\text{C}-\text{NH}_2$ Glycine methylester

$\longrightarrow$ (4.13)

N-*tert*-Butyloxycarbonylalanyl glycine methyl ester

$\xrightarrow[\text{catalyst}]{\text{H}_2}$

Alanyl glycine methyl ester

$$
\overset{\text{CH}_3}{\underset{\text{CH}_3}{\text{CH}_3\!-\!\text{CH}}} \;+\; \text{CO}_2 \;+\; \text{NH}_2\!-\!\text{CH}\cdots
$$

Isobutane

The amino group blocker is removed from the blocked peptide by mild hydrogenation, and the methyl ester group can be split by mild alkaline hydrolysis. The process of synthesizing large peptides and small proteins, pioneered by Bruce Merrifield, has been automated using a solid support medium rather than the classic organic synthetic procedure shown in Equation (4.13). The principle, however, remains the same.

4.4 PROTEINS

Proteins are large polypeptides with molecular weights ranging from a few thousand into the millions. They contain 16% N on the average. Because some 20 amino acids are present in most proteins and there is no limitation to the size and amount of each amino acid a protein may contain, the number and types of proteins found in nature are almost limitless. Each protein has certain physical and chemical properties that are uniquely suited to its role in the living organism. The properties a protein may exhibit are ultimately a result of its amino acid content. Amino acid side chains determine whether the protein is water soluble, whether it is acidic or basic, and the shape it assumes. It is thus extremely important to study the amino acid content and sequences in proteins, as well as to ascertain their shapes and sizes. To exhibit a specific biologic property, a protein must not only contain the correct amino acid sequence but it must also have the appropriate size and shape.

For the sake of convenience, the different aspects of protein structure have been divided into four categories: primary, secondary, tertiary, and quaternary structures. When we speak of the *primary* structure of a protein, we are concerned with the amino acid sequence of its component polypeptide chains. A protein may have a single polypeptide chain with one N and one C terminus, or it may have two or more polypeptide chains, often termed *subunits*, with multiple N and C termini. *Secondary* structure problems address themselves to whether the polypeptide chains of a protein exhibit any sort of periodicity of structure in three dimensions: that is, is the polypeptide chain simply an extended ribbon, or is it present in the form of a spring or a folded structure? Secondary structure has also been referred to as *conformation*. *Tertiary* structure is concerned with the overall three-dimensional appearance of the protein: for example, is the shape of the protein molecule best approximated by a sphere or by a disk? Last, *quaternary* structure refers to the number, size, and shape of component polypeptide chains in a protein.

Proteins may be classified on the basis of the properties they possess. We may, for instance, distinguish simple and conjugated proteins. The latter, in contrast to simple proteins, possess components other than amino acids. Such proteins are often described on the basis of their non–amino acid components: lipoproteins are those containing lipid; glycoproteins contain carbohydrate; nucleoproteins contain nucleic acid; and heme proteins contain heme as prosthetic groups. Metalloproteins contain metals. They may be heme proteins, such as *hemoglobins*, iron-sulfur proteins, often termed *ferredoxins*, or enzymes with metal prosthetic groups. Classification may also exist on the basis of solubility: *albumins* are proteins soluble in water, whereas *globulins* require some salt to go into solution, for example 0.005–0.1 M NaCl. The terms "albumin" and "globulin" are used by clinical biochemists. Shapes of protein molecules may also serve as a basis for classification. Thus, *globular proteins* are usually soluble in aqueous media and are relatively symmetric. Fibrous proteins, on the other hand, are less soluble and are quite asymmetric. Among fibrous proteins are *collagen*, the most abundant protein of the human organism; hair *keratin*; *silk fibroin*; and the muscle protein *myosin*. Function may also serve as a basis classifying proteins. Proteins may function as structural entities, to perform contraction (contractile proteins), biologic catalysts (enzymes), or as means of transport or binding of small molecules. Other classification schemes are also possible.

4.4.1 Molecular Weights of Proteins

An investigation of the properties of a protein usually begins with the determination of its molecular weight. Historically, methodologies involving osmotic pressure, viscosity, light scattering, and especially ultracentrifugal measurements have been used for molecular weight determinations. The more modern techniques involve molecular sieve (gel) chromatography and gel electrophoresis, not because these are more accurate, but because they are relatively rapid and do not require elaborate instrumentation. The procedure of *gel filtration* is based upon the fact that certain materials manufactured in the bead form, which have porosities of known size, permit smaller proteins to penetrate the beads while allowing the larger proteins to bypass the bead altogether. Small proteins thus take a longer route through the column than larger proteins. This is illustrated in Figure 4.2. By

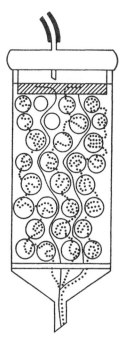

Figure 4.2 Gel filtration of a large-molecular-weight protein (solid line) and a small-molecular-weight protein (dotted line). The latter penetrates the beads and takes a longer route through the column. The large-molecular-weight protein passes among the beads, taking a shorter route through the column.

noting the elution volume from a standardized column, such as that shown in Figure 4.3, the molecular weight of an unknown protein may be estimated. It is assumed that the unknown protein has approximately the same shape as the proteins used to standardize the column. Separation can then be presumed to have occurred on the basis of protein size. A relatively asymmetric protein migrates faster (small elution volume) down a molecular sieve column than a relatively symmetric (globular) protein of the same molecular weight; hence it is important to keep the shapes of proteins in mind when performing gel filtration experiments.

Another widely used procedure for molecular weight determinations is *gel electrophoresis*, in which the migration of proteins is accomplished through an electrical field. To avoid shape effects on the rate of migration, as well as differences in net charge, most proteins may be rendered into a random coil con-

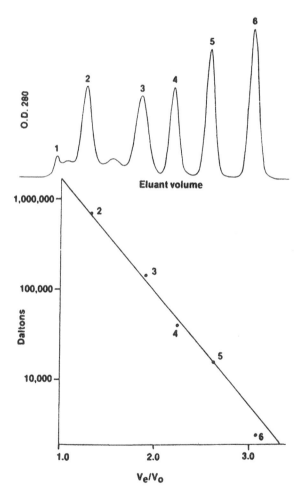

Figure 4.3 Gel filtration of a set of standard proteins on BioRad Biogel A 1.5 M column. The y scale is logarithmic. The x scale is the ratio of protein eluted volume to void volume. Point 2 is thyroglobulin (MW 670,000), 3 is bovine IgG (MW 158,000), 4 is ovalbumin (MW 44,000), 5 is myoglobin (MW 17,000), and 6 is cyanocobalamin (vitamin B_{12}, MW 1350). (Reproduced by permission of BioRad Laboratories.)

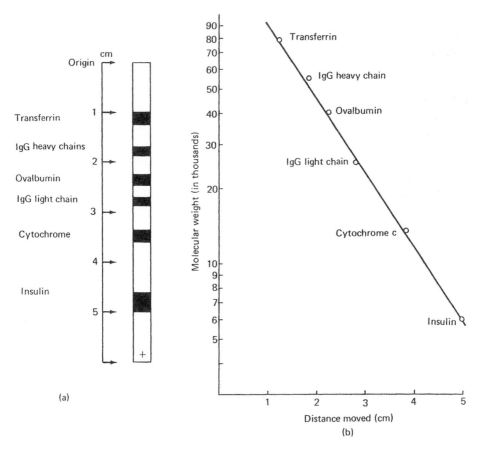

Figure 4.4 Polyacrylamide gel electrophoresis of a standard mixture of proteins. (a) Gel stained with a dye after electrophoresis. (b) Distance moved versus log of the molecular weight. (Adapted from Bezkorovainy A, Grohlich DA. Comparative study of several proteins of the transferrin class. Comp Biochem Physiol 47B:787–797, 1974.)

formation through the action of urea and mercaptoethanol (see later). An anionic detergent, such as sodium dodecyl sulfate (SDS), is then added, which binds to the protein, giving it an overwhelmingly net negative charge. Thus, all proteins in a standard mixture, as well as the unknown protein, are negatively charged and are in the random coil conformation, and their migration through the porous gel is solely a function of their molecular weights. This holds true as long as the proteins consist of single polypeptide chains. If there are proteins with two or more subunits, these subunits then become separated, and the gel gives molecular weights of the subunits, not the native protein. Figure 4.4 illustrates the essentials of this method.

4.4.2 Primary Structures of Proteins

One of the first tasks in elucidating the primary structure of a protein is to determine its amino acid content. To accomplish this, the protein must first be hydrolyzed to break the peptide linkages. This is generally accomplished with 6

N HCl for 24–72 h. Alkaline hydrolysis is used to liberate tryptophan, because it is destroyed by acid hydrolysis. Amino acids can then be detected qualitatively by the method of partition chromatography. Quantitation is done by liquid chromatography using various types of *ion-exchange resins*. This method has been automated and is conveniently done in high-performance liquid chromatography (HPLC) systems. The amino acid content of a protein may be expressed in terms of percentage by weight or, if the molecular weight is known, as the number of amino acid residues per molecule of protein.

The amino acid sequence of a protein can be determined directly by the Edman degradative procedure. Proteins larger than 30–60 amino acid residues in length do not lend themselves well to this procedure, however, and must first be fragmented. A number of fragmenting agents break specific peptide linkages. Among these are the digestive endopeptidases trypsin and chymotrypsin. Trypsin breaks those peptide linkages in which the basic amino acids contribute the carboxyl group, whereas chymotrypsin breaks those linkages in which the aromatic amino acids contribute the carboxyl groups. Cyanogen bromide (CNBr) breaks those peptide bonds in which methionine contributes carboxyl groups. There are some bacterial proteinases whose specificities are known, and these have also been utilized for fragmenting proteins. Amino acid sequences in each fragment are then determined.

When a protein has been fragmented and sequenced, it then becomes necessary to determine the order in which each fragment appears in the original protein. One can begin by determining the N-terminal and the C-terminal residues of each fragment obtained and comparing these with the N- and C-terminal groups of the native protein. End-group analysis has been described. If the identification of the amino- and carboxyl-terminal fragments is not sufficient to arrange all the fragments obtained in their proper order, then the protein must be fragmented with another agent, so that the investigator can find fragments with overlapping amino acid sequences and thus fit them into the native protein structure.

Determining amino acid sequences of proteins by classic procedures is a tedious process. In addition, proteins are often insoluble (e.g., membrane proteins) or cannot be easily purified. However, if the protein's gene, mRNA, or cDNA of the mRNA are available, the amino acid sequence of the protein can be determined from nucleotide sequences rapidly and unambiguously using the universal genetic code. In this code, each amino acid in correlated with one or more nucleotide triplets in mRNA (see Chapter 12). mRNA is "transcribed" from DNA and can be used to synthesize complementary (cDNA) via an enzyme called *reverse transcriptase*. In many cases it is easier to isolate the mRNA or cDNA of a protein than the protein itself.

It is frequently necessary to compare the primary structures of several related proteins without going through the enormous task of determining their entire amino acid sequences. This may be accomplished by a method called *fingerprinting*, whereby the proteins are first subjected to fragmentation with trypsin or another agent and then the fragment mixture is subjected to two-dimensional *partition chromatography*. This is a technique that separates peptides, amino acids, and other compounds by partitioning them between an aqueous (stationary) and an organic (mobile) phase on a supporting medium, such as paper or silica gel. In closely related proteins, all fragments (peptides) are in identical positions, except for perhaps one or two peptides. These can then be eluted from the supporting medium and studied more thoroughly. Fingerprinting was the method whereby the difference between the normal and *sickle cell hemoglobin* (HbS) was discovered. The difference was within 1 peptide of 27 obtained, which proved to be the N-terminal peptide of the β chain. In HbS, a valyl residue replaces a glutamate group in position 6 of the β chain. See Chapter 7 for a discussion of HbS disease.

Proteins with analogous functions, isolated from different life forms, often contain sections with identical amino acid sequences. Such proteins are believed to have originated by a gene duplication process and subsequent divergence. But for acceptable point mutations (amino acid substitutions) that have occurred during the course of evolution, such proteins would have had identical amino acid sequences. It is believed that those amino acid sequences that have been retained throughout the course of evolution are essential for the function of the protein, and had a mutation occurred resulting in a substitution of an amino acid in these crucial protein sections, the mutation would have been lethal to the animal. Proteins that show similarities in their amino acid sequences are *homologous proteins*.

It is possible to construct a phylogenetic tree on the basis of amino acid sequence studies of homologous proteins possessing the same function in a series of species. The basic principle is that the closer two animals are on the evolutionary scale, the fewer amino acid substitutions are found in their proteins having the same function. The first such tree was worked out by Margoliash and his colleagues on the basis of amino acid sequence studies in cytochrome c of a number of species. Cytochrome c is an enzyme involved in electron transport, which has 104 amino acid residues. Table 4.3 shows the number of amino acid substitutions in this protein in a number of species compared with humans. In general, phylogenetic trees constructed on the basis of the primary structure of proteins correspond rather well to those constructed on the basis of paleontologic and geologic data.

Homologous proteins also exist within a single animal species, and they may actually have different functions. Examples of such homologous proteins

Table 4.3 Amino Acid Substitutions in Cytochrome c from the Following Species Compared with the Human

Species	No. amino acid substitutions
Chimpanzee	0
Rhesus monkey	1
Dog	11
Horse	12
Dogfish	23
Moth	31
Wheat	35
Neurospora (fungus)	43
Yeast	44

include the enzyme lysozyme and the milk protein α-lactalbumin; the hydrophobic small molecule binding proteins β-lactoglobulin (a milk protein), retinol binding protein, and lipoprotein D (serum proteins) and the BG protein (secretory protein from olfactory epithelium); and the serine proteinase/esterase group: trypsin, chymotrypsin, elastase, acetylcholine esterase, plasmin, and thrombin. This last group of enzymes has a highly conserved amino acid sequence that stretches around the active serine and histidine residues, and all are inhibited by diisopropylfluorophosphate (DFP), a nerve gas that combines with the active-site serine residue.

The homology phenomenon has also been observed in the subunits (component polypeptide chains) of various protein molecules. The best example is provided by the hemoglobin series, a group of O_2 binding proteins, largely from red-blood cells. The oldest protein of this group from an evolutionary point of view is *myoglobin*, a muscle protein with a molecular weight near 18,000. An ancestral gene coding for a primitive heme protein may have undergone a duplication process some 475 million years ago to give ancestors of modern myoglobins, on the one hand, and a precursor of modern *globins* (protein portion of hemoglobin), on the other. The various polypeptide chains of *hemoglobin* have then arisen by duplications of genes, in which the gene coding for the α chain is the most primitive. Protein homology is also observed in single-chain proteins, which are products of the gene fusion process. Thus in *transferrin*, the iron-carrying protein of human plasma, the two halves (*domains*), residues 1–336 and 337–678, show an extensive internal homology of nearly 40%.

4.4.4 Secondary Structure of Proteins

In most proteins, the constituent polypeptide chain(s) does not exist in the extended unordered form. This was appreciated through the examination of x-ray diffraction patterns of both fibrous and crystalline soluble proteins (e.g., hemoglobin). X-rays (wavelength 1.54 Å) are diffracted by fibers or crystals because of the periodicity (repeated orderliness) of their structures. Diffracted x-rays may be captured on film in the form of symmetric smudges (in fibers) or an array of dots (with crystals), from which bond lengths, folding and coiling, and the overall three-dimensional structure in proteins may be deduced. Such x-ray diffraction patterns are illustrated in Figure 4.5.

Pauling and Corey were pioneers in interpreting such protein x-ray diffraction patterns. By studying x-ray diffraction patterns of model amino acid and peptide crystals, they were able to establish bond lengths and angles in peptides, that the peptide bond was essentially planar, and that the carbon atoms attached to the amide (–N–C=O) group were trans with respect to each other. In extrapolating these data to proteins, Pauling and coworkers proposed that the dimensions of the peptide bond were universal, that all peptide bonds in a protein were identical, and that *hydrogen bonds* existed between the N–H and the C=O groups of peptide bonds that were located in close proximity to each other. Such hydrogen bonds were proposed to be 2.68–2.92 Å long and could not deviate from the axis of the N–H bond by more than 30°. With these limitations in mind, Pauling's group could construct two helical polypeptide chain structures. One contained 5.1 residues per turn, each amide residue being hydrogen bonded to

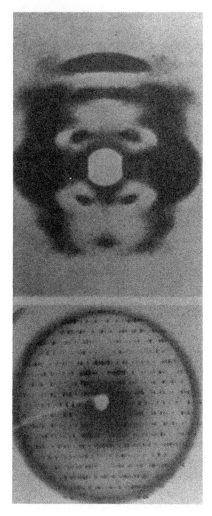

Figure 4.5 X-ray diffraction patterns of fibrous collagen (upper pattern) and hemoglobin crystal (lower pattern). Positions of smudges or dots may be related to molecular parameters of the protein molecule. (Reproduced with permission from Kartha G. Picture of proteins by x-ray diffraction. Acct Chem Res 1:374–381, 1968.)

the fifth amide residue above and below the starting peptide bond. The hydrogen bond was at 25° relative to the axis of the N–H bond. This structure was termed the γ helix, and it has not yet been found in nature. The second possibility was a helix with 3.6–3.7 amino acid residues per turn with 1.45–1.53 Å per residue. Each amide residue was hydrogen bonded to the third peptide linkage above and below the starting amide bond. The hydrogen bonds were found to exist at an angle of 10° relative to the N–H bond. This structure was termed the α helix.

The α-helical structure was predicted to give meridional (vertical axis of Figure 4.5) x-ray reflections with spacings at 1.45–1.53 Å and at 5.22–5.62 Å, representing the translational length of each amino acid residue and the translational length of each turn of the α helix, respectively (3.6–3.7 residues at 1.45–1.53 Å each). These two very typical reflections have indeed been observed in a number of fibrous proteins of the α-keratin type (α-myosin, fibrinogen, porcupine quill, bacterial flagella, hair keratin, and synthetic poly-γ-benzyl glutamate). The α helix is illustrated in Figure 4.6, and it is almost universally found in native proteins.

As stated earlier, the α helix structure is stabilized by hydrogen bonds; these are interactions of 1–7 kcal/M, stabilized by ΔH effects, between hydrogen atoms with a partial positive charge, on the one hand, and oxygen atoms, on the other (see Chapter 3). Hydrogen bonds stabilizing the α helix involve the N–H group of one peptide linkage and the C=O group of another. Figure 4.7 shows that the α helix-stabilizing hydrogen bonds form 13-atom rings (3.6_{13} helix).

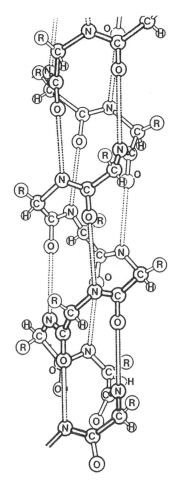

Figure 4.6 The right-handed α helix. The darkened bonds delineate the polypeptide backbone. Dotted bonds are hydrogen bonds, where the H atoms normally present on the N atoms have been omitted. Notice the location of amino acid side chains (R) on the outside periphery of the α helix. (Reproduced with permission from Kendrew JC. The three-dimensional structure of a protein molecule. Sci Am December:10, 1961.)

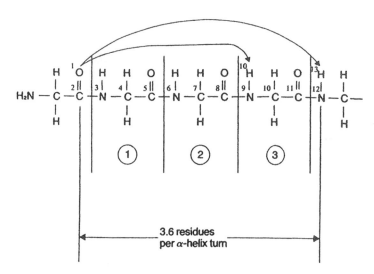

Figure 4.7 Formation of the hydrogen bond in the α helix between =O (1) and –H (13) to give a 13-atom ring. A 10-atom ring is also shown. The =O and H–N are not shown in a transconfiguration for cosmetic reasons of appearance. (Reproduced with permission from Melius P. Alpha-helix revisited. Trends Biochem Sci August, 1980.)

Other structures are also possible, such as the 10-atom ring (3_{10}) or the 16-atom ring (π) helix; however, these do not occur to any great extent in nature. Another feature of α helix geometry is that the amino acid side chains are located outside the α-helical core in planes perpendicular to the α helix axis. The core of the α helix is hydrophobic.

The α helix is an important component of *integral membrane proteins*. These are proteins that traverse the hydrophobic plasma and organelle membranes (see Chapter 9) and perform important biologic functions. The portion of the protein that is embedded in the membrane is α-helical because the α helix provides for a maximum number of hydrogen bonds, which serve to reduce the hydrophilic nature of peptide linkages. The side chains of such trans-membrane α helices are also hydrophobic, even though under normal circumstances, such amino acids would prefer to form other secondary structures.

The second type of secondary structure recognized by the x-ray crystallographers is the pleated sheet structure, formerly called the β helix. It comes in two forms, the *parallel* and the *antiparallel* structures. These are shown in Figure 4.8. The most prominent features of the pleated sheet structures are that, in the parallel type, each amino acid residue accounts for a spacing of 3.25 Å, whereas the antiparallel sheet spacing is 3.51 Å. Because in a fully extended polypeptide chain this distance is 3.65 Å, the pleated sheet structures are only slightly folded. Another feature is that, in the parallel sheet, all polypeptide chains run in the same direction, whereas in the antiparallel type, contiguous chains run in opposite directions. Proteins that contain extensive pleated sheet structures are stretched hair keratin, silk fiber, and many soluble globular proteins. Table 4.4 lists percentages of amino acid residues present in the α-helical, pleated sheet, and β turn conformations for some representative proteins.

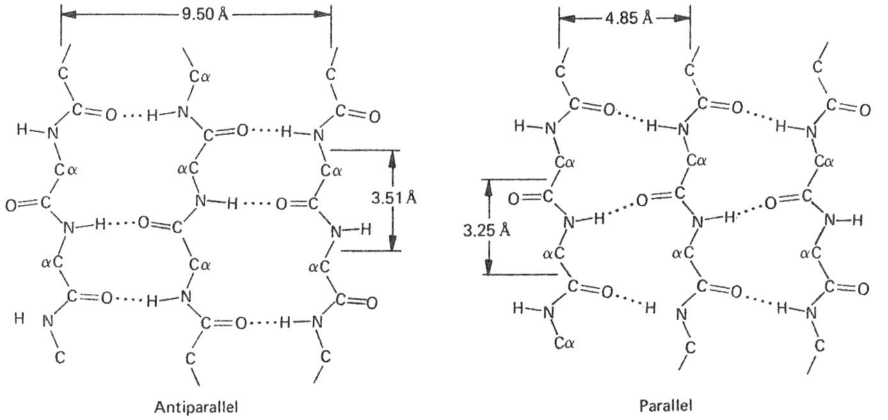

Figure 4.8 Parallel and antiparallel pleated sheet structures. Dotted lines indicate hydrogen bonds. (Reproduced with permission from Bezkorovainy A. Basic Protein Chemistry. Springfield, IL: Thomas, p. 114, 1970.)

Table 4.4 Types of Secondary Structures Found in Some Representative Proteins and Fidelity of the Chou-Fasman Prediction (P)

Protein	% α	No.[a]	P_α[b]	% B[c]	P_β[b]	No. turns
Carboxy peptidase A	38	9	65	17	62	13
Chymotrypsin	14	3	46	45	70	17
Concanavalin A	2	1	100	57	64	—
Cytochrome b_5	52	6	81	25	70	2
Cytochrome c	39	5	—	—	—	6
Insulin A	52	3	50	6	—	—
Lactate dehydrogenase	45	10	58	20	68	10
Lysozyme	40	6	72	12	35	6
Myoglobin	79	8	88	0	—	6
Pancreatic trypsin inhibitor	28	2	47	33	64	—
Ribonuclease	26	3	89	35	68	2
Thermolysin	38	7	73	22	64	1

[a]Number of helical segments, mostly α-helical.
[b]Percentage of helical or pleated sheet structures predicted correctly.
[c]Pleated sheet structures.
Source: Data from Liljas A, Rossmann MG. X-ray studies of protein interactions. Annu Rev Biochem 43:475–505, 1974; Argos P, Schwarz JS, Schwarz J. An assessment of protein secondary structure prediction methods based on amino acid sequence. Biochim Biophys Acta 439:261–273, 1976.

A third type of ordered structure giving x-ray patterns is the collagen helix. The basic collagen unit consists of three intertwined chains, in which one twist accounts for a distance of 9 Å, with three amino acid residues present in each twist.

A commonly occurring secondary structure type, which was not considered by Pauling and his associates, is the β turn (also called the tight turn). The

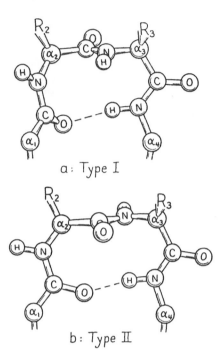

Figure 4.9 Two major types of β (tight) turns. In type II, R₃ is usually glycine. (Reproduced with permission from Richardson JS. The anatomy and taxonomy of protein structure. Adv Prot Chem 34:167–339, 1981.)

two major types of β turns are shown in Figure 4.9. Note that they differ from each other on the basis of the R_2 and R_3 orientations: in type I these are trans to each other, whereas in type II they are cis. Although both types of turns are stabilized by hydrogen bonds creating 10-atom rings, neither is helical. Other types of tight turns are also found, although less frequently than types I and II. A structure related to the β turn is the β bulge, which most often occurs as an irregularity in pleated sheet structures.

The random coil is the extended polypeptide chain, which shows no orderliness or periodicity whatever. It does not yield x-ray diffraction patterns. Each amino acid accounts for 3.65 Å in the random coil.

The reason proteins assume secondary structures has to do with their thermodynamic stability. It has already been stated that the geometry of the peptide bond permits the formation of hydrogen bonds in the α helix. Another reason is the interaction of the various residues associated with a polypeptide chain: those conformations in which interference with free rotation is minimal are most stable. Consider two peptide linkages with a central α carbon, illustrated in Figure 4.10. Free rotation of the essential planar peptide groupings is permitted about the two bonds on either side of the α carbon atom. Such rotation cannot proceed freely, however, because the –H and =O groupings interfere with each other. Hence, to minimize overlap of these groups, the protein chain assumes a conformation such that these groups leave a maximum amount of space with respect to each other, thus minimizing the energies of interaction. The

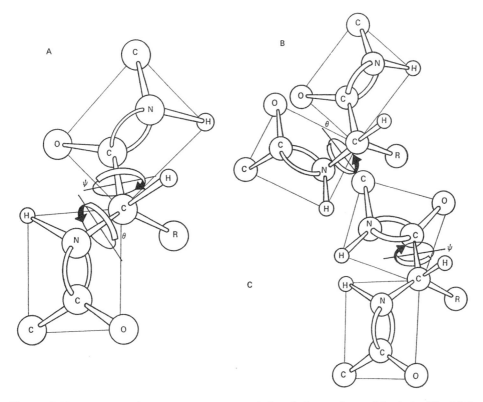

Figure 4.10 Rotation of two contiguous peptide bonds in a polypeptide chain. The N-C linkage is indicated as a double bond to emphasize its partial double-bond character and planarity. The values of angles ϕ and ψ are taken as 0 when the two peptide bonds are coplanar (structure A). Structure B indicates positions of the two peptide bonds when $\psi = 0°$ and $\phi = 180°$, whereas structure C indicates $\psi = 180°$ and $\phi 0°$ (Drawn by Dr. H. Sky-Peck, Rush Medical College, Chicago, IL.)

various positions of the two peptide groupings shown in Figure 4.9 may be represented by the magnitude of angles subtended when these groups rotate about the two bonds on either side of the α carbon atom. These angles are termed ϕ and ψ. If the various combinations of ϕ and ψ are examined, only a limited number of such combinations are found to give stable peptide conformations. These relationships are shown in Figure 4.11, which is termed a *Ramachandran plot*, in honor of its discoverer. Note that when the properties of the α helix, the pleated sheet, and collagen structures are examined, they happen to fall in the "permissible" areas of the Ramachandran plot.

Ramachandran plots serve to answer the question of why the α-helical or the pleated sheet structures have the properties that they do; however, the plots do not serve to predict whether a given polypeptide chain will assume the α-helical, the pleated sheet, or a random conformation. Anfinsen and his colleagues have proposed that it is the amino acid composition and sequence in a given peptide chain that determine the conformation the chain assumes. Ideally, we should be able to look at an amino acid sequence of a protein and then

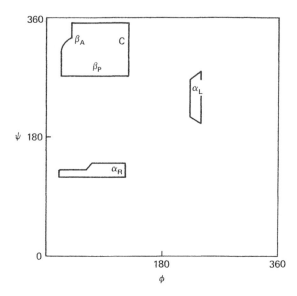

Figure 4.11 Ramachandran plot showing permissible conformational regions. α_R and α_L indicate positions of the right- and left-handed α helices; β_A and β_P indicate the positions of the anti-parallel and parallel pleated sheet structures, respectively. C indicates collagen.

predict where the α helix, pleated sheet, and turn structures are located. By examining the occurrence of all amino acids in the secondary structures of proteins with known conformations (x-ray diffraction patterns!), it has been possible to determine that some amino acids occur more frequently in α helix; others tend to the pleated sheet structures or turns. Quantitatively, it is possible to assign a probability factor P to each amino acid that characterizes its occurrence in one of the secondary structure forms. Randomness (no preference) is indicated by a P value of 1. This is characteristic of Arg. On the other hand, for Met and Glu, the P_α values are 1.47 and 1.44, respectively, and their P_β values are 0.97 and 0.75. These two amino acids thus tend to be associated with the α helix. Pro and Gly have P_α values of 0.50 and 0.56, respectively, and P_β values of 0.64 and 0.92. Their turn P values, however, are 1.91 and 1.64, respectively, and hence they tend to be located in turns. Amino acids with bulky side chains, Val, Leu, Ile, Trp, Tyr, Thr, and Phe tend to pleated sheets: their P_β values are 1.49, 1.02, 1.45, 1.14, 1.25, 1.21, and 1.32, respectively. Pro, Gly, Ser, Asp, and Asn are present in turns, the rest of the amino acids in the α helix.

The most frequently used predictive method for secondary structures was developed by Chou and Fasman. They proposed that an α helix is present where four of six adjacent amino acids are α helix formers and if their average $P_\alpha > 1.0$ and their $P_\beta < 1$. The α helix continues until a Pro residue is reached or the average P_α of four consecutive residues is less than 1. A pleated sheet is preferred when three of five consecutive residues are pleated sheet formers, where their average $P_\beta > 1.04$ and their $P_\alpha < 1$. Again, this conformation is continued until the average P_β of four adjacent residues is less than one. A turn is encountered where four adjacent amino acids are turn formers. The Chou-Fasman method, as well as others, are not perfect, but they do provide a starting point from which we can get an idea of what a protein looks like. Table 4.4 indicates the predictive values for several proteins, based on the Chou-Fasman predictive approach.

4.4.4 Tertiary Structure of Proteins

Various hydrodynamic studies of proteins, for example viscosimetry and diffusion, have shown that proteins behave in solution as fairly compact and symmetric particles. In time, equations were developed to describe the overall size and shape of proteins in terms of ellipsoids of revolution. Two basic types of ellipsoids of revolution, the *prolate* and *oblate*, are used to depict the approximate three-dimensional shapes of protein molecules. These are shown in Figure 4.12. Each ellipsoid of revolution may also be described by an *axial ratio*, that is, the ratio of the short axis to the long axis. A spherical protein molecule has an axial ratio of 1:1, whereas an asymmetric molecule, such as fibrinogen, may have an axial ratio of 1:10.

The exact three-dimensional appearance a protein assumes is governed by a number of factors, including the amino acid content of proteins. Proteins soluble in aqueous solutions have a very specific distribution of amino acid side chains: the polar side chains are located on the surface in contact with the aqueous environment, whereas the hydrophobic side chains are in the protein particle interior, in a hydrophobic environment. Occasionally, polar groups may be present in the protein particle interior; these are said to be buried and may be exposed only upon denaturing the protein. It is thus clear that the higher the number of polar residues in a protein molecule, the greater is the protein surface area: the protein is more asymmetric as the number of polar residues increases. On the other hand, the higher the number of hydrophobic residues, the smaller is the protein surface area. Minimum surface area is achieved with a spherical particle. This may not be sufficient to keep away all the hydrophobic groups

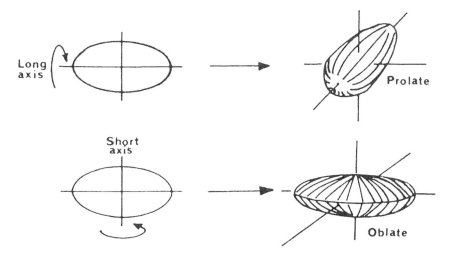

Figure 4.12 Three-dimensional appearance of prolate and oblate ellipsoids of revolution representing three-dimensional protein structures. (Reproduced with permission from Bezkorovainy A. Basic Protein Chemistry. Springfield, IL: Thomas, p. 83, 1970.)

from the aqueous environment, and the protein may then aggregate to form a larger multisubunit particle. We may illustrate this principle using the following approximations for accessible protein surface areas, where A is the surface area, $Å^2$ is square angstroms, and M is the molecular weight:

> For native globular proteins, $A = 11.116M^{2/3}Å^2$
> For denatured proteins (maximum surface area), $A = 1.44MÅ^2$.
> For dimers (per subunit), $A = 0.857 \times 11.116 \times M^{2/3}\ Å^2$.
> For tetramers (per subunit), $A = 0.714 \times 11.116 \times M^{2/3}\ Å^2$.

These relationships clearly indicate that the water-accessible surface area per subunit decreases as the protein molecules aggregate to form larger particles.

Although various hydrodynamic studies have shown that most soluble protein particles have relatively simple shapes that can be approximated by ellipsoids of revolution with axial ratios not too far from 1, the anatomy of such protein particles is far from simple, if we look at their constituent secondary structures and the interactions required to maintain their three-dimensional appearance. A given protein molecule may consist only of packed segments of α helix, but then again, several other types of secondary structures may also be present. Each protein molecule has a unique secondary structural anatomy, all such structures being packed into a relatively compact and symmetric particle. Figure 4.13 illustrates the anatomy of some proteins. The hemoglobin β subunit is illustrated in Figure 4.13A; it shows only α helix with a number of turns, in which the constituent heme molecule can be observed in the upper left-hand portion of the molecule. In Figure 4.13B is the structure of triose phosphate isomerase, a glycolysis pathway enzyme, showing sections of α helix, parallel pleated sheet structures, turns, and disordered structures. In Figure 4.13C we see *β-lactoglobulin*, a bovine milk protein that binds hydrophobic substances. It contains an α helix segment, disordered structures, and antiparallel pleated sheets. The pleated sheet structures in Figure 4.13B and C are arranged to form *barrel* structures. The barrel in β-lactoglobulin also contains the binding site for hydrophobic substances; in this case, vitamin A is shown within this barrel.

Structurally, proteins have been divided by Chothia and colleagues into five classes: class I has only α helix (e.g., Figure 4.13A); class II has only pleated sheet structures (e.g., soybean trypsin inhibitor); class III has both α helix and β pleated sheets, but these are segregated away from each other (e.g., lysozyme); class IV has others in the primary structure (e.g., Figure 4.13B and C); and class V has little secondary structure. The latter are generally small and heavily interlinked with −S–S− bonds or contain metal. The packing of the various secondary structures is apparently governed by the arrangement of hydrophobic amino acid residues therein. On a higher organizational level, large single-chain protein molecules may assume forms in which they appear to consist of several independent units, each with its own secondary structure packing patterns. These are *domains*. An example is the transferrin molecule, which consists of the N- and C- terminal domains, each with its own iron binding site. The two domains are connected by an octapeptide bridge.

The bonds that serve to maintain proteins in their native tertiary conformations may be covalent or physical in nature. The only covalent linkage serving this purpose is the *disulfide bond*. It may join several polypeptide chains

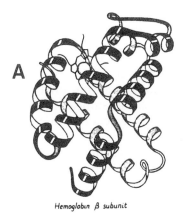

Hemoglobın β subunit

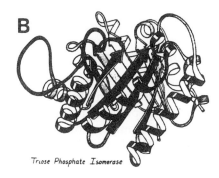

Triose Phosphate Isomerase

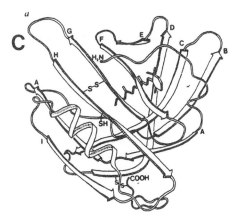

Figure 4.13 Anatomy of selected proteins. (A) The β subunit of hemoglobin carrying a heme molecule; (B) triose isomerase; and (C) β-lactoglobulin carrying a molecule of vitamin A. Spirals represent helix segments, and the broad arrows are pleated sheet polypeptide segments showing the direction from the N to the C terminus. (A and B reproduced with permission from Richardson JS. The anatomy and taxonomy of protein structure. Adv Prot Chem 34:168–339, 1981. C reproduced with permission from Papiz MZ, Sawyer L, Eliopoulos EE, North ACT, Findlay JBC, Sivaprasadarao R, Jones TA, Newcomer ME, Kraulis PJ. The structure of beta-lactoglobulin and its similarity to plasma retinol-binding protein. Nature 324:383–385, 1986.)

together, as in insulin and immunoglobulins, or it may join two segments of the same polypeptide chain, as in vasopressin, oxytocin, and β-lactoglobulin (Figure 4.13C). A disulfide bond, $-S-S-$, is formed by oxidation of two SH residues; thus, two cysteine molecules can be oxidized to form one cystine molecule.

Hydrophobic interactions are formed when two or more hydrophobic groups (for example, side chains of valine, leucine, phenylalanine, and so on) in an aqueous environment find themselves sufficiently close to exclude water molecules from their vicinity. These interactions are primarily a result of entropy effects and are believed to be of major importance in the maintenance of the tertiary structures of proteins. Scheraga and coworkers have also proposed that hydrophobic interactions may be involved in the stabilization of the α helix and the pleated sheet structures.

The *electrostatic* bond (salt linkage) is formed between two oppositely charged polar groups, for example between a γ-glutamyl group and an ϵ-amino group. They are also believed to be stabilized by entropy effects. Tertiary structures may also be stabilized by hydrogen bonds. However, hydrogen bonds are normally associated with secondary structures.

4.4.5 Quaternary Structure of Proteins

The term "quaternary structure" refers to the interaction of several polypeptide chains in a noncovalent manner to form multisubunit protein particles termed *oligomers*. Individual subunit polypeptide chains are also referred to as *protomers*. Oligomers usually have an even number of subunits (two or more). The noncovalent interactions may be of the hydrophobic, hydrogen bond, or the polar type. Examples are hemoglobin and lactate dehydrogenase (four protomers each) and many allosteric enzymes.

In many instances, one sees multisubunit proteins whose individual polypeptide chains are held together via disulfide bonds in addition to physical interactions. Examples are insulin and the immunoglobulins. However, the nature of their subunit interactions is not referred to as quaternary structure.

4.4.6 Protein Denaturation

Although most proteins are relatively stable compounds, their secondary, tertiary, and quaternary structures may be disrupted by a number of agents. Treatment with such agents may be so drastic as to cause a loss in the α-helical or pleated sheet structure, which may be converted into the random coil state. The protein would no longer behave as a compact particle when examined by hydrodynamic methods. If a protein contains $-S-S-$ linkages, random coil state (complete denaturation) is achieved if these are broken as well. Denaturation is then a process whereby all physical bonds in a protein are broken without the splitting of any peptide linkages. Denaturation may also be partial, in which certain aspects of the secondary and/or tertiary structure are broken, others being left intact. The unfolding of protein chains during denaturation has been studied by kinetic techniques, and certain proteins have been shown to unfold and refold more rapidly than others. These rate differences have been related to the proline content of proteins; proteins containing proline unfold and refold more slowly than proline-poor proteins. Apparently this is caused by a slow transition of the peptide bonds involving proline from the trans to the cis configuration during refolding. In native proteins, all peptide bonds are in the trans configuration. Denaturation is always accompanied by a loss of biologic function.

Partial or complete protein denaturation can be accomplished by a variety of agents. Thus, organic solvents serve to break the hydrophobic interactions, and acids and bases serve to break electrostatic linkages. Trichloroacetic acid is of special importance in the laboratory, because it can rapidly denature and precipitate proteins. High concentrations of urea or guanidine hydrochloride may break hydrogen, especially the hydrophobic interactions. Among physical agents causing denaturation are heat, irradiation, and surface tension.

Disulfide linkages may be broken either oxidatively or reductively. The former method involves the treatment of the protein with performic acid, which converts all disulfide bonds into cysteic acid residues. This procedure is usually performed before a protein is hydrolyzed for amino acid analysis. Cystine and cysteine are then determined as cysteic acid. The reductive cleavage of disulfide bonds involves the treatment of the protein with mercaptoethanol ($SH-CH_2-CH_2-OH$), followed by the alkylation of the newly formed $-SH$ groups. The complete disruption of all secondary interactions (that is, complete denaturation) can be achieved in most proteins with 6 M guanidine hydrochloride and 0.1 M mercaptoethanol or 8 M urea and 0.1 M mercaptoethanol.

A number of physical parameters of the protein change because of complete or partial denaturation. As the protein becomes much less symmetric, it exerts a greater resistance to various types of movement, and in many cases it precipitates. In denatured proteins, compared with their native counterparts, one generally finds lower sedimentation and diffusion rates, higher intrinsic viscosity, and a more negative optical rotation. This last phenomenon requires explanation: the optical rotation of a protein can be divided into two components. The first is provided by the optical rotation of the constituent amino acids. These are, of course, L-amino acids, and it so happens that most of them are levorotatory. Because the free rotation about the various bonds present in a protein is restricted owing to the constraints in the secondary and tertiary structures, however, a dextrorotatory contribution is superimposed. When the physical bonds are disrupted and the dextrorotatory contribution is thus eliminated, the denatured protein acts largely as a mixture of its constituent amino acids in regard to optical rotation. The specific rotation of native proteins is between -20 and $-40°$, whereas that of denatured proteins is near $-100°$.

When a protein consisting of two or more polypeptide chains is completely denatured, including the disruption of the disulfide bonds, the protein dissociates into subunits, each with a random coil conformation. When studied in the gel electrophoresis system in the presence of SDS (Figure 4.4), the constituent subunits separate according to their molecular weights (MW). Thus, immunoglobulin (MW 160,000), consisting of two light and two heavy chains (MW 25,000 and 55,000, respectively), shows two bands upon electrophoresis in a buffer containing 0.1 M mercaptoethanol, 6 M urea, and SDS. Hemoglobin (MW 67,000) shows only one band, because all four of its subunits have a molecular weight near 16,000. A single-chain protein, although completely denatured, also migrates as a single band with a molecular weight equal to that of its native counterpart. The molecular weights of native multisubunit proteins are best determined by gel filtration (Figure 4.3) or ultracentrifuge techniques.

4.4.7 Ionic Properties of Proteins

Proteins are *polyelectrolytes*: they carry positive and negative charges, and this property is ascribed to their polar amino acid side chains. Thus, proteins can be titrated, and the number of acidic and basic residues present can thereby be estimated. In addition, proteins migrate in an electrical field, and this movement is termed *electrophoresis*. Such migration, of course, depends on the net charge of the protein at the time of electrophoresis, which in turn depends on the pH of the medium.

Proteins may be positively charged, negatively charged, or carry no net charge. In the last case, the number of positive charges is exactly equal to the number of negative charges, and the pH at which this situation occurs is the *isoelectric point* (p*I*). At their p*I* values, proteins should not move in an electrical field. If a protein has a large number of acidic amino acid side chains, its p*I* will be rather low, for example in the pH 3–5 region. These are acidic proteins. On the other hand, those proteins that contain an abundance of basic amino acid side chains have high p*I*, in the pH range 9–11. They are basic proteins, and histones are an example. Most proteins have p*I* values somewhere between these extremes. When the pH of the medium in which the protein is dissolved is below its p*I*, the protein has a net positive charge, whereas if the pH is above the p*I*, the net charge is negative. The p*I* of a protein may be estimated experimentally by performing electrophoresis at pH values above and below its p*I*, as shown in Figure 4.14.

The p*I* of a protein depends of the sum total of the p*K* values of its constituent amino acid side chains. Although the p*K* values of each amino acid functional group are known (Table 4.2), if these were incorporated into a protein,

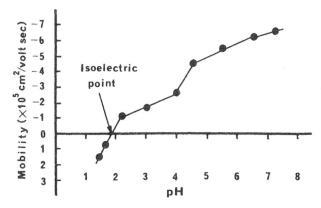

Figure 4.14 Estimation of the isoelectric point of human α-acid glycoprotein (orosomucoid), an acid glycoprotein from plasma. p*I* is the point at which the mobility curve intersects the *x* axis. (Reproduced with permission from Bezkorovainy A. Basic Protein Chemistry. Springfield, IL: Thomas, p. 22, 1970.)

their pK values could become quite different. Such internal pK values of protein side chains depend greatly on neighboring group effects. For instance, the pK of a γ- or β-COOH group may be as high as 7 in a protein, where it is around 4 in a free amino acid. It is impossible to predict the internal pK values of protein side chains, and they must be determined experimentally.

Because proteins have different isoelectric points, their mixtures can be separated by the method of electrophoresis. For maximum separation, a pH is chosen at which maximum diversity among the net charges of the constituent proteins is expected. Thus, pH 8.6 has been chosen as most suitable for the separation of human serum proteins. Human serum contains a mixture of proteins, which when subjected to electrophoresis can be separated into five groups. In the order of their migration toward the anode (positive pole), these are the τ-globulin, β-globulin, α_2-globulin, α_1-globulin, and albumin. The pattern obtained by the method of *moving boundary electrophoresis* (also called *Tiselius electrophoresis* after its discoverer) is illustrated in Figure 4.15. It can be seen from this figure that, whereas τ-globulin moved slightly toward the cathode at pH 8.6, all the other fractions moved toward the anode. At pH 8.6, τ-globulin is expected to have a slightly net positive charge, whereas all the other fractions have a net negative charge.

Today electrophoresis is most often performed on a supporting medium rather than by the moving boundary method. The medium may be paper, a

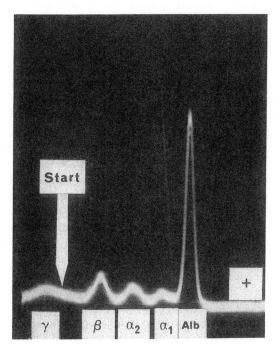

Figure 4.15 Moving boundary electrophoresis pattern of normal human serum (Reproduced with permission from Bezkorovainy A. Basic Protein Chemistry. Springfield, IL: Thomas, p. 20, 1970.)

membrane of cellulose acetate, an agarose gel film, or a polyacrylamide column. The protein mixture is applied to the medium, and the electrical field is then turned on. After an appropriate time interval, the medium is stained by a dye that has an avidity for proteins, and protein fractions are thus visualized. The stained strip can be passed through a densitometer, which converts the band pattern into a plot that looks very similar to that in Figure 4.15. The area under each peak is proportional to the intensity of its corresponding band. It can be integrated by the densitometer, so that quantitative information on each serum component can be obtained.

Note that electrophoresis separates proteins on the basis of their net charge. If the electrophoretic picture shows only one protein component, and this is observed at several pH values, it may be suspected that the protein is homogeneous. To establish homogeneity more firmly, the protein should also be subjected to a procedure that analyzes it according to size, for example ultracentrifugation and/or electrophoresis in a polyacrylamide gel in the presence of urea and sodium dodecyl sulfate.

Preparative separation of proteins can be achieved on the basis of charge differences by a method termed *ion-exchange chromatography*. This procedure involves the packing of a column with a material, such as cellulose, to which have been chemically attached charged groups, such as diethylaminoethyl. The latter are protonated and have a positive charge associated with a negatively charged counterion, such as chloride. This particular system is termed *diethylaminoethyl-cellulose* (DEAE-cellulose) chromatography. If a protein solution at a specific pH is applied to this column, all negatively charged proteins replace the Cl^- and associate with the positively charged diethylaminoethyl residues. This is *anion exchange*. The positively charged or uncharged proteins are not retained by the column. The absorbed proteins can now be eluted stepwise either by decreasing the pH of the eluant buffer or increasing its salt concentration, or both. The protein with the weakest negative charge (most basic) elutes first, whereas the most acidic protein elutes last. The column may also be packed with cellulose to which negatively charged groups (e.g., carboxymethyl groups in carboxymethyl-cellulose) are attached with Na^+ as counterions. The Na^+ exchanges with any positively charged proteins (*cation exchange*), and the absorbed proteins are then eluted stepwise with buffers of increasing pH or increasing salt concentration or both. Again, the negatively charged or uncharged proteins are not retained by the cation-exchange column. Separation of protein mixtures can also be accomplished by molecular sieve chromatography (see earlier) or on the basis of protein hydrophobicity (*reversed-phase chromatography*). Last, the analytic technique of *isoelectric focusing* can be mentioned. The basis for this protein separation technique is the creation of a pH gradient across a supporting medium, along with electrophoresis of the protein mixture through this gradient. The various proteins stop moving at the locations where the pH is equal to their respective p*I* values. This extremely sensitive technique, in combination with polyacrylamide gel electrophoresis, was applied by N. G. Anderson and coworkers to map out proteins in such complex biologic fluids as human plasma, milk, urine, and various cell extracts. Thus, more than 250 proteins have been identified in human urine and a minimum of 100 in whole saliva, and 275 proteins in addition to hemoglobin were detected in red cell lysates.

QUESTIONS

For Questions 4.1–4.8, mark as follows:
  a. If 1, 2 and 3 are correct
  b. If 1 and 3 are correct
  c. If 2 and 4 are correct
  d. If 4 only is correct
  e. If all are correct

4.1. Denatured proteins
  1. Have higher viscosities than their native counterparts.
  2. Have a higher water-accessible surface area compared with their native counterparts.
  3. Usually have lost their biologic activities.
  4. May have more titrable residues per molecule than their native counterparts.

4.2. The bonds broken during the process of denaturation are
  1. Hydrogen bonds.
  2. Electrostatic bonds.
  3. Hydrophobic bonds.
  4. Peptide bonds.

4.3. To move electrophoretically in a gel according to size only, the protein solvent must contain
  1. Buffer at a very high or low pH.
  2. Anionic detergent, such as sodium dodecyl sulfate.
  3. Salt, such as NaCl, at least at $1\ M$ concentration.
  4. Reducing agent, such as mercaptoethanol.

4.4. The α helix
  1. Can be disrupted by high concentrations of urea.
  2. Is left-handed in most naturally occurring proteins.
  3. Is terminated by proline residues.
  4. Exists only in combination with pleated sheet structures.

4.5. Which analytic or preparative technique is based on acid-base properties of proteins?
  1. Isoelectric focusing.
  2. Electrophoresis in nondenaturing solvents.
  3. Chromatography on DEAE-cellulose.
  4. Molecular sieve (gel filtration) chromatography.

4.6. Properties of disulfide bonds include
  1. Cleavage only through reduction by mercaptoethanol, for example.
  2. Stabilization of tertiary structures of proteins.
  3. Stabilization of secondary structure of proteins.
  4. The joining of polypeptide chains in many multisubunit proteins.

4.7. Properties of a zwitterionic amino acid include
  1. Ability to migrate in an electrical field.
  2. Maximum buffering capacity when in solution.
  3. All residues are protonated.
  4. Net charge in zero.

4.8. Factors that are of importance in the maintenance of the right-handed α helix are
  1. Constituent amino acids are of the L conformation.
  2. Peptide bonds have a partially planar character.
  3. The =O and –H residues present in each peptide bond are trans with respect to each other.

4. In three dimensions, the =O of the first peptide bond is sufficiently close to the –H residue of the fourth peptide bond in the carboxyl-terminal direction to form a hydrogen bond.

Answer Questions 4.9–4.13 using the following choices:
a. Diisopropyl fluorophosphate
b. Ninhydrin
c. Cyanogen bromide
d. Phenylisothiocyanate
e. Fluorodinitrobenzene

4.9. Splits peptide bonds where methionine contributes the carboxyl group
4.10. Reacts with the –OH groups of serine in certain esterases
4.11. Reagent that deaminates amino acids
4.12. Reagent that allows the determination of the N-terminal amino acid in proteins without hydrolysis with strong mineral acids
4.13. In the following table, which is *incorrect*?

		Amino acids per repeating stretch (Å)	Pitch rise (Å)	Distance per each amino acid (Å)
a.	α helix	3.6	5.4	1.5
b.	Parallel pleated sheet	2	6.5	3.25
c.	Antiparallel pleated sheet	2	6.95	3.51
d.	Collagen	3	9	3.0
e.	Random coil	3	11.0	3.65

For Questions 4.14–4.17, use the following information. You have isolated an unknown peptide whose titration curve is presented in Figure 4.16. The peptide absorbed ultraviolet light at 280 nm. Treatment with trypsin released free alanine and arginine. Treatment with chymotrypsin resulted in quantitative production of a neutral tripeptide and an alkaline dipeptide.

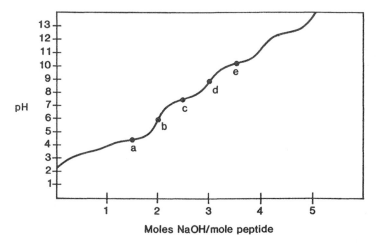

4.14. The most likely structure of the peptide is
a. Arg-Glu-Trp-Lys-Ala

    b. Ala-Lys-Trp-Glu-Arg
    c. Arg-Trp-Lys-Glu-Ala
    d. Arg-Glu-Lys-Trp-Arg-Ala
    e. Lys-Arg-Ala-Trp-Glu-Ala

4.15. The isoelectric point of the peptide is near pH
    a. 3.8   b. 6.0
    c. 7.6   d. 9.0
    e. 11.4

4.16. The peptide will have a net charge of 1.5 at which point on the titration curve?

4.17. If you had 100 ml of 1 M peptide, what must you add to adjust the pH from point d on the titration curve to 4.0? Assume you have available 1 M NaOH and 1 M HCl.
    a. 200 ml HCl   b. 167 ml HCl
    c. 67 ml HCl   d. 33 ml HCl
    e. 67 ml NaOH

Answers

4.1. (e) Denatured proteins are more asymmetric with a larger surface area than native proteins; they are biologically inactive and may contain more titrable groups as buried groups are exposed to the environment.

4.2. (a) Denaturation involves the breaking of physical bonds, not peptide bonds.

4.3. (c) To determine molecular weights of proteins by gel electrophoresis, a protein must be rendered into the random coil conformation by breaking disulfide bonds (mercaptoethanol) and physical bonds (urea), and the charge must be made overwhelmingly negative with SDS. Electrophoresis may be performed at a neutral pH.

4.4. (b) There are proteins with α-helical conformations only (e.g., myoglobin), and α helix is right-handed in naturally occurring proteins (L-amino acids).

4.5. (a) The only method not based on acid–base properties of proteins is gel filtration chromatography, which takes advantage of protein size.

4.6. (c) Disulfide bonds may also be cleaved oxidatively (performic acid); they play no role in stabilizing secondary structures (H bonds), yet they join subunits and stabilize tertiary structures of proteins.

4.7. (d) A zwitterion has a net charge of 0, with deprotonated carboxyl groups and protonated amino groups. In solution, zwitterions have minimal buffering capacities, because the pH is isoelectric.

4.8. (e) A polypeptide chain assumes the α-helical conformation because this is where H bonds can be formed most effectively. The planar conformations of peptide bonds with the =O and –H groups trans to each other contributes to the stability of the α helix.

4.9. (c) Methionine peptide bonds are broken by CNBr.

4.10. (a) DFP inhibits serum proteinase group of enzymes, including choline esterase.

4.11. (b) Ninhydrin deaminates amino acids and forms a blue complex with the NH_3 released.

4.12. (d) Phenylisothiocyanate is used to sequence proteins from the N terminus, because no destruction of the protein during the determination is necessary.

4.13. (e) A random coil has no repeating pattern. That is why it does not give x-ray diffraction patterns.

4.14. (a) Trypsin breaks all peptide bonds in which basic amino acids contribute the –COOH group: Arg-Glu and Lys-Ala. Chymotrypsin splits those peptide bonds in which an aromatic (ultraviolet-absorbing) amino acid contributes the –COOH group (Trp-Lys). Because it produces a dipeptide and a tripeptide, the original peptide must be a pentapeptide. The titration curve indicates that Lys, Arg, and Glu are components.

4.15. (d) By inspection, it is clear that at pH 9, the carboxyl and the N-terminal groups are deprotonated, whereas the amino and guanido groups are protonated, to give −2 and 2 charges for a net of 0.

4.16. (a) Because the isoelectric point is at point d, the 1 charge is at point b, and at point a, half of the γ-carboxyl group is protonated to give a net charge of 1½.

4.17. (b) We know that we must use 100 ml HCl to go from point d to point b. Beyond this, we must use the Henderson–Hasselbalch equation: 4 = 4.3 + log prot/unprot, where unprot/prot = 2. Hence two of three α-carboxyl groups are unprotonated at pH 4. This is two-thirds of 100 mmol, requiring 67 ml HCl to accomplish the protonation from point b to pH 4.0. Therefore, a total of 167 ml of 1 M HCl is required.

PROBLEMS

4.1. If you had a peptide with the following probable structure, how would you proceed to prove it? Be sure to indicate all separation procedures that are likely to work in any specific instance, as well as cleavage reagents. Do not use the Edman reagent or the carboxypeptidases beyond the C terminus of any peptide.

Leu–Glu–Met–Cys–Tyr–Asp–Ala
                    |
Ser–Lys–Ala–Cys–Lys–Ala–Tyr

4.2. What is the isoelectric point of γ-carboxyglutamate? Assume that the pK values of the two γ-carboxyl groups are identical at 4.1. Draw a titration curve for γ-carboxyglutamate.

4.3. Indicate how you would prepare 1 L of 0.1 M glutamate buffer at pH 3.7. Assume that you have solid monosodium glutamate and 10 M HCl. Use the following pK values: α-carboxyl, 2.0; γ-carboxyl, 4.1; and α-amino, 9.5. The molecular weight of monosodium glutamate is 169.

4.4. The following polar amino acid compositions with their internal pK values have been determined for two small proteins, lysozyme and calmodulin. Estimate their isoelectric points.

Amino acid residue	pK	Lysozyme	Calmodulin	
C terminus	3.4	1	1	
β-Carboxyl (Asp)	3.9	7	16	
γ-Carboxyl (Glu)	4.3	2	21	
Imidazole (His)	6.5	1	1	
N terminus	7.6	1	0	(blocked)
Phenolic (Tyr)	9.9	3	2	
ε-Amino (Lys)	10.3	6	8	
Guanido (Arg)	12.5	11	6	

BIBLIOGRAPHY

Anderson NG, Anderson L. The human protein index. Clin Chem 28:739–748, 1982.
Blake CCF, Johnson LN. Protein structure. Trends Biochem Sci April:147–151, 1987.
Branden C, Tooze J. Introduction to Protein Structure. New York: Garland, 1991.

Chotia C. Structural invariants in protein folding. Nature 254:304–308, 1975.

Creighton TE. Proteins. New York: WH Freeman, 1984.

Duncan R, McConkey EH. How many proteins are there in a typical mammalian cell? Clin Chem 28:749–755, 1982.

Levitt M, Chotia C. Structural patterns in globular proteins. Nature 261:552–558, 1976.

Richardson JH. The anatomy and taxonomy of protein structure. Adv Prot Chem 34:167–339, 1981.

Teller DC. Accessible area, packing volumes and interaction surfaces of globular proteins. Nature 260:729–731, 1976.

5

Proteins with Biological Activity: Enzymes

After completing this chapter, the student should

1. Be able to classify an enzyme into its correct class and know the type of reaction catalyzed by each class.
2. Be able to classify a reaction by reaction order.
3. Understand the concepts of catalytic site and enzyme–substrate complex and the major processes by which enzymes enhance reaction rates.
4. Understand the Michaelis-Menten equation, its derivation, and its transformations.
5. Recognize competitive, noncompetitive, and uncompetitive inhibitions by their kinetic effects.
6. Understand the mechanisms of two-substrate reactions.
7. Understand the basis for allosterism, the mode of action of allosteric activators and inhibitors, and the Hill equation.
8. Understand the two models for allosteric enzyme function.
9. Understand the effects of pH, ionic strength, and temperature on enzyme reactions.
10. Understand enzyme regulation via cellular enzyme levels, compartmentation, metabolic pathway regulation, and covalent modifications.
11. Understand the role of coenzymes and cofactors in enzymatic catalysis.
12. Be familiar with the most useful enzyme determinations in the clinical biochemistry laboratory, understand the importance of timing in the determination of enzyme activity for diagnostic purposes, and know the utility of isozyme determinations.

5.1 INTRODUCTION

Enzymes are complex protein catalysts found in all living cells that increase the rate at which reactions approach equilibrium. They do not change the equilibrium constant of a reaction, and therefore they do not change its thermodynamic properties. At the temperature and pH usually present in the cells, most chemical reactions would not proceed in the absence of enzymes at rates sufficient to support cell viability.

Two of the most important properties of enzymes are their specificity of action and their effectiveness. Enzymes are not only very specific for the type of reaction they catalyze but may also be very specific for the substrate they utilize. As a result, there are virtually no side reactions or by-products. Equally important is their effectiveness: enzymes can increase reaction rates by 10^6–10^{12}-fold.

We will consider in this chapter the general processes by which enzymes achieve enhancement of reaction rates, basic chemical and enzymatic kinetics and inhibition, the roles of cofactors and coenzymes, the effects of environmental factors, the regulation of enzyme activity, and some clinical applications of enzymology.

5.2 NAMING AND CLASSIFICATION OF ENZYMES

Enzymes have been given various trivial names as they were discovered. Some of these names were informative, and some were not. To establish an unambiguous system for enzyme classification and nomenclature, the International Union of Biochemists proposed a system in which enzymes are grouped into six major classes.

Class 1. Oxidoreductases catalyze oxidation and reduction reactions. They include the dehydrogenases, oxidases, reductases, peroxidases, oxygenases, hydroxylases, and catalases.

Class 2. Transferases transfer chemical groups from one molecule to another, or within a single molecule. They include amino, acyl, methyl, glucosyl, and phosphoryl transferases, kinases, phosphomutases, transaldolase, and transketolase.

Class 3. Hydrolases make use of water to cleave a single molecule into two molecules. They include esterases, glycosidases, peptidases, thiolases, phospholipases, amidases, ribonuclease, and deoxyribonuclease.

Class 4. Lyases split a molecule by a nonhydrolytic process, leaving double bonds (or alternatively, by adding groups to double bonds). They include decarboxylases, aldolases, hydratases, dehydratases, and synthases (synthetic enzymes).

Class 5. Isomerases interconvert isomeric structures by intramolecular rearrangements. They include racemases, epimerases, *cis-* and *trans-*isomerases, intramolecular transferases (mutases), and intermolecular lyases.

Class 6. Ligases join two separate molecules by creating a new chemical bond at the expense of nucleoside triphosphate (e.g., ATP) hydrolysis. They include enzymes that form C–O, C–S, C–N, and C–C bonds. Synthetases are ligases.

Each of the preceding major classes is divided into subclasses by the nature of the molecular substituent or chemical bond involved, and these are further divided into sub-subclasses by a variety of criteria. Each class, subclass, and sub-

subclass is assigned a number. A fourth digit is the serial number of the enzyme in its sub-subclass.

Individual enzymes are assigned a four-digit number, a systematic name, and a trivial name more commonly used by biochemists. For example, EC (Enzyme Commission) 2.7.1.2 denotes a transferase (major class 2) and indicates that a phosphate group is transferred (subclass 7) and that an alcohol group accepts the phosphate (sub-subclass 1). The final digit denotes that the enzyme is ATP:D-glucose-6-phosphotransferase (glucokinase). For the most part, we will use the trivial names accepted by the IUB in our subsequent discussion of enzymes that participate in metabolic pathways.

5.3 CHEMICAL KINETICS

5.3.1 Chemical Reaction Order

Because the general principles of chemical kinetics apply to enzyme-catalyzed reactions, a brief discussion of basic chemical kinetics is useful at this point. Chemical reactions may be classified on the basis of the number of molecules that react to form the products. Monomolecular, bimolecular, and termolecular reactions are reactions involving one, two, or three molecules, respectively.

Reactions may also be classified on a kinetic basis by reaction order, which may be zeroth-order, first-order, second-order, third-order, or pseudo-first-order, contingent on how the reaction rate is affected by the concentration of the reactants. The rate equation for the reaction $A \rightarrow P$ may be written as

$$\frac{-dA}{dt} = kA^n \tag{5.1}$$

in which k is the rate constant with the dimensions of reciprocal time and the exponent n is a number required to make the equation valid. In this case $n = 1$. The rate of the reaction is equivalent to the product of the constant k and the time-dependent concentration of reactant A. Thus, the rate becomes slower as more A is converted to P. Reactions described by the rate law in Equation (5.1) are first-order reactions, because the right-hand side of the equation contains the concentration of a single substance raised to the first power ($n = 1$). Integration of Equation (5.1) gives

$$\log \frac{A_0}{A} = \frac{kt}{2.3} \tag{5.2}$$

in which A_0 is the concentration of A at zero time and A is the concentration of A at time t.

The *half-time* ($t_{1/2}$) is the time required for the transformation of 50% of the initial amount of the reactant to the product. Thus, $\log [A_0/(\frac{1}{2})A_0] = kt_{1/2}/2.3$, and $2.3 \log 2 = kt_{1/2}$. Completing the calculations, we get

$$t_{1/2} = \frac{0.69}{k} \tag{5.3}$$

In first-order reactions, $t_{1/2}$ is independent of the initial concentration of reactant A_0. It should be noted that $t_{1/2}$ is not one-half the time required for the reaction to be completed. It is the time required for one-half of the reactant to disappear. The half-time relationship is a useful concept in the determination of drug clearances from the human organism or to determine protein turnover rates (see Chapter 20), provided that first-order kinetics are applicable.

For the reaction $A + A \rightarrow P$, we can write $-dA/dt = k(A)(A) = k\,A^2$. In this case, the rate involves a higher power of the concentration ($n = 1 + 1 = 2$) and the reaction is second-order. For the reaction $A + B \rightarrow P$, the rate is proportional to the first power of each reactant and $-d(A)(B)/dt = k(A)(B)$. The reaction is first-order with respect to A or B, but the overall reaction is second-order, because the right-hand side of the equation contains the product of two concentrations. The value of $t_{1/2}$ will depend on the initial reactant concentration(s), and the second-order rate constants have the dimensions of reciprocal concentration times time. Reactions of higher order, such as third order, are relatively rare, and their rates are proportional to the product of three concentration terms.

Whenever a reactant is present in large excess, its concentration is virtually constant during the course of the reaction. Thus, in a second-order reaction $A + B \rightarrow P$ in which the concentration of B is very high and that of A is low, the reaction may appear to be first-order, because its rate will be nearly proportional to the concentration of A. This is an apparent or pseudo-first-order reaction. Pseudo-first-order reactions are common among biochemical reactions in which water is one of the reactants. Since the concentration of water is 55.5 M and far in excess of everything else, the reaction appears to behave like a first-order reaction. An example is the hydrolysis of an ester,

$$
\begin{array}{c}
\quad\ \ \overset{\displaystyle O}{\underset{\displaystyle \|}{}} \\
CH_3\text{-}C\text{-}O\text{-}CH_3 + H_2O \rightarrow CH_3\text{-}COOH + CH_3OH
\end{array}
\tag{5.4}
$$

which is a typical pseudo-first-order reaction.

Zeroth-order reactions are those in which the rate is independent of the concentration of any reactants. The zeroth-order equation is

$$
\frac{-dc}{dt} = V = k_0
\tag{5.5}
$$

in which c is the concentration of the reactant and k_0 is the zeroth-order rate constant. Because the reaction is independent of concentration, there is no concentration term in the equation, and addition of more reactant will not increase the rate. With enzymes, this occurs at very high reactant (substrate) concentrations. The disappearance of reactant or appearance of product proceeds at a constant rate independent of reactant concentration. When this occurs, the reaction rate depends on the concentration of the catalyst (enzyme) or on some factor other than the concentration of the reactant. All catalytic sites are filled, so addition of more reactant cannot increase the rate.

5.3.2 The Arrhenius Activation Energy

For a reversible reaction such as

$$
A + B \underset{k_2}{\overset{k_1}{\rightleftarrows}} C + D
\tag{5.6}
$$

with rate constants k_1 and k_2, the thermodynamic equilibrium constant K_t is

$$K_t = \frac{[C][D]}{[A][B]} \tag{5.7}$$

A kinetic equilibrium constant can also be calculated from the rate constants of the forward and reverse reactions as follows:

$$K_k = \frac{k_1}{k_2} \tag{5.8}$$

In most cases, $K_t = K_k$. It should be noted that K_t is a thermodynamic expression of the state of the system, whereas k_1 and k_2, and hence K_k, are kinetic expressions related to the rate at which the thermodynamic state is attained. Note also that at equilibrium the rates are equal; the rate constants do not change.

At a given temperature, K_k, k_1, and k_2 are constants. They all change when the temperature is altered. If the forward reaction proceeds faster (k_1 increases faster than k_2), K_k will increase. The relationship between k_1 and temperature is given by the *Arrhenius equation*:

$$\ln k_1 = \ln A - \frac{E_a}{RT} \tag{5.9}$$

in which A is a constant referred to as the collision factor and E_a is also a constant, the *Arrhenius activation energy*. E_a is the amount of energy that one must put into the system to produce a transition state and bring about a reaction. This may be represented graphically as shown in Figure 5.1 for the uncatalyzed reaction. Thus, a chemical reaction will take place when some fraction of the reactant molecules are raised to a higher energy level, a transition state. This energy

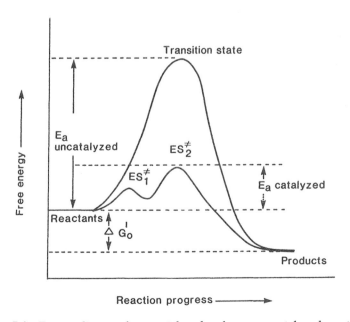

Figure 5.1 Energy diagram for uncatalyzed and enzyme-catalyzed reactions.

barrier can be overcome by heating to provide additional kinetic energy or by the addition of a catalyst (an enzyme in biologic systems), which produces a transition state with lower E_a. Low activation energies mean relatively fast reactions, whereas high activation energies signify relatively slow reactions.

Both E_a and A can be determined graphically by plotting $\log k_1$ against $1/T$ (T is in kelvins), because Equation (5.9) has a linear form. Within limits, a linear plot results with a slope of $-E_a/2.3R$ and a y intercept of $\log A$.

5.3.3   Nature of Enzyme Catalysis

As noted earlier, enzymes usually increase reaction velocities by 10^6–10^{12}-fold over the uncatalyzed rate. All enzymes appear to use the same principles to increase reaction rates. It seems evident from the Arrhenius equation that enzymes could increase reaction rates by decreasing E_a or by increasing A by orienting the reactants appropriately, or by doing both. A comparison of the reaction progress curves for the uncatalyzed and enzyme-catalyzed reactions in Figure 5.1 shows that E_a (the energy barrier) is considerably lower in the enzyme-catalyzed reaction. This reduction in E_a is probably brought about by stabilizing the transition states $ES_1\#$ and $ES_2\#$ by specific binding. The combination of enzyme and substrate produces a new pathway in which the transition state energy is lower than that of the uncatalyzed reaction. Note, however, that the equilibrium and the ΔG_0 are the same for both the catalyzed and uncatalyzed reactions. Enzymes do not change the thermodynamics of the system; they only affect the rate of approach to equilibrium. There may be several hills and valleys in the energy diagram for the enzyme-catalyzed reaction; this allows the enzyme to break up one large energy barrier into two or more smaller transition states. The enzyme–substrate complex, ES, is not a transition state and is usually found in the valleys of the reaction progress diagram.

5.4   CHEMICAL BASIS FOR ENZYME ACTION

5.4.1   Formation of the Enzyme–Substrate Complex

It is clear that the formation of an enzyme–substrate complex is required for both the catalytic action of an enzyme and its substrate specificity. Substrates are bound to a relatively small region of the enzyme called the *active* or *catalytic site*, which contains specific residues directly responsible for catalytic action. The active site is three-dimensional and is formed by groups from different areas of the linear polypeptide sequence. Activity therefore depends on the integrity of the three-dimensional structure of the enzyme. The specificity of binding depends upon a complementary relationship between the enzyme active site and the substrate.

Several models have been proposed to explain the fit of the substrate into the active site. The first of these was the *lock-and-key model*, in which the substrate fits the binding site as a key fits its lock. This model did not explain the fact that the shapes of the active sites of some enzymes were changed by binding with substrates. Subsequently, the *induced-fit model* was proposed. In this model the substrate creates its own site on a suitable portion of the enzyme (Figure 5.2). A

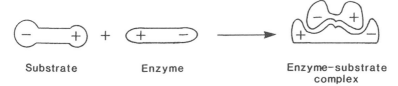

Substrate   Enzyme   Enzyme–substrate
complex

Figure 5.2 Schematic model for induced fit.

strain is imparted to specific bonds of the substrate, increasing its ground-state energy level and its reactivity. An induced conformational change in the enzyme often accompanies the binding of substrate.

5.4.2 Mechanisms of Enzyme Action

There are several processes that account for the enhancement of reaction rates by enzymes. The major mechanisms are proximity-entropy effects, substrate strain, covalent catalysis, and acid–base catalysis.

When a substrate binds to an enzyme, it is both concentrated in a localized zone and aligned so that participating amino acyl side chains of the enzyme and the interacting groups of the substrate have the proper orientation to achieve the maximal reaction rate. In addition, the state of randomness of the substrate is decreased, thus decreasing its entropy (Chapter 2). The result is that the entropy difference between reactants and products is less and the activation energy is decreased, so the reaction can occur more rapidly. *Proximity effect* is the name given to the ability of the enzyme to hold its substrates close together and properly oriented to each other and to the participating moieties of the enzyme in preparation for the reaction. All of these conditions will enhance the reaction rate. The proximity effect and the decrease in entropy each contribute some 10^3–10^4-fold to the increased rate achieved by enzymes.

As noted earlier, the binding of the substrate to the enzyme can induce strain in specific bonds of the substrate, increasing its ground-state energy level and its reactivity. The substrate assumes bond angles and lengths more closely approximating those of the transition state. This approximation of the transition state lowers the activation energy primarily by increasing the ground-state energy level of the substrate. Because an enzyme's binding site is designed for a molecule approaching the transition state and not for the substrate per se, it was expected that compounds closely resembling a transition state might bind more avidly to the enzyme than the natural substrate and be potent enzyme inhibitors. This has been found to be true in certain instances, which opens the way for the synthesis of powerful inhibitors that may prove to be of considerable importance in medicine.

Many enzymes form covalent bonds with their substrates to form true intermediates. Enzyme-bound coenzymes (prosthetic groups) can also form covalent bonds with the substrate. Enzyme effects involving such formation of covalent bonds with the substrate are referred to as *covalent catalysis*. The enzyme-bound or coenzyme-bound substrate is more reactive than the original substrate. An example is transamination (Chapter 20), where the amino acid forms a Schiff's base with the coenzyme pyridoxal phosphate. Chymotrypsin forms such an intermediate via its serine active sites. The mechanism is shown in Figure 5.3, in which His-57 removes a proton from the hydroxyl group of Ser-195. The alkoxide formed acts upon the carbonyl carbon of the peptide bond, releasing the amino-terminal end of the polypeptide chain and forming an acylated enzyme via Ser-195. The acylated enzyme (which has been isolated) is then cleaved by water. This deacylation step is much slower than the acylation step, because deacylation must occur before the next substrate molecule can be hydrolyzed.

The general acid–base catalysis mechanism often involves the two forms of the imidazole residue of histidine: the protonated acid and the unprotonated base. The acid donates a proton, and the base accepts a proton, both resulting in appropriate shifting of electrons. In ribonuclease, specific histidine residues act as general acid–base catalysts in the cleavage of the RNA chain at 3'-phosphodiester linkages of pyrimidine nucleotides. A pyrimidine-2'-3'-phosphoribose is formed as an intermediate. Figure 5.4 shows the mechanism for this reaction, in which His-119 serves as an acid to protonate the phosphodiester link and His-12 acts as a base to generate an alkoxide on the pyrimidine nucleotide 3'-hydroxyl group. This alkoxide attacks the phosphorus atom, producing a cyclic phosphate intermediate and a shorter RNA fragment (product 1). The cyclic intermediate is then cleaved by His-12 acting as an acid and His-119 acting as a base, plus H_2O, to yield product 2, an RNA fragment terminating in a pyrmidine nucleoside 3'-phosphate. In this mechanism, His-119 first acts as an acid, then as a base, whereas His-12 acts first as a base, then as an acid.

The pK of the histidine imidazole residue is about 6.0. At or near this pH, the rates of protonation and deprotonation are not only equal but also very rapid. Such a mechanism probably increases reaction rates by 10^2–10^3-fold.

In many cases, a combination of mechanisms will exist, proximity-entropy effects, covalent modification, and general acid–base effects as well as other processes that we may not have discussed.

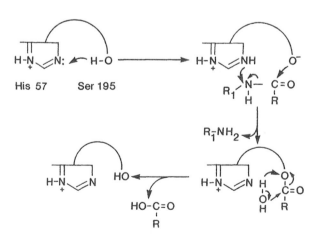

Figure 5.3 Covalent catalysis by chymotrypsin.

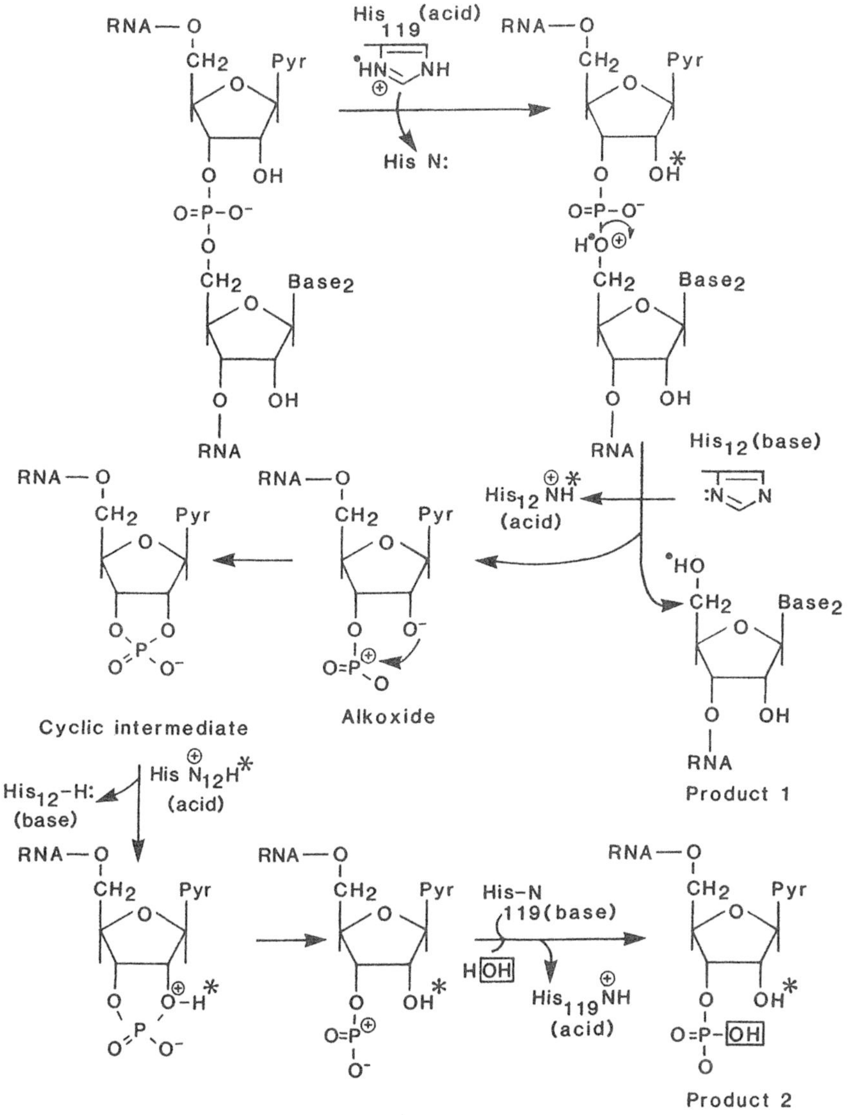

Figure 5.4 Acid and base catalysis by ribonuclease.

5.5 KINETICS OF ENZYME-CATALYZED REACTIONS

5.5.1 Units of Enzyme Activity

The most commonly used unit of enzyme activity has been defined as the amount of activity that catalyzes the transformation of 1 μmol of substrate per minute under specified assay conditions. *Specific activity* is the number of enzyme units per milligram of protein (μmol/min per milligram of protein). The *turnover number* or catalytic constant is equal to the units of enzyme activity per μmole of enzyme (μmol/min per μmol of enzyme).

A new international unit has been recommended. The *katal* (kat) is defined as the amount of enzyme activity that transforms 1 mole of substrate per second. Activities can also be given in millikatals (mkat), microkatals (µkat), nanokatals (nkat), etc. Both specific activity and turnover number can also be expressed in these units.

5.5.2 General Remarks

Although chemical kinetics apply in general to enzyme-catalyzed reactions, a feature that distinguishes them from chemical reactions is saturation with substrate. When the initial velocity V_0 of an enzyme-catalyzed reaction is plotted against substrate concentration [S], a hyperbolic curve is obtained as shown in Figure 5.5. At low [S], the initial velocity is nearly proportional to [S] and the reaction is first-order with respect to substrate. At higher [S], the initial velocity tapers off and is no longer proportional to [S]. With further increases in [S], initial velocity becomes independent of [S] and V_0 asymptotically approaches a limiting value. The reaction becomes zeroth-order with respect to [S], and the enzyme is considered to be saturated with substrate. This limiting value is com-

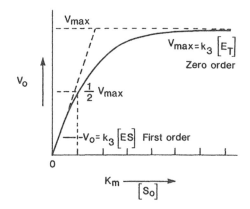

Figure 5.5 Effect of substrate concentration [S] on the velocity (V_0) of an enzyme-catalyzed reaction.

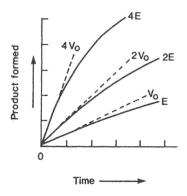

Figure 5.6 Progress curves for increasing concentration of enzyme and saturating levels of substrate.

monly given the name *maximum velocity* (V_{max}), although there is no maximum value of V_0 in the mathematical sense; that is, there is no point at which the slope of the plot of V_0 vs. [S] is zero. However, we will follow the common convention and use the designation V_{max} in our subsequent discussions.

The V_0 of an enzyme-catalyzed reaction depends not only on [S] but also on the enzyme concentration. When [S] is sufficient to saturate the enzyme, doubling the amount of enzyme will double V_0; increasing the enzyme by fourfold will correspondingly increase V_0 by fourfold, and so on. Figure 5.6 shows progress curves for increasing concentration of enzyme with saturating levels of substrate. The final equilibrium position is the same for all enzyme concentrations, but the velocities at which it is attained will be different.

5.5.3 Michaelis–Menten Kinetics

In 1913, Michaelis and Menten presented a general theory for enzyme kinetics, extended later by Briggs and Haldane, which accounts for the velocity curve shown in Figure 5.5. This theory for reactions catalyzed by enzymes having a single substrate assumes that the substrate S binds to the active site of the enzyme E to form the enzyme–substrate complex ES, which yields the product P and the free enzyme E:

$$E + S \underset{k_2}{\overset{k_1}{\rightleftharpoons}} ES \tag{5.10}$$

$$ES \underset{k_4}{\overset{k_3}{\rightleftharpoons}} E + P \tag{5.11}$$

In this formulation, the k's are the specific rate constants for the two reversible reactions. The velocity of a reaction is equal to the rate of formation of P minus the rate of disappearance of P and is given by

$$V_0 = \frac{dP}{dt} = k_3 [ES] = k_4 [E][P] \tag{5.12}$$

However, when the initial velocity (V_0) is measured, the concentration of P will be very low so that $k_4 [E][P] << [ES]$, and V_0 may be approximated by the first-order relationship

$$V_0 = k_3 [ES] \tag{5.13}$$

A second assumption is now made that the concentration of ES is constant during the time V_0 is determined. With this steady-state provision, the rate of formation of ES must be equal to the rate of breakdown of ES. The rate of formation of ES is

$$\frac{d\,ES}{dt} = k_4 [E][P] \tag{5.14}$$

and because we are dealing with initial velocities, where [P] << [S], we can use the approximation

$$\frac{d\,ES}{dt} = k_1 [E][S] \tag{5.15}$$

for Equation (5.14).

The rate of breakdown of ES is given by

$$\frac{-d\,\text{ES}}{dt} = k_2\,[\text{ES}] + k_3\,[\text{ES}] \tag{5.16}$$

and in the steady state, $d\,\text{ES}/dt = -d\,\text{ES}/dt$. Therefore, $k_1\,[\text{E}][\text{S}] = k_2\,[\text{ES}] + k_3\,[\text{S}]$, or

$$\frac{[\text{E}][\text{S}]}{[\text{ES}]} = \frac{k_2 + k_3}{k_1} = K_m \tag{5.17}$$

In Equation (5.17), the ratio of constants $(k_2 + k_3)/k_1$ has been replaced by a single constant, the *Michaelis-Menten constant*, K_m. K_m is therefore approximately equal to the dissociation constant of the enzyme–substrate complex (ES).

The total enzyme concentration $[\text{E}_T]$ is equal to the concentration of the free enzyme E plus the concentration of ES, or $[\text{E}_T] = [\text{E}] + [\text{ES}]$. This is rewritten as

$$[\text{E}] = [\text{E}_T] - [\text{ES}] \tag{5.18}$$

Substituting Equation 5.18 into Equation (5.17), we get

$$K_m = \frac{([\text{E}_T] - [\text{ES}])[\text{S}]}{[\text{ES}]} \tag{5.19}$$

and solving for [ES] we get

$$[\text{ES}] = \frac{[\text{E}_T][\text{S}]}{K_m + [\text{S}]} \tag{5.20}$$

Substituting Equation (5.13) into Equation (5.20), we get

$$V_0 = \frac{k_3[\text{E}_T][\text{S}]}{K_m + [\text{S}]} \tag{5.21}$$

When V_0 is measured, the concentration of S is essentially equal to the initial concentration of substrate, $[\text{S}_0]$, and Equation (5.21) may be approximated by

$$V_0 = \frac{k_3[\text{E}_T][\text{S}_0]}{K_m + [\text{S}_0]} \tag{5.22}$$

When the substrate concentration is so high that all the enzyme is present in the form of ES, that is, $[\text{ES}] = [\text{E}_T]$, we reach the maximum velocity, V_{max}, given by a form of Equation (5.13),

$$V_{max} = k_3[\text{E}_T] \tag{5.23}$$

Substituting V_{max} for its value in Equation (5.22), we get

$$V_0 = \frac{V_{max}[\text{S}_0]}{K_m + [\text{S}_0]} \tag{5.24}$$

which is termed the *Michaelis-Menten equation*. This rate equation relates the initial velocity V_0 to maximum velocity V_{max} through the Michaelis-Menten constant K_m. The two constants of this equation, K_m and V_{max}, are unique to each enzyme under specific conditions of temperature, pH, substrate concentration, solution parameters, etc. For any enzyme–substrate system, the K_m will have a characteristic value (in moles per liter) independent of the concentration of the enzyme. If the enzyme acts on several substrates, it will have a characteristic K_m for each substrate. Remember that V_{max} will increase with increasing enzyme concentration, as shown in Figure 5.6.

A special numerical relationship arises from the Michaelis-Menten equation when the initial velocity is equal to half the maximal velocity, that, is $V_0 = (\frac{1}{2})V_{max}$. Equation 5.24 then reduces to $K_m = [S_0]$. This means that K_m is equal to the substrate concentration in moles per liter at which the reaction velocity is half its maximum value.

It was stated above the K_m is the dissociation constant of the enzyme–substrate complex. This is true only if $k_3 << k_2$. Since $K_m = (k_2 + k_3)/k_1$ [Equation (5.17)], and the dissociation constant $K_d = k_2/k_1$, K_m is larger than K_d, and approximation that $K_m = K_d$ is valid only if k_3 is much smaller than k_2.

5.5.4 Transformations of the Michaelis-Menten Equation

Because V_{max} is approached asymptotically in the saturation curve shown in Figure 5.5, the estimation of K_m and V_{max} is not very accurate. Equation (5.24) can be algebraically transformed into a linear form more suitable for plotting experimental data and obtaining K_m and V_{max}.

One common transformation of the Michaelis-Menten equation is the double-reciprocal plot of Lineweaver and Burk, which is obtained by taking the reciprocal of both sides of Equation (5.24) to yield

$$\frac{1}{V_0} = \frac{K_m + [S_0]}{V_{max}[S_0]} \tag{5.25}$$

Rearranging Equation 5.25, we get

$$\frac{1}{V_0} = \frac{K_m}{V_{max}[S_0]} + \frac{1}{V_{max}} \tag{5.26}$$

A plot of $1/V_0$ vs $1/[S_0]$ yields a straight line with a slope of K_m/V_{max}, an intercept of $1/V_{max}$ on the $1/V_0$ axis, and an intercept of $-1/K_m$ on the $1/[S_0]$ axis (Figure 5.7). The main advantage of this plot over that of Figure 5.5 is that determination of K_m and

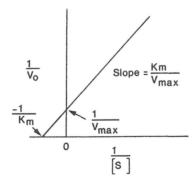

Figure 5.7 Double-reciprocal Lineweaver-Burk plot.

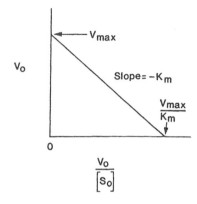

Figure 5.8 Eadie-Hofstee plot.

V_{max} does not require estimation of an asymptote. Although this plot is very widespread in the literature, it does distort the appearance of any experimental error in the primary observations of V_0, so it is not possible to judge which points are most accurate when drawing a straight line through the set of points. Nevertheless, this plot can provide valuable information in enzyme inhibition (see below).

A second and perhaps more useful transformation is obtained by multiplying both sides of Equation (5.26) by V_{max} and rearranging to get

$$V_0 = \frac{-K_m V_0}{[S_0]} + V_{max} \tag{5.27}$$

this is the *Eadie-Hofstee equation*. A plot of V_0 vs $V_0/[S_0]$ yields a straight line with a slope of $-K_m$ and intercepts on the V_0 and $V_0/[S_0]$ axes of V_{max} and V_{max}/K_m, respectively. This plot magnifies departures from linearity, which might not be seen in the double-reciprocal plots (Figure 5.8).

5.6 ENZYME INHIBITION

5.6.1 Introduction

Substances that cause enzyme-catalyzed reactions to proceed more slowly are termed *inhibitors,* and the phenomenon is termed *inhibition.* When an enzyme is subject to inhibition, the reaction still may obey Michaelis-Menten kinetics but with apparent K_m and V_{max} values that vary with the inhibitor concentration. If the inhibitor acts only on the apparent K_m, it is a *competitive inhibitor*; if it affects only the apparent V_{max}, it is a *noncompetitive* inhibitor; and if it affects both constants, it is an *uncompetitive inhibitor*.

5.6.2 Competitive Inhibition

In the simplest case of competitive inhibition, the substrate and inhibitor compete for the same site on the enzyme. The combination of a competitive inhibitor (I) with the enzyme can be written in the same manner as the combination of enzyme with substrate: E + I $\rightleftarrows$ EI, where K_i is the dissociation constant of EI and is equal to [E][I]/[EI]. Since the formation of EI depends upon [I] just as the formation of ES is dependent on [S], the rate of a competitively inhibited reaction is strictly dependent upon the relative concentrations of S and I at fixed concentrations of E. In the presence of a competitive inhibitor, Equation (5.26) is replaced by

$$\frac{1}{V_0} = \frac{K_m}{V_{max}}(1 + \frac{[I]}{K_i})(\frac{1}{[S_0]}) + \frac{1}{V_{max}}$$ (5.28)

in which [I] is the concentration of I and K_i is the dissociation constant of the EI complex. All other terms are identical to those of Equation (5.26). The slope of the inhibited reaction is increased by a factor of $1 + [I]/K_i$, thus increasing the apparent K_m. V_{max} is not altered by a competitive inhibitor, indicating that it does not interfere with the breakdown of the ES complex. Graphical analysis of Equation 5.28 is shown in Figure 5.9A.

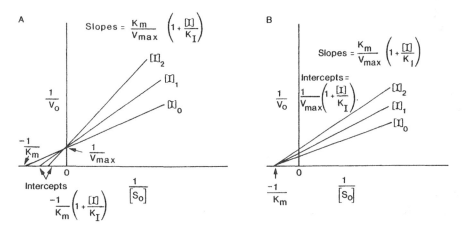

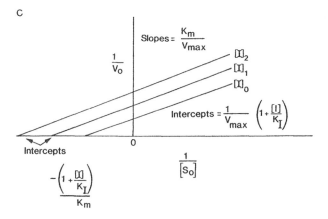

Figure 5.9 Double-reciprocal plots showing different types of inhibition. (A) Competitive inhibition [Equation (5.28)]; (B) noncompetitive inhibition [Equation (5.29)]; (C) uncompetitive inhibition (Equation 5.30). K_m and V_{max} are estimated from the slopes of uninhibited reactions, and K_I from the slopes and/or intercepts of the inhibited reactions.

A classic example of competitive inhibition is the inhibition of succinate dehydrogenase by malonate, a structural analogue of succinate. Competitive inhibitors are usually structural analogues of the substrate, the molecule with which they are competing. They bind to the active site but either do not have a structure that is conducive to enzymatic modification or do not induce the proper orientation of catalytic amino acyl residues required to affect catalysis. Consequently, they displace the substrate from the active site and thereby depress the velocity of the reaction. Increasing [S] will displace the inhibitor.

5.6.3 Noncompetitive Inhibition

In noncompetitive inhibition, the inhibitor binds to the enzyme at a site other than the substrate-binding site and binds in the same manner to the ES complex, producing two inactive forms, EI and ESI: $E + I \rightleftarrows EI$ and $ES + I \rightleftarrows ESI$. There are two inhibitor constants:

$$K_i^{EI} = \frac{[E][I]}{[EI]} \quad \text{and} \quad K_i^{ES} = \frac{[ES][I]}{[ESI]}$$

These constants may or may not be equal, but for our purposes we will assume that they are and they can then be designated simply as K_i. We can then write the double-reciprocal expression for noncompetitive inhibition as follows:

$$\frac{1}{V_0} = \frac{K_m}{V_{max}}\left(1 + \frac{[I]}{K_i}\right)\left(\frac{1}{[S_0]}\right) + \frac{1}{V_{max}}\left(1 + \frac{[I]}{K_i}\right) \tag{5.29}$$

All terms are identical to those of Equation (5.28). Graphical analysis of Equation (5.29) is shown in Figure 5.9B. Both the slope and the intercept on the $1/V_0$ axis are increased by the factor $(1 + [I]/K_i)$. If both increase by the same amount, the intercept on the $1/[S_0]$ axis will remain the same and K_m is unchanged. V_{max} is reduced because part of E and ES are bound as EI and ESI. Because ES can bind I, V_{max} cannot be restored to its value in the presence of inhibitor, regardless of how high the level of substrate may be. It should be noted that classical noncompetitive inhibition is attained only under rapid equilibrium conditions, where $K_m = K_d$.

Examples of noncompetitive inhibitors are heavy-metal ions, such as Hg^{2+}, Ag^+, and Pb^{2+}, which react reversibly with thiol groups of enzymes, and chelating agents such as ethylenediaminetetraacetic acid (EDTA). The latter can chelate metals requisite for the activity of some enzymes. Provided that the inhibitor has not formed a covalent bond with the enzyme, inhibition can often be reversed by dialysis. Dialysis will not reverse those situations in which the inhibitor is permanently covalently bound to the enzyme. Examples of such irreversible inhibitions are those produced by diisopropylfluorophosphate, which irreversibly binds to active serine residues of some hydrolytic enzymes, and p-chloromercuribenzoate, which binds to thiol groups of certain enzymes. Irreversible inhibition may be distinguished from classic noncompetitive inhibition by plotting V_{max} against increasing [E]. For noncompetitive inhibition the plot will go through the origin, whereas in the case of irreversible inhibition the plot will have a finite intercept on the [E] axis.

5.6.4   Uncompetitive Inhibition

Uncompetitive inhibition results when an inhibitor combines reversibly with ES
to yield an inactive ESI complex, ES + I $\rightleftarrows$ ESI, and K_i = [ESI]/[ES][I]. The
double-reciprocal equation is then

$$\frac{1}{V_0} = \frac{K_m}{V_{max}}\left(\frac{1}{[S_0]}\right) + \frac{1}{V_{max}}\left(1 + \frac{[I]}{K_i}\right)$$
(5.30)

where all terms are the same as in Equations (5.28) and (5.29). Graphical analysis
(Figure 5.9C) shows a decrease in both K_m and V_{max}, resulting in lines parallel to
that given in the absence of inhibitor. Uncompetitive inhibitors may bind at a site
distant from the active site or at a site different from but overlapping with the
active site. In either case, the result is to lower both the catalytic efficiency of the
enzyme and its apparent binding efficiency for the substrate. Infinitely high [S]
will not convert all of the enzyme to ES, and some ESI will always be present.
Uncompetitive inhibition is common in two-substrate reactions (see below) and
probably relates to the sequential addition of two enzyme ligands in an obligate
order. It is rare in single-substrate reactions.

5.7   TWO-SUBSTRATE REACTIONS

Many enzymes catalyze reactions with two interacting substrates, and although
the kinetics of these reactions are more complex than those of one-substrate
reactions, they still obey Michaelis-Menten kinetics. Reactions of the type A + B
$\rightleftarrows$ P + Q usually fall within either of two classes with respect to kinetic behavior
and mechanism of action.

   In the first general class, both substrates are bound to the enzyme at the
same time. The order of binding may be A or B first, or random. This implies that
the enzyme has distinct, nonoverlapping binding sites at the active site for the
two substrates. Double-reciprocal plots ($1/V_0$ vs $1/A_0$) at constant but different
concentrations of B yield intersecting straight lines as shown in Figure 5.10A.
This type of kinetic result implies that both substrates must be bound to the
enzyme before the reaction can occur and is called the *sequential* or *single-
displacement mechanism*.

   An example of a random type of reaction is creatine + ATP $\rightleftarrows$ creatine
phosphate + ADP, which is catalyzed by creatine kinase (see Chapter 20). In this
case, creatine and ATP are bound to the active site in either sequence, and after
the transfer of the phosphate group of the bound ATP to the bound creatine both
products are released in either sequence.

   For an *ordered mechanism*, the reaction catalyzed by alcohol dehydrogenase
is an appropriate example:

   Enzyme + NAD^+ $\rightarrow$ enzyme-NAD^+

   Enzyme-NAD^+ + ethanol $\rightarrow$ enzyme-NAD^+-ethanol

   Enzyme-NAD^+-ethanol $\rightarrow$ enzyme-NADH + acetaldehyde

   Enzyme-NADH $\rightarrow$ enzyme + NADH + H^+

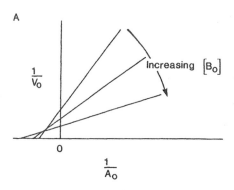

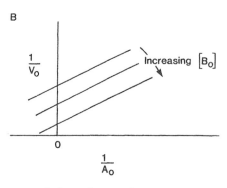

Figure 5.10 Double-reciprocal plots of two-substrate reactions at three different concentrations of B. (A) Sequential reaction mechanism; (B) ping-pong mechanism.

Thus, NAD^+ must be bound first, and as a consequence an excess of NADH will inhibit the reaction by competing only with the binding of the first substrate to the enzyme.

In the second general class of two-substrate reactions, the *ping-pong* or *double-displacement mechanism*, the two substrates do not bind to the enzyme simultaneously, usually because a single binding site is used for both substrates. In such reactions, one substrate must be bound and the product released before the second substrate can be bound and the second product released. The first substrate reacts with the enzyme to modify it covalently, usually by the transfer of a functional group. This functional group is then transferred to the second substrate and restores the enzyme to its original state. Thus, we have

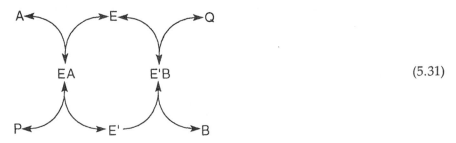

(5.31)

Double-reciprocal plots in ping-pong reactions ($1/V_0$ vs $1/[A_0]$) at constant but different concentrations of B give parallel straight lines that never intersect (Figure 5.10B). An example of such reactions are those catalyzed by transaminases (Chapter 20):

$$\text{Amino acid-1} + \alpha\text{-keto acid-2} \rightleftarrows \text{amino acid-2} + \alpha\text{-keto acid-1} \qquad (5.32)$$

Amino acid-1, the first substrate, combines with the enzyme, and its amino group is then transferred to the pyridoxal phosphate prosthetic group of the enzyme. The first product, α-keto acid-1, is released from the active site and is replaced by the second substrate, α-keto acid-2, to which the amino acid is then transferred from the enzyme to form amino acid-2. Amino acid-2 is then released from the active site of the enzyme, restoring the enzyme to its original form.

5.8 ALLOSTERIC ENZYMES

In the kinetic considerations discussed above, a plot of $1/V_0$ vs $1/[S_0]$ yields a straight line, and the enzyme exhibits Michaelis-Menten (hyperbolic or saturation) kinetics. It is implicit in this result that all the enzyme-binding sites have the same affinity for the substrate and operate independently of each other. However, many enzymes exist as oligomers containing subunits or domains that function in the regulation of the catalytic site. Such enzymes do not exhibit classic Michaelis-Menten saturation kinetics.

Allosteric enzymes are enzymes whose activity at the catalytic site is modified by the reversible noncovalent binding of specific metabolites, termed effectors or modulators. *Effectors* are bound at specific sites, allosteric sites, which are different from catalytic sites. Effectors may be stimulatory (positive) or inhibitory (negative). Positive effectors increase the rate of an enzyme reaction by reducing the apparent K_m, increasing V_{max}, or both. Conversely, negative effectors increase the apparent K_m, decrease V_{max}, or both. Allosteric enzymes that respond to positive or negative effectors with a change in the apparent K_m but not in V_{max} are *K enzymes*. *M enzymes* or *V enzymes* are those that respond with an alteration of V_{max} but not K_m. There are a few allosteric enzymes in which both K_m and V_{max} are altered. Both positive and negative effectors achieve their effects on the catalytic site of the enzyme by altering the three-dimensional structure of the enzyme protein, that is, they change the conformation of the enzyme.

Most allosteric enzymes are oligomeric, consisting of several subunits. Identical subunits are termed *protomers*. The binding of a ligand (any molecule that binds to a macromolecule) to one protomer can have an effect, either positive or negative, on the binding of the ligand to other protomers in the oligomer. The influence that the binding of a ligand to one protomer has on the binding of a ligand to other protomers of an oligomeric protein is termed *cooperativity*. *Homotropic* interactions are those that involve homologous substances, for example substrate influencing substrate binding, inhibitor influencing inhibitor binding, or activator influencing activator binding, and usually have a positive effect. *Heterotropic* interactions, which may be either positive or negative, are those in which the effect of one ligand influences the binding of a different ligand. Both types of interactions are achieved by cooperativity between subunits. It may be noted that the oxygen-induced conformational change in hemoglobin (Chapter 7) is often termed an allosteric effect. Because it is produced by the substrate O_2, it is actually a homotropic cooperative interaction. We will, however, presume that any ligand-induced change in conformation is an allosteric effect.

Figures 5.11A and B show the characteristic sigmoid curves obtained as a result of interaction between the substrate site, the stimulating modulator site, and the inhibitory modulator site for K and M classes of enzymes. The curves in the absence of modulators are homotropic effects caused by cooperative binding of the substrate. Heterotropic modulators, which can be either positive or negative in their actions, are molecules other than the substrate.

Increasing concentrations of negative modulators act like a competitive inhibitor (increase K_m) in K-class enzymes and like noncompetitive inhibitor in M-class enzymes.

Aspartate carbamoyl transferase (ACTase) from *Escherichi coli* has been studied in great detail. It catalyzes the first reaction unique to pyrimidine biosynthesis:

$$\text{Carbamoyl phosphate} + \text{L-aspartate} \xrightarrow{\text{ATCase}} N\text{-carbamoyl-L-aspartate} + P_i \qquad (5.33)$$

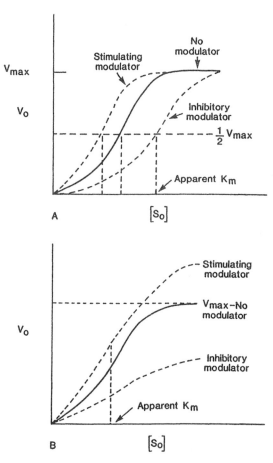

Figure 5.11 Effects of stimulating and negative modulators (effectors) on K and M classes of enzymes. (A) K class; (B) M class.

and can be used as an example of one class of allosteric enzymes. It has two catalytic protomers and three regulatory protomers. Figure 5.11A shows the effect of substrate (aspartate) concentration on the activity of ACTase alone, in the presence of a positive modulator such as ATP, and in the presence of a negative modulator, cytidine triphosphate (CTP), the end product of the pyrimidine biosynthetic pathway (Chapter 10).

It was noted earlier that Michaelis-Menten kinetics and its linear transformations are not valid for allosteric enzymes. Instead, the Hill equation, an equation originally empirically developed to describe the cooperative binding of O_2 to hemoglobin (Chapter 7), is used. The expression describing such a straight-line plot is

$$\log[V_0/(V_{max} - V_0)] = n \log [S_0] - K' \qquad (5.34),$$

in which n is the *Hill coefficient*, which is indicative of cooperativity, and K' is a complex constant that equals K_m if $n = 1$. A plot of $\log [V_0/(V_{max} - V_0)]$ vs $\log [S_0]$ on a linear scale yields a straight line with a slope of n. For a Michaelis-Menten enzyme, $n = 1$. For an allosteric enzyme with four protomers, n may approach 3, indicating strong cooperative binding. If $n < 1$, the sites exhibit negative cooperativity. When $V_0 = (½)V_{max}$, $\log [V_0/(V_{max} - V_0)] = 0$ and $n \log [S_0] = \log K'$. This allows the determination of the substrate concentration that produces half-maximal velocity when saturation kinetics are sigmoid (Figure 5.12).

Two of the more popular models to explain cooperativity are the concerted transition or symmetry model proposed by J. Monod, J. Wyman, and J.-P. Changeux in 1965, and the sequential interaction model proposed by D.L. Koshland, G. Nemethy, and D. Filmer in 1966. The *concerted model* proposes that the oligomer exists in two different states only, the T (tight) and the R (relaxed), which are in equilibrium. The transition between one conformation and the other is an all-or-none process with no hybrids. Some ligands bind preferentially to one oligomer conformation, whereas other ligands bind preferentially to the other. Activators and substrates are assumed to bind preferentially to the R state, shifting T $\rightleftarrows$ R equilibrium to the right. At infinitely high concentrations of

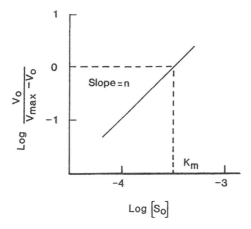

Figure 5.12 Graphic evaluation of Hill equation for determination of substrate concentration yielding V_{max}.

activator, the enzyme will be converted completely to the R state and a plot of V_0 vs $[S_0]$ becomes hyperbolic. Allosteric inhibitors are presumed to bind preferentially to the T state, shifting the T $\rightleftarrows$ R equilibrium to the left. This model does not explain negative cooperativity, because the nature of the sites does not change. The substrate changes only the distribution of sites, and a reduction in binding affinity when a site is occupied by substrate is not possible.

In the *sequential model*, two conformational states are also proposed. However, many intermediate hybrid states between all-on and all-off are postulated, each with its own catalytic activity. The effect of substrate or ligand binding is transmitted sequentially in the oligomer from one subunit to another. Binding of additional molecules of substrate or ligand binding is transmitted sequentially in the oligomer from one subunit to another. Binding of additional molecules of substrate or modulator may be either stronger (positive cooperativity) or weaker (negative cooperativity). This model offers more delicate modulation of the activity of allosteric enzymes than does the symmetry model.

5.9 ENVIRONMENTAL EFFECTS ON ENZYME ACTION

5.9.1 Introduction

Environmental factors such as pH, ionic strength, and temperature affect enzyme activity. They must be controlled when making in vitro measurements of enzyme activity and heeded in vivo when abnormal conditions such as acidosis, alkalosis, and fevers may exist.

5.9.2 Proton Concentration (pH)

Because active sites of enzymes frequently have ionizable groups that must be in a specific ionic form to maintain the conformation of the active site, bind the substrate, or catalyze the reaction, it follows that pH will influence the velocity of enzyme-catalyzed reactions. In addition, the substrate may contain ionizable groups, and only a specific ionic form can bind to the enzyme or undergo catalysis.

Most enzymes show a bell-shaped pH–velocity profile and a characteristic pH at which their activity is maximal. Figure 5.13 shows V_0 vs pH curves for three enzymes. Note that both the pH optimum and the form of the velocity profile vary with the enzyme. Such curves must be interpreted with caution, as they give no indication why the velocity declines above and below the pH optimum. The decline in rate may be due to the formation of improper forms of the enzyme or substrate (or both) or inactivation of the enzyme, or it may be due to a combination of these factors. The possibility of enzyme inactivation is frequently overlooked, although a pH stability curve is necessary for enzyme characterization. A pH stability curve is readily obtained by preincubating the enzyme at a specified pH for a period of time equal to the assay incubation time and then assaying activity at the optimum pH.

The pH optimum is not necessarily identical with intracellular pH. Many other factors determine the pH stability of an enzyme. These include ionic strength and temperature, enzyme concentration, and substrate and cofactor concentrations among others. Despite these constraints, the pH vs V_0 profiles are

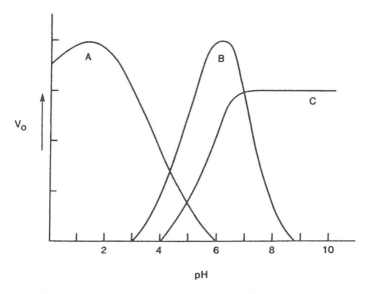

Figure 5.13 Velocity vs pH profiles of three enzymes.

useful for suggesting which amino acids may be involved in the catalytic action. For example, enzyme B in Figure 5.13 has half-maximal velocity at pH 4.5 and pH 7.0. The pK value of the side-chain carboxyl group of an aspartic acid or glutamic acid residue in a protein is 4.5, and that of histidine is 7.0. Assuming that the pH–velocity profile reflects the ionization state of aspartate or glutamate and histidine residues, one can infer that the aspartate or glutamate residue must be in the anionic form (ionized, negatively charged) and histidine residues must be protonated (positively charged) for the reaction to occur. The values for K_m and V_{max} may vary with pH.

5.9.3 Ionic Strength

Neutral salts have a significant effect on the solubility of proteins. The effects of salts can be expressed in terms of their ionic strength (u) when they are in solution. Ionic strength can be calculated as

$$u = \frac{1}{2} \Sigma \, MZ^2 \tag{5.35}$$

where M is the molarity of each ionic species and Z is the charge of the ion regardless of sign. Thus, the ionic strength of 0.1 M KCl is 0.1, whereas that of 0.1 M Na$_2$SO$_4$ is 0.3. It is important when determining the effect of pH on a reaction that all buffers used be of the same ionic strength, because any given buffer may have a different ionic strength at different pH values, and two different buffers may have different ionic strengths at the same pH.

5.9.4 Temperature

Figure 5.14 shows the typical curve for the temperature dependence of the rate of an enzyme-catalyzed reaction. The initial increase in rate is followed by a

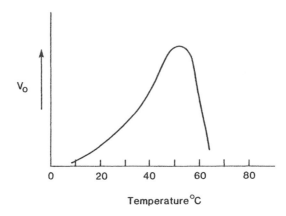

Figure 5.14 Effect of temperature on enzyme activity.

precipitous drop that is due to thermal denaturation of the enzyme. The precise, highly ordered tertiary structure necessary for catalysis has been disrupted. This occurs for most enzymes in the range of 55–60°C. Enzymes from thermophilic bacteria living in hot springs may tolerate temperatures of 90°C or more. Some enzymes, usually those that are membrane associated, are known to be denatured at low temperatures and are said to be cold sensitive.

Most enzymes show a 50–300% increase in reaction rate when the temperature is increased by 10°, and the ratio of rate constants at two temperatures 10° apart is usually between 1.5 and 4.0 for most enzymes. This value is termed Q_{10} and is derived from the Arrhenius equation [Equation (5.9)], which can be integrated to give

$$E_a = \frac{2.3\,R\,T_1\,T_2}{T_2 - T_1} \log \frac{k_2}{k_1} \tag{5.36}$$

where k_1 and k_2 are rate constants (V_{max} values) of the reaction at the two temperatures. If $T_2 - T_1 = 10°C$, then k_2/k_1 becomes Q_{10} and

$$E_a = \frac{2.3\,R\,T_2\,T_1 \log Q_{10}}{10} \tag{5.37}$$

Q_{10} is also V_{max2}/V_{max1}. A Q_{10} of 2 (rate increases twofold) is equivalent to an E_a of about 12,600 cal/mol for a temperature increase from 25 to 35°C.

5.10   REGULATION OF ENZYME ACTIVITY

5.10.1   Introduction

In the preceding discussion of enzyme activity, little was said about the overall regulation and coordination of these activities within a smoothly functioning cell. Clearly, the flow of metabolites through anabolic and catabolic pathways must be consistent with the requirements of the cell (and the organism) and effectively respond to both short- and long-term perturbations in the intracellular and extracellular environment. There are many mechanisms that affect enzyme activity, and the more important ones are summarized below.

5.10.2 Level of Enzymes

As noted earlier, the velocity of any enzyme-catalyzed reaction is dependent upon the amount of effective enzyme present. Enzyme biosynthesis, like that of all proteins, is under genetic control, a long-term process. Biosynthesis of enzymes may be increased or decreased at the genome level. Various hormones can activate or repress the mechanisms controlling gene expression. Enzyme levels are the result of the balance between synthesis and degradation. This enzyme turnover may be altered by diverse physiological conditions, by hormone effects, and by the level of metabolites.

5.10.3 Compartmentation of Enzymes and Enzyme Systems

In eukaryotic cells, different enzymes and enzyme systems are segregated into the various organelles and intracellular structures. This facilitates regulation of various processes independently of others. Table 5.1 lists the intracellular distribution of some important enzymes and metabolic sequences in a model mammalian cell. Some processes, such as urea biosynthesis and gluconeogenesis, depend on the interplay of reactions occurring in more than one compartment. A further extension of spatial organization occurs in multicellular organisms in which different tissues have their distinctive metabolic characteristics that are subject to control in response to special needs of the organism.

5.10.4 Metabolic Pathway Regulation

A metabolic pathway consists of a sequence of enzyme-catalyzed steps. The pathway usually has a *rate-limiting step,* the reaction in the sequence with the lowest velocity. This may be due to the enzyme having a high K_m for its substrate or to the enzyme being subject to inhibition by a negative effector, usually a product of the pathway. In the latter case, an allosteric enzyme is involved.

Table 5.1 Compartmentation of Some Major Enzymes and Metabolic Processes

Plasma membrane	Amino acid transport systems, Na^+-K^+ ATPase
Cytosol	Glycolysis, glycogenesis and glycogenolysis, hexose monophosphate pathway, fatty acid synthesis, purine and pyrimidine catabolism, aminoacyl-tRNA synthetases
Mitochondria	Tricarboxylic acid cycle, electron transport and oxidative phosphorylation, fatty acid oxidation, urea synthesis
Nucleus	DNA and RNA synthesis
Endoplasmic reticulum (rough and smooth)	Protein synthesis, steroid synthesis, glycosylation, detoxification
Lysosomes	Hydrolases
Golgi apparatus	Glycosyl transferases, glucose-5-phosphatase, formation of plasma membrane and secretory vesicles
Peroxisomes	Catalase, D-amino acid oxidase, urate oxidase

Consider the reaction sequence

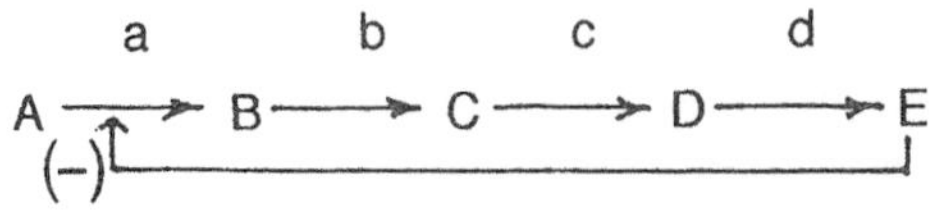

(5.38)

in which the capital letters B, C, and D indicate intermediates in the synthesis of E and each intermediate is formed by enzyme a, b, or c. When an appreciable amount of E has been synthesized, it acts to inhibit enzyme a, and further synthesis of E is halted at the beginning of the reaction sequence. This *feedback inhibition* usually involves virtually irreversible enzyme steps.

Now consider the branched sequence

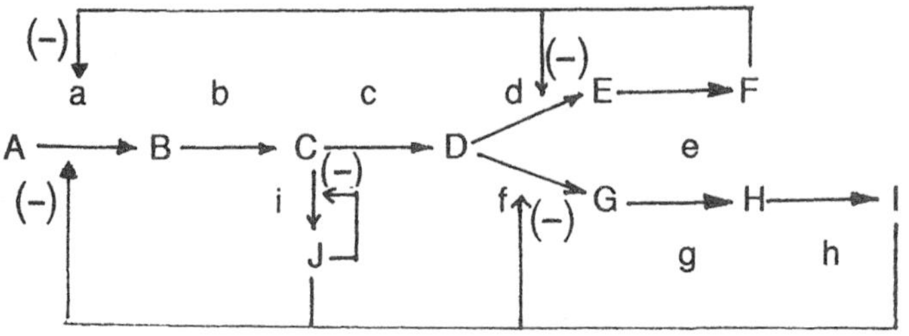

(5.39)

End products F and I may inhibit two enzymes each. The rate-limiting reaction for all products (F, I, and J) is A → B; for A → F, rate-limiting reactions are A → B and D → E; for A → I, they are A → B and D → G; and for J, they are A → B and C → J.

Each metabolic pathway has a committing reaction, which may or may not be identical to the rate-limiting reaction. This committing reaction designates the fate of an intermediate. In Equation (5.39), it is D → G for I and D → E for F.

There may also be feedback activators, especially where cross-regulation occurs: the product of one pathway activates another pathway. Thus, in purine biosynthesis (Chapter 10),

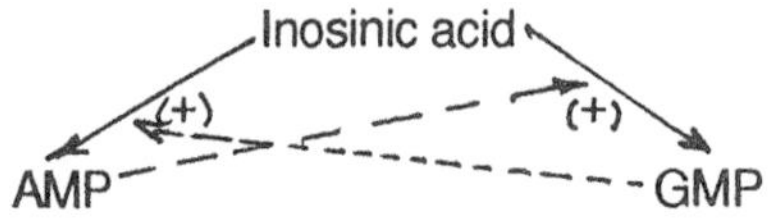

(5.40)

AMP activates the synthesis of GMP, and GMP activates the synthesis of AMP. At the same time, AMP inhibits its own synthesis, and GMP does the same.

5.11.5 Covalent Modification

There are two general types of covalent modification of enzymes that regulate their activity. These are the irreversible activation of inactive enzyme precursors, the *zymogens*, and the reversible interconversion of active and inactive forms of an enzyme.

Many enzymes are synthesized as inactive zymogens and are activated only after secretion from their site of synthesis and storage. Activation is achieved by cleavage of one or more peptide bonds. A standard example is the secretion of trypsinogen and chymotrypsinogen from the pancreas into the gastrointestinal tract and their subsequent conversion to active trypsin and active chymotrypsin. These endopeptidases are very potent enzymes, and if released in the pancreas they produce extensive autolysis, which probably accounts for the severe pain experienced by patients with acute pancreatitis.

The first recognized example of a reversible covalent modification in enzymes was seen in animal tissue glycogen phosphorylases, where the active and inactive forms of the enzyme were found to be phosphorylated and dephosphorylated, respectively. Although other types of covalent enzyme modification exist, the most common mode of covalent modification is via reversible phosphorylation–dephosphorylation. This is associated with the *second messenger* concept. When an extracellular ligand (first messenger) binds to cell surface receptors, the receptors undergo a conformational change that leads to the generation of an intracellular signaling molecule (second messenger) that alters the behavior of the target cell. Two of the more important second messengers are cyclic AMP (cAMP) and calcium ions. Cyclic AMP is synthesized from ATP by the plasma membrane–bound enzyme adenylate cyclase and is destroyed by enzymes called phosphodiesterases. Increasing cAMP levels stimulate cAMP-dependent protein kinases to phosphorylate specific serine or threonine residues in enzymes. This covalent phosphorylation in turn regulates the activity of these enzymes either positively or negatively. The proteins that have been phosphorylated by cAMP-dependent protein kinases are dephosphorylated by a phosphoprotein phosphatase, which itself is regulated by cAMP. A simplified version of these events is shown in Figure 5.15.

The protein kinase is tetrameric, consisting of two regulatory and two catalytic subunits. The latter are inactive as long as the complex still exists. Cyclic AMP reacts with the regulatory subunits, changing their conformations and causing the release of now active catalytic subunits.

Some protein kinases are cAMP-independent and respond instead to increased free Ca^{2+} levels. Some of these kinases contain the calcium-binding subunit calmodulin. Binding of Ca^{2+} to calmodulin induces an allosteric activation analogous to the activation of protein kinases by cAMP. Some protein kinases, such as phosphorylase kinase, are regulated by both cAMP and Ca^{2+}.

Second messengers not only allow the transduction of extracellular signals to intracellular ones but also provide a means for greatly amplifying the initial

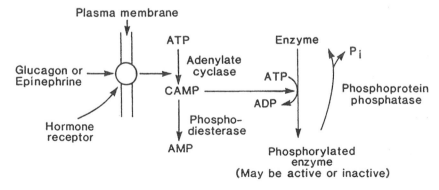

Figure 5.15 Role of cAMP in covalent modification of enzyme activity.

signal. Each receptor protein activates many molecules of adenylate cyclase, which in turn catalyze the formation of a large number of cAMP molecules, each of which in turn activates a large number of protein kinase molecules, and so forth. The result is that one extracellular signaling molecule can generate many thousands of molecules of the product. A similar mechanism is present in the blood coagulation cascade system (Chapter 7), though it is unidirectional in this case.

5.11 COFACTORS, COENZYMES, AND PROSTHETIC GROUPS

The terms *cofactor*, *coenzymes*, and *prosthetic group* are used to describe the nonprotein moieties of the enzyme active center. The distinction between these terms is not sharp. Some of the cofactors are derivatives of vitamins that form either covalent or noncovalent linkages at or near the active site of the enzyme, and some are metal ions. If a cofactor (coenzyme) is tightly bound to the protein moiety (the *apoenzyme*), it is often referred to as a prosthetic group. A coenzyme that is easily removed from the holoenzyme, leaving behind the apoenzyme, is often regarded as a second substrate.

Many enzymes require metal ion cofactors for their activity. Such enzymes are either metalloenzymes, in which case the metal ion is tightly bound, or metal-activated enzymes, in which case the bound metal ion is retained in an equilibrium with free metal ions.

Many of the coenzymes are derivatives of vitamins. A coenzyme function is known for each of the water-soluble vitamins except vitamin C. A detailed discussion of the water-soluble vitamins and their conversion to coenzymes is found in Chapter 6. The biochemical functions of fat-soluble vitamins (A, D, E, K) are, with exception, less clearly understood. They are also further considered in Chapter 6.

5.12 ENZYMES IN CLINICAL DIAGNOSIS

Determination of the activity of various enzymes normally at low levels or absent from plasma is an important aid for diagnosis, differential diagnosis, and prognosis in numerous disease states, especially those involving the heart, liver, and pancreas. The plasma levels of intracellular enzymes are normally low to zero and vary only within narrow limits in healthy individuals. However, in many organic diseases, the release of cellular enzymes is increased, either by enhanced permeability of cell membranes or by cell destruction. The rate of appearance of intracellular enzymes in plasma depends on their molecular size, their compartmentation (cytosol or mitochondria, for example), and their concentration gradient between intra- and extracellular levels. Although the relationship is not necessarily direct, the greater the extent of damage to the tissue, the greater the increase in the plasma level of the enzyme. The rate of elimination of an enzyme depends on its stability and on its destruction by the cells of the reticuloendothelial system. The half-life of "diagnostic enzymes" can range from several hours to several days, thus making the time of their measurement of critical importance.

Because the intermediary metabolism of various organs is virtually the same, organ-specific enzymes are very rare. One example usually cited is the acid phosphatase of the prostate. However, the enzyme complement of the various organs may differ with respect to relative activities of the enzymes, the time dependence of their appearance in plasma, and the pattern of their isoenzymes (see below). Table 5.2 presents a list of enzymes commonly used for organ- and disease-specific diagnoses.

The importance of timing is shown in Figure 5.16, in which the time-course curves for creatine kinase (CK), lactate dehydrogenase (LDH), and aspartate

Table 5.2 Commonly Assayed Enzymes for Organ- and Disease-Specific Diagnoses

Enzyme	Organ or disease
Acid phosphatase	Prostatic carcinoma
Alkaline phosphatase	Liver, bone disease
Aspartate aminotransferase (AST)	Liver, heart disease
Lactate dehydrogenase (LDH)	Liver, heart
Creatine kinase (CK)	Heart, muscle
Amylase	Pancreatic disease
Lipase	Pancreatic disease

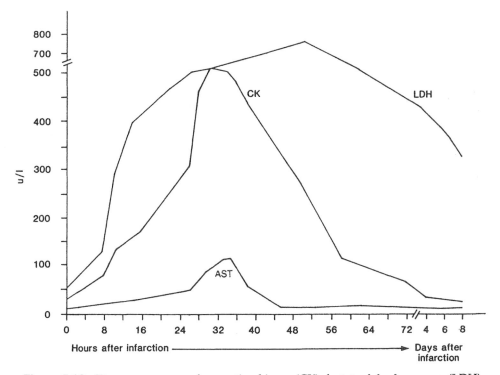

Figure 5.16 Time-course curve for creatine kinase (CK), lactate dehydrogenase (LDH), and aspartate aminotransferase (AST) in myocardial infarction.

aminotransferase (AST) are shown for a case of myocardial infarction. CK is elevated by 4–8 h, reaches a maximum at 16–36 h, and returns to normal on about the fourth or fifth day. At the other extreme is LDH, which is elevated by 5–12 h, reaches a maximum in 24–60 h, and returns to normal after a week or two. It is obvious that an assay of CK after the third or fourth day would be of little use for early diagnosis, and that of LDH is much more useful for a late-diagnosed infarction. AST behaves similarly to CK.

Isoenzymes or *isozymes* are enzymes from a single species that have the same kind of enzymatic activity but differ in chemical structure. In addition, they may differ in quantitative characteristics such as possessing different K_m's with the same substrate and may differ in response to temperature and effectors. Isozymes of more than 100 enzymes have been demonstrated in humans. The most important of these for diagnostic purposes are the isozymes of LDH, CK, alkaline phosphatase, leucine aminopeptidase, acid phosphatase, and aldolase. These have been exploited for differential organ diagnosis.

Lactate dehydrogenase occurs as a tetramer with two kinds of subunits designated H for heart and M for muscle. Five different LDHs are separable and identifiable by electrophoresis. The composition of these and their major tissue locations are as follows:

LDH 1 H_4 Heart, kidney, erythrocyte
LDH 2 H_3M Heart, kidney, erythrocyte
LDH 3 H_2M_2 Brain, pancreas
LDH 4 HM_3 Lung, spleen
LDH 5 M_4 Skeletal muscle, liver

Creatine kinase (CK) is a dimeric enzyme with two subunits, M (muscle type) and B (brain type). Three isozymes are distinguished: CK 1-BB (brain), CK 2-MB (heart), and CK 3-MM (skeletal muscle). The total CK activity found in skeletal muscle is almost entirely of the CK 3 type, that in heart muscle is 15–20% CK 2 and the remainder CK 3, and that in brain is all CK 1. In the human being, the only significant source of blood CK 2 is the heart muscle. Because the intact blood-brain barrier appears to be impermeable to CK, the occurrence of CK 1 in blood is unlikely. The total serum CK activity in healthy individuals is almost exclusively that of CK 3.

For the diagnosis of myocardial infarction, it is not only the detection of CK 2-MB that is important but also the contribution of the CK 2 fraction to the total CK activity. Activities of CK 2 in excess of 5% of the total CK activity should be regarded with suspicion. CK 2 as well as total CK activity will increase within a few hours of the acute episode. Maximum activity of CK 2 may precede that of total CK and remain elevated until the third or fourth day. LDH 1 release occurs 1–2 days after the appearance of CK (Figure 5.16). LDH 2 activity is normally higher than that of LDH 1. However, in myocardial infarction, the activity of LDH 1 will exceed that of LDH 2 near the time the CK 2 returns to normal levels. Thus, the judicious choices of the proper enzymes and the appropriate time, coupled with isozyme determinations, can provide a considerable degree of diagnostic certainty.

QUESTIONS

5.1. An enzyme
  a. Changes the equilibrium constant of a reaction
  b. Increases the standard free energy of the reaction
  c. Hastens the attainment of equilibrium of a chemical reaction
  d. Redistributes the concentrations of reactants and products at equilibrium compared to the uncatalyzed reaction
  e. Raises the activation energy for a chemical reaction

5.2. If one wanted to determine the activation energy of a chemical reaction, one would do which of the following?
  a. Measure rate constants as a function of temperature
  b. Measure equilibrium constants as a function of time
  c. Measure velocities as a function of pH
  d. Measure rate constants as a function of time
  e. Measure equilibrium constants as a function of temperature

5.3. A bell-shaped curve is obtained when one plots enzyme activity on the y axis against which parameter(s) on the x axis?
  a. Temperature
  b. Substrate concentration
  c. Inhibitor concentration
  d. pH
  e. Two of the above

5.4. Why do we use initial velocities when determining K_m values?
  a. Equilibrium is reached very rapidly.
  b. Measurements are most accurate at the beginning of a reaction.
  c. The forward reaction is unopposed by the reverse reaction, because little, if any, product is present.
  d. Rate constants change as the reaction progresses.
  e. K_m changes during the course of the reaction; the convention is to use the K_m of the initial velocity.

For questions 5.5–5.8, use the following information. An enzyme, molecular weight 100,000, converts 50 µg/mL of a substrate (molecular weight 100) to the product per minute at an enzyme concentration of 5 µg/mL.

5.5. The specific activity of the enzyme in international units per milligram is
  a. 0.1
  b. 1.0
  c. 10
  d. 100
  e. 1000

5.6. The turnover number of the enzyme is:
  a. 10,000
  b. 100,000
  c. 1000
  d. 100
  e. 0.1

5.7. How many milligrams of the enzyme are in one international unit?
  a. 0.01
  b. 1.0
  c. 5.0

    d. 10

    e. 100

5.8. What is the time required for one catalytic cycle, that is, how long does it take for one molecule of the substrate to be converted to the product?

    a. 1 min

    b. 0.1 min

    c. 0.01 min

    d. 0.001 min

    e. 0.0001 min

5.9. The apparent K_m of an allosteric enzyme can be estimated from a

    a. Lineweaver-Burk plot

    b. Eadie-Hofstee plot

    c. Michaelis-Menten expression

    d. The Hill equation

    e. Two of the above

5.10. When the velocity of an enzymatic reaction is equal to its V_{max}, then the rate of substrate conversion to the product may be increased by

    a. Increasing the temperature

    b. Adding more substrate

    c. Adding more enzyme

    d. Adding more product

    e. Two of the above

5.11. At maximum velocity, which is/are correct?

    a. The kinetics are first-order.

    b. $V = k_3[ES]$

    c. $k_1 = k_2$

    d. $k_1 = 0$

    e. Two of the above

5.12. Which is not a property of allosteric enzymes?

    a. Greatest velocity change is observed at about $(\frac{1}{2})V_{max}$.

    b. A substance not related to either the product or the substrate may increase enzyme activity.

    c. A substance not related to either the product or the substrate may decrease enzyme activity.

    d. In the symmetrical model, there are molecules that may contain half the subunits in the T and half in the R conformation.

    e. An allosteric enzyme is usually found at the beginning of a metabolic pathway.

5.13. What is the ionic strength of a solution containing 0.2 M NaCl and 0.5 M $CaCl_2$?

    a. 1.7 M

    b. 1.4 M

    c. 0.7 M

    d. 0.35 M

    e. 0.2 M

5.14. What is the Q_{10} of a reaction catalyzed by an enzyme with an activation energy of 3000 cal? Assume that the enzyme activities have been measured at 15, 20, and 25°C.

    a. 1.20

    b. 1.88

    c. 2.01

    d. 2.25

    e. 35

5.15. In the metabolic pathway given below, which reaction is most likely to be rate-determining for the product of G via the feedback effect?

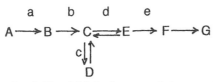

5.16. In question 5.15, which is the committing reaction for the production of D?

5.17. In a metabolic pathway that does not contain any allosteric enzymes, of the enzymes involved, the rate-limiting reaction enzyme will have the
   a. Highest V_{max}
   b. Lowest V_{max}
   c. Highest K_m
   d. Lowest K_m
   e. Highest activation energy

5.18. Regulation of enzyme activity in vivo involves all of the following, except
   a. Conversion of a zymogen to an enzyme
   b. Reaction of the active site with diisopropylfluorophosphate
   c. Changing the K_m of an allosteric enzyme
   d. Breaking certain covalent interactions in the enzyme with phosphatases
   e. Dissociation of the enzyme into subunits

5.19. A cofactor in an enzyme reaction may do all of the following, except
   a. Catalyze the activation of the enzyme by breaking peptide bonds, such as the conversion of a zymogen to an enzyme
   b. Act as an electron acceptor or donor with respect to the substrate
   c. Covalently bind the substrate
   d. Chelate the substrate by sharing electrons with specific functional groups of the substrate
   e. All of the above

5.20. Isozymes
   a. May have different K_m values while catalyzing the same reaction
   b. Are enzymes of similar or identical structures catalyzing different reactions
   c. Are enzymes inhibited by the same inhibitor(s)
   d. Always have the same V_{max} but different K_m's
   e. Are enzymes with the same optimum pH and temperature

5.21. The following diseases may be diagnosed by enzyme assays indicated, except:
   a. Prostatic cancer—alkaline phosphatase
   b. Myocardial infarction—aspartate aminotransferase (AST)
   c. Acute pancreatitis—amylase and lipase
   d. Bone cancer—alkaline phosphatase
   e. Liver disease—alkaline phosphatase and alanine aminotransferase (ALT)

In questions 5.22–5.26, choose answers from the following:
   a. Lactate dehydrogenase (LDH)
   b. Creatine kinase
   c. Both
   d. Neither

5.22. Occur(s) in the form of isozymes
5.23. May be used in the diagnosis of myocardial infarction
5.24. May be used in the diagnosis of skeletal muscle disorders

5.25. In a heart enzyme, a mixture of tetramers
5.26. Will not be observed in the bloodstream some 40 h following myocardial infarction
5.27. Methotrexate is an antitumor agent whose structure resembles that of folic acid. It inhibits the enzyme that converts folic acid to tetrahydrofolic acid. The inhibition most likely involves which of the following?
   a. Lowered K_m and V_{max}
   b. Increased K_m
   c. Lowered V_{max}
   d. Increased K_m and lowered V_{max}
   e. Increased K_m and V_{max}
5.28. The constant that reflects the affinity of an enzyme for its substrate is
   a. V_{max}
   b. Activation energy
   c. The first-order rate constant
   d. K_m
   e. The free energy of the reaction catalyzed
5.29. An enzyme catalyzing the reaction lecithin + cholesterol → fatty acid cholesterol ester + lysolecithin may be classified as a(n)
   a. Oxidoreductase
   b. Ligase
   c. Hydrolase
   d. Transferase
   e. Lyase
5.30. Which consideration or assumption does not enter into the derivation of the Michaelis-Menten equation?
   a. The enzyme E and substrate S form an enzyme–substrate complex ES.
   b. Each active site works independently of the others.
   c. The rate-limiting reaction is the formation of the enzyme–substrate complex ES.
   d. When substrate concentration is very high, all enzyme is present in the form of ES, and then the velocity is V_{max}.
   e. The velocity of the reaction is determined by the rate of conversion of ES to E + product.
5.31. The K_i for an inhibitor of an enzyme is
   a. The dissociation constant of the enzyme–inhibitor complex, EI → E + I
   b. The K_m of the enzyme in the presence of the inhibitor
   c. Activation energy of the inhibited enzyme
   d. The dissociation constant of the enzyme–substrate complex, ES → E + S, in the presence of the inhibitor
   e. The affinity constant of the enzyme for the substrate in the presence of the inhibitor
5.32. Hydrolytic activity of pepsin is maximal at pH 2–3, the stomach pH, and aspartate is an essential component of the active site. Pepsin is inactive at pH 7. Which enzymatic reaction mechanisms is most likely of major importance in the action of pepsin?
   a. Acid–base catalysis
   b. Covalent modification
   c. Proximity–entropy effects
   d. Substrate strain
   e. Zymogen activation
5.33. Which is not a correct description or property of K_m?
   a. It is the substrate concentration at half-maximal velocity of the enzyme reaction.
   b. It can be estimated accurately from plots of velocity versus $[S_0]$.

    c. It can be obtained from the x intercept of the Lineweaver-Burk plot.

    d. It is the dissociation constant of the enzyme–substrate complex, ES → E + S.

    e. It can be calculated from the slope of the Eadie-Hofstee plot.

Answers

5.1. (c) An enzyme simply decreases the time it takes to reach equilibrium (by lowering the activation energy). It does not change the equilibrium constant or distribution of reactants and products at equilibrium.

5.2. (a) The equation one uses for the determination of activation energy is the Arrhenius equation, $\ln k_1 = \ln A - E_a/RT$, where $\ln k_1$ is plotted against $1/T$, the slope is then $-E_a/R$, and E_a is the activation energy.

5.3. (e) This could be either the optimum pH or optimum temperature.

5.4. (c) The initial velocity is maximal because there is little if any product to oppose the forward reaction via mass action or other effects.

5.5. (d) Fifty micrograms of substrate is 0.5 μmol. Therefore, activity is 0.5 IU/mL. If we define specific activity (sp act) as the amount of enzyme that exhibits 1 IU of activity per milligram, then sp act = (0.5 IU/mL)/(0.005 mg/mL) = 10^4 IU/mg.

5.6. (a) *Five micrograms of the enzyme is 5/100,000 = 5×10^{-5} μmol. Turnover number (TN) is moles of substrate converted by 1 mol of enzyme per unit time. Therefore,*

$$\frac{0.5 \text{ μmol/mL} \times \text{min}}{5 \times 10^{-5} \text{ μmol/mL}} = 10^4$$

5.7. (a) Since 0.5 μmol of substrate is converted to product per minute by 5 μg of enzyme, 10 μg of enzyme will convert 1 μmol of substrate per minute, which is 1 IU.

5.8. (e) Catalytic cycle is nothing but the reciprocal of the turnover number. Therefore, one catalytic cycle will be $1/10^4 = 10^{-4}$ min.

5.9. (d) The Hill equation is used to estimate K_m for allosteric enzymes. Equations based on classic Michaelis-Menten kinetics are not applicable.

5.10. (e) Rate will be increased by adding more enzyme or increasing the temperature. Adding more substrate will not work, because all enzyme molecules are already saturated with substrates.

5.11. (b) At V_{max}, kinetics are of the zeroth order, and as all enzyme molecules are saturated with substrate, V will equal $k_1[ES]$.

5.12. (d) In the symmetrical model, there are no T and R hybrids. The T form changes to all R form, and vice versa. The sequential model provides for such hybrids.

5.13. (a) 0.2 M NaCl dissociates into $[Na^+] = 0.2$ M and $Cl^- = 0.2$ M, and 0.5 M $CaCl_2$ dissociates into $[Ca^{2+}] = 0.5$ M and $[Cl^-] = 1.0$ M. Total $[Cl^-] = 1.0 + 0.2 = 1.2$ M. $u = (1/2)[(0.2 \times 1^2) + (1.2 \times 1^2) + (0.5 \times 2^2)] = 1.7$ M.

5.14. (a) Using Equation 5.37, we get $\log Q_{10} = 30,000/(2.3 \times 1987 \times 288 \times 298) = 0.077$. Antilog of 0.077 is 1.20. It is an unusually low Q_{10}.

5.15. (e) The answer is not d because the conversion of C to E is reversible, and neither can it be a or b, because the intermediate C can also be diverted to D.

5.16. (c) Answer b will not work, because intermediate C can be diverted to E and on to G.

5.17. (c) The enzyme with the highest K_m will be rate-limiting, because high K_m indicates low substrate binding affinity. Reaction cannot proceed unless substrate is bound to the enzyme.

5.18. (b) Diisopropylfluorophosphate (DFP) is an artifically produced (nerve gas–like) compound that inhibits serine proteases and esterases. Inactive enzymes may be activated by dissociation into subunits such as is the case with cAMP-dependent protein kinases.

5.19. (a) Conversion of a zymogen to an enzyme does not usually involve a cofactor used in the enzyme reaction.

5.20. (a) *Isozymes* are enzymes from different organs of the organism that perform the same function. They may have different K_m's for the substrate they use.

5.21. (a) Prostatic cancer is diagnosed by acid phosphatase measurements (see Table 5.2).

5.22. (c) Both enzymes are present as isozymes: LDH as a tetramer of the H and M subunits, and CK as a dimer of the M and B subunits.

5.23. (c) Both are used to detect myocardial infarction.

5.24. (c) Both enzymes are increased in plasma in skeletal muscle disorder, but the isozyme pattern will differ from that seen in myocardial infarction.

5.25. (a) LDH is a tetrameric enzyme. In the heart enzyme the H subunits predominate, whereas in skeletal muscle the M subunits predominate.

5.26. (b) CK will disappear after about 40 h following myocardial infarction, whereas LDH will linger for days.

5.27. (b) Methotrexate is a competitive inhibitor of dihydrofolate reductase because its structure is similar to those of folic acid and dihydrofolic acid. Competitive inhibitors are characterized by an increase in the K_m of the enzyme (lowered affinity for the substrate) while V_{max} remains unchanged.

5.28. (d) A low K_m reflects a high affinity for the substrate, and a high K_m, a low affinity.

5.29. (d) Lecithin-cholesterol acyl transferase is a transferase; it transfers the fatty acyl group from lecithin to cholesterol.

5.30. (c) Formation of the enzyme–substrate complex is not rate-limiting; it is the dissociation of the enzyme–substrate complex, ES → E + P, that is.

5.31. (a) As K_m is the dissociation constant for the ES complex, K_i is the dissociation constant for the EI complex, EI → E + I.

5.32. (a) Data presented suggest that acid–base catalysis is of major importance in the hydrolytic action of pepsin. The pK of the beat carboxyl group of aspartate is around 4 in the free acid and may very well be lower in the protein molecule due to neighboring group effects. A pH optimum near the pK of aspartic acid suggests that the ability of aspartate to accept and donate protons is of major importance in its mode of action.

5.33. (b) Accurate determination of the K_m by plotting velocities against substrate concentrations is usually not possible, because such a plot cannot estimate V_{max} very effectively. A Lineweaver-Burk or Eadie-Hofstee plot is much more effective.

PROBLEMS

5.1. In an enzyme-catalyzed reaction S → P, derive the expression for the first-order constant k in terms of K_m and V_{max}.

5.2. Allopurinol is a drug given to gout sufferers. It inhibits an enzyme of the purine degradation pathway called xanthine oxidase by acting in the capacity of a substrate. However, its product, oxidized allopurinol, is not able to leave the active site of the enzyme, thus blocking it. Is there a name for this type of substrate? What inhibition kinetics would you observe with a Lineweaver-Burk plot, and why?

5.3. At what substrate concentration are enzymes most effective and respond best to the needs of the cells, and why?

5.4. The following data were obtained for a Michaelis-Menten enzyme with and without an inhibitor:

	Initial velocity (arbitrary units)	
[S] (mM)	Without inhibitor	With inhibitor
2	9	—
4	17	14
6	23	18
8	29	22
10	34	24
14	42	28
18	50	—
25	59	34
30	67	—

Determine the V_{max} and K_m of the native enzyme. Identify the type of inhibitor that is shown, and determine the K_m and V_{max} of the inhibited enzyme. How do you explain the difference in K_m values?

5.5. The following data were obtained for an allosteric enzyme:

[S] (mM)	Velocity (% of V_{max})
1.00	10
1.38	20
1.58	25
3.16	50
6.31	75
7.90	80
12.60	90

Show that this enzyme is indeed allosteric; determine its cooperativity coefficient (Hill coefficient). Is the cooperativity positive, or is it negative? What is K'? Is K' equal to K_m? If not, why not? When is $K' = K_m$?

BIBLIOGRAPHY

Adolph L, Lorenz R. Enzyme Diagnosis in Disease of the Heart, Liver, and Pancreas. Basel: S. Karger, 1982.
Hammes CG. Enzyme Catalysis and Regulations. New York: Academic Press, 1982.
Saier MH. Enzymes in Metabolic Pathways. New York: Harper & Row, 1987.
Tietz NW. Textbook of Clinical Chemistry. Philadelphia: WB Saunders, 1986.

6

Vitamins and Minerals

After completing this chapter, the student should

1. Recognize the structure of each vitamin and its coenzyme.
2. Know the type of reaction catalyzed by each coenzyme and be able to identify the active site of the coenzyme.
3. Know the etiology of various vitamin deficiency diseases.
4. Understand the action of coenzyme antagonists such as methotrexate.
5. Know the mechanisms of fat-soluble vitamin transport throughout the organism.
6. Understand the role of vitamin A in the visual process and be able to explain the metabolisms of vitamin A and related compounds.
7. Know how provitamins D are converted to their active counterparts and how this process is controlled.
8. Understand the physiologic actions of vitamin D and its role in calcium and phosphate metabolism.
9. Understand the role of vitamin K in the organism and how its antagonists affect blood coagulation.
10. Know the physiologic action of vitamin E and its connection to selenium.
11. Know the following aspects of Cu, Zn, Mo, Cr, Mg, Se, and Ca physiology, wherever applicable: mode of transport, mechanism of absorption, mechanism of action, deficiency diseases with their symptoms, diagnostic aspects.

6.1 INTRODUCTION

Vitamins are physiologically important dietary components that cannot be manufactured by the organism. Dietary vitamin deficiencies may result in pathology and even death. Pellagra is a good example: it is a niacin deficiency disease that was a major cause of death in the southern United States because corn, the staple foodstuff in that area, is niacin-deficient. Moreover, corn is tryptophan-deficient, which magnifies the damage because tryptophan gives rise to niacin coenzymes in the human organism (see Chapter 20). Pellagra was not eradicated until niacin was discovered in the 1930s by Elvehjem and his associates. Vitamin deficiencies are rare today in the United States. Nevertheless, they do occur in patients living on total parenteral nutrition (TPN), in vegetarians, in alcoholics, and in persons on prolonged fad diets.

Vitamins are essential in mammalian physiology because their coenzyme forms are prosthetic groups or cofactors in many enzyme reactions or because they can perform certain specialized functions in the human organism. Vitamin A and its role in the visual process is an example. The biology of vitamins may be examined from the nutritional or biochemical points of view. The former is concerned with minimum daily requirements, dietary sources, bioavailability, and deficiency syndromes. The biochemist looks for structures, functional groups, conversion to coenzymes, mechanisms of action, mode of transport, and storage. Both aspects will be addressed in this chapter, though the emphasis will be on the biochemical properties of vitamins.

It should be noted that deficiency states for some vitamins (e.g., pantothenic acid) are practically unknown in human beings. In such cases, deficiency states may be simulated by feeding the subject an appropriate vitamin antagonist. In another series of situations, vitamin deficiencies can be brought about by interfering with their absorption intentionally or may be the result of a disease process. Thus, fat-soluble vitamin deficiency may develop in cases of fat malabsorption syndromes (steatorrhea): sprue, pancreatic insufficiency, and bile duct obstruction.

Vitamins have been variously classified and categorized, for example, on the basis of their solubilities. The fat (lipid)-soluble vitamins are A, D, E, and K, and the rest are said to be water-soluble. With some exceptions, the latter are converted to physiologically active forms called *coenzymes* in the organism. The coenzymes act either as *prosthetic* (firmly protein-bound) *groups* of enzymes or as loosely bound cofactors or cosubstrates. A number of water-soluble vitamins have been grouped into the so-called B-complex because they occur together in the same food sources. They are thiamine, riboflavin, niacin, pantothenic acid, pyridoxine, folic acid, and vitamin B_{12}. Thiamine, niacin, riboflavin, and pantothenic acid have been referred to as *energy-releasing* vitamins because they participate in metabolic reaction sequences (pathways) that serve to oxidize carbohydrates, fats, and amino acids to yield energy in the form of ATP. Sometimes, the term *energy-releasing* and *B-complex* are used interchangeably.

Table 6.1 lists the water-soluble vitamins with their structures and coenzyme forms. Certain portions of the coenzymes are especially important in their biological activities, and they are indicated by arrows. For example, in case of coenzyme A, a thiol ester is formed between its –SH residue and the acyl group being transferred. And in the case of pyridoxal phosphate, its carbonyl residue forms a Schiff base with the amino group of the amino acid that is being decarboxylated. Fat-soluble vitamins (Table 6.2) are also transformed into biologically active substances. However, with the possible exception of vitamin K, these do not operate as prosthetic groups or cosubstrates in specific enzyme reactions.

Both Tables 6.1 and 6.2 list the recommended dietary allowances (RDA) for each vitamin. These are recommended by the Food and Nutrition Board of the National Academy of Sciences. The values given are designed to maintain a

Table 6.1 Water-Soluble Vitamins and Their Coenzymes[a]

Name	Structure	Coenzyme name and structure	Function	Deficiency disease	Daily requirement
Riboflavin, vitamin B$_2$	Ribityl / Isoalloxazine residue	Flavin mononucleotide (FMN) / Flavin adenine dinucleotide (FAD)	Redox reactions	Ariboflavinosis (rare)	1.1–1.5 mg
Niacin, vitamin B$_3$	Nicotinic acid / Nicotinamide	Nicotinamide-adenine dinucleotide (NAD)	Redox reactions; as glucose tolerance factor (GTF) in conjunction with Cr	Pellagra	12–20 mg

Table 6.1 Continued

Name	Structure	Coenzyme name and structure	Function	Deficiency disease	Daily requirement
		Nicotinamide-adenine dinucleotide phosphate (NADP)			
Pyridoxine,[b] vitamin B_6	Pyrimidine residue	Pyridoxal phosphate	Decarboxylation and transamination reactions in amino acids	Rare	2 mg
Thiamine, vitamin B_1	Pyrimidine residue / Thiazole residue	Thiamine pyrophosphate (TPP)	Decarboxylation and transketolation reactions	Beri-beri and Wernicke-Korsakoff syndrome	1.0–1.5 mg
Pantothenic acid	β-Alanine residue	Coenzyme A (CoA)	Activates carboxyl groups; acyl group transfer	Rare	5–10 mg

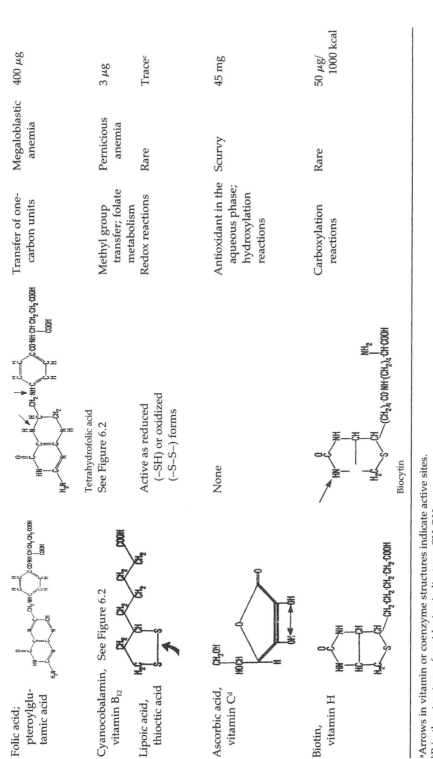

Folic acid; pteroylglutamic acid	Tetrahydrofolic acid See Figure 6.2	Transfer of one-carbon units	Megaloblastic anemia	400 μg
Cyanocobalamin, vitamin B_{12}	See Figure 6.2	Methyl group transfer; folate metabolism	Pernicious anemia	3 μg
Lipoic acid, thioctic acid	Active as reduced (–SH) or oxidized (–S–S–) forms	Redox reactions	Rare	Trace[c]
Ascorbic acid, vitamin C[d]	None	Antioxidant in the aqueous phase; hydroxylation reactions	Scurvy	45 mg
Biotin, vitamin H	Biocytin	Carboxylation reactions	Rare	50 μg/ 1000 kcal

[a]Arrows in vitamin or coenzyme structures indicate active sites.

[b]R in the structure of pyridoxine indicates –CH$_2$OH.

[c]Lipoic acid may be synthesized in the human organism in sufficient quantities to meet its daily requirement. Hence many authorities do not consider it to be a vitamin.

[d]When ascorbic acid is oxidized, the two vicinal –OH groups are converted to keto residues, =O.

TABLE 6.2 The Fat-Soluble Vitamins and Provitamins

Name	Structure	Function	Deficiency disease	Daily requirement (adult)	Sources
Vitamin A	α-Carotene β-Carotene Vitamin A$_1$ (all-trans) (retinol*),	Visual cycle; bone formation; epithelial cell differentiation	Night blindness; skin lesions	4.5 g Carotene from green vegetables; or 750 mg vitamin A$_1$	Plants, fruit, berries, vegetables for the carotenes; fish liver oil for vitamin A$_1$
Vitamin D	Ergosterol 7-Dehydrocholesterol	Calcium absorption and metabolism	Rickets in children, osteomalacia in adults	400 IU (10 µg vitamin D$_3$)	Yeast and hen's egg for ergosterol; animal products for 7-dehydrocholesterol; irradiated ergosterol for vitamin D$_2$; fish liver oil, milk, egg yolk, irradiated 7-dehydrocholesterol for vitamin D$_3$.

Vitamin D$_2$ (ergocalciferol*)

Vitamin D$_3$ (cholecalciferol*)

5,7,8-Trimethyltocol (α-tocopherol)

Vitamin K$_1$ (phylloquinone*)

Menadione (Vitamin K$_3$, methyl-naphthoquinone)

Vitamin E[a] (tocopherols)	Antioxidant in the lipid phase; free radical trap	Liver atrophy; red blood cell hemolysis; heurologic disorders	10–30 mg	Vegetable oils; animal products; eggs.
Vitamin K	Blood coagulation; biosynthesis of calcium-binding proteins	Bleeding (increased prothrombin time)	1 μg/kg (est.)	Green plants and tomatoes; menadione is synthetic

[a]When R$_1$ and R$_3$ are methyl groups, the compound is called alpha-tocopherol. Several other tocopherols, where R$_1$, R$_2$, or R$_3$ are H-residues, are found in nature; they may not be as active biologically as alpha-tocopherol.

131

healthy state in an average human being with a safety margin factored in. They are the best approximation on the basis of turnover studies, blood vitamin levels, and other pertinent data.

6.2 WATER-SOLUBLE VITAMINS AND COFACTORS

6.2.1 Redox Vitamins and Cofactors

Niacin, riboflavin, and lipoic acid give rise to coenzymes that participate in redox reactions. Niacin and riboflavin are essential in the human diet, whereas lipoic acid may be synthesized within the human organism. Lipoic acid is a required growth factor in many microorganisms and protozoa. It reacts covalently with the ϵ-amino groups of apoenzymes to give the active holoenzymes:

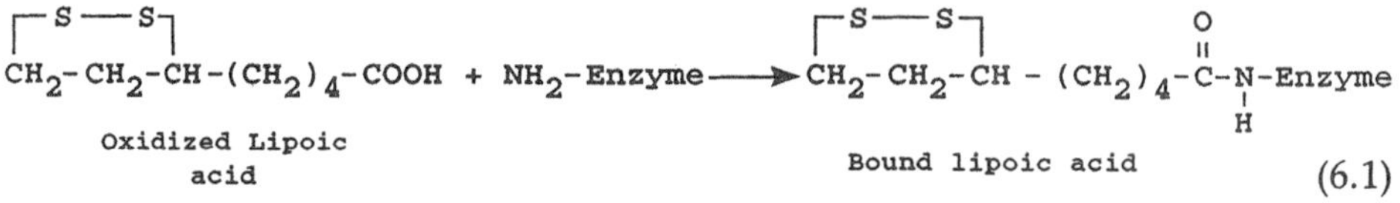

$$
\underset{\substack{\text{Oxidized Lipoic} \\ \text{acid}}}{\overset{\lceil S - S \rceil}{CH_2\text{-}CH_2\text{-}CH\text{-}(CH_2)_4\text{-}COOH}} + NH_2\text{-}Enzyme \longrightarrow \underset{\text{Bound lipoic acid}}{\overset{\lceil S - S \rceil}{CH_2\text{-}CH_2\text{-}CH - (CH_2)_4\text{-}\underset{H}{\overset{O}{\overset{\|}{C}}\text{-}N\text{-}Enzyme}}}
$$

$$(6.1)$$

Niacin and riboflavin are converted to their respective coenzymes, NAD$^+$ and NADP$^+$ on the one hand and flavin munonucleotide (FMN) and flavin adenine dinucleotide (FAD) on the other, as described in Chapter 10. Some NAD$^+$ can be synthesized from tryptophan, as described in Chapter 20. Tryptophan, however, provides only a fraction of our daily NAD$^+$ requirements.

Niacin ia a nutritional term applied to both nicotinic acid and nicotinamide and to a mixture of the two. Their structures and those of their coenzymes are given in Table 6.1. Numerous redox reactions use NAD$^+$ and NADP$^+$ or NADH and NADPH. The latter are used largely in reactions designed to reductively synthesize various substances, mostly in the extramitochondrial areas of the cell. NAD$^+$, on the other hand, is used largely in its oxidized form in catabolic redox reactions. The rat liver cytosol NADPH/NADP$^+$ ratio is about 80, whereas its NADH/NAD$^+$ ratio is only 8×10^{-4}. Table 6.3 lists some biochemical reactions in which these cofactors participate. It shows that they are of crucial importance in the metabolism of carbohydrates, fats, and amino acids.

When biological substances are oxidized they generally lose two electrons and two hydrogen atoms to the oxidizing agent. Although NAD$^+$ and NADP$^+$ do indeed accept two electrons each, they can bind only one hydrogen atom, releasing the other as a proton. The nicotinamide ring accepts the electrons, and the hydrogen atom reacts in the form of a hydride ion, as shown in Figure 6.1. The

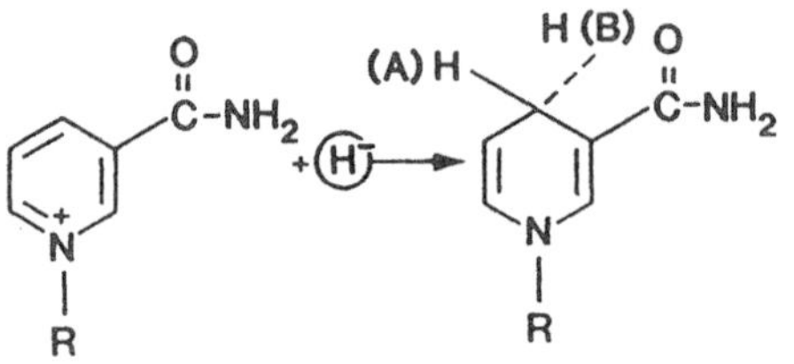

Figure 6.1 Reduction of the nicotinamide ring in NAD$^+$ and NADP$^+$. R represents the adenine nucleotide portion of the molecule.

Table 6.3 Typical Biochemical Redox Reactions That Utilize Cofactors Derived from Niacin and Riboflavin

Cofactor	Biochemical reaction	Enzyme
FMN	Amino acid → α-keto acid + NH_3	L-Amino acid oxidases
FAD	Succinate → furmarate[a]	Succinate dehydrogenase
	Fatty acyl CoA → enoyl CoA[b]	Fatty acyl CoA dehydrogenase
	Glycerol-3-phosphate → dihydroxyacetone phosphate (mitochondrial)[c]	Glycerol-3-phosphate dehydrogenase
$FADH_2$	UQ → UQH_2[d]	Complex II system
NAD	Glutamate → α-ketoglutarate	Glutamate dehydrogenase
	Pyruvate → acetyl CoA + CO_2	Pyruvate dehydrogenase complex
	Lactate → pyruvate	Lactate dehydrogenase
	Malate → oxaloacetate[a]	Malate dehydrogenase
	Glyceraldehyde-3-phosphate → 1,3-diphosphoglyceric acid[e]	Glyceraldehyde-3-phosphate dehydrogenase
	α-Ketoglutarate → succinyl CoA[a]	α-Ketoglutarate dehydrogenase
NADH	UQ → UQH_2[d]	Complex I system
	Acetoacetate → β-hydroxybutyrate	β-Hydroxybutyrate dehydrogenase
NADPH	Glucose-6-phosphate → 6-phosphogluconic acid[f]	Glucose-6-phosphate dehydrogenase
	Acetyl CoA → palmitate	Fatty acid synthetase
	Steroids $\xrightarrow{O_2}$ hydroxysteroids	Cytochrome P-450 system

[a]A Krebs cycle reaction (Chapter 18).
[b]A β-oxidation reaction (fatty acid metabolism) (Chapter 19).
[c]A mechanism for transporting reducing equivalents from cytosol into the mitochondria (Chapters 17 and 18).
[d]An oxidative phosphorylation reaction (Chapter 17).
[e]A glycolysis reaction (Chapter 18).
[f]A hexose monophosphate shunt reaction (Chapter 18).

hydrogen atom is not bound to the NAD^+ or $NADP^+$ randomly. Depending on the specificity of the redox enzyme involved, it appears either on the top face (face A) of the ring structure or on its bottom face (face B). Dehydrogenases that catalyze the NAD^+/NADH interconversions may thus be classified into A and B types.

Riboflavin is a combination of the isoalloxazine ring and ribitol. Conversion of the vitamin to FMN and FAD occurs via phosphorylation and adenylation, respectively, as indicated in Table 6.1. In the case of FAD or FMN, both the electrons and the hydrogen atoms are bound by the isoalloxazine ring structure of the riboflavin portion. The site of this reduction is pointed out in Table 6.1. FAD is often bound very tightly to the enzyme. For both the NAD^+ and FAD-type coenzymes, the adenylate portion of the coenzyme is necessary for binding to the enzyme. Table 6.3 also lists some representative reactions in which FAD and FMN are cofactors.

6.2.2 Biotin

Biotin is a vitamin that, among other things, catalyzes the fixation of CO_2 onto organic molecules. It is generally bound to lysine residues of apoenzymes by means of its carboxyl group. Such a complex is referred to as *biocytin*. It is released from dietary protein in the gut by normal digestive processes and is absorbed into the organism. It is cleaved into biotin and lysine by the ubiquitous enzyme biotinidase (also called biocytinase). It is noteworthy that an egg white protein, avidin, binds biotin rather tightly and prevents its utilization in the diet. A biotin deficiency can develop from the consumption of large amounts of raw egg white. Avidin is inactivated by cooking.

6.2.3 Vitamin B$_{12}$

Various vitamin B$_{12}$ derivatives are shown in Figure 6.2, where the R group is usually taken as CN$^-$. This form of vitamin B$_{12}$ is cyanocobalamin. In the active coenzyme, the CN$^-$ is replaced by a 5'-deoxyriboadenosyl residue or by –CH$_3$. Vitamin B$_{12}$ seems to be the only mammalian substance that contains cobalt. It also has a unique corrin ring structure, which is very similar to that of heme. Metabolic reactions requiring vitamin B$_{12}$ are discussed in Chapters 19 and 20.

In the stomach, dietary vitamin B$_{12}$ is bound by a glycoprotein called the *intrinsic factor*, which is produced by the stomach's parietal cells and has a molecular weight of 42,000–45,000. The vitamin B$_{12}$–intrinsic factor complex travels to the ileum, where the vitamin is absorbed, leaving the intrinsic factor behind. Vitamin B$_{12}$ deficiency results in pernicious anemia, a disorder of DNA biosynthesis. This is due in part to the fact that folic acid coenzymes cannot be used for DNA biosynthesis. The metabolism of vitamin B$_{12}$ and that of folic acid are thus closely linked (see Chapter 20). Nutritional vitamin B$_{12}$ deficiency is seen in strict vegetarians, but it can also be brought about by an absence of the intrinsic factor, as is the case with gastrectomized patients. In the bloodstream, vitamin B$_{12}$ is transported in combination with three serum proteins called transcobalamins. Transcobalamin II is best known: it is responsible for transporting cobalamin across cell membranes. Transcobalamin II is a protein with a molecular weight of 38,000. Transcobalamins are also found in the gastrointestinal tract, though their precise role in vitamin B$_{12}$ absorption, if any, is unknown.

6.2.4 Folic Acid

Folate in the human organism is converted to tetrahydrofolate (THF or FH$_4$) by a reductive process. The reduction reaction is a stepwise one: folate to dihydrofolate, then to THF. A single enzyme, dihydrofolate reductase, catalyzes both steps. The reaction is inhibited by folate analogues and the antitumor agents methotrexate and aminopterin (Figure 6.3). Because THF is required for DNA biosynthesis (Chapter 10) and tumors have a very high level of DNA biosynthetic activity, even modest decreases in THF availability will inhibit tumor growth.

Many microorganisms do not require folate for growth. They can make their own folate as long as another growth factor, para-aminobenzoic acid, is present in the growth medium. One can observe this compound in the folate structure in Table 6.1. The growth of such organisms, which are often pathogens, can be inhibited by para-aminobenzoic acid analogues called sulfa drugs. One of the first sulfa drugs was the dye prontosil, which in vivo produces sulfanilamide, an analogue of para-aminobenzoic acid, as shown in Figure 6.4.

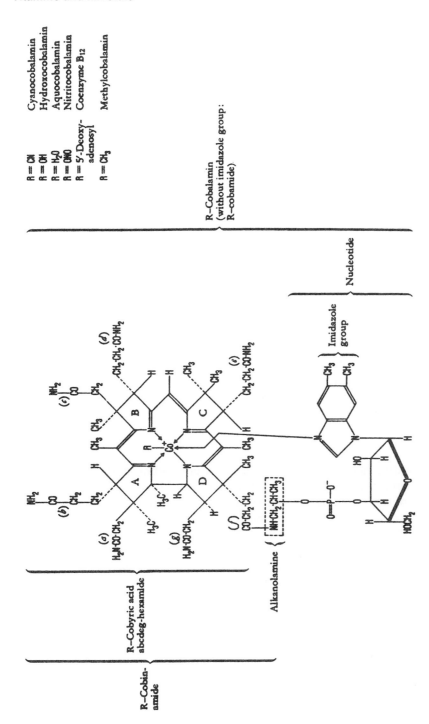

Figure 6.2 Forms of vitamin B_{12} and its derivatives. The central ring structure is called the corrin ring. The R group is usually associated with CN^- in the vitamin, but other groups are also found. (Reproduced by permission from Diem K, Leutner C. Scientific Tables. Basel: Ciba-Geigy, 1971, p. 482.)

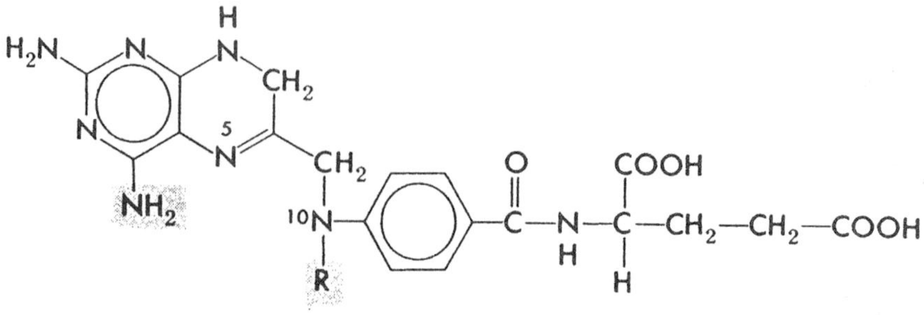

Structures of aminopterin (R=H)
and amethopterin (R=CH$_3$)

Figure 6.3 Antitumor agents methotrexate (amethopterin) and aminopterin. They inhibit dihydrofolate reductase competitively.

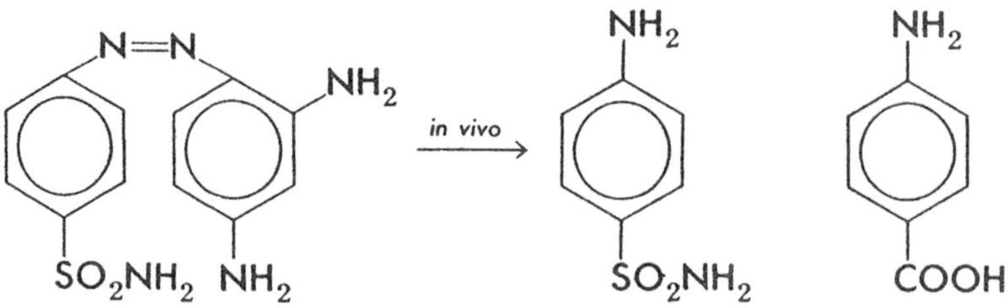

Prontosil   Sulfanilamide   PABA

Figure 6.4 Structure of prontosil and sulfanilamide. PABA is para-aminobenzoic acid.

Sulfa drugs are effective in many infections, especially those involving the genitourinary tract.

Tetrahydrofolate functions as a carrier of one-carbon units. There are numerous metabolic reactions that require either the addition or removal of a one-carbon unit of some specific oxidation state. THF binds one-carbon units of three oxidation levels: the methanol, formaldehyde, and formate states. These are shown in Table 6.4 along with their origins and uses. The various one-carbon units are interconvertible, as shown in Figure 6.5. Nicotinamide coenzymes are involved. In addition, the one-carbon unit may be released as CO_2. The methanol-level THF-bound one-carbon unit 5-methyl-THF is the storage and transport form. Once formed, its main pathway of metabolism is to form methionine from homocysteine, a reaction that requires vitamin B_{12} in the form of methylcobalamin (see Figure 6.2 and Chapter 20):

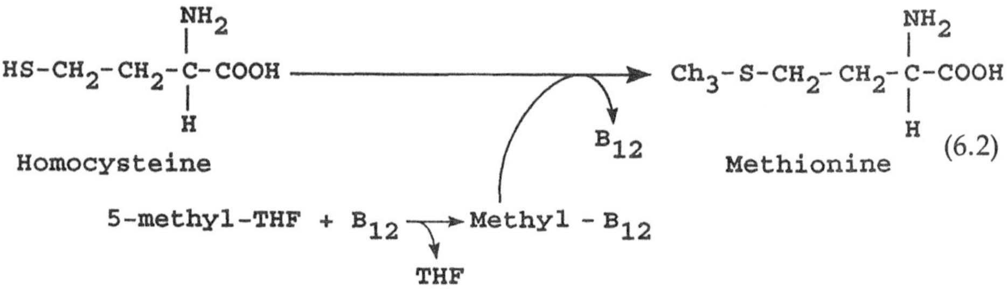

Table 6.4 One-Carbon Tetrahydrofolic Acid Complexes[a]

Oxidation level	Structure	Source	Used in the biosynthesis of:
Methanol	 N_5-methyl-FH$_4$	5,10-Methylene-FH$_4$. This is also the storage and circulatory form of folic acid	Methionine from homocysteine
Formaldehyde	 5,10-methylene-FH$_4$	Glycine, sarcosine, dimethyl-glycine, serine, formaldehyde, N_5-methyl-FH$_4$, 5,10-methenyl-FH$_4$	Serine, thymine
Formate	 N_{10}-formyl-FH$_4$	Formate, N_5-formyl-FH$_4$, 5,10- methenyl-FH$_4$	Purines, formyl methionine-tRNA, CO$_2$
	 5,10-methenyl-FH$_4$	5,10-Methylene-FH$_4$, formimino-FH$_4$	Purines
	 N_5-formyl-FH$_4$	N_{10}-Formyl-FH$_4$, formyl glutamate	
	 N_5-formimino-FH$_4$	Histidine, 5,10-methenyl-FH$_4$	Histidine

[a]Tetrahydrofolic acid is designated by FH$_4$; only the region of the one-carbon unit attachment, which involves nitrogens 5 and 10 of the FH$_4$ molecule, is shown.

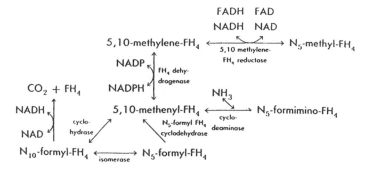

Figure 6.5 Interconversions among various forms of tetrahydrofolate-bound one-carbon units. FH$_4$ designates tetrahydrofolate.

In vitamin B$_{12}$ deficiency, a functional folate deficiency is observed because folate is "trapped" in the form of 5-methyl-THF. Both folate and vitamin B$_{12}$ deficiencies result in megaloblastic anemia. Actual folate deficiency is often observed in alcoholics and pregnant women.

6.2.5 Ascorbic Acid

Ascorbic acid is a vitamin in primates. In most other animals, it can be synthesized by a branch of the glucoronic acid pathway (Chapter 18). It is apparently not changed into any coenzyme in the human being and participates as a vitamin in a reducing capacity in several biochemical reactions. These include the posttranslational hydroxylation of proline in collagen biosynthesis (Chapter 8) and in tyrosine metabolism (Chapter 20). Ascorbic acid is oxidized to dehydroascorbic acid, a diketo derivative of ascorbate. *Scurvy* is a deficiency disease caused by a shortage of dietary ascorbic acid. In children, this results in defective bone formation; in adults, extensive bleeding occurs in a number of locations. Scurvy is to be suspected if serum ascorbic acid levels fall below 1 μg/mL.

6.3 FAT-SOLUBLE VITAMINS

6.3.1 Fat-Soluble Vitamin Transport

Fat-soluble vitamins, A, D, E, and K, or their precursors (provitamins) are absorbed into the intestinal mucosal cells along with other dietary lipids or their digestion products. Thus, any aberrations in lipid absorption also affect the absorption of fat-soluble vitamins. In the intestinal mucosal cells, fat-soluble vitamins are incorporated into a lipoprotein particle called the *chylomicron*. This lipoprotein consists largely of diet-derived triglyceride, though it also contains protein and other lipids (Chapter 19). Chylomicrons travel via the lymphatic system to the systemic circulation and thence to adipose and other tissues, where their triglycerides are removed through the action of lipoprotein lipase. What remains of the chylomicrons are the chylomicron remnants, which, along with their fat-soluble vitamins, are cleared by the liver.

The liver distributes fat-soluble vitamins or their precursors throughout the organism. Whereas vitamins A and D are transported away from the liver in combination with their specific binding proteins, vitamins E and K leave the liver in combination with another lipoprotein, very low density lipoprotein (VLDL). It too loses its triglyceride in various tissues by the action of lipoprotein lipase. The triglyceride-depleted VLDL, following additional modifications such as acquisition of cholesterol, is known as low-density lipoprotein (LDL). Some 50% of LDL is cleared by the liver, but the other 50% is internalized by other tissues, thus providing such tissues with vitamins E and K.

The avidity of VLDL and LDL for vitamins E and K is very high. In fact, in persons with very high blood VLDL or LDL levels, these vitamins may move from the tissues to the bloodstream. Vitamin E deficiency has been observed in children with hereditary hypercholesterolemia (very high blood LDL levels).

6.3.2 Vitamin A

The main dietary precursors of vitamin A-type compounds are the carotenes, chiefly β-carotene. Compounds derived from this isoprenoid substance (Table 6.2) are involved in the visual process, maintenance of epithelial cell integrity, and even protection against neoplasms. Vitamin A-related compounds may be toxic if ingested in excessive amounts.

In the intestinal mucosal cells, β-carotene is cleaved via an *oxygenase* (an enzyme that introduces molecular O_2 into organic compounds) to *trans*-retinal (aldehyde form of *trans*-retinol, as shown in Table 6.2), which in turn is reduced to *trans*-retinol, vitamin A_1. Retinol is then esterified with a fatty acid, becomes incorporated into chylomicrons, and eventually enters the liver, where it is stored in the ester form until it is required elsewhere in the organism. The ester is then hydrolyzed, and vitamin A_1 is transported to its target tissue bound to retinol-binding protein (RBP). Since RBP has a molecular weight of only 20,000 and would be easily cleared by the kidneys, it is associated in the bloodstream with another plasma protein, prealbumin.

Figure 6.6 indicates the various reactions typical of vitamin A_1. Retinoic acid, oxidized *trans*-retinal, is apparently involved in epithelial cell physiology. Retinol phosphate, *trans*-retinol esterified with a phosphate residue, associates with various membrane structures through its hydrophobic isoprenoid residue, leaving its hydrophilic phosphate group in contact with the aqueous environment. It serves as an anchor for growing oligosaccharide chains in the same manner as dolichol phosphate does (see Chapter 18).

The most thoroughly studied area of vitamin A physiology is its role in the visual process. In the retina, vitamin A_1 is oxidized to *trans*-retinal, which then isomerizes to *cis*-retinal (see Figure 6.6). The latter, in the rod cells, combines with the membrane protein opsin to form rhodopsin (visual purple). In the cone cells, opsin is somewhat different, and the rhodopsin equivalent there is iodopsin. The combination of opsin and *cis*-retinal involves the formation of a Schiff base and a polar interaction that stabilizes *cis*-rhodopsin. When light strikes the latter, it is converted through a series of rather unstable intermediates back to *trans*-retinal and opsin (bleached rhodopsin). Such intermediates are designated by the term activated rhodopsin in Figures 6.6 and 6.7, their instability being due to a charge separation phenomenon.

The "activated rhodopsin," shown in Figure 6.6, is what generates the visual impulse. This rather complex process is illustrated in Figure 6.7 and in-

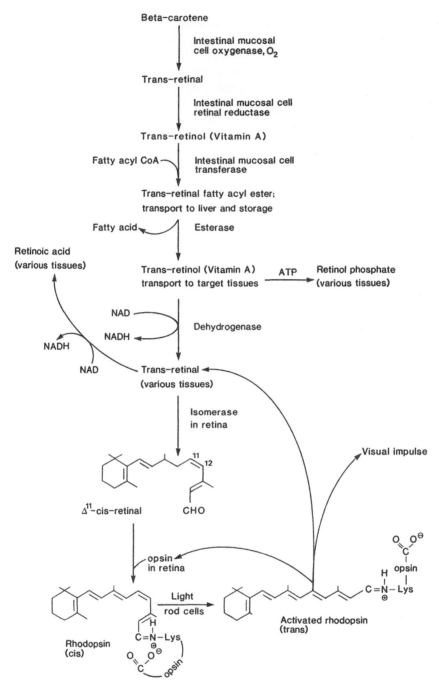

Figure 6.6 Biosynthesis of various vitamin A derivatives from β-carotene and their role in human physiology.

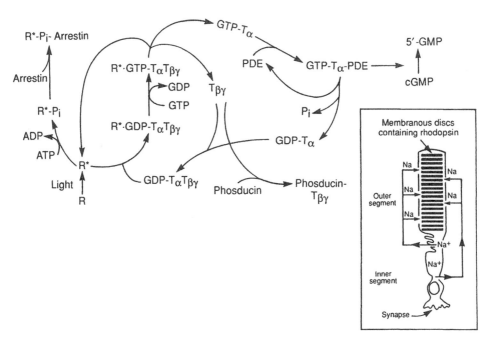

Figure 6.7 The rhodopsin–transducin cascade resulting in cGMP hydrolysis. R is rhodopsin; R* is "activated rhodopsin"; $T_{\beta\gamma}$ is the transducin $\beta\gamma$-subunit complex; T_{α} is the transducin α subunit. Inset: A rod cell showing entry of Na^+ ions into the outer segment of the cell through cGMP-sensitive channels and existing from the inner segment via an ATPase pump. (Based, in part, on Lolley RN, Lee RH. Cyclic GMP and photoreceptor function. FASEB J 4:3001–3008, 1990, and partly on Zurer PS. Chemistry of vision. Chem Eng News November, 1983, p. 34.)

volves the participation of the G-type protein called transducin. A G-type protein functions by binding GTP or GDP, thus activating certain enzymes or metabolic events. G-proteins are also involved in the second messenger phenomenon (Chapter 16). Transducin consists of three subunits, α, β, and γ, and binds GDP. It interacts with activated rhodopsin, GDP is replaced by GTP, and the whole complex dissociates into activated rhodopsin, the $\beta\gamma$ ($T_{\beta\gamma}$) complex, and the α-subunit–GTP complex (GTP–T_{α}).

GTP–T_{α} activates a phosphodiesterase (PDE) whose job it is to hydrolyze cyclic guanosine monophosphate (cGMP), a guanosine phosphate in which the phosphate group is esterified to the –OH groups of both positions 3' and 5' of the ribose residue. The product of this reaction is guanosine-5'-phosphate (GMP) (Chapter 10). It is said that one photon can result in the hydrolysis of as many as 100,000 cGMP molecules. Thus, the transducin-based cascade has an extraordinarily high amplifying power. The GTP–T_{α}–PDE complex is readily dissociated through GTP hydrolysis to GDP and P_i, resulting in an inactivation of PDE. The T_{α}–GDP complex may then combine with $T_{\beta\gamma}$ to form the transducin–GDP complex, thus completing the cycle.

The rod cells consist of outer and inner segments (Figure 6.7). The rhodopsin is bound to membranous disks located in the outer segments. These disks also contain channels that admit Na^+ ions into the cell. The Na^+ is then pumped out of the cell by an ATPase located in the inner segment of the cell. This movement of sodium ions is called the *dark current*, because it takes place in the absence of light. The sodium ion channels are maintained in the open position by cGMP. When light strikes the rhodopsin and the cascade described above is set in motion, the cGMP is hydrolyzed by the activated PDE, the channels are closed, and the dark current ceases. This leads to a polarization of the cell membrane and generation of an electric current resulting in a visual impulse.

Limitation (quenching) of the effects of light becomes a serious consideration in view of the extraordinary efficiency of the transducin cascade. Though little is known about such quenching mechanisms, two proteins have been recognized as being involved in this process. Phosducin is known to combine with $T_{\beta\gamma}$, the result of which is a limited regeneration of transducin–GDP from GDP–T_α and $T_{\beta\gamma}$. Arrestin is known to combine with a phosphorylated form of activated rhodopsin, thus making the latter unavailable for combination with transducin–GDP. A specific protein kinase is known to phosphorylate activated rhodopsin. In both cases, the result is the lowering of cGMP hydrolysis, limiting the closure of the Na^+ channels and dampening of the magnitude of the visual impulse.

6.3.3 Vitamin D

Vitamin D-active substances are required in the diets of growing children and pregnant women, but normal adults receiving sufficient doses of sunshine can manufacture sufficient amounts of these compounds to meet their needs. Active vitamin D compounds can by synthesized in such individuals from 7-dehydro-cholesterol (see Table 6.2), an intermediate in cholesterol biosynthesis. Dietary sources also include cholecalciferol, which is produced from 7-dehydrocholesterol and ergosterol (Table 6.2). 7-Dehydrocholesterol and ergosterol are often referred to as *provitamins*.

Biologically active forms of vitamin D are derived from their provitamins as shown in Figure 6.8. It is seen that the provitamins are changed by sunlight to either vitamin D_3 or vitamin D_2. This occurs in the skin. Vitamin D_3 is then picked up by the vitamin D-binding protein of serum and carried to the liver, where it is hydroxylated by an endoplasmic reticulum hydroxylase (a form of oxygenase) to 25-hydroxycholecalciferol. The latter enters the bloodstream (it is the most common circulating vitamin D-like compound), from which it is extracted principally by the kidney and hydroxylated at position 1 or 24. In the former case, 1,25-dihydroxycholecalciferol is the active form of vitamin D. It is often referred to as a hormone. 24,25-Dihydroxycholecalciferol is inactive. Both the 1- and 24-hydroxylases are mitochondrial enzymes that use molecular oxygen. When cellular levels of 1,25-dihydroxycholecalciferol are high, the 1-hydroxylase is inhibited and the 24-hydroxylase is stimulated. The reverse occurs when cellular levels of 1,25-dihydroxycholecalciferol are low. This is an example of the feedback inhibitory phenomenon.

1,25-Dihydroxycholecalciferol acts primarily on three tissues: bone, kidney, and intestine. The effect is to increase blood calcium levels. Thus, Ca^{2+} (and phosphate) are mobilized from bone through the action of 1,25-dihydroxycholecalciferol, Ca^{2+} reabsorption by the kidney is increased, and the intestinal

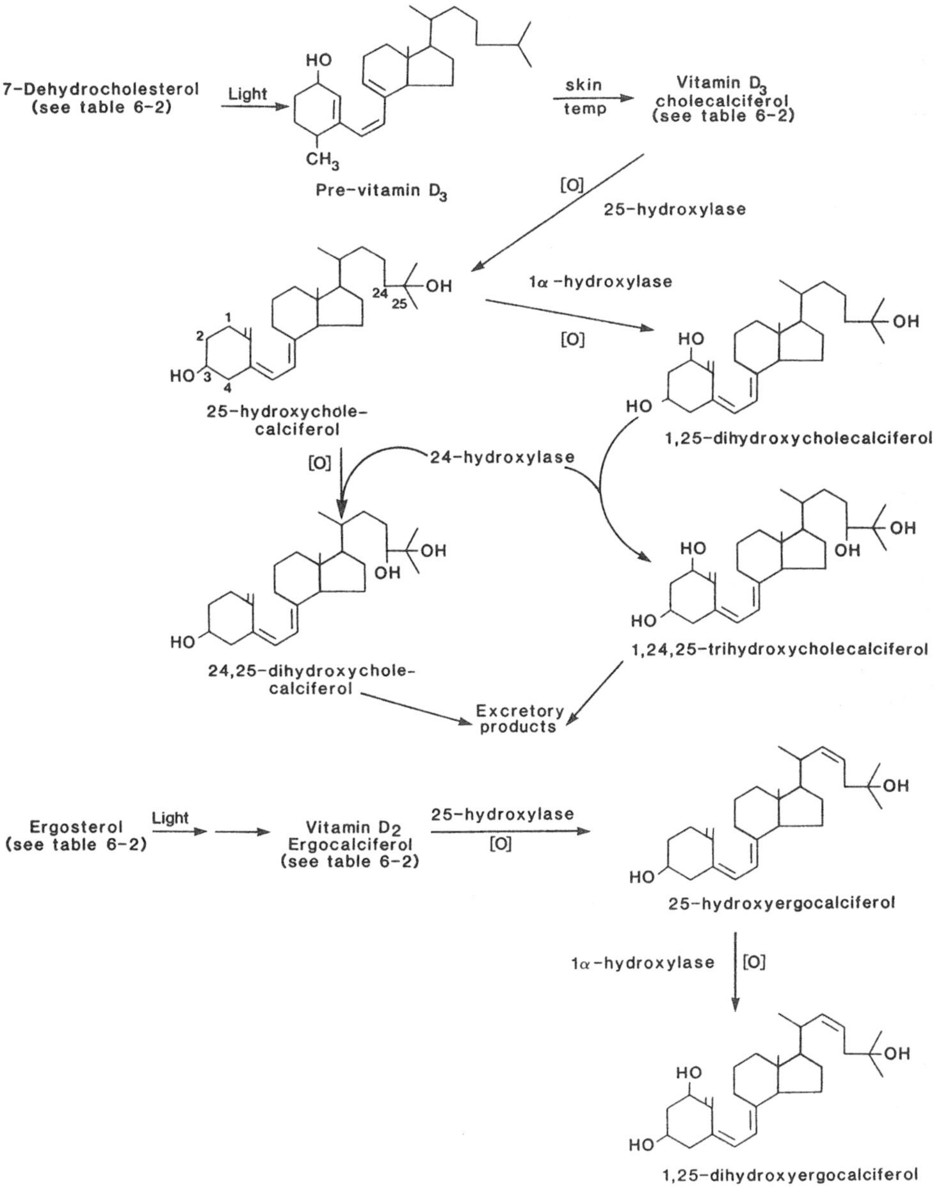

Figure 6.8 Biosynthesis of biologically active vitamin D compounds from their pro-vitamin precursors.

mucosal cells increase the production of a calcium-binding protein (MW 8800 in the rat), which facilitates the transcellular movement of calcium in the intestine. Serum Ca^{2+} levels have an influence on the biosynthesis of 1,25-dihydroxy-cholecalciferol, though it is not clear if the effect is a direct one. It is known that low serum Ca^{2+} levels will induce the secretion of parathyroid hormone (para-thormone), which increases the 1-hydroxylase activity and decreases the 24-

hydroxylase activity. Low phosphate levels are also known to increase the 1-hydroxylase activity.

Parathormone is produced in the parathyroid glands. It is synthesized as a prohormone, which is converted to the active 84-amino acid protein (MW 9500). It has a direct effect on those bone cells that destroy (resorb) bone. It also has a direct effect on kidney tubules, increasing Ca^{2+} reabsorption but also increasing the excretion of phosphate. In hypocalcemic situations, the Ca^{2+}/P_i ratio is initially lower than normal, and parathormone thus serves to restore the balance. In rickets, a disease brought about by a simple dietary vitamin D deficiency, parathormone levels are high, which results in bone resorption and the typical bone lesions seen in these patients. The peptide hormone calcitonin is produced by the thyroid gland when serum Ca^{2+} levels are high. It decreases bone resorption and thus tends to lower serum Ca^{2+} levels. Both parathormone and calcitonin increase cAMP levels in their target tissues.

6.3.4   Vitamin K

Compounds with vitamin K activity (Table 6.2) are required in our diets for γ-carboxyglutamate biosynthesis (Table 4.1). This amino acid is produced from certain protein glutamyl residues by carboxylation. Proteins that contain γ-carboxyglutamate are blood prothrombin and coagulation factors VII, IX, and X (see Chapter 7). Other proteins of this type are osteocalcin from bone and several kidney and muscle calcium-binding proteins.

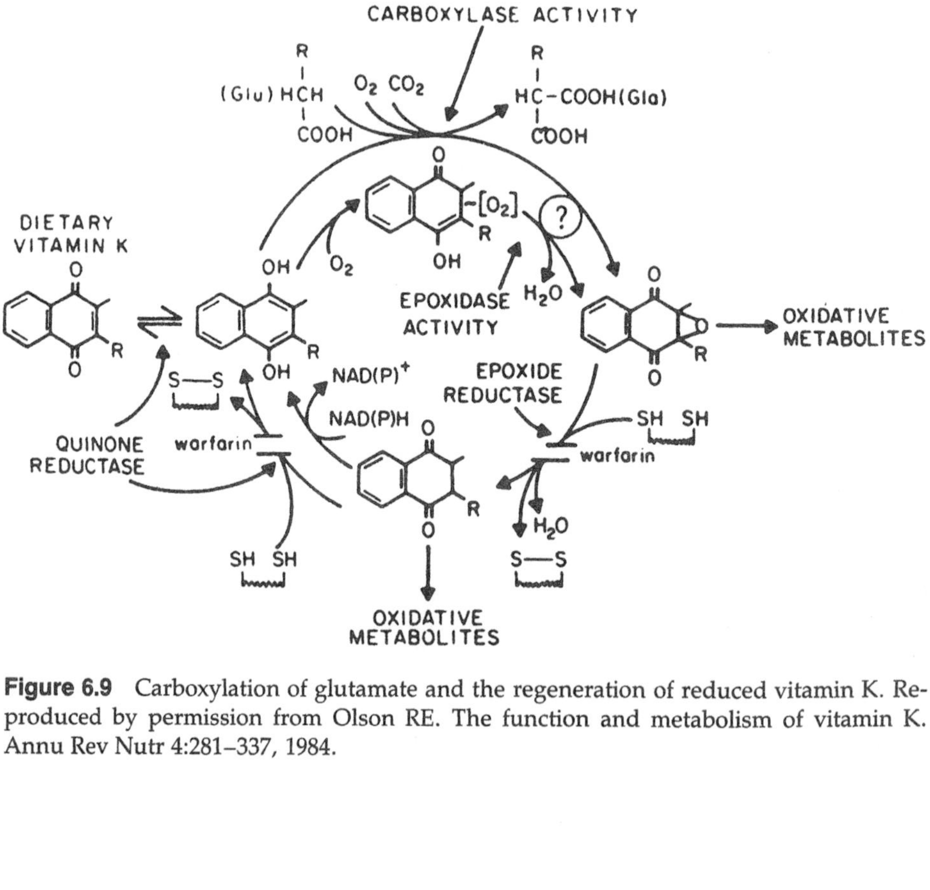

Figure 6.9   Carboxylation of glutamate and the regeneration of reduced vitamin K. Reproduced by permission from Olson RE. The function and metabolism of vitamin K. Annu Rev Nutr 4:281–337, 1984.

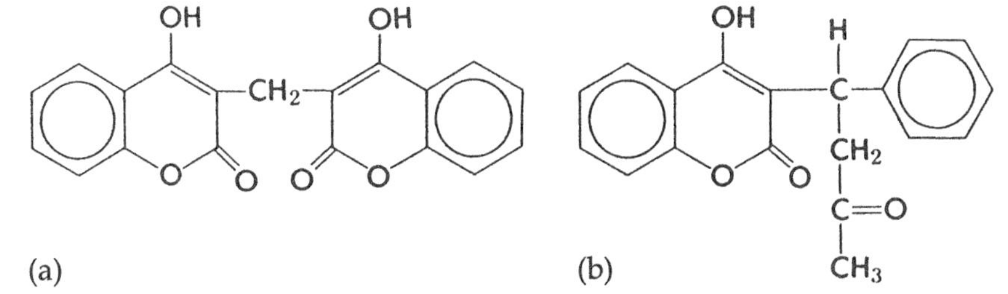

Figure 6.10 Structures of (a) dicoumarin and (b) warfarin, antagonists of vitamin K.

The carboxylation reaction is catalyzed by γ-glutamylcarboxylase, whose substrates are peptide-bound glutamate, O_2, CO_2, and reduced (hydroquinone form) vitamin K. The mechanism of action most likely involves activation of the γ-methylene residue of glutamate to a carbanion, which then interacts with the CO_2. Vitamin K is oxidized in the process and is then reconverted to the hydroquinone form via an epoxide intermediate with the participation of NADPH, sulfhydryl groups, and various enzymes. These reactions are summarized in Figure 6.9.

Deficiency of vitamin K increases the time for blood coagulation. In the laboratory, a vitamin K-deficient blood sample shows an increased prothrombin time. Vitamin K deficiency can also be generated by its antagonists such as dicoumarin or warfarin (Figure 6.10). Dicoumarin was first isolated from spoiled clover that was causing a hemorrhagic disease in cattle. Warfarin is a synthetic compound that is used as rat poison. Derivative of these compounds, for example, 4-hydroxycoumarin are used as anticoagulants in human beings. These compounds act by blocking the reduction of oxidized vitamin K as shown in Figure 6.9.

6.4 METAL COFACTORS

Like coenzymes, metals often serve as prosthetic groups or cofactors in various enzyme reactions and are therefore required in our diets. Sodium and potassium are found in greatest abundance in the human organism. Na^+ is the principal cation in extracellular fluids, whereas K^+ is the principal intercellular cation. Though these metals are extremely important in cell physiology, muscle physicology, transmission of biological messages, and other biological phenomena, they are not commonly found in enzyme reactions as prosthetic groups. Iron is a very important dietary component because it is required for oxygen transport and a number of enzyme reactions. Its biochemistry will be discussed in Chapter 7. Table 6.5 lists other biologically important metals with their dietary requirements and biological functions. The latter may include redox or electron relay functions or the chelation of nucleophilic substrates during the enzymatic transmutation.

Several metals, for example Cu, Zn, and Mn, are associated with a group of enzymes called superoxide dismutases. These enzymes scavenge the superoxide anion, O_2^-, which may be a by-product of various redox reactions or the electron transport system (Chapter 17). The superoxide anion gives rise to the very de-

Table 6.5 Essential Metals in the Human Being

Metal	Ionic form	Daily requirement	Some enzyme(s) in which the metal is found	Notes
Zn	Zn^{2+}	16 mg	Over 200; e.g., carbonic anhydrase, carboxypeptidases	Sickle cell anemia causes a Zn deficiency
Cu	Cu^+, Cu^{2+}	2 mg	Cytochrome c oxidase, tyrosinase, lysyl oxidase, superoxide dismutases	Cu deficiency has been associated with atherosclerosis in animals
Se	—	50–200 μg	Glutathione peroxidase	Associated with vitamin E metabolism; may be considered to be a nonmetal
Cr	Cr^{3+}	50–200 μg	Glucose tolerance factor (GTF)	Deficiency causes a diabetes-like syndrome, esp. in the elderly
Mn	Mn^{2+}, Mn^{3+}	2.5–5 mg	Superoxide dismutase	Can replace Mg^{2+} in many reactions
Mg	Mg^{2+}	300–400 mg	Most ATP-requiring enzyme reactions	—
Mo	—	0.15–0.5 mg	Xanthine dehydrogenase, sulfite, aldehyde oxidases	Mo seems to be always bound to a cofactor—a compound containing a pterin ring
Ca	Ca^{2+}	800 mg	Coagulation factors, e.g., prothrombin	Important second messenger in hormone action and the visual process
Fe	Fe^{2+}, Fe^{3+}	1–2 mg	Proline hydroxylase, diphosphoribonucleoside dehydrogenase, peroxidases	Component of hemoglobin and all other heme proteins; component of iron-sulfur proteins (ferredoxins)

structive ·OH radical, so it is only prudent to have a system in place for its removal. Superoxide dismutases convert O_2^- to H_2O_2 as follows:

$$2\,O_2^- + 2\,H^+ \rightarrow H_2O_2 + O_2 \tag{6.3}$$

Hydrogen peroxide is degraded by a group of enzymes called peroxidases, which are located in the peroxisome subcellular particles. There may be various electron acceptors involved, such as glutathione, designated as G below:

$$H_2O_2 + 2\,G\text{–SH} \xrightarrow{\text{Glutathione peroxidase}} G\text{–S–S–G} + 2\,H_2O \tag{6.4}$$

Glutathione peroxidase is a selenium-containing enzyme. A special form of peroxidase is catalse, an enzyme with one of the highest known turnover numbers (vicinity of 44,000 H_2O_2 molecules per molecule of catalase per second), which uses H_2O_2 as both an oxidizing and reducing agent:

$$2 H_2O_2 \xrightarrow{\text{Catalase}} 2 H_2O + O_2 \tag{6.5}$$

The above reactions may be considered to be detoxification reactions that permit various life forms to survive in an oxygen atmosphere. Strictly anaerobic microorganisms lack superoxide dismutases and cannot survive long in air. To them, oxygen is toxic.

Nutritional metal deficiencies, except for iron, are relatively uncommon in the United States. Deficiencies are more often brought about by various pathological conditions, iatrogenically (e.g., as a result of total parenteral nutrition), or by unwholesome habits. For instance, geophagia, the eating of clay, will elicit a severe Zn deficiency. Alcoholism will result in Mg deficiency. A genetic absorption defect, acrodermatitis enteropathica, is observed most often in bottle-fed infants. This syndrome does not develop in breast-fed infants. It may be treated with megadoses of $ZnSO_4$. Another genetic disease, Menke's syndrome, results in severe Cu deficiency in many organs. Copper absorption, excretion, storage, and transport are all abnormal in patients with this condition. Deficiencies of Zn and other metals (especial Ca) may also develop if the diet contains excessive amounts of fiber and phytate (hexaphosphoinositol). Such substances lower the bioavailability of metals. A serious condition that may be accompanied by metal deficiencies (because of lowered absorption) is inflammatory bowel disease, which includes ulcerative colitis and Crohn's disease. The absorption of Zn and Mg is especially affected. Metals may also interfere with the absorption of other metals. Thus, dietary Zn supplementation is known to significantly lower the absorption of Cu and may elicit Cu deficiency symptoms.

Metal deficiency symptoms are usually multifaceted. Zinc deficiency results in stunted growth, interference with wound healing, hypogonadism, loss of taste and smell acuities, and skin lesions. Diagnosis can be made by analyzing serum Zn levels or by measuring serum alkaline phosphatase, which is a Zn enzyme that is severely depressed in Zn deficiency. Selenium deficiency is associated with increased cancer risks in some areas. Copper deficiency is associated with anemia, neutropenia, failure to form disulfide bonds in hair keratin, and depigmentation, because the synthesis of melanin (hair, skin, and eye pigment) depends upon the copper-containing enzyme tyrosinase (Chapter 20). Magnesium deficiency results in hypocalcemia and hypokalemia (mechanism unknown), tetany, and convulsions.

Transport and storage of metals are still not completely understood. It is believed that Cu is transported from the intestinal tract to the liver bound to serum albumin, though its entry into hepatocytes occurs via Cu–histidine complexes. From the liver, Cu is exported by the serum protein ceruloplasmin. Ceruloplasmin also has monoamine oxidase and ferroxidase activities (Chapter 7). Copper deficiency can be detected by measuring serum ceruloplasmin, as 80–90% of the Cu in peripheral blood is bound to this protein. Recent evidence has indicated that factor V (proaccelerin) of the coagulation cascade (Chapter 7) is ceruloplasmin or a similar protein. Zinc is apparently transported throughout the organism bound to serum albumin, though a small amount is also bound to α-2-macroglobulin.

Wilson's disease is a copper storage disorder that is apparently due to an inherited lesion in the copper excretion mechanism. One in 200–400 persons is a carrier of the disease. Diagnosis may be made by measuring serum ceruloplasmin levels. Whereas normal serum ceruloplasmin is 200–400 mg/L, in Wilson's disease patients it is well below 200 mg/L. Liver copper in these patients (determined by biopsy) is more than 250 μg/g, whereas normal individuals show a value of only 20–45 μg/g. Liver function deterioration is the most prominent symptom of Wilson's disease. Treatment includes chelation therapy with penicillamine.

Both Zn and Cu are stored in tissues bound to a small protein called metallothionein (MW 7000). This protein contains 61 amino acids, of which 20 are cysteine residues. The –SH groups serve as excellent metal binders. Metallothionein binds Cu most avidly, but it is the Zn that has the greatest influence on its biosynthesis. It is argued that the reason excessive amounts of dietary Zn can inhibit Cu absorption is that Cu becomes "trapped" by the intestinal mucosal cell metallothionein, which is present in increased quantities because of the Zn. The trapped Cu remains in the intestinal mucosal cells until it is lost in the feces through the normal process of mucosal cell exfoliation.

Two metals, both apparently essential, act in the human being in conjunction with organic cofactors. These metals are chromium and molybdenum. A deficiency of Cr produces an abnormal glucose tolerance curve resembling that of insulin-dependent diabetes. It is believed that Cr somehow helps insulin to interact with its cellular receptors. The nature of the organic Cr mediator, the glucose tolerance factor (GTF), has not been completely elucidated. It was first detected in the 1960s by Mertz and associates, and recent evidence indicates that it may be a peptide with a molecular weight of 1500 containing Asp, Glu, Gly, and Cys in a 5:4:2:1 ratio.

Molybdenum is a component of at least three enzymes: aldehyde oxidase, xanthine dehydrogenase, and sulfite oxidase. The first two contain FAD, whereas the last is a heme protein similar to cytochrome c. Xanthine dehydrogenase can also act as an oxidase, that is, it can use O_2 as an electron acceptor. Physiologically, however, it uses NAD^+ as an electron acceptor when it converts hypoxanthine to xanthine and the latter to uric acid (see Chapter 10). Aldehyde and sulfite oxidases are true oxidases physiologically; they both use O_2 as an electron acceptor. Molybdenum in all three enzymes is associated with a pterin-like cofactor whose structure is shown in Figure 6.11. The Mo cofactor cannot be

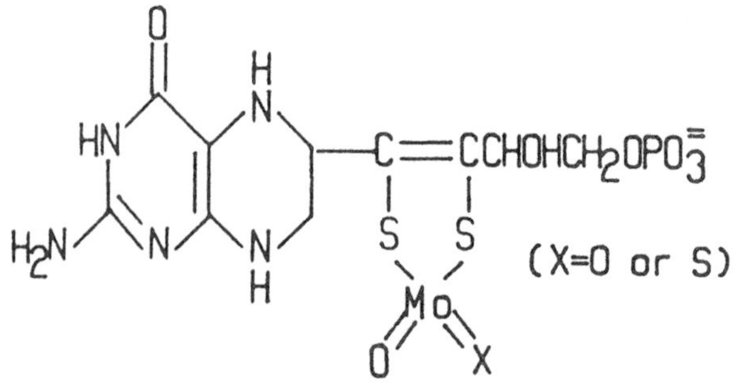

Figure 6.11 Structure of the pterin cofactor, which binds molybdenum in aldehyde oxidase, xanthine oxidase, and sulfite oxidase. [Reproduced by permission from Rajagopalan, KV. Molybdenum, an essential trace element. *Nutr. Rev.*, 45:321–328 (1987).]

synthesized in newborns with a pertinent genetic lesion. Such infants show severe neurologic pathologies, and the activities of their sulfite oxidase and xanthine dehydrogenase are nil.

QUESTIONS

Certain types of reactions that are necessary to convert vitamins to their respective coenzymes are listed below (a–e). In Questions 6.1–6.4, match the vitamin with its corresponding reaction.

    a. Reduction
    b. Phosphorylation only
    c. Hydroxylation
    d. Oxidation and phosphorylation
    e. Reaction with an adenine-containing nucleotide

6.1.   Thiamine
6.2.   Pantothenic acid
6.3.   Riboflavin
6.4.   Pyridoxine
6.5.   Which is not true of dihydrofolate reductase?
    a. Uses folate as a substrate
    b. Uses dihydrofolate as a substrate
    c. Activates folate to tetrahydrofolate coenzyme
    d. Is inhibited by methotrexate
    e. Attaches reduced one-carbon units to tetrahydrofolate
6.6.   Each NADH is capable of generating three ATP molecules. How many ATP molecules can be generated when 5-methyltetrahydrofolate is converted to tetrahydrofolate and CO_2?
    a. 0   c. 6   e. 12
    b. 3   d. 9
6.7.   In the visual impulse, all of the following take place *except*
    a. Transducin activates a phosphodiesterase.
    b. Sodium current is initiated in the rod cell.
    c. Calcium ions are released from intracellular storage.
    d. Cyclic GMP is hydrolyzed.
    e. The light "bleaches" rhodopsin.
6.8.   Low serum calcium levels will result in
    a. Activation of 25-hydroxycholecalciferol-24-hydroxylase
    b. Activation of 25-hydroxycholecalciferol-1-hydroxylase
    c. Increase in serum calcitonin levels
    d. Decrease in reabsorption of phosphate by the kidney tubules
    e. Lowering of serum parathormone levels
6.9.   Which of the following can alleviate rickets?
    a. Administration of   c. Eating green vegetables
        24,25-dihydroxycholecalciferol   d. Sunshine
    b. Administration of fish oil   e. Two of the above

For Questions 6.10–6.12, use the following code:
    a. Biotin   c. Both
    b. Vitamin K   d. Neither

6.10. Mode of action involves O_2
6.11. Participate(s) in carboxylation reactions
6.12. Present in large quantity in egg white

For Questions 6.13–6.15, use the following code:
> a. NAD   c. Both
> b. FAD   d. Neither

6.13. Accept(s) two electrons
6.14. Accept(s) one hydrogen atom
6.15. Accept(s) two hydrogen atoms

For Questions 6.16–6.18, use the following code:
> a. Vitamin A   c. Both
> b. Vitamin D   d. Neither

6.16. Liver plays an important role in metabolism.
6.17. Target tissue for active form(s) is intestine.
6.18. Kidney plays an important role in metabolism.

In Questions 6.19–6.23, use the following key:
> a. 1, 2, and 3 are correct.
> b. 1 and 3 are correct.
> c. 2 and 4 are correct.
> d. 4 only is correct.
> e. All are correct.

6.19. Absorption of vitamin B_{12}
> 1. Takes place in the stomach
> 2. Is drastically decreased in patients with gastrectomy
> 3. Does not take place unless the vitamin is in the oxidized state
> 4. Does not take place unless bound to a glycoprotein produced by stomach cells

6.20. Zinc deficiency
> 1. May be caused by prolonged parenteral nutrition
> 2. May be present in cases of ulcerative colitis
> 3. May result in skin lesions
> 4. May be detected by measuring serum alkaline phosphatase

6.21. Copper deficiency
> 1. May be detected by measuring serum ceruloplasmin
> 2. May be elicited by excessive intake of zinc
> 3. Is present in Menke's syndrome
> 4. May be caused by a decrease in circulating metallothionein

6.22. Superoxide dismutases
> 1. Are metalloenzymes that have Zn, Cu, or Mn as prosthetic groups
> 2. Are localized entirely in peroxisomes
> 3. React to produce hydrogen peroxide
> 4. Are present in all strict anaerobes

6.23. Copper metabolism is associated with
> 1. Geriatric diabetes
> 2. Acrodermatitis enteropathica
> 3. Sickle cell disease
> 4. Wilson's disease

Answers

6.1. (b) Thiamine is phosphorylated to thiamine pyrophosphate.
6.2. (e) Pantothenic acid is activated to coenzyme A using ATP.
6.3. (e) Riboflavin is activated to FAD.
6.4. (d) Pyridoxine is activated to pyridoxal phosphate.

6.5. (e) Dihydrofolate reductase activates folate to tetrahydrofolate with dihydrofolate as an intermediate. Methotrexate, an antitumor agent, inhibits this enzyme.

6.6. (d) The 5-methyl group is first oxidized to the formaldehyde level, then to the formate level, then to CO_2. Three steps require three molecules of NAD or an equivalent, for a total of $3 \times 3 = 9$ ATP molecules.

6.7. (b) In the visual process, the flow of sodium ions (dark current) is interrupted when cGMP is hydrolyzed.

6.8. (b) Low serum Ca^{2+} levels increase parathoromone production, which stimulates the 1-hydroxylase and inhibits the 24-hydroxylase activities.

6.9. (e) Rickets is caused by shortages of vitamin D. Vitamin D may be generated by sunlight striking 7-dehydrocholesterol in the skin, or it may be supplied in fish oil.

6.10. (b) Vitamin K utilizes O_2 and CO_2 when glutamate residues are carboxylated.

6.11. (c) Both biotin and vitamin K are involved in fixation of CO_2.

6.12. (d) Egg white contains avidin, a biotin-binding protein, but little if any vitamin K or biotin.

6.13. (c) Both coenzymes are reduced by accepting two electrons.

6.14. (a) NAD accepts only one hydrogen atom and releases the other as a proton into the medium.

6.15. (b) FAD binds two hydrogen atoms along with two electrons. Under some circumstances, however, it may bind only one hydrogen atom.

6.16. (c) Vitamin A is stored in the liver as a fatty acyl ester; vitamin D is hydroxylated in the liver in the 25-position.

6.17. (b) Target tissue for 1,25-dihydroxycholecalciferol, among others, is the intestine, where a Ca^{2+}-binding protein is synthesized under its influence.

6.18. (b) 25-Hydroxycholecalciferol is hydroxylated in both the 1- and 24-positions in the kidney.

6.19. (c) Absorption of vitamin B_{12} takes place in the small intestine. It must be bound to the intrinsic factor to be absorbed in any quantity.

6.20. (e) All are correct.

6.21. (a) Metallothionein is a metal storage protein, not a circulating protein.

6.22. (b) Superoxide dismutases are present in various subcellular particles, for example mitochondria. Peroxisomes contain peroxidases such as catalase. Superoxide dismutases convert the superoxide anion to H_2O_2 and are absent from anaerobic microorganisms.

6.23. (d) Only Wilson's disease is associated with copper metabolism. Sickle cell anemia and acrodermatitis enteropathica are associated with Zn metabolism, and geriatric diabetes, with Cr deficiency.

PROBLEMS

6.1. A 6-month-old child was breast-fed exclusively by a mother who had been a strict vegetarian for at least 7 years. He was totally unresponsive to stimuli. His hemoglobin was 5.7 g/dL, and his bone marrow aspirates showed megaloblastic changes in blood cells. His serum folate and iron were normal. His urine contained increased amounts of homocystine, methylmalonic acid, and glycine. Propose a reason for this infant's illness, and discuss its biochemical etiology. Discuss other possible reasons for the same or similar symptoms in a patient. Explain the abnormal serum and urine chemistries.

6.2. A 9-month-old boy was breast-fed, then changed to a soymilk, fruit, and vegetable regimen. His parents were strict vegetarians and did not take their son outside too often. He came to the hospital's attention because of a broken femur. X-rays showed that he had another, older femur fracture and, in addition, his legs showed prominent bowing. His serum alkaline phosphatase was highly elevated, whereas phosphorus was below normal and calcium was normal. Propose a reason for this boy being prone to develop fractures of his bones, and give the biochemical etiology of this disorder. Explain the abnormal blood chemistries. Propose a mode of treatment for this child.

6.3. A 27-year-old man developed a bronze hue to his skin, became jaundiced, and showed signs of disorientation. His liver enzymes were grossly elevated. Ceruloplasmin level was a low normal, but he excreted large amounts of copper in his urine. Propose a reason for this patient's illness, and give the biochemical details. Why is there such severe liver damage? What can be done for the patient?

6.4. A 72-year-old man who was living alone and subsisted on soups, milk, and bread presented with muscular weakness, chronic fatigue, a depressed mental state, occasional vomiting of blood, and occult blood in the stool. Gastroscopy showed an extensive lesion in the stomach, and the man was diagnosed as having a gastric tumor. In addition, he was slightly anemic and bruised easily. Gastric resection was scheduled, but when the patient was given vitamin supplements, he immediately showed dramatic improvement. Surgery was canceled, and the gastric lesion disappeared. Propose a reason for this person's illness, and provide a biochemical explanation for his signs and symptoms.

BIBLIOGRAPHY

Danks DM. Copper deficiency in humans. Annu Rev Nutr 8:235–257, 1988.

Hendricks KM. Zinc deficiency in inflammatory bowel diseases. Annu Rev Nutr 46:401–408, 1988.

Henry HL, Norman AW. Vitamin D: metabolism and biologic actions. Annu Rev Nutr 4:493–520, 1984.

Olson RE. The function and metabolism of vitamin K. Annu Rev Nutr 4:281–337, 1984.

Shills ME. Magnesium in health and disease. Annu Rev Nutr 8:429–460, 1988.

7

Proteins with Biological Activity: Blood Proteins

After completing this chapter, the student should

1. Know the general properties of blood: the functions of its cellular elements and the meaning of the terms *plasma, serum, hematocrit, plasma proteins, hemoglobin, coagulation*.
2. Know the general properties of hemoglobin and myoglobin—what heme is and its structure, what the various globin chains consist of, oxidation forms of iron, how the iron molecule is held in hemoglobin, mode of oxygen binding by hemoglobins, binding of charged and uncharged compounds and ions—and the significance of glycosylated hemoglobin.
3. Know what the embryonic and fetal hemoglobins are, their structural and functional peculiarities, and their appearance during the life cycle of the human being.
4. Be able to derive and use the Hill equation and know the meaning of the Hill coefficient P_{50} and the Hill plot.
5. Be able to interpret oxygen saturation curves of various types of hemoglobins by relating such curves to their properties and describe how the release of O_2 is affected.
6. Be able to recite the function of hemoglobin as a buffer and its role in CO_2 disposal.
7. Understand the various models that explain the behavior of hemoglobin as an allosteric O_2 binder.
8. Know the molecular etiology for the various types of abnormal hemoglobins and their O_2-binding peculiarities, including sickle cell hemoglobins.
9. Know the metabolic pathway leading to the biosynthesis of heme: enzymes, intermediates, controls, and the etiology of the various porphyrias.
10. Know the heme degradation pathway leading to bilirubin: intermediates (recognize structures), enzymes, and controls.
11. Know the biochemistry and physiology of bilirubin and urobilinogen, be able to describe their use as diagnostic tools in liver diseases, and recognize the various disorders of bilirubin metabolism.

12. Know the general concepts of iron metabolism: absorption, transport, storage, daily fluxes.
13. Know the function and diagnostic utility of transferrin and ferritin and be able to solve problems involving total iron and total iron binding capacity.
14. Be familiar with, know the function of, and know the diagnostic significance of the following plasma proteins: haptoglobin, hemopexin, albumin, fibrinogen, immunoglobulins, α-1-antitrypsin, and complement.
15. Know the components and the operation of the blood coagulation cascade.
16. Know the utility of total serum protein and A/G ratio determinations and be able to solve problems involving these parameters and the results of serum protein electrophoresis determinations.

7.1 GENERAL PROPERTIES OF BLOOD

The various tissues and organs of the organism are connected with the outside environment as well as with each other, through circulation, and it is through the medium of blood that nutrients are transported to cells and waste products are removed. The general composition of blood remains remarkably constant despite the fact that numerous biochemical substances and cellular elements are constantly leaving and entering it. This steady state is maintained by biochemical and physiologic regulatory processes that result in equal rates of destruction and formation, or output and input, of cellular elements and biochemical substances.

Cells in the higher organism are bathed in interstitial fluid to which waste products are added and from which substances are removed by processes of diffusion. Regulation of the composition of interstitial fluid is achieved by diffusion through the capillary walls to and from the circulating blood. Through these mechanisms, cells are able to maintain their cellular environment within certain limits and are protected temporarily from large external physical and chemical variations.

The primary functions of the blood may be considered in a broad sense to be the following: (1) metabolic regulation—transport of oxygen, carbon dioxide, metabolites, hormones; (2) physical and chemical regulation—temperature, acid–base balance, and osmotic pressure and fluid balance; and (3) regulation of body defenses—protection against infection by the action of antibodies, leukocytes, and other mechanisms and prevention of hemorrhage.

Normal values for total blood volume vary depending on the methods used for its determination and the basis of reference (sex, age, weight, surface area). In a healthy adult or normal body habitus, the circulating blood comprises 6–8% of the body weight, or 63–80 mL/kg. Blood consists of cellular elements suspended in a solution containing a host of proteins and low molecular weight substances. There are three types of cells in blood: the red cells (*erythrocytes*), the white cells (*leukocytes*), and *platelets* (thrombocytes). Only the white cells possess

Table 7.1 Some Normal Serum Constituents

Constituent	Normal range
Serum proteins	6–8 g/100 mL
Glucose (fasting)	70–115 mg/100 mL
Urea nitrogen	8–20 mg/100 mL
Nonprotein nitrogen	18–30 mg/100 mL
Uric acid	3.0–6.5 mg/100 mL (male)
	2.5–5.5 mg/100 mL (female)
Creatinine	0.6–1.1 mg/100 mL
Cholesterol (total)	140–280 mg/100 mL
Cholesterol esters	72–78% of total
Bilirubin (total)	0.3–1.0 mg/100 mL
Bilirubin (conjugated or "direct")	0.1–0.4 mg/100 mL
Sodium	137–148 meq/L
Chloride	98–110 meq/L
Potassium	3.5–5.3 meq/L
Total CO_2	21–29 mmol/L
Calcium	8.7–10.7 mg/100 mL
Phosphorus (inorganic)	2.5–4.8 mg/100 mL (adult)
	4.0–6.5 mg/100 mL (child)
Magnesium	1.6–2.2 meq/L
Lactate	6–16 mg/100 mL

nuclei. The red cells are concerned with the transport of oxygen and carbon dioxide and the buffering capacity of blood. The white cells are concerned with the resistance of the organism against disease and the removal and destruction of certain types of waste and foreign material from the organism. Platelets are concerned with blood coagulation. It is believed that an abnormal triggering of platelet aggregation may initiate myocardial infarction and thrombus formation in peripheral tissues.

When blood clots, a plasma protein called fibrinogen is converted to fibrin, which forms a network of threads. Blood cells become enmeshed in this network and form the clot. The clear fluid formed as the clot retracts is the *serum*. When citrate, heparin, or some other anticoagulant is added to blood to prevent clotting and the cells are removed by centrifugation, the fluid remaining is *plasma*. Plasma differs from serum in that it contains fibrinogen and certain other coagulation factors not contained in serum.

As pointed out above, serum contains a host of components that are present in solution. These are listed in Table 7.1. The quantitative determination of these constituents can provide useful information on the nature and extent of a number of pathologic conditions.

7.2 HEMOGLOBIN

7.2.1 Introduction

One cubic millimeter of human blood contains some 5 million red blood cells. Their principal component is the protein hemoglobin, which accounts for about

32% of the total red blood cell weight and for over 90% of total red blood cell solids. Its broad function is to bind molecular oxygen for transport to tissues (there is 1.34 mL of O_2 bound per gram of hemoglobin) and to act as a buffer and transporter of carbon dioxide and protons. Hemoglobin is frequently quantitated in a clinical hematology laboratory, because its level in the blood often reflects disease processes. Normal hemoglobin levels in adult humans are 16 ± 2 g/100 mL of blood in males and 14 ± 2 g/100 mL in females. Lower values generally indicate the presence of an anemic condition, and higher values generally indicate erythrocytosis, such as is found in the disease polycythemia vera. In this disease, hemoglobin levels may reach 18–24 g/100 mL blood, so the blood becomes extremely viscous.

Other ways of measuring the red cell status of blood include counting the red cells and measuring the hematocrit value. *Hematocrit value* is obtained by centrifuging blood in the presence of an anticoagulant in a graduated capillary tube and determining the fraction of the volume occupied by the red cells. If red cell packing were perfect, the hematocrit would be 30% of the blood volume for males. Since the packing of cells is not complete, normal hematocrit values are usually given as 47% for males and 42% for females.

Individual types of hemoglobin may also be studied in greater detail by methods such as electrophoresis, by observing their propensity to become denatured, and by determining their ability to take up or give up oxygen. These studies are valuable if a patient is suspected of having an abnormal hemoglobin in his or her red cells. Such abnormal forms of hemoglobin may be the cause of severe clinical symptoms.

Hemoglobin is bright red when saturated with oxygen (oxyhemoglobin) and dark red with a purplish tinge when the oxygen is removed (deoxyhemoglobin). Hemoglobin has several absorption maxima, the major band being at about 400 nm. This is also called the Soret absorption band. In the oxygen-saturated form, hemoglobin has additional absorption maxima at 578 nm (also called the α band) and at 540 nm (β band). The α and β bands are replaced by a single band at 555 nm when oxygen is removed from the hemoglobin. Other types of hemoglobins have characteristic absorption bands in the 500–700-nm range, and these have been used as convenient identification criteria. The hemoglobins, like other proteins, will also have absorption maxima in the ultraviolet range of the spectrum. Visible spectra of some hemoglobins are shown in Figure 7.1.

7.2.2 Structure and Composition

The reason hemoglobin is red is that, in addition to its polypeptide portion, globin, it contains the O_2-bonding heme molecules, which have a highly coordinated set of double bonds. Red blood cell hemoglobin has a molecular weight of 64,450. It consists of two α-polypeptide chains with a molecular weight of 15,126 each (141 amino acids) and two β-polypeptide chains with a molecular weight of 15,867 each (146 amino acids). Each polypeptide chain (α or β) binds one heme molecule with a molecular weight of 616. The overall shape of horse hemoglobin is almost spherical with the dimensions $64 \times 55 \times 50$ Å.

Of all hemoglobin-type proteins known, the simplest one from a structural point of view is myoglobin. This sperm whale protein consists of a single

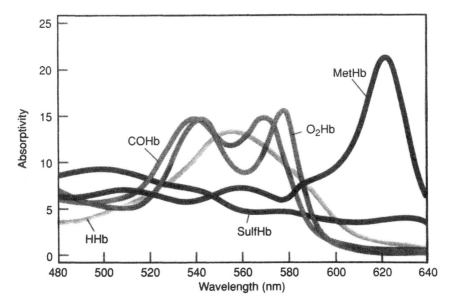

Figure 7.1 Absorption spectra of various hemoglobins in the 480–640 nm range. Met Hb, O₂Hb, COHb, HHb and SulfHb designates methemoglobin, oxygenated hemoglobin, carbon monoxide hemoglobin (carboxyhemoglobin), deoxyhemoglobin and sulfhemoglobin, respectively. (Reproduced with permission from Moran RF, Fallon KD. Oxygen saturation, content and the dyshemoglobins: Part I. Clin Chem News January:11, 1990.)

polypeptide chain with 153 amino acids and a single heme molecule for a total molecular weight of about 18,000. It is quite compact, measuring 44 × 44 × 25 Å. Myoglobin is the most primitive hemoglobin-like protein from an evolutionary point of view. It is an intracellular protein whose function is to store oxygen in the cells for metabolic purposes.

The structure of heme is illustrated in Figure 7.2. The molecule consists of four pyrrole-like ring structures (see structure I, Figure 7.2) joined by methene bridges (=C–), plus various side chains: methyl, vinyl, and propyl. It is a planar molecule. Associated with nitrogen atoms of the ring is a ferrous iron ion (Fe^{2+}); two nitrogen atoms have lost their protons, thus carrying one negative charge each, and these then form electrostatic interactions with the positively charged iron. The other two nitrogen atoms form coordinate-covalent bonds with iron. If iron is removed from heme, the result is protoporphyrin IX (structure IV, Figure 7.2). The chemical prototype of all porphyrin-type compounds is porphin (structure III, Figure 7.2). Though porphyrin IX is planar, iron is located somewhat above that plane to accommodate its octahedral bonding geometry. When hemoglobin binds O_2, the Fe^{2+} is pulled back into the plane of the porphyrin ring.

The iron in heme may be oxidized to the ferric form, and the molecule then acquires a net positive charge (heme is neutral). A negative counterion must be associated with the oxidized heme. If the counterion is Cl^-, then the compound is hemin. If it is OH^-, the compound is hematin.

Like most soluble proteins, hemoglobin has a relatively hydrophilic surface and a hydrophobic interior. Heme is located in the hydrophobic interior of each α

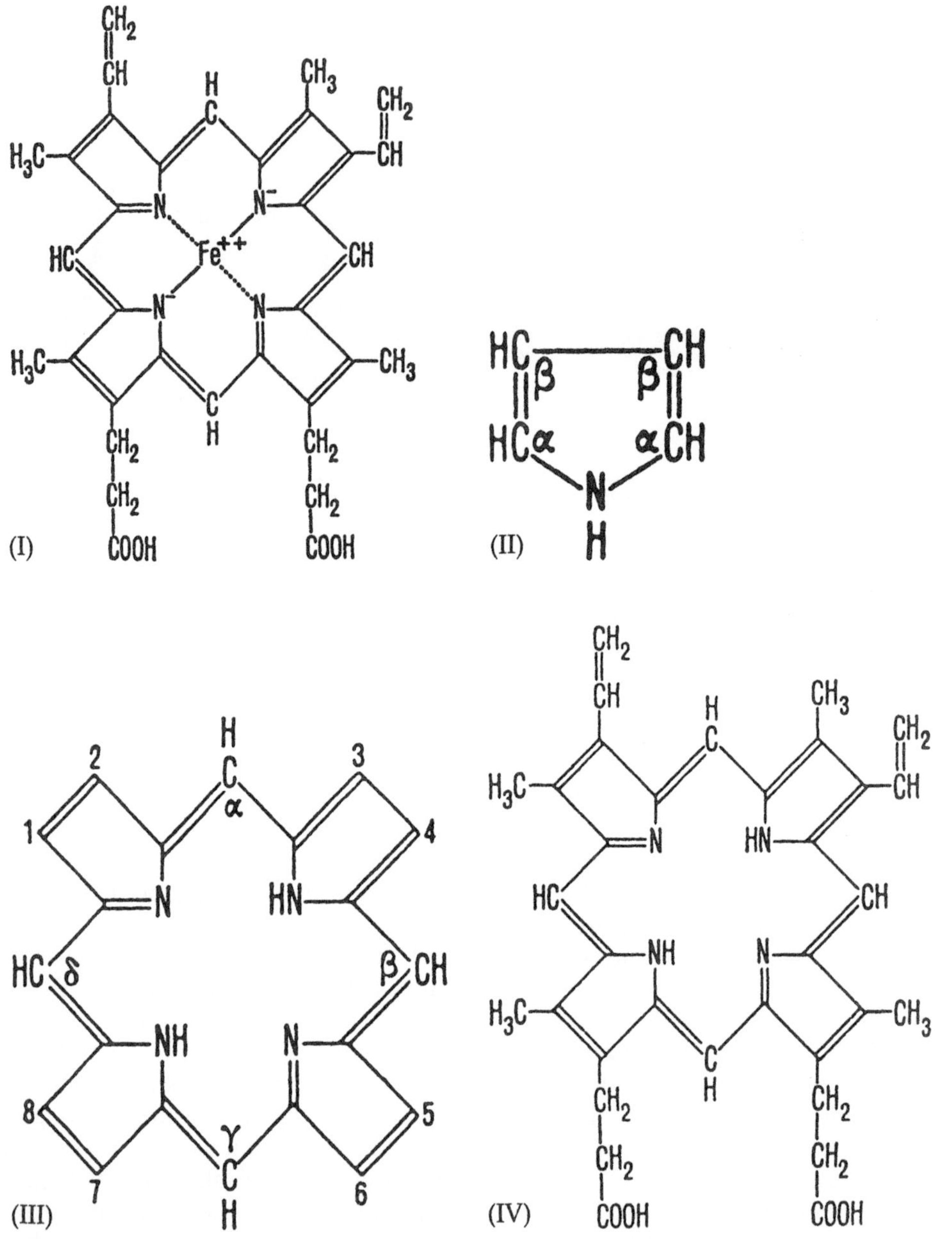

Figure 7.2 Structures of various compounds associated with heme chemistry. I, heme; II, pyrrole; III, porphin; IV, protoporphyrin IX, which is heme with the iron removed. (Reproduced with permission from Diem K, Lentner C. Scientific Tables. Basel: Ciba-Geigy, 1971, pp. 355–362.)

or β domain, the interaction being, in part, through hydrophobic bonding. Its precise location is sometimes referred to as the hydrophobic pocket. The position of the heme residue is shown for both the α and β subunits in Figure 7.3. The ferrous iron portion of heme is also associated with certain residues of the globin molecule. The so-called proximal imidazole residues (No. 87 in the α chains and No. 92 in the β chains) form coordinate-covalent interactions with iron. These histidine residues are also termed F8 residues because they are present in the F helix of hemoglobin. An oxygen molecule interacts with the iron atom and the distal histidine residue, which is No. 58 in the α chain and No. 63 in the β chain. The latter residues are also termed E7 imidazole residues because they occur in the E helix of hemoglobin. Iron in oxyhemoglobin has an octahedral geometry and is attached to six ligands. In deoxyhemoglobin, the sixth position (oxygen-binding) remains empty. Heme molecules are well separated from each other in hemoglobin, their iron atoms being at least 25 Å apart. This is necessary to make the oxygen–heme interaction relatively weak and reversible. The presence of the proximal and distal imidazole residues also contributes to this phenomenon. Since the F8 and E7 histidyl residues are essential for normal oxygen binding, they have been highly conserved through the course of evolution.

The secondary structure of the hemoglobins consists largely of α-helical segments and short stretches of various bends and interhelical segments. In sperm whale myoglobin, there are nine helical regions with a total of 131 amino acids out of a total of 153. The helixes are labeled A (N-terminal) through H (plus F'). The F helix contains the proximal histidyl residue (F8, No. 93). The E helix contains the distal residue (E7, No. 64) as well as the E11 valine residue (No. 68), which apparently controls access to the hydrophobic pocket where heme is situated. The E11 residue is in position 62 of the α chain and position 67 of the β chain of hemoglobin.

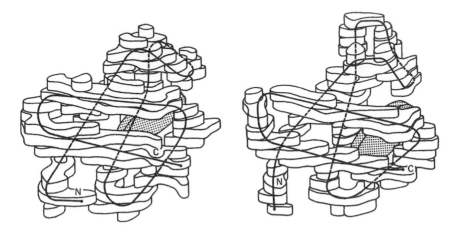

Figure 7.3 Three-dimensional appearance of the α (left) and β (right) chains of hemoglobin. The lines from the N- to the C-terminal ends follow the pathway of the polypeptide chains (dotted sections are the plane of the paper). The shaded disks are heme molecules. (Reproduced by permission from Perutz MF. Biophysical Chemistry. San Francisco: Freeman, 1975, pp. 40–52.)

Heme iron in either myoglobin or hemoglobin can be oxidized to the ferric form by a variety of substances. Oxidized myoglobin and hemoglobin are termed metmyoglobin and methemoglobin, respectively. Oxidized hemoglobins do not bind oxygen; instead they bind water, which is also capable of making a bridge between iron and the distal imidazole residue. Methemoglobin has a net positive charge on each of the heme constituents and is therefore associated with negative counterions such as Cl^-. An especially stable complex is formed between the cyanide ion (CN^-) and methemoglobin, and this complex is used in the laboratory quantitation of hemoglobin. The latter is first oxidized by ferricyanide, then NaCN is added to create cyanomethemoglobin, which is determined colorimetrically. There are other substances that can combine with hemoglobins. Because the heme residue in hemoglobin is not charged, it will form complexes with such neutral molecules as NO (nitric oxide) and CO (carbon monoxide). The latter has an affinity for hemoglobin some 200 times that of O_2. The carbon monoxide–hemoglobin complex is carboxyhemoglobin.

Normal hemoglobin is often abbreviated as HbA, or if one wants to designate its component polypeptide chains, as $\alpha_2^A \beta_2^A$. When electrophoresis is performed on a normal human red blood cell lysate, one finds, in addition to HbA, a small quantity of another hemoglobin, HbA_2. HbA_2 accounts for about 2.5% of total hemoglobin of red cells and consists of two α chains and two δ chains. The δ chains thus replace β chains in HbA_2. HbA_2 is also associated with four heme residues and functions perfectly normally. Its composition may be designated as $\alpha_2^A \delta_2^A$.

The human organism, during the course of its development, contains hemoglobin varieties with polypeptide chains other than the α, β, and δ. Thus, there are the γ chains, components of fetal hemoglobin (HbF). There are also the ϵ and the ζ chains, which appear only during the embryonic stage of development. Figure 7.4 illustrates the appearance of various non-adult hemo-

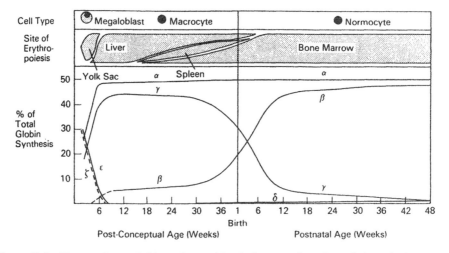

Figure 7.4 Human hemoglobin polypeptide chains as a function of time during gestation and postnatal development. (Reproduced with permission from Weatherall DJ, Clegg JB. The Thalassemia Syndromes. Boston: Blackwell, 1981.)

globin subunits during gestation and up to 48 weeks of age. Aberrant adult hemoglobins may also exist because of various types of genetic lesions. Most often, this is the result of point mutations in which a single amino acid, either in the α or, more often, the β chain is replaced by another amino acid. This may cause a profound change in the physiologic behavior of hemoglobin. For example, in sickle cell hemoglobin, a valine residue replaces the normal glutamate residue in position 6 of the β chain. This causes a solidification of the deoxy sickle cell hemoglobin (HbS) in peripheral blood vessels with attendant physical symptoms. Various hemoglobins and their component polypeptide chains are listed in Table 7.2. It should be noted that all hemoglobin polypeptide chains, including the myoglobins, are homologous proteins, having arisen from the same ancestral gene. Many hemoglobins can be separated from each other electrophoretically, which provides a convenient laboratory identification tool for the physician. Their relative mobilities are illustrated in Figure 7.5.

Another use of the electrophoretic method in the realm of hemoglobin biochemistry is in monitoring patient compliance in the diabetic state or even in diagnosing diabetes. A certain percentage of hemoglobin (mean is 6.5%) exists in the glycosylated form, the glycohemoglobins. The major fraction of this group of proteins is glycosylated HbA, termed HbA_{1C}. The N-terminal valine residues of the β chains are associated with glucose molecules in the ketoamine form ($Glc-CO-CH_2-NH-Val$). As glucose levels rise, HbA_{1C} levels also rise to as much as 20% of total Hb. HbA_{1C}, unlike blood glucose, remains elevated for the life of the red blood cell even if blood glucose levels decline to normal. HbA_{1C} thus provides a history of blood sugar level in a patient over a long period of time—about 8 weeks. If blood glucose history for the past 2–3 weeks is desired, a "fructosamine" determination can be made. This is a quantitation of glycosylated serum proteins, largely serum albumin. The half-lives of serum proteins are much shorter than that of Hb. "Fructosamine" determination is done colorimetrically and determines a fructosamine-like adduct formed when glucose reacts with the $-NH_2$ residues of serum proteins.

Table 7.2 Various Polypeptide Chains Found in Hemoglobins

| Hemoglobin | Number of polypeptide chains | | | | | | Notation |
	α	β	γ	δ	ζ	ϵ	
HbA	2	2					$\alpha_2^A \beta_2^A$
HbA$_2$	2			2			$\alpha_2^A \delta_2^A$
Fetal Hb (HbF)	2		2				$\alpha_2^A \gamma_2^F$
HbH[a]		4					β_4^A
Hb$_{Barts}$[a]			4				γ_4^F
Hb$_{GowersI}$[b]					2	2	$\zeta_2 \epsilon_2$
Hb$_{GowersII}$[b]	2					2	$\alpha_2^A \epsilon_2$
Hb$_{Portland}$[b]			2		2		$\zeta_2 \gamma_2^F$
Sickle cell Hb (HbS)[a]	2	2(S)					$\alpha_2^A \beta_2^S$

[a]Pathologic.
[b]Embryonic.

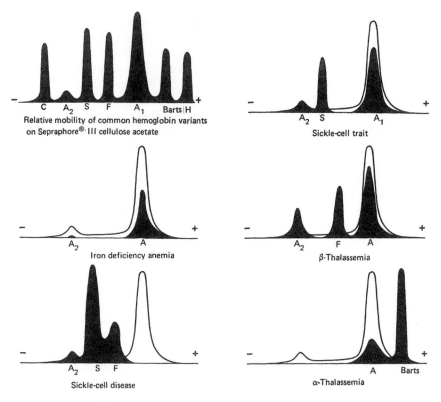

Figure 7.5 Electrophoretic patterns of erythrocyte lysates bearing abnormal hemoglobins. C, A_2, S, F, A_1, Barts, and H are hemoglobins C, A_2, S (sickle), A_1 (normal), Barts and H, respectively. Electrophoresis was done at pH 8.6, the medium was stained with a protein-specific dye, and the bound dye was quantitated densitometrically. Absorbance is on the y axis, distance moved, on the x axis, Shaded areas represent abnormal patterns. (From a circular by Gelman Instrument Co., Ann Arbor, MI, by permission of the copyright holder.)

7.2.3 Function of Hemoglobin

Myoglobin reacts with O_2 according to the equation

$$\text{Myoglobin} + O_2 \rightleftharpoons \text{myoglobin-}O_2 \tag{7.1}$$

or

$$\text{Mb} + O_2 \rightleftharpoons \text{Mb-}O_2$$

For this reaction, we can write an equilibrium constant expression as follows:

$$K = \frac{[\text{MbO}_2]}{[\text{Mb}][O_2]} \quad \text{or} \quad \frac{[\text{MbO}_2]}{[\text{Mb}]} = K[O_2] \tag{7.2}$$

Oxygen is usually measured in terms of its partial pressure, pO_2, expressed as millimeters of mercury (mm Hg). pO_2 will, of course, be proportional to $[O_2]$, and we may then rewrite Equation 7.2 as

$$\frac{[MbO_2]}{[Mb]} = K'(pO_2) \tag{7.3}$$

Most hemoglobins, however, do not obey the simple mass action equation (Equation 7.2) and instead obey the empirical *Hill equation*:

$$\frac{[HbO_2]}{[Hb]} = K' \times (pO_2)^n \tag{7.4}$$

where n is the Hill coefficient, which is characteristic of each hemoglobin. For myoglobin, $n = 1$, whereas for human hemoglobin $n = 2.8$. Taking logarithms of both sides of Equation 7.4 and letting $[HbO_2]/[Hb] = Y$, we have

$$\log Y = \log K' + n \log pO_2 \tag{7.5}$$

When this equation is plotted as $\log Y$ against $\log pO_2$, the result is a straight line with n as the slope and K' the y intercept. This is the *Hill plot* and is shown in Figure 7.6a. For myoglobin, the Hill plot passes through the origin with a slope (Hill coefficient) of 1, whereas the plot for hemoglobin has a slope of 2.8. The Hill plot also defines another constant that is characteristic of each hemoglobin: P_{50}, the pO_2 at which the hemoglobin is 50% saturated with O_2. In such a case, $Y = 1$, and Equation 7.5 reduces to

$$-\log K' = n \log P_{50} \tag{7.6}$$

This means that the value of P_{50} may be determined from the Hill plot's y intercept or x inercept. For example, the y intercept in the case of myoglobin is 0, and since $n = 1$, $P_{50} = 1$ mm Hg. For hemoglobin, the y intercept is -4.0. Using Equation 7.6, we get $4 = 2.8 \log P_{50} = 26.8$ mm Hg. Likewise, one can look at where the Hill plot intersects the x axis ($y = 0$); for myoglobin this is at 0, and hence $P_{50} = 1$ mm. For hemoglobin, the intersection is at -1.42, which is the log of 26.3 mm, a figure very close to the 26.8 mm calculated above.

The difference in the behavior of hemoglobins may be shown graphically in another way: by plotting percent saturation with oxygen against pO_2, as is shown in Figure 7.6b. Mathematically, this plot may be represented by the equation

$$\% \text{ saturation with } O_2 = \frac{(pO_2)^n}{(pO_2)^n + (P_{50})^n} \tag{7.7}$$

where n is the Hill coefficient. It is seen in Figure 7.6b that myoglobin picks up oxygen extremely rapidly and becomes saturated at a very low pO_2. The behavior of hemoglobin, however, resembles the behavior of allosteric enzymes discussed in Chapter 5: the curve is sigmoidal with a considerable lag period at low pO_2, but as O_2 interacts with the hemoglobin, an enhancement (positive cooperativity), of O_2 uptake is observed. In fact, the most dramatic response to small changes in pO_2 occurs at the P_{50} mark, around 26–27 mm Hg. The Hill coefficient is indicative of cooperativity among the various subunits of hemoglobin. A value of $n = 1$ indicates no cooperativity whatever, as is the case with myoglobin. A value of $n > 1$ indicates positive cooperativity, whereas if $n < 1$ there is negative cooperativity.

The molecular basis for the cooperativity effects in hemoglobins has been worked out in some detail. However, before delving into that, it is necessary to

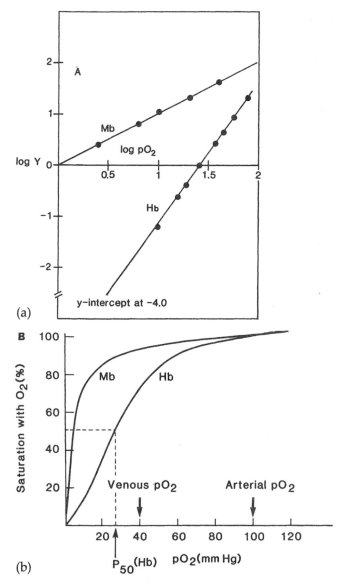

Figure 7.6 Oxygen association with myoglobin (Mb) and human hemoglobin (Hb). (a) The Hill plot; (b) a plot of oxygen partial pressure against the degree of hemoglobin saturation with oxygen.

point out two phenomena that under physiological conditions affect the binding of O_2 by hemoglobins. These are the effects of pCO_2/H^+ and 2,3-diphosphoglycerate (2,3-DPG). It has been observed that as pCO_2 increases, the binding of O_2 by hemoglobin decreased. This has been shown to be due to an increase in $[H^+]$ rather than $[CO_2]$ because in solution there exist the equilibria

$$CO_2 + H_2O \leftrightarrows H_2CO_3 \leftrightarrows H^+ + HCO_3^- \tag{7.8}$$

These reactions are enhanced in the red blood cells through the action of car-bonic anhydrase. Thus, a decrease in pH will cause a loss of O_2 from oxyhemo-globin. The other factor that affects the binding of O_2 by hemoglobin is the presence in the red blood cells of nearly stoichiometric amounts of 2,3-DPG (Figure 7.7). 2,3-DPG stabilizes deoxyhemoglobin by forming electrostatic inter-actions between its phosphate residues on the one hand and the following amino acid residues of the β chain on the other: N-terminal groups, His-2 and His-143 (H21). It is significant to note that in the γ chains (HbF), the H21 His is replaced by Ser. This results in weaker binding of 2,3-DPG by HbF and stabiliza-tion of the O_2-containing forms. Thus, the affinity of HbF for O_2 is greater than that of HbA. The carboxyl group of 2,3-DPG is associated with the ϵ-amino group of βLys82 in deoxyhemoglobin. Persons living at high altitudes have greater quantities of 2,3-DPG in their red blood cells. This helps in the delivery of oxygen to peripheral tissues. Oxyhemoglobin too binds 2,3-DPG at the same sites, but such interaction is much weaker than it is in deoxyhemoglobin, be-cause the conformations of oxy- and deoxyhemoglobins are different and be-cause the interrelationships among the four subunits are different.

The models that have been proposed to explain the allosteric behavior of hemoglobin toward O_2 all assume that the subunits of hemoglobin can take on either one of two conformations: the R (relaxed) form and the T (tight) form. The R forms have a high affinity for O_2, whereas the T forms have a low affinity. The sequential (Adair–Koshland) model proposed that as deoxyhemoglobin (all T forms) was exposed to increasing pO_2, there would be a lag period at the begin-ning, but as the first subunit bound a molecule of O_2 and changed its con-formation to the R form, the conformational change would exert an influence on a neighboring subunit to change its shape to the R form, which then would pick up O_2 more easily than the first subunit did. The sequential model thus proposed that partially oxygenated hemoglobin molecules would consist of mixtures of the R and T forms. The symmetrical (Monod) model, on the other hand, proposed that any given hemoglobin molecule was either in all R or all T conformations and a sudden transition would occur as increasing quantities of O_2 became bound to hemoglobin.

Perutz has presented the most comprehensive allosteric model for the func-tion of hemoglobin. It is of the symmetrical type and is presented in Figure 7.8. This model provides for the binding of 2,3-DPG by the T forms but not by the R

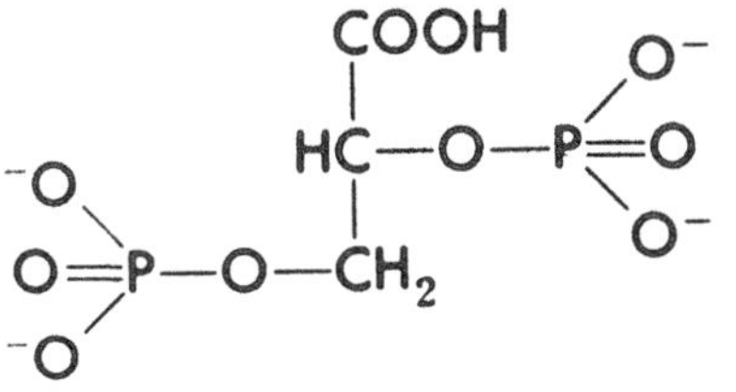

2,3-Diphosphoglyceric
acid (DPG)

Figure 7.7   Structure of 2,3-diphosphoglyceric acid (2,3-DPG).

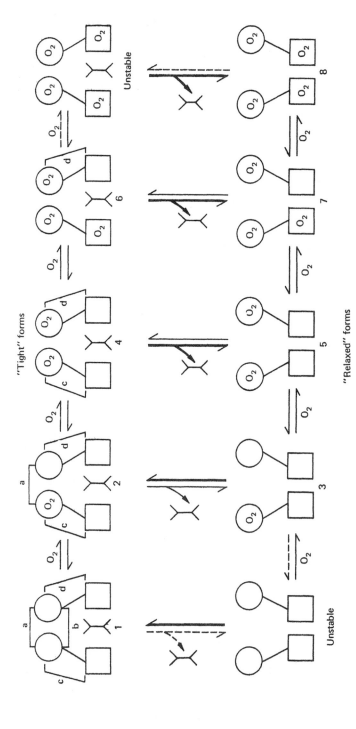

Figure 7.8 Equilibria among the R and T forms of hemoglobins: α-chains are represented by circles, β-chains by squares. The clamps represent electrostatic interactions. $\rightarrowtail$ represents 2,3-diphosphoglycerate. a, b, c and d represent electrostatic linkages that are broken or formed in the processes of interconversion between the reversible tight to relaxed conformation.

forms, and it provides for the effect of increasing proton concentration, which also favors the T forms and thus the release of O_2 by oxyhemoglobin. In the process of converting the R to the T forms, a portion of the protons produced by the carbonic anhydrase reaction (Equation 7.8) is bound by hemoglobin and is thus buffered. This is the *Bohr effect*. Such protons interact with certain histidyl and amino residues of oxyhemoglobin to make these residues positively charged. In effect, this increases the pK values of such residues and increases the pI of hemoglobin from 6.7 in oxyhemoglobin to 7.6 in deoxyhemoglobin. The protonated, positively charged residues then proceed to form electrostatic interactions with negatively charged residues, thus converting the R forms into the T forms and releasing O_2. Some such electrostatic interactions are indicated by a–d in Figure 7.8. More precisely, they are as follows: $\alpha_1$40 Lys–β_2-C-terminus; $\alpha_2$40 Lys–β_2-C-terminus; and intrasubunit interactions in the β-chains between His-146 and Asp-94. These electrostatic interactions do not exist in the more acidic oxyhemoglobin. For every equivalent of O_2 released from hemoglobin, about 0.3 equivalent of $[H^+]$ is bound. The bound H^+ are called the *Bohr protons*. They are released in the lung, where pO_2 is high and pCO_2 is low, and the T forms change back to the R forms.

In addition to binding and delivering oxygen, hemoglobin also plays a role in transporting CO_2 from peripheral tissues to the lungs. Most of the CO_2 that diffuses into the blood cells is converted to H^+ and HCO_3^- by the carbonic anhydrase reaction. Some protons are buffered by hemoglobin via the Bohr effect (40%); others (50%) are buffered nonspecifically by various residues of hemoglobin; and the remainder are buffered by other means (e.g., phosphate). The HCO_3^- diffuses from the red blood cells into plasma and is replaced by Cl^-. This chloride shift is shown in Figure 7.9. Not all the CO_2 that diffuses into the red cells from peripheral tissue is converted to HCO_3^-. Some interacts with the N-terminal groups of hemoglobin to give carbamino complexes:

$$\underset{}{RNH_2} + CO_2 \rightleftharpoons R\text{--}\overset{\displaystyle H}{\underset{\displaystyle |}{N}}\text{--}\overset{\displaystyle O}{\underset{\displaystyle \|}{C}}\text{--}O^- + H^+ \tag{7.9}$$

Deoxyhemoglobin, because of its higher pI, has a greater affinity for CO_2 than oxyhemoglobin. It should also be noted that the formation of carbamino complexes (Equation 7.9) results in the generation of protons, which are added to the proton pool that must be buffered by hemoglobin in the peripheral tissue. N-terminal groups of hemoglobin thus compete for CO_2, 2,3-DPG binding, and electrostatic bond formation that is part of the Bohr effect.

Venous blood has a pO_2 of about 40 mm Hg, as opposed to 100 mm Hg for arterial blood. Hemoglobin in the latter is almost 100% saturated with O_2, whereas in venous blood it may be 75% saturated. In some peripheral tissues such as the muscle, where pO_2 may be as low as 20 mm Hg and $[H^+]$ very high, O_2 saturation level of hemoglobin may become as low as 20–30%. Venous blood hemoglobin thus has a greater concentration of T forms than of R forms. Compared to arterial blood, venous blood also has about 1.7 meq/L more bicarbonate, 0.3 meq/L more carbamino-type CO_2, and 0.2 meq/L more dissolved CO_2, for a total CO_2 differential of about 2.2 meq/L. In the lungs, where pCO_2 is low and pO_2 is high, the HCO_3^- and carbamino residues are reconverted to CO_2, which results in the removal of protons from the T forms of partially deoxygenated hemoglo-

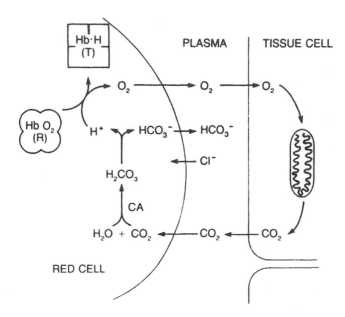

Figure 7.9 Delivery of oxygen to peripheral tissue by oxyhemoglobin. Production of protons from CO_2 and H_2O, catalyzed by carbonic anhydrase (CA) and their uptake by hemoglobin are also shown. The pCO_2 in peripheral tissues is high and pO_2 is low, causing the conversion of hemoglobin R forms into the T forms with the concomitant release of O_2. (Reproduced by permission from Bunn HF, Forget BG. Hemoglobin: Molecular, Genetic, and Clinical Aspects. Philadelphia: WB Saunders, 1986, p. 41.)

bin, the release of 2,3-DPG, and the reconversion of the hemoglobin into the R type, which can now bind O_2.

7.2.4 Evolution of Hemoglobins

Hemoglobin-type proteins are widely distributed in nature. Even some plants and bacteria have hemoglobins. The evolution of hemoglobins has been traced by a number of investigators, including Goodman and colleagues, whose work product appears in Figure 7.10. There are several notable points that can be brought out. Thus, some 200 million years ago, there was a β-gene duplication event that gave rise to the modern β genes on the one hand and α genes on the other. The ϵ and τ genes diverged some 100 million years ago. In the α-gene group, a divergence took place some 350 million years ago to generate the α and the ζ genes. Gene duplication giving rise to the α and the β ancestral genes took place some 450 million years ago, and the myoglobins diverged from hemoglobins about 475–500 million years ago. On the other hand, the differences between the β and δ chains are very small, a divergence having occurred only some 40 million years ago. It is thus clear that myoglobin is the oldest hemoglobin from an evolutionary point of view, followed by the α chains, then the β chains.

Globin genes in human beings are located on chromosomes 11 and 16. The α-family genes (α and ζ) are located on chromosome 16, whereas the β-family

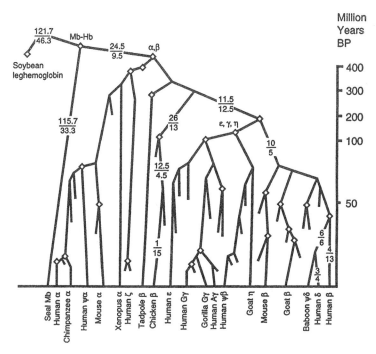

Figure 7.10 Phylogenetic tree of various hemoglobin subunits constructed on the basis of the respective gene nucleotide sequences. Numerators of numbers along some lines indicate nucleotide substitutions (mutations) resulting in changes in amino acid composition, whereas the denominators indicate silent changes. Diamonds indicate gene duplication locations, whereas other branch points are the result of specialization. The prefix ψ indicates pseudogenes. Note that globins indicated by α, ϵ, ζ belong to the α-group, whereas those indicated by β, γ, δ belong to the β-group. The η-gene is an ancestral gene for the human beings and appears as a pseudogene designated as $\psi\beta$ in human chromosomes. (Adapted from Goodman HM, Koop BF, Czelusuiak J, Weiss ML, Slighton JL. The η-globin gene. J Mol Biol 180:803–823, 1984.)

genes (β, δ, γ, ϵ) are located on chromosome 11. Several α or β pseudogenes are also located on chromosomes 16 and 11, respectively.

7.2.5 Abnormal Hemoglobins

Almost 200 abnormal hemoglobins are known. Some of these are listed in Table 7.3. Most of them have arisen by way of the point mutation process, where an amino acid in either the α or, more frequently, the β chain is substituted by another amino acid. This, more likely than not, will result in abnormal physiologic function of the hemoglobin. In other situations, the genetic basis for hemoglobin abnormality may be more complex. For instance, in Lepore-type hemoglobin, an unequal crossover between two chromosomes No. 11 results in a recombinant $\delta\beta$ gene and a gene product that carries the characteristics of both the δ and β chains. Thus, in Hb Boston, an Hb Lepore-type protein, the crossover occurs between residues δ 87 and β 116. Abnormal hemoglobins are classified below on the basis of their physiological effects.

Table 7.3 A Representative List of Abnormal Hemoglobins

Category	Hemoglobin name	Amino acid substitution(s)	Notes
High O_2 affinity	Hb Rainier[a]	β145Tyr →Cys	Disulfide bridges present
	Hb Little Rock	β143 His→Gln	2,3-DPG binding decreased[b]
	Hb Zurich	β63 His→Arg	Heme pocket opened, stability decreased[b]
	Hb St. Etienne	β92 His→Gln	Proximal histidine group lost; stability decreased
	Hb Hiroshima	β146 His→Asp	Salt bridge stabilizing T form impossible to make
Low O_2 affinity	Hb Kansas	β102 Asn→Thr	T form stabilized
	Hb Moabit	α86 Leu→Arg	Stability lowered because a hydrophobic group of heme pocket is replaced by a polar one
	Hb Hammersmith	β42 Phe→Ser	T form favored
Methemo-globinemias	Hb St. Louis	β28 Leu→Gln	Heme pocket opened, stability decreased
	Hb Milwaukee	β67 Val→Gln	Decreased O_2 affinity, Fe^{2+} oxidized through negative charges
	Hb Chicago	β63 His→Tyr	Increased stability for Fe^{3+} by the tyrosine residue
α-Helix disruptors[c]	Hb Bicetre	β63 His→Pro	Helix E disrupted, heme pocket opened; Met Hb forms
	Hb Duarte	β62 Ala→Pro	Helix E disrupted; stability decreased; increased O_2 affinity
	Hb Abraham Lincoln	β32 Leu→Pro	Interrupts helix B
	Hb Bibba	β136 Leu→Pro	Interrupts helix H
Decreased solubility	HbS	β6 Glu→Val	Sickling of red cells
	HbC	β6 Glu→Lys	Sickling, especially in S/C heterozygote
	HbD	β6 Glu→Glu	Sickling, especially in S/D heterozygote
Stability of Hb decreased	Hb Torino	β43 Phe→Val	Heme pocket destabilized
	Hb St. Luke's	α95 Pro→Arg	Subunits dissociate
	Hb Bristol	β67 Val→Asp	Heme pocket destabilized
	Hb Baylor	β81 Leu→Arg	Heme pocket destabilized

[a]Many hemoglobin variants show several abnormalities, e.g., O_2-binding defect plus a decrease in stability.
[b]When stability is lowered, hemoglobins precipitate more easily than HbA.
[c]These destabilize the hemoglobin, causing it to precipitate.
Source: Most information in this table has been distilled from Dickerson RE., Geis I, Hemoglobin: Structure, Function, Evolution, and Pathology. Menlo Park, CA: Benjamin/Cummings, 1983, pp. 151–157.

High Oxygen Affinity Hemoglobins

Generally, patients with high oxygen affinity hemoglobin are discovered because they have higher than normal hematocrit; that is, they have increased levels of red blood cells. This presumably occurs because the abnormal hemoglobin cannot give up sufficient amounts of oxygen to the peripheral tissues, and the organism tries to compensate for this defect by producing more red cells. In most cases this works out well, and the patient can usually lead a normal life.

Figure 7.11 shows the oxygen dissociation curve of one such hemoglobin, Hb Rainier, where it is seen that this hemoglobin is still 50% saturated with oxygen at a pO_2 of about 12 mm Hg compared to 27 mm Hg in normal hemoglobin. The value of n in the Hill equation is 1.5 for this hemoglobin.

On the molecular level, Hb Rainier differs from Hb A in that the penultimate tyrosyl residues of the β chains (in position 145) are replaced by cysteinyl residues. In shorthand, we designate this substitution by the code β145Tyr$\rightarrow$Cys. This substitution (point mutation) results in a destabilization of the T form of Hb Rainier, so the R forms are preferred and oxygen is not likely to leave the Hb Rainier molecule.

In Hb Little Rock, we have a β143His$\rightarrow$Gln replacement. The effect of this replacement is that DPG cannot be bound by the Hb Little Rock molecule, which therefore results in the predominance of the R forms of the hemoglobin. In general, then, amino acid substitutions in the high oxygen affinity hemoglobins interfere with the subunit interactions in such a way that either T forms are destabilized or R forms are stabilized.

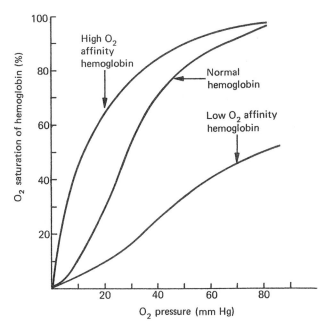

Figure 7.11 Oxygen affinity curves of a high O_2 affinity hemoglobin (e.g., Hb Rainier) and a low O_2 affinity hemoglobin (e.g., Hb Kansas), compared to that of normal hemoglobin.

In connection with hemoglobin mutants that possess a high affinity for oxygen, it would be appropriate to mention the properties of three hemoglobins that may be considered to be normal under some circumstances. These are the HbF (see above), hemoglobin H (HbH), and hemoglobin Barts (Hb Barts). HbH is a β-chain tetramer, whereas Hb Barts is a γ-chain tetramer. The latter two have higher than normal oxygen-binding activity. The reason HbF binds O_2 more avidly than HbA was discussed above. In a 1-day-old child, where HbF makes up about 77% of total hemoglobin, the P_{50} value is about 19 mm Hg compared to 27 mm Hg for HbA. Normally, HbF disappears soon after birth; however, a hereditary HbF disease exists, where HbF persists throughout life. HbF is also present as a secondary phenomenon in the red cells of certain anemic individuals.

Hemoglobin H and Hb Barts are usually found in pathologic conditions, where normal hemoglobin biosynthesis is diminished. This occurs, for instance, in certain types of thalassemias (see Chapter 14).

Hemoglobins with Low Oxygen Affinity

Hemoglobins with low oxygen affinity are encountered less frequently than those described in the previous section and are generally detected in persons with unexplained cyanosis. A typical example, Hb Kansas, is presented in Figure 7.11. In this mutant, we have a replacement characterized by β102Asn$\rightarrow$Thr. This results in interference with a normal interaction between the α_1 and the β_2 subunits so that the T form is stabilized, and the hemoglobin has a lesser chance to bind oxygen. In these types of mutants, we have stabilization or favoring of the T forms and/or a destabilization of the R forms of hemoglobin.

Hereditary Methemoglobins

When an amino acid substitution involves the heme-containing pocket of globin, one effect may be that the globin can no longer protect the ferrous iron of heme from becoming oxidized to the ferric form. The result is a formation of methemoglobin, which cannot bind oxygen. The most common symptoms in such cases are cyanosis and a brownish coloration of the blood.

Hemoglobins with Heme-Binding Anomalies

It is said that members of the largest group of abnormal hemoglobins are characterized by their inability to bind heme properly. This anomaly may be brought about by amino acid substitutions in the hydrophobic pocket of the globin polypeptide chain, so that the heme molecule is unable to form one of the normal bonds linking it with the globin. Thus, in Hb St. Etienne, the histidyl group normally coordinated with the heme iron is replaced by glutamine (β92His$\rightarrow$Gln), whereas in Hb Hammersmith, a phenylalanine residue is replaced by serine (β42Phe$\rightarrow$Ser), with the result that a hydrophobic bond is no longer formed between heme and globin. Clinically, such hemoglobins are very susceptible to denaturation, which in turn results in red cell hemolysis with the symptoms of hemolytic anemia.

Hemoglobins with Altered α-Helix Content

The stability of the hemoglobins depends in great part on the α-helical conformation of their polypeptide chains. If an amino acid in the α-helical region of the protein is replaced by proline, the α helix is broken at that point. When this happens in hemoglobin, it easily becomes denatured. These conditions are again characterized by red cell lysis and the clinical symptoms of hemolytic anemia. Example is Hb Abraham Lincoln, where β32Leu→Pro.

Hemoglobins with Solubility Abnormalities

There are several instances of abnormal hemoglobins that cannot fit precisely into any of the preceding categories. The best known among these is sickle cell hemoglobin, or hemoglobin S (HbS). It is found largely in the black populations of the world. In the United States, it is estimated that one black individual in 70–300 has the disease (a homozygote), whereas about 10% are carriers (they are said to have the sickle cell anemia trait). Hemoglobin S arises out of a substitution of the hydrophilic glutamic acid residue in position 6 of the β chain with the hydrophobic valine residue (β6Glu→Val). This substitution makes the deoxy form of the protein less soluble in aqueous medium so that it tends to form gels while in the peripheral tissue, causing tissue hypoxia. The red cells then assume a characteristic sickle shape shown in Figure 7.12.

A disorder related to sickle cell anemia is the HbC disease, which is also found mostly among persons of African ancestry. Its symptoms, however, are less severe than those with the HbS disorder. HbC is a hemoglobin with a β6Glu→Lys substitution. It is believed that HbS and HbC arose as a means of combating malaria, because red cells containing HbS and HbC are more resistant to the invasion of the malarial parasite than are normal red cells.

7.3   HEME METABOLISM

7.3.1   Heme Biosynthesis

Heme, a component of hemoglobins (see Figure 7.1), is assembled in the organism from relatively simple substances: glycine and succinyl CoA. The entire process is depicted in Figure 7.13. The pathway is initiated in the mitochondria. The first intermediate, δ-aminolevulinate (ALA), then diffuses into the cytosol, where the pyrrole ring structure is formed to give porphobilinogen (PBG). Four PBG units condense to form the linear molecule hydroxymethyl bilane, which, in the presence of uroporphyrinogen III cosynthase, is condensed to form uroporphyrinogen III, the first compound containing a porphyrin-like ring structure. Uroporphyrinogen III is then decarboxylated to coproporphyrinogen III, and the latter diffuses into mitochondria where it is further decarboxylated to protoporhyrinogen IX. An oxidation step then produces protoporphyrin IX, which accepts ferrous iron in the presence of ferrochelatase, also known as heme synthase.

It is important to note that uroporphyrinogen III is an asymmetric compound with respect to its side chains. In the absence of uroporphyrinogen III cosynthase, hydroxymethyl bilane is converted nonenzymatically to the symmet-

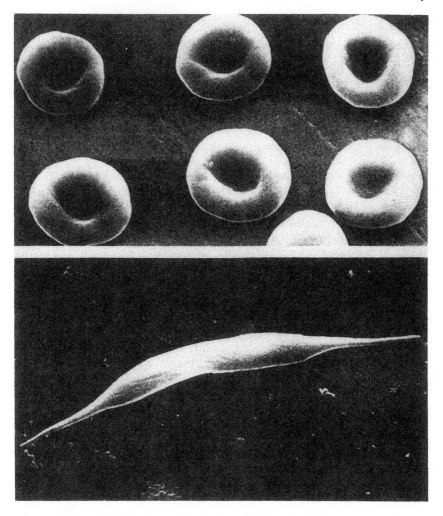

Figure 7.12 Normal and sickled red blood cells. (Reproduced by permission from Chem Eng News, January 6, 1975.)

rical uroporphyrinogen I. All porphyrins found in nature come from either uroporphyrinogen I or uroporphyrinogen III. As seen above, uroporphyrinogen III gives rise to heme in animals and to chlorophyll in plants, where Mg^{2+} is the metal rather than Fe^{2+}. In bacteria, uroporphyrinogen III may also be converted to vitamin B_{12} (see Chapter 6). Porphyrinogens can be oxidized enzymatically to porphyrins. These relationships are shown in Figure 7.14.

In iron deficiency anemia, Zn^{2+} may be used instead of iron by ferrochelatase in the biosynthesis of heme. Red blood cell lysates in such instances contain increased quantities of Zn-hemoglobin. In addition, red cells from iron-deficient patients also contain increased amounts of protoporphyrin IX. Zinc-hemoglobin and protoporphyrin IX determinations are thus used in the diagnosis of iron deficiency anemia.

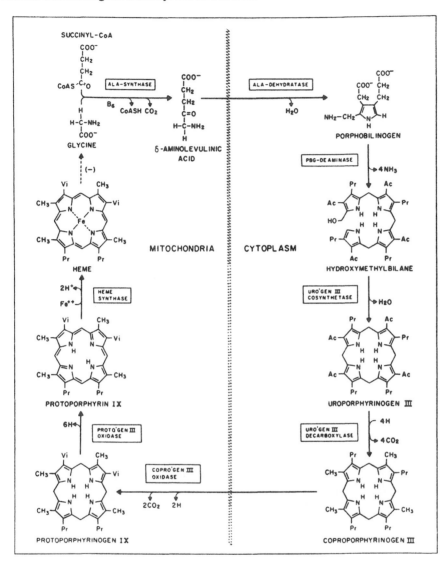

Figure 7.13 The heme biosynthesis pathway. ALA, δ-aminolevulinic acid; PBG, porphobilinogen; uro'gen, uroporphyrinogen; copro'gen, coproporphyrinogen; prot'gen, protoporphyrinogen; Ac, acetate; Pr, propionate; vi, vinyl. (Reproduced by permission from Preface. *Enzyme* 28:91–93, 1982.)

Control of heme biosynthesis revolves around the initial enzyme, ALA-synthase. Heme, the end product of this pathway, exerts an inhibitory effect on ALA-synthase through several mechanisms. Heme, or its oxidation product hematin, activates a repressor protein that turns off ALA-synthase biosynthesis at the translation level. Erythropoietin, a protein produced by the kidneys and found in larger than normal amounts in high-altitude dwellers, counteracts the effects of the repressor protein. Erythropoietin deficiency exists in chronic kid-

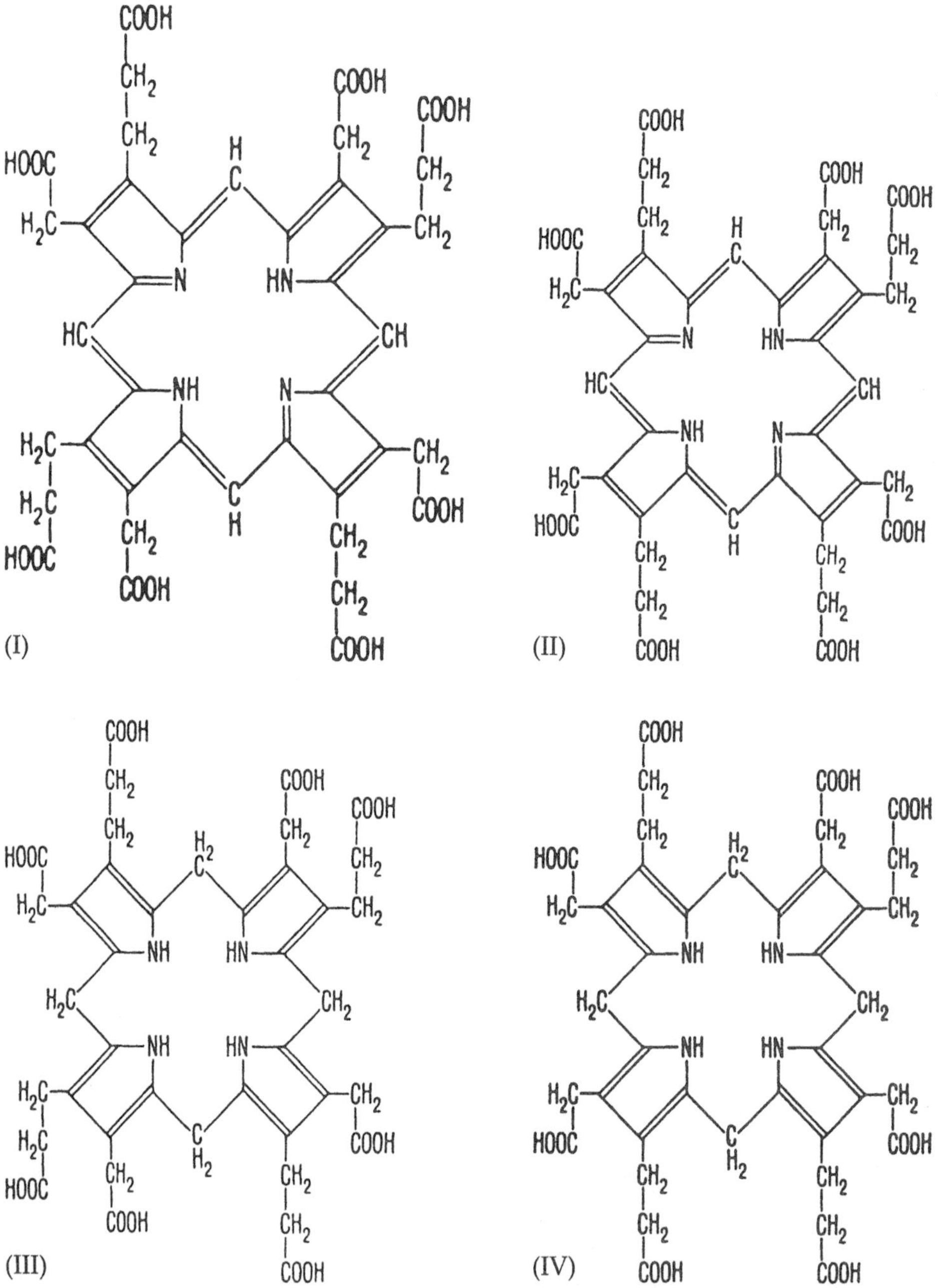

Figure 7.14 Structures of uroporphyrinogens I and III (structures I and II) and their oxidation products, uroporphyrin I and III (structures III and IV). (Reproduced by permission from Diem K, Lentner C. Scientific Tables. Basel: Ciba-Geigy, 1971, pp. 355–362.)

ney failure patients, hence the observed anemia condition in such patients. Heme also inhibits the translocation of ALA-synthase from the cytosol into the mitochondria. Additional controls include direct allosteric inhibition of ALA-synthase by heme and the fact that among all heme biosynthetic enzymes, ALA-synthase has the highest K_m and for that reason is rate-limiting. Heme also regulates globin biosynthesis; the lower the cell heme level, the lower the rate of globin synthesis. ALA-synthase is stimulated by steroids resulting from the reduction of 5β-dehydro steroids, such as testosterone. This enzyme appears in human beings at puberty.

Porphyrias are diseases brought about by deficiencies of enzymes that participate in the biosynthesis of heme. They are usually hereditary and may affect the liver or the blood-forming tissues. All prophyrias are characterized by the excretion in the urine and/or feces of heme biosynthesis intermediates. ALA-synthase is derepressed in porphyrias, because cellular heme levels are lower than normal. Hereditary porphyrias have been classified, on the basis of their symptomatic effects, into the neurologic, cutaneous, and mixed varieties. Acute intermittent porphyria is a neurologic porphyria. It is caused by an inadequate functioning of the PBG deaminase enzyme. The result is an extraordinarily high production of ALA and PBG and their excretion in urine. Acute intermittent porphyria patients, especially when stressed by fasting or drug intake, may lapse into a coma and die. This type of porphyria is especially prevalent among Laplanders. Treatment is via parenteral glucose administration, which seems to depress ALA-synthase activity.

Cutaneous porphyrias are disorders characterized by an extreme skin sensitivity to light. This may be due to the accumulation in the skin of various heme biosynthesis intermediate porphyrins. In congenital erythropoietic porphyria, which largely affects erythropoietic tissue, uroporphyrinogen III cosynthase activity is severely depressed. Instead of being converted to uroporphyrinogen III, hydroxymethyl bilane is converted to uroporphyrinogen I, which, under the influence of uroporphynogen III decarboxylase, may be converted to coproporphyrinogen I. Both the uroporphyrinogen I and coproporphyrinogen I are oxidized to their corresponding porphyrins, which are then accumulated in the tissues and excreted in the urine. Porphyria cutanea tarda is said to be the most common porphyria. It is caused by a decreased activity of liver uroporphyrinogen III decarboxylase. In this case, the patient's urine contains large quantities of uroporphyrin III and some uroporphyrin I. Erythropoietic protoporphyria, characterized by high fecal protoporphyrin IX levels, is due to depressed levels of ferrochelatase.

Among the mixed protoporphyrias are variegate porphyria and hereditary coproporphyria, both of which affect the liver. In the former, protoporphyrinogen III oxidase seems to be defective. Urine contains increased levels of coproporphyrin III and protoporphyrin IX. Variegate porphyria is especially prevalent among white South Africans. In hereditary coproporphyria, coproporphyrinogen III decarboxylase is depressed, resulting in the excretion of the coproporphyrin III in the urine and feces. There are a number of acquired porphyrias, the most common being the lead poisoning variety. The existence of an acquired porphyria results in the excretion in the urine and feces of coproporphyrins and protoporphyrins. The latter are excreted, in part, because lead inhibits the uptake of iron by immature red blood cells and has a direct inhibitory effect on ferrochelatase.

It may be noted that although the human organism is capable of degrading metal-containing porphyrins such as heme, it has no means of degrading porphyrins containing no metal, for example coproporphyrins and uroporphyrins. These must be excreted as such. The latter two are water-soluble and are thus found in urine and to some extent in the feces. Protoporphyrins, however, are largely water-insoluble and are excreted in the feces. Finally, it may be mentioned that porphyrias make their appearance after puberty. This has been associated with the appearance of 5β-steroid reductases, as discussed above.

7.3.2 Heme Degradation

As senescent red blood cells are removed from circulation and destroyed by reticuloendothelial cell systems (e.g., splenocytes and Kupffer cells), heme too is degraded. The first step in heme degradation appears to be the oxidation of iron from the ferrous to the ferric state to yield methemoglobin. Then, under the influence of microsomal heme oxidase, hematin is hydroxylated to hydroxyheme and the ring is opened to yield CO (carbon monoxide) and the bilverdin–iron complex. The latter loses iron to yield the green biliverdin (see Figure 7.15). Biliverdin is reduced to the orange-yellow water-insoluble bilirubin, which is picked up by serum albumin and transported into liver cells. In the hepatocyte, bilirubin is conjugated with one or two molecules of glucoronic acid to make it water-soluble and then transported across the cell membrane into bile canaliculi to be exported into the small intestine via the bile duct.

In the small intestine, bilirubin is deconjugated and reduced to three substances collectively called urobilinogens that differ from each other in their degrees of oxidation (double bonds). Urobilinogens are to some extent absorbed from the small intestine. In the lower intestinal tract, urobilinogens may be reoxidized into urobilins, which give the stool its characteristic brown color. Figure 7.16 illustrates the movement of bilirubin and urobilinogen throughout the organism.

The rate of heme degradation is controlled by the levels of active heme oxidase. Its activity is dependent upon cellular heme levels: the higher the heme content, the more active is heme oxidase.

The human bloodstream contains both unconjugated (albumin-bound) and conjugated bilirubin. Their total concentration ranges from 0.2 to 1.0 mg/dL, of which conjugated bilirubin accounts for 0–0.2 mg/dL. Normally, little if any conjugated bilirubin is found in the urine. But a 24-hr urine sample may contain 0.5–4 mg of urobilinogen. Feces normally produce 250–350 mg of urobilin and urobilinogen per day. These values are drastically changed in liver or hemolytic disease, so their determination serves as a valuable diagnostic tool.

Conjugated and unconjugated bilirubin concentrations in serum may be measured via the van den Bergh reaction. The conjugated bilirubin reacts directly with diazotized sulfanylic acid and is thus termed "direct bilirubin." Unconjugated (albumin-bound) bilirubin does not react with the reagent unless the serum is treated with alcohol, and its concentration is thus termed "indirect bilirubin." The determination of direct and indirect serum bilirubin, as well as

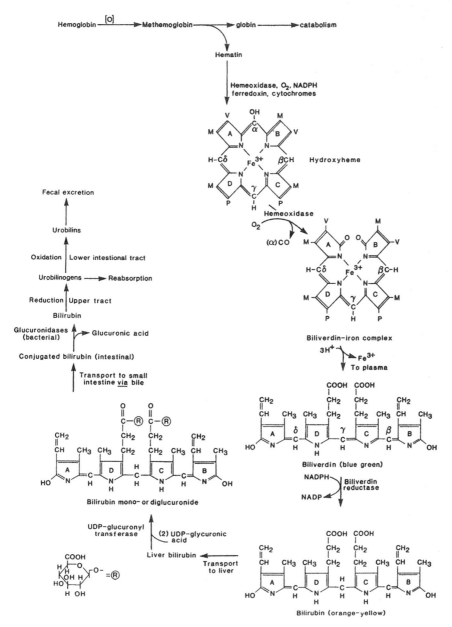

Figure 7.15 Degradation of heme and bilirubin metabolism. M, methyl; V, vinyl; P, propyl.

urine bilirubin and urobilinogen, can give valuable information with respect to liver and other diseases. In prehepatic jaundice, which may be caused by increased rates of red cell destruction such as are found in hemolytic anemia and erythroblastosis fetalis (Rh disease), a large amount of indirect bilirubin is present in serum. It is conjugated in the liver at a rapid pace and is excreted into the bile duct. As a result, fecal urobilinogen will be high, as will be urine uro-

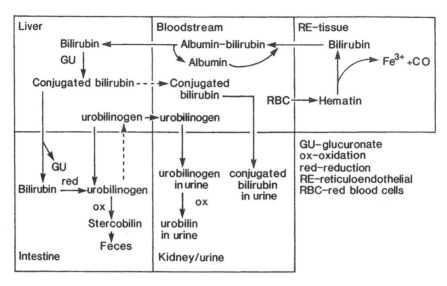

Figure 7.16 Movement of bilirubin and its metabolic products through the various tissues. GU is glucuronic acid, red is reduction, ox is oxidation, and RBC is red blood cells.

bilinogen. In posthepatic jaundice, caused by obstruction of the bile duct by a stone or tumor, direct bilirubin in the serum is high, and fecal and urinary urobilinogens are low. Urinary bilirubin will also be high.

Hepatic jaundice is more complex than either pre- or posthepatic jaundice. It is caused by liver disease, and the bilirubin–urobilinogen profile may depend on the stage of the disease. In the early stages of hepatitis, for instance, the hepatocyte is not capable of internalizing all the reabsorbed urobilinogen, and the latter appears in large quantities in the bloodstream and urine. As the disease progresses and liver swells, thus shutting off bile drainage, no conjugated bilirubin gets into the intestinal tract. The result is a dearth of urobilinogen in the feces (clay-colored stool) and large quantities of conjugated bilirubin in the bloodstream and urine. As the swelling subsides, conjugated bilirubin enters the intestine and urobilinogen is produced in large amounts. The urine once again contains higher then normal urobilinogen levels.

There are three congenital anomalies of bilirubin metabolism that cause bilirubin levels in the bloodstream to be abnormally high. In Gilbert's disease, unconjugated bilirubin is increased in the bloodstream. It is believed that there is some defect in the mechanism of bilirubin transport into the liver cells in this disease. In the case of the Crigler-Najjar syndrome, the level of the enzyme catalyzing the conjugation of bilirubin, that is, liver uridine diphosphate (UDP): glucuronyl transferase, is very low, so that large amounts of unconjugated bilirubin are present in the bloodstream. In the Dubin-Johnson syndrome, there is a defect in the conjugated bilirubin excretion into the bile canaliculi. The result is a mild increase in plasma conjugated bilirubin levels.

A condition similar to the Crigler-Najjar syndrome, though of only a temporary nature, is neonatal jaundice, which exists when the newborn (especially a

premature newborn) does not have a functional liver UDP-glucuronyl transferase. Indirect bilirubin may rise to 15–20 mg/dL or higher. Immediate treatment involves putting the patient under an ultraviolet light lamp. This induces
the isomerization of water-insoluble bilirubin (termed the Z-isomer) to the water-
soluble E-isomer. The latter can then be cleared by the kidneys. Blood exchange
transfusion is required if bilirubin levels exceed 15–20 mg/dL. If untreated,
bilirubin in such cases enters the brain cells, causing the condition kernicterus,
which results in nerve cell degeneration.

7.4 PLASMA PROTEINS ASSOCIATED WITH HEMOGLOBIN PHYSIOLOGY

7.4.1 Haptoglobin and Hemopexin

Haptoglobin is a glycoprotein that combines avidly with hemoglobin released
from hemolyzed red blood cells according to the equation

$$\alpha_2^A \beta_2^A \rightarrow 2\ \alpha^A \beta^A \xrightarrow{Hp} Hp - \alpha^A \beta^A \xrightarrow{\alpha^A \beta^A} \alpha^A\ \beta^A - Hp - \alpha^A \beta^A \tag{7.10}$$

Here, Hp designates haptoglobin and $\alpha_2^A \beta_2^A$ designates hemoglobin. This
shows that hemoglobin dissociates into dimers before it can combine with
haptoglobin. The hemoglobin–haptoglobin complex is rapidly taken up by
hepatocytes and is catabolized. Plasma haptoglobin levels are drastically decreased in hemolytic disease because of the combination of haptoglobin with
hemoglobin and is increased in various inflammatory conditions. The latter
acute phase response involves several other plasma glycoproteins. Acute phase
response is generated by such conditions as infectious disease (e.g., tuberculo-
sis), cancer, and arthritis. Physiologically, the combination of haptoglobin with
hemoglobin is an antimicrobial device. By removing hemoglobin from plasma,
haptoglobin ensures that heme iron is made unavailable for any microorganisms
whose virulence may be increased by the availability of heme or iron. Hemopexin, a plasma glycoprotein with a molecular weight of 57,000, binds free
hematin for the same antimicrobial purposes. Hematin may find its way into
plasma from reticuloendothelial cells, where it is generated when methemoglobin is degraded to bilirubin.

In 1955, Smithies noted that purified haptoglobin samples moved as a
series of components when subjected to electrophoresis in starch gel. These are
now referred to as protein polymorphs. All haptoglobins can be categorized into
the three groups 1-1 (homozygous), 2-2 (homozygous), and 2-1 (heterozygous).
Their electrophoretic patterns are shown in Figure 7.17. Genetically, haptoglobin
biosynthesis is controlled by two allelic genes. Chemically, there are three types
of polypeptide chains associated with haptoglobins: α^1 (MW 9000), α^2 (MW
18,000), and β (MW 41,000). The α^2 chain is a product of the fusion of two α^1
genes. Haptoglobin 1-1 consists of two α^1 and two β chains; haptoglobin 2-1 is a
series of $\alpha^1\beta \cdot \alpha^2\beta$ oligomers; and haptoglobin 2-2 is a series of $\alpha^1\beta$ oligomers. Such
oligomers are held together by disulfide bonds. Since haptoglobin types are an
inherited characteristic, haptoglobins can be used for forensic purposes. Most
plasma proteins show polymorphism in gel electrophoretic systems.

Figure 7.17 Gel electrophoresis of haptoglobins. Haptoglobin 1-1 moves as a single component, whereas the other two types show genetically derived polymorphisms. Hemoglobin-binding activity is identical in the three types.

7.4.2 Transferrin and Iron Metabolism

Transferrin is a single-chain glycoprotein that binds 2 g-atoms of ferric iron per mole of protein. The iron is chelated via tyrosyl and histidyl residues, and the complex is extremely stable at physiologic pH. The function of transferrin is to transport iron throughout the human organism, especially to the immature red cells, which cannot effectively acquire iron for the biosynthesis of hemoglobin unless it is presented to them in combination with transferrin. Specific transferrin receptors are present on the surface of such immature red cells as well as in all other tissues. Receptor-mediated endocytosis (see Chapter 9) is believed to be the main means of transferrin-bound iron entry into cells. Transferrin is also believed to be antimicrobial because it withholds iron from microorganisms.

Under normal circumstances, transferrin is one-fourth to one-third saturated with iron. The level of saturation may decrease in systemic infection or cancer and in iron deficiency anemia, the most common nutritional deficiency in the United States. In individuals with iron deficiency anemia, transferrin levels are increased. The level of saturation with iron increases in iron overload syndromes such as hereditary hemochromatosis or as a result of repeated blood transfusions, as is the case in thalassemia patients. Determinations of total plasma iron (TI) and plasma total iron binding capacity (TIBC) are routinely performed in the clinical biochemistry laboratory. The TIBC value reflects transferrin levels in plasma: the amount of iron that can be bound by transferrin is equal to TIBC × 0.7. Total plasma iron levels in iron deficiency anemia become abnormal before hemoglobin levels show any change.

Iron is best absorbed in the ferrous form or as heme. It is believed that transferrin, transported into the small intestine from the liver via bile, carries iron into the intestinal mucosal cells. Though about 16 mg of iron enter these cells every day, only 1–2 mg finds its way into the bloodstream. The rest remains bound to an iron storage protein called ferritin and is eventually lost in the feces in the normal sloughing-off process. Iron absorption also depends on its bioavailability, for example its ability to be released from other food substances with which it is associated. Phytate, for example, which is a common component of plant foods, inhibits metal absorption and lowers iron bioavailability.

During a 24-hr period, a total of about 35 mg of iron is turned over through the plasma compartment, even though total plasma iron amounts to only about 4 mg. Most of the iron (about 28 mg/day) goes to the blood-forming tissues for hemoglobin synthesis. At the same time, about 28 mg of iron is returned to the plasma from the reticuloendothelial tissues. About 4 mg/day is exchanged with iron storage sites, especially the liver, 3 mg/day is exchanged with various other extracellular fluids, and 1–2 mg/day is absorbed and excreted. The human organism has about 4 g of iron distributed as follows: about 70% in hemoglobin, 20% in storage combined with ferritin, and 5% in myoglobin. It is also present in various cytochromes and numerous heme and nonheme enzymes and proteins. Among the latter are the iron-sulfur proteins, the ferredoxins. Iron is associated with cysteine residues and elemental sulfur in ferredoxins. These proteins are used in various redox reactions.

Ferritin is an iron storage protein present in all tissues. It consists of 24 subunits of two types that differ from each other in amino acid content and size and are present in different combinations. The molecular weights are 19,000 and 21,000, and the entire molecule (less iron) has a molecular weight ranging from 400,000 to 500,000, depending on its tissue of origin. Iron can add as much as 20% to this molecular weight value. Iron in ferritin is present in the form of ferric hydroxide–phosphate micelles. Ferritin is present in the circulation in nanogram amounts. It is of considerable diagnostic importance because its plasma levels reflect iron stores (ferritin bound). Ferritin levels are high in patients with iron overload syndrome and low in those with iron deficiency anemia. Serum ferritin determinations are especially useful in determining early stages of iron deficiency anemia; they change downward before the TI or hemoglobin level shows any change. Iron parameters in the iron-overloaded and iron-deficient organism are summarized in Table 7.4.

Table 7.4 Iron Parameters in Iron Deficiency and Overload

Parameter	Normal range	Iron deficiency	Idiopathic hemochromatosis
Iron stones	0.5–1.5 g	None	Up to 50 g
Iron absorption (mg/day)	1–2	10–20	High
Serum total iron (μg/dL)	120	15	250
Serum total iron-binding capacity[a] (μ/dL)	350	475[b]	263[c]
Serum ferritin (ng/mL)	12–250	<10	>1000

[a]These are average values.
[b]Reflects increased serum transferrin levels.
[c]It is almost equal to TI. The low TIBC reflects lower serum transferrin level because of possible liver damage.
Source: Data mostly from Pollycove M, Hemochromatosis. In The Metabolic Basis of Inherited Disease, 4th ed. Stanbury JB, Wyngardeu JB, Frederickson DS, Eds. New York: McGraw-Hill, 1978, pp. 1127–1164.

7.5   PLASMA PROTEINS

7.5.1   Introduction

Human plasma contains over 200 individual proteins. Some of these have been discussed above, and Table 7.5 summarizes the properties of the major plasma proteins. The most convenient way of looking at plasma proteins is by employing the various types of electrophoresis (Chapter 4). The moving-boundary system is shown in Figure 4.12, which indicates that serum may be separated into five protein components. Only one, albumin, is a pure protein. The others are mixtures of proteins. Electrophoretic mobilities of various plasma proteins are also indicated in Table 7.5. Thus, the γ-globulin component consists of a variety of immunoglobulins of the IgG type. Taken together, these immunoglobulins consti-

Table 7.5   Properties of Some Plasma Proteins[a]

Protein	Concentration in plasma (mg/dL)	Molecular weight	Electrophoretic mobility at pH of 8.6	Function
Albumin	3500–5500	66,000	Albumin	Osmotic pressure; transport
Prealbumin	10–40	61,000	Albumin	Binds thyroxine
α_1-Antitrypsin	210–500	45,000	α_1-Globulin	Inhibits elastase
Orosomucoid	75–100	42,000	α_1-Globulin	Binds some steroids
TBG	1–2	58,000	α_1-Globulin	Binds thyroxine
Transcortin	7	52,000	α_1-Globulin	Binds steroids
Haptoglobin				
Type 1-1	95–212	90,000	α_2-Globulin	Binds hemoglobin
Type 2-2	95–212	360,000	α_2-Globulin	Binds hemoglobin
Ceruloplasmin	20–45	140,000	α_2-Globulin	Binds copper, amine, and iron oxidase
α_2-Macroglobulin	150–420	820,000	α_2-Globulin	Inhibits trypsin and plasmin
Transferrin	200–400	80,000	β-Globulin	Binds iron
Hemopexin	70–130	57,000	β-Globulin	Binds free hematin
Plasminogen	20–40	87,000	β-Globulin	Activated to plasmin, which lyses fibrin
Prothrombin	150	72,000	β-Globulin	Activated in thrombin, which clots fibrinogen
Complement[b]	100–200	—	β-Globulin	Enters into immune reactions
Fibrinogen	200–450	340,000	β-Globulin	Clots to give fibrin
Immunoglobulin A	90–450	$\geq$ 160,000	β-Globulin	Immunity
Immunoglobulin M	60–280	10^6	β-Globulin	Immunity
Immunoglobulin G	800–1800	160,000	γ-Globulin	Immunity

[a]Does not include lipoproteins. Their properties are discussed in Chapter 19.
[b]Consists of nine components.

tute the second most abundant component of serum proteins. Other immuno-globulin types, IgA and IgM, have β-globulin mobility. The β-globulin group also contains transferrin, a lipoprotein called LDL (Chapter 19), plasminogen, and prothrombin. Among the α_2-globulins are ceruloplasmin and haptoglobin, while α_1-globulins include some hormone-carrying proteins and α_1-antitrypsin.

Most serum proteins as well as fibrinogen (a plasma protein) have been isolated and thoroughly characterized. Individual serum proteins can be isolated by an array of procedures that depend on their size, shape, net charge, and solubility under a variety of conditions. Among such techniques are the stepwise precipitation of proteins with salts ("salting out"), chromatography on cation and anion exchangers, fractionation with organic solvents such as ethanol or ether, and gel filtration on media of specific porosities. All plasma proteins except the immunoglobulins are synthesized in the liver.

7.5.2   Albumin

Albumin is the most abundant serum protein. Its main function is to serve as a regulator of blood osmotic pressure and to act as a carrier of small water-insoluble molecules. About 75% of the total osmotic pressure of serum is attribut-able to albumin. Due to its low molecular weight, albumin is one of the first serum proteins to appear in the urine after kidney damage, and in some forms of serious kidney diseases serum albumin levels may fall to as low as 0.8 g/dL, with up to 60 g of albumin being excreted in the urine in 1 day. When such albumin losses occur, the patient will develop a condition termed edema, in which, owing to the decreased osmotic pressure of blood, water will move into intersti-tial spaces of the extremities and other parts of the organism, causing swelling. Edema also occurs during malnutrition, because albumin is preferentially broken down to provide essential amino acids for the maintenance of the organism's vital processes. Serum albumin level are determined to assess a patient's protein nutritional state.

Albumin also acts as a transport medium for a variety of substances. It is the principal, if not the only, means of transport for free bilirubin (breakdown product of heme) and free fatty acids. It also binds calcium ions, hematin, ste-roids, thyroxine, and various drugs and dyes.

The biosynthesis of serum albumin takes place in the liver. Normally, its half-life in the human being is 19 days, though this may change in response to disease or dietary availability of essential amino acids. It is interesting to note that rat serum albumin is biosynthesized in the form of "proalbumin," that is, the basic albumin molecule has attached to its N-terminus a peptide, Arg-Gly-Val-Phe-Arg-Arg, which is lost upon the secretion of the protein into the ex-tracellular compartment.

7.5.3   Fibrinogen, Blood Coagulation, and Fibrinolysis

Fibrinogen is a rather asymmetric molecule that consists of three pairs of identi-cal polypeptide chains, called the α, β, and γ chains (MW 63,500, 56,000, and 47,000, respectively). Blood coagulation is initiated by the action of thrombin on fibrinogen, whereby two small peptides are removed from the fibrinogen. This permits fibrinogen molecules to aggregate via physical interactions to form fibrin. This aggregate is linear (head-to-head) and has the properties of a soft gel. Further polymerization to form tough insoluble clots is accomplished by a specific enzyme called factor XIII, which forms peptide linkages between the ε-amino groups of one fibrin monomer and the τ-carboxyl groups of another. This serves to join a number of linear fibrin polymers to form cross-linked fibrin lattices.

Thrombin (MW 39,000) is a proteolytic enzyme of the serine protease group. It is derived from prothrombin, a circulating plasma protein, through the proteolytic action of a complex consisting of the proteolytic enzyme factor X (or factor X_a), another protein called factor V (accelerator protein), calcium, and phospholipid. Factor V has recently been identified as the plasma copper protein ceruloplasmin or a similar protein (see Chapter 6).

Factor X (Stuart factor) is present in plasma in the inactive form. It may be activated by the proteolytic removal of a peptide by a tissue protein–phospholipid complex (often called thromboplastin) and the activated form of factor VII in the presence of Ca^{2+}. This means of activating factor X is termed the extrinsic coagulation system. Factor X may also be activated by a complex between activated factor IX (factor IX_a) and factor VIII (the antihemophilic factor). Factor IX (Christmas factor) is activated by active factor XI, and factor XI is activated by active factor XII (Hageman factor). The latter series of events is termed the *intrinsic coagulation system*. Thus, the entire blood coagulation cascade consists of a series of proteolytic steps, and most of the inactive coagulation factors are really zymogens. Exceptions are factors V and VIII, which are called *accessory proteins*. Absence of factor VIII causes classic hemophilia, which accounts for about 80% of all hemophilias known. Absence of factor IX is the cause of hemophilia B (Christmas disease), which accounts for 10–20% of all hemophilias. Hemophilia C, the absence of factor XI, accounts for the rest of hemophilias. A number of coagulation factors bind Ca^{2+} and therefore contain τ-carboxyglutamic acid. Their biosynthesis requires vitamin K (see Chapter 6). These are prothrombin (factor II) and factors VII, IX, and X. The rationale for giving vitamin K antagonists (e.g., warfarin) to patients to prevent the formation of blood clots is that they partially inhibit the biosynthesis of these coagulation factors. Coagulation may be prevented in vitro by Ca^{2+} chelators such as citrate, ethylenediaminetetraacetic acid (EDTA), and heparin. These are used to collect plasma rather than serum samples after the blood is drawn.

Once fibrin is formed, the coagulation factors are removed from the bloodstream via rapid catabolism by liver cells and the presence of coagulation factor inhibitors in plasma. Of special importance is the thrombin inhibitor, which is a protein with a molecular weight of 65,000. Fibrin clots themselves are gradually removed by the proteolytic enzyme plasmin, which is a serine protease. It is produced from a circulating precursor called plasminogen by the proteolytic removal of a peptide though the action of the tissue plasminogen activating factor, which is produced largely by endothelial cells. This factor is now used to dissolve clots in coronary arteries in myocardial infarction patients. Other substances that can activate plasminogen to plasmin are urokinase, produced by the kidneys and excreted in the urine, and streptokinase of bacterial origin. Plasmin digests fibrin clots into fragments with molecular weights of 55,000–85,000. It is eventually inactivated by plasma α_2-antiplasmin, a potent

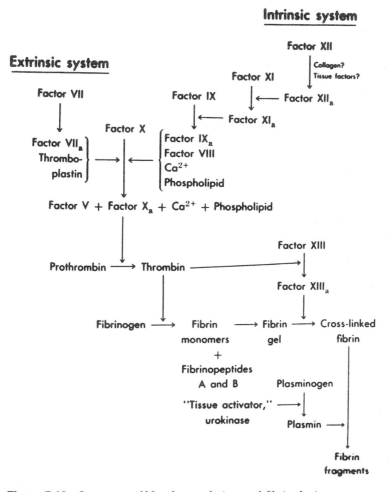

Figure 7.18 Summary of blood coagulation and fibrinolysis processes.

plasma proteolytic enzyme inhibitor. The dissolution of fibrin clots is called fibrinolysis. The blood coagulation cascade and fibrinolysis are summarized in Figure 7.18.

7.5.4 Miscellaneous Notes on Plasma Proteins

Several of the major plasma proteins listed in Table 7.5 have been discussed in this chapter, and others (e.g., prealbumin and ceruloplasmin) were discussed in Chapter 6. Immunoglobulins will be dealt with in Chapter 14. It should be mentioned that plasma contains a number of hormone-binding proteins, examples being the thyroxine-binding globulin (TBG) and the steroid-binding proteins transcortin and α-1 acid glycoprotein (orosomucoid). A very important glycoprotein from a diagnostic point of view is α_1-antitrypsin, whose job is to protect lung tissue against proteolytic damage. It is especially active against the enzyme *elastase* released by neutrophils. Smoking increases neutrophil levels in the lung and hence the release of elastase. At the same time, smoking decreases

α_1-antitrypsin levels in the bloodstream. Smokers are thus especially susceptible to lung damage by elastase, the result being the development of emphysema. α_1-Antitrypsin levels of emphysema patients are almost always below normal and can serve as a diagnostic tool for this disease. Lipoproteins are an important group of plasma proteins that will be discussed in Chapter 19.

Plasma (serum) contains a number of enzymes released by various tissues of the organism. Such enzyme levels are increased in specific disease processes when organ damage occurs. Serum enzyme determinations are therefore valuable diagnostic tools; they were discussed in Chapter 5. Another cellular component that appears in the bloodstream is myoglobin (Mb). It is commonly determined when myocardial infarction is suspected in a patient. Normal blood myoglobin levels are 10–70 μg/L, whereas in an infarcted patient it rises to 500–1000 μg/L. Maximum levels of blood Mb are seen between 8 and 12 hr following infarction, which is sooner than the peaking of creatine phosphokinase (see Chapter 5).

A series of proteins collectively called the complement participate in the immune response to the entry of foreign cellular or viral material into the organism. This group of proteins consists of about 20 entities, some of which are enzymes. Complement was first associated with the lysis of foreign red blood cells in the nineteenth century; it also participates in the lysis of bacterial cells. The complement activation cascade, very similar to the blood coagulation cascade, involves the stepwise activation, via proteolysis, of various components of the complement system until a final protein complex, the membrane attack unit (also called the C5b-9 complex), is generated. It then punches holes in the membrane to which it is bound.

The complement cascade (Figure 17.19) is initiated in two ways: by the classic pathway and by the alternative pathway. In the former, as immunoglobulins of the G or M type (see Chapter 14) are bound to an antigen, the complement-binding site on the CH2 domain of IgG is exposed to the environment and binds a subunit of the C1 component of the complement series. This subunit is called the C1q protein; it has a molecular weight of about 460,000, and it has a collagen-like amino acid sequence and helical arrangement (see Chapter 8). The IgG (or IgM)-bound C1q leads to the activation of another subunit of C1, namely C1r, which initiates a stepwise process leading to the activation of C5. The alternative pathway also leads to the activation of C5; however, it is initiated nonspecifically without an IgG– or IgM–antigen complex. The alternative pathway is activated by polysaccharides (e.g., on bacterial cell walls), by bacterial endotoxins, and by IgA complexes. C1 components are not involved in this process. The pathway from activated C5 to the formation of the C5b-9 complex is termed the terminal or final pathway.

Activated components of complement are also involved in attracting neutrophils and macrophages to the area where the foreign material is located. Some activated complement components, when bound to the foreign cell membrane, will favor phagocytosis by phagocytes. A more detailed discussion of the complement system is beyond the scope of this book, and the interested student is directed to standard immunology texts for more information.

The clinical biochemistry laboratory often determines total serum protein content and the albumin/globulin (A/G) ratio. A normal ambulatory adult will

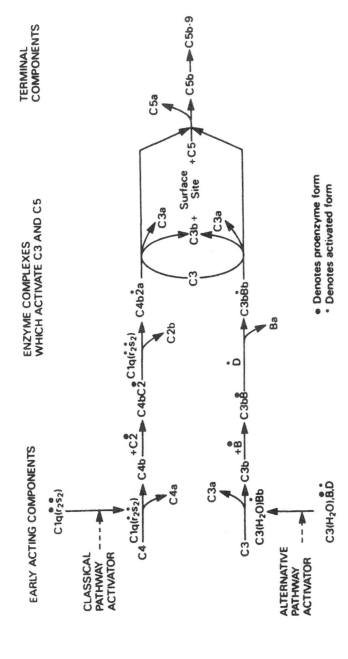

Figure 7.19 The complement cascade. r and s denote C1r and C1s components of the C1 protein complex. (Reproduced by permission from Campbell RD, Law SKA, Reid KBM, Sim RB. Structure, organization, and regulation of the complement genes. Annu Rev Immunol 6:161–195, 1988.)

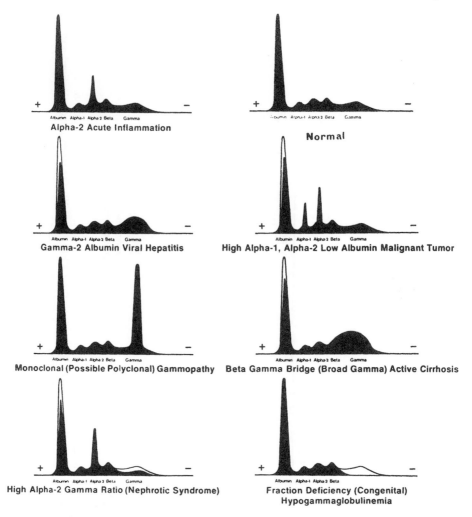

Figure 7.20 Serum protein electrophoresis in the normal state and in some disease states. (Reproduced by permission from a circular by the Gelman Instrument Co., Ann Arbor, MI.)

show a total protein value (determined by the biuret reaction) of 6.4–8.3 g/dL. Serum albumin accounts for 3.5–5.0 g/dL, and the rest is "globulin," which may be calculated by subtracting the albumin value from the total protein value if albumin has been determined independently. More often, the serum protein profile is arrived at by determining total protein and the electrophoretic distribution of the five serum fractions: albumin and α_1-, α_2-, β-, and γ-globulins. Normal mean values are, in percent of total protein, 58%, 3%, 11%, 12%, and 16%, respectively. The mean normal A/G ratio is therefore 1.36, with a normal range of 1.2–1.6. These values will change in various disease processes, for instance in the nephrotic syndrome, where albumin levels are low and α_2-globulin levels are high. This will result in a low A/G ratio. Serum protein patterns in some disease states are illustrated in Figure 7.20.

QUESTIONS

For Questions 7.1 and 7.2, refer to the following information. A patient had a total protein of 6.4 g/dL, and serum electrophoresis shows the following distributions for albumin and α_1-, α_2-, β-, and γ-globulins: 66%, 1%, 11%, 13%, 9%.

7.1. What is the A/G ratio of the patient's serum?
  a. 1.5
  b. 1.9
  c. 0.52
  d. 1.2
  e. 7.3

7.2. Which are the proteins that are most likely lacking or are in excess in the patient's serum? (Refer to Table 7.5.)
  a. Albumin is in excess, Ig G low, other proteins normal.
  b. All proteins are too low (protein-losing syndrome).
  c. Albumin is high, other proteins are normal.
  d. Transferrin and albumin are high, all other proteins are normal.
  e. α_1-Antitrypsin is low, Ig G low, other proteins normal.

7.3. A patient has highly elevated serum indirect bilirubin and urine urobilinogen and a very slightly elevated serum direct bilirubin. What is the most likely diagnosis?
  a. Neonatal jaundice
  b. Posthepatic jaundice
  c. Hemolytic jaundice
  d. Acute stage of viral hepatitis
  e. Crigler-Najjar syndrome

7.4. Venous blood has greater quantities of certain chemicals than arterial blood. Which is *not* present in greater quantity in venous blood?
  a. Carbamino hemoglobin
  b. Glycosylated hemoglobin
  c. Bicarbonate
  d. Dissolved CO_2
  e. T-forms of hemoglobin

7.5. Which statement is not correct for heme oxidase?
  a. Is controlled by cellular heme levels
  b. Splits the heme ring to biliverdin-Fe^{3+} and CO_2
  c. Is present in reticuloendothelial cells
  d. Introduces oxygen into the hematin ring structure
  e. Does not degrade protoporphyrin IX

7.6. Iron deficiency anemia can be detected by measuring which of the following in the red blood cells?
  a. Zinc hemoglobin
  b. Copper hemoglobin
  c. Protoporphyrin IX
  d. a and b
  e. a and c

7.7. Which porphyrin is found in urine and/or feces if uroporphyrinogen III cosynthase is defective in a patient?
  a. Protoporphyrinogen IX
  b. Uroporphyrin III
  c. Uroporphyrin I
  d. Coproporphyrin I
  e. Two of the above

7.8.   Cellular heme levels control the biosynthesis of heme. Which is an incorrect state-
       ment in regard to this process?
   a.   The action of heme can be counteracted to some extent by erythropoietin.
   b.   Heme inhibits the transport of δ-aminolevulinate synthase into mitochondria.
   c.   The action of heme may be counteracted to some extent by certain 4,5-
        dihydrosteroids.
   d.   Heme activates a repressor protein that inhibits δ-minolevulinate synthase
        translation.
   e.   High levels of heme channel porphyrin biosynthesis toward uroporphyrinogen
        I (symmetric), which is then excreted in the urine.

Suppose you get the following data for a hemoglobin that you have isolated from a
patient.

$Y(HbO_2/Hb)$	pO_2
25.1	39.8
6.3	15.8
1.6	6.3
0.40	2.5

Answer Questions 7.9–7.11.

7.9.   The Hill coefficient is
   a. 1.0   d. 2.8
   b. 1.5   e. 3.5
   c. 20

7.10. What is the P_{50}?
   a. 4.6   d. 24
   b. 5.8   e. 29.8
   c. 10.8

7.11. What type of hemoglobin have you isolated?
   a.   Negative subunit cooperativity, higher than normal O_2 affinity
   b.   Normal hemoglobin
   c.   Positive subunit cooperativity, lower than normal O_2 affinity
   d.   Positive subunit cooperativity, higher than normal O_2 affinity
   e.   Little or no subunit cooperativity, higher than normal O_2 affinity

7.12. If coprophyrinogen III decarboxylase (oxidase) were defective in a porphyria pa-
       tient, which compound would be least likely to be found in the feces or urine of the
       patient?
   a. Uroporphyrin I   d. Porphobilinogen
   b. Coproporphyrin III   e. Protoporphyrin IX
   c. Uroporphyrin III

7.13. A patient's serum sample has a TI of 55 mg/dL and a TIBC of 657 mg/dL. What is
       the transferrin content (mg/dL) of the sample and what is its percent saturation
       with iron? Molecular weight of transferrin is 80,000; atomic weight of iron is 56.
   a. 328 mg/dL and 12%   d. 293 mg/dL and 33%
   b. 293 mg/dL and 25%   e. 328 mg/dL and 45%
   c. 243 mg/dL and 33%

7.14. Interpretation of the results in Question 7.13 is that
   a.   The patient is normal.
   b.   The patient is iron-overloaded.
   c.   The patient is iron-deficient.

d. The patient is normal, though he is synthesizing too much transferrin.

e. None of the above.

In Questions 7.15–7.21 use the following key:

a. 1, 2, and 3 are correct.

b. 1 and 3 are correct.

c. 2 and 4 are correct.

d. 4 is correct.

e. All are correct.

7.15. The Bohr effect in hemoglobin physiology is associated with

1. $CO_2 + H_2O \rightarrow H_2CO_3 \rightarrow H^+ + HCO_3^-$

2. The buffering capacity of hemoglobin

3. The reversible ionization of certain amino and imidazole residues

4. Combination of CO_2 with hemoglobin to form carbamino adducts

7.16. Carbon dioxide generated in peripheral tissue is transported to the lungs via the bloodstream as

1. Carbamino residues

2. "Dissolved" CO_2

3. Bicarbonate ions

4. Carbonate ions

7.17. Differences between oxy- and deoxyhemoglobins:

		Oxy-Hb	Deoxy Hb
1.	2,3-DPG	Bound	Not bound
2.	R forms	Predominating	Rare
3.	Form of iron	Fe^{3+}	Fe^{2+}
4.	Isoelectric point	6.7	7.6

7.18. Potential antimicrobial proteins are

1. Haptoglobin

2. Hemopexin

3. Transferrin

4. Ferritin

7.19. In sickle cell anemia

1. Glutamate in position 6 of the β-chain of HbA is substituted by valine.

2. HbS is present in red cells, which electrophoretically moves more slowly than HbA.

3. Red cell shapes are distorted and asymmetric.

4. HbS forms gel polymers in oxygenated form.

7.20. Iron absorption

1. Involves the production of transferrin by the intestinal mucosal cell, which sequesters iron in the gut and brings it to the cells.

2. Occurs equally well from ferrous and ferric salts.

3. Is controlled mainly at the point of entry into the mucosal cells; of 16 mg Fe ingested daily, only 1–2 mg enter the intestinal mucosal cell.

4. May depend on iron "bioavailability"; though iron may be present in the diet, it may not be absorbed because of the presence of various binding agents such as phytate.

7.21. The uptake of iron by erythropoietic tissue involves

1. The transport of Fe^{2+} sequestered to amino acids across the cell membranes

2. Iron-saturated transferrin

3. Largely iron bound to circulating ferritin
4. The process of receptor-mediated endocytosis

In Questions 7.22 and 7.23, mark as follows:
    a. Transferrin   c. Both
    b. Ferritin   d. Neither

7.22.   Serum levels increased in iron deficiency anemia
7.23.   Bind(s) iron in the ferric state

In Questions 7.24–7.27 mark as follows:
    a. Hemoglobin   c. Both
    b. Myoglobin   d. Neither

7.24.   Binds oxygen and iron changes from Fe^{2+} to Fe^{3+}
7.25.   Oxygen is bound by iron component and the proximal histidyl residue
7.26.   The ancestral gene evolved at least 475 million years ago
7.27.   Bohr effect observed in

Answers

7.1.   (b)   If albumin represents 66% of total protein, then albumin is 4.2 g/dL and globulin is $6.4 - 4.2 = 2.2$ g/dL. A/G = 4.2/2.2 = 1.9.
7.2.   (e)   Comparing the values given to normal ranges, it is seen that α_1- and γ-globulins are low. IgG is a component of the γ-globulin group, and α_1-antitrypsin is a component of the α_1-globulin group. Albumin, as calculated in Question 7.1, is normal.
7.3.   (c)   As there is a lot of urine urobilinogen, the liver must be conjugating the bilirubin, and it is moved into the intestinal tract where urobilinogen is formed. An increase in serum indirect (unconjugated) bilirubin indicates hemolytic disease.
7.4.   (b)   By elimination; dissolved CO_2, bicarbonate, and carbamino groups are higher in venous blood, because CO_2 is being transported from the peripheral tissue to lungs via these vehicles. Venous blood, containing more deoxyhemoglobin than arterial blood, will have more T-forms.
7.5.   (b)   Heme oxidase produces CO, not CO_2, from heme.
7.6.   (e)   In iron deficiency anemia, red blood cells contained increased quantities of Zn-hemoglobin and protoporphyrin IX.
7.7.   (e)   Uroporphyrin I and coproporphyrin I will be present in the urine. In the absence of uroporphyrinogen cosynthase, hydroxymethyl bilane will spontaneously cyclyze into uroporphyrinogen I. Some of it will be oxidized to uroporphyrin I. Some will be decarboxylated by uroporphyrinogen decarboxylase to coproporphyrinogen I and then oxidized to coproporphyrin I. None of these will be degraded by heme oxidase.
7.8.   (e)   High levels of heme shut down ALA-synthase activity. Answer e is totally incorrect.

For Questions 7.9–7.11, first take logs of Y and pO_2 and plot log Y against pO_2. You will see a straight line.

7.9.   (b)   Calculate the Hill coefficient from the slope of the curve. For example,

$$n = \frac{y_1 - y_2}{x_1 - x_2} = \frac{1.4 - 0.2}{1.6 - 0.8} = \frac{1.2}{0.8} = 1.5$$

The Hill coefficient is 1.5.

7.10. (a) Determine P_{50} from the x intercept; it is 0.66, and the antilog of 0.66 = P_{50} = 4.6. Alternatively, the y intercept is -1. Since

$$-K' = n \log P_{50}, \quad \log P_{50} = -\frac{K'}{n} = \frac{1}{1.5} = 0.67, \quad \text{and } P_{50} = 4.6.$$

7.11. (d) As $n > 1$, there is positive cooperativity, but not to the same extent as in hemoglobin. As $P_{50} = 4.6$, which is between that of hemoglobin and myoglobin, the new hemoglobin has a high oxygen affinity.

7.12. (e) If coproporphyrinogen III decarboxylase (oxidase) was not functioning normally, there would be a shortage of protoporphyrinogen IX. Hence its oxidation product, protoporphyrin IX, would not be excreted. The four other compounds would be found in abnormal amounts in blood or feces.

7.13. (a) Iron that can be bound by transferrin is $657 \times 0.7 = 460$ μg/dL. Percent saturation with iron is therefore $55/460 \times 100 = 12\%$. Now, the amount of iron that can be bound by transferrin is $460/56 = 8.2$ μmol/dL. As transferrin binds a maximum of two atoms of Fe^{2+} per molecule, there must be $8.2/2 = 4.1$ μmol transferrin/dL. This is $4.1/1000 \times 80,000 = 328$ mg/dL.

7.14. (c) Normal range for TI is 50–160 μg/dL in males; TIBC is 250–400 μg/dL, and transferrin is 200–400 mg/dL (mean is 295). Even though TI is a low normal and transferrin is a high normal, saturation is only 12%, and we can conclude that the patient is mildly iron-deficient.

7.15. (a) 1, 2, and 3 are correct. Carbamino groups are not associated in any major way with the buffering of protons by hemoglobin.

7.16. (a) 1, 2, and 3 are correct. Carbonate is not found in the human bloodstream.

7.17. (c) 2 and 4 are correct. Oxyhemoglobin has a pI of 6.7, does not bind 2,3-DPG, and is largely in the R conformation. Neither hemoglobin contains Fe^{3+}.

7.18. (a) 1, 2, and 3 are correct. Haptoglobin removes hemoglobin, and transferrin mops up Fe^{3+} and even Fe^{2+}. These can increase bacterial virulence if not rapidly sequestered. Ferritin is not associated with antibacterial action.

7.19. (a) 1, 2, and 3 are correct. HbS forms gels with deoxygenated hemoglobin, making 4 wrong.

7.20. (d) Only 4 is correct. Transferrin used for iron absorption is produced in the liver. The ferrous form is absorbed best, and most available dietary iron may enter the intestinal mucosal cell. However, only 1–2 mg/day is transferred to the bloodstream.

7.21. (c) 2 and 4 are correct. Iron enters cells by the receptor-mediated endocytosis mechanism still bound to transferrin. In the cells, iron is separated from transferrin and the latter is exocytosed back into the medium.

7.22. (a) Transferrin levels increase in iron deficiency anemia. Ferritin levels decrease.

7.23. (c) Transferrin binds Fe^{3+} to its amino acid side-chains, while ferritin binds Fe^{3+} as ferric hydroxide micelles.

7.24. (d) In a normal oxygen-binding process, the valence of Fe does not change.

7.25. (d) Oxygen is bound up with iron and the distal histidyl group.

7.26. (b) Myoglobin is the oldest hemoglobin from an evolutionary point of view.

7.27. (a) The Bohr effect is not observed in myoglobin, because there are no subunits to interact with each other.

PROBLEMS

7.1. A 24-year-old female developed blistering sun-sensitive dermatosis. A medical history revealed that she was taking birth control pills and consumed moderate amounts of alcohol. Analysis of urine showed the presence of uroporphyrins, and the enzyme profile of her red blood cell lysates revealed a 50% deficiency in uroporphyrinogen III decarboxylase. Her serum iron levels were elevated. Address the following issues:

a. What disorder do you see in this patient?
b. Would you expect other analytes to be elevated in serum or urine?
c. What is the significance of birth control medication and alcohol consumption? What about serum iron?
d. To what are the skin lesions due?

7.2. A 27-year-old male had a high hematocrit and a high blood uric acid level. Though electrophoresis of red blood cell lysates showed no abnormality, isoelectric focusing indicated the presence of two kinds of hemoglobin in equal amounts. One of these was normal HbA, whereas the other was one not normally seen in red blood cells. Isolation of the latter showed that serine in the β-89 position was replaced by asparagine. A Hill plot of the unknown hemoglobin showed an x intercept of 1.20. The patient was treated with phlebotomy resulting in a marked improvement of his physical symptoms. Answer the following questions:

a. Why did isoelectric focusing separate the two hemoglobins, but electrophoresis did not?
b. Explain the differences in oxygen-binding properties of the normal and abnormal hemoglobins.
c. What are some of the causes of the observed behavior of the abnormal hemoglobin? Which is the most likely possibility here?

7.3. A 39-year-old woman developed progressive weakness in her muscles, fatigue, and headaches. Her blood hemoglobin was only 4 g/dL, her hematocrit at 15%, and her red cells contained high amounts of protoporphyrin IX. Her hemoglobin was normal. Total serum iron was 207 μg/dL. Her IgM and IgA were elevated, though not of the "monoclonal" type. Staining bone marrow cells for iron showed little if any iron. Administration of iron did not result in improvement. In spite of blood transfusions and other therapy, the patient deteriorated rapidly and even developed insulin-dependent diabetes. As "a last resort," she was treated with azathiopine, an immunosuppressor. She thereupon showed marked improvement and was eventually discharged with a supply of an immunosuppressant. Answer the following questions:

a. What did the serum iron determinations show?
b. What did negative staining of bone marrow results indicate?
c. What was indicated when she did not respond to iron supplementation?
d. What was the connection between her diabetes and the blood problem?
e. Pull it all together, and formulate a hypothesis of why this woman became ill.

BIBLIOGRAPHY

Brock JH, Halliday JW, Pippard MJ, Powell LW. Iron Metabolism in Health and Disease. London: WB Saunders, 1994.

Bunn HF, Forget BG. Hemoglobin: Molecular, Genetic, and Clinical Aspects. Philadelphia: WB Saunders, 1986.

Dickerson RE, Geis I. Hemoglobin: Structure, Function, Evolution, and Pathology. Menlo Park: Benjamin/Cummings, 1983.

8

Proteins with Biological Activity:
Fibrous Proteins

After completing this chapter, the student should

1. Understand the basic primary and secondary structures of collagen, including modes of cross-linking.
2. Know the biosynthetic sequence of events leading to tropocollagen and the collagen fibrils.
3. Know the different types of collagens, their properties, and where they occur.
4. Know the molecular basis of the various collagen diseases and deficiency diseases affecting collagen integrity.
5. Know the properties of elastin, mode of cross-linking, and the energetics for elastin stretching and relaxation.
6. Know the basic structures, functions, and occurrence of fibronectin and laminin.
7. Know the basic structure and organization of keratin and keratin filaments.
8. Understand the anatomy of the skeletal muscle cell, including all its components.
9. Understand the microscopic structure of the myofibril.
10. Know the structures of myosin and the thin filament and its components.
11. Understand the muscle contraction mechanism.
12. Know the energy sources for muscle contraction.
13. Understand the composition, structure, and function of microfilaments and microtubules.

8.1 COLLAGEN

8.1.1 Introduction

Connective tissue is a term applied to a conglomeration of substances that constitute the extracellular nonvascular space in various tissues of the organism. It serves to bind the cells together, to provide resiliency to tissues, and sometimes to serve as a vehicle for nutrient delivery to various types of cells. The connective tissue consists of ground substance in which are embedded blood vessels and the fibrous proteins collagen and elastin. There are a number of other proteins as well, for example fibronectin. The ground substance is made up of proteo-glycans, which are high molecular weight polysaccharides combined with pro-teins that account for as much as 30% of connective tissue weight. The nature of this material will be discussed in Chapter 9. In this chapter, we will examine the properties of connective tissue proteins and other proteins.

8.1.2 Collagen Structure

Collagen is the most abundant protein of the human organism, comprising about 30% of all body protein. It is present in large quantities in tissues that are high in "white" connective tissue—skin, cartilage, and bone—and is intimately associated with proteoglycans. In many ways, it is a very atypical protein. Its amino acid composition and secondary structure are, with some exceptions, unlike those of any other protein known. Native collagen is a relatively insoluble fibrous protein.

The basic unit, tropocollagen, can be prepared from native insoluble colla-gen by prolonged acid extraction. Tropocollagen is 3000 Å long and 14 Å thick and has a molecular weight of about 300,000. It consists of three polypeptide chains, each having over 1000 amino acid residues. The most prominent amino acid is glycine, which accounts for about one-third of all the amino acids in collagen. Proline and hydroxypoline (22%) and alanine (11%) are the next most abundant amino acids. In addition to hydroxyproline, collagen contains another amino acid, hydroxylysine, which rarely, if ever, occurs in other proteins. The typical amino acid sequence in a collagen polypeptide chain is Gly-X-Y, where proline may occupy positions X or Y but hydroxyproline may occupy position Y only. For example, the N-terminus of the α_1 chain of tropocollagen (see below) contains the following amino acid sequence: Gly-Pro-Met-Gly-Pro-Ser-Gly-Pro-Arg-Gly-Leu-Hyp-Gly-Pro-Hyp-Gly-Ala-Hyp-Gly-Pro-Glu-, etc.

The secondary structure of tropocollagen is helical on two levels: each polypeptide chain has a left-handed helical sense, with 3.3 amino acids per turn and a total linear distance of 9.6 Å per turn. This gives a pitch of 9.6/3.3 = 2.91 Å for each amino acid. Three such helical polypeptide chains are assembled into tropocollagen cables consisting of three intertwined polypeptide chains, forming a superhelix with a right-handed sense. The superhelix, and each subhelical component, has a total of about 29 turns (104 Å per turn). Each turn consists of 36 amino acids, giving a total of about 1044 amino acids per strand and a total of about 3100 amino acids per tropocollagen molecule. Moreover, the subhelices are arranged in the superhelix in such a way that the glycine residues are on the interior of the superhelix and in contact with each other. The X and Y residues face the environment and are therefore able to accommodate any bulky side chains. A cross section of the superhelix is illustrated in Figure 8.1.

In native collagen, individual tropocollagen molecules are assembled into microfibrils. Individual tropocollagen molecules interact laterally, not end to end. In fact, there is a 400 Å gap between tropocollagen molecules when they are aligned in a linear (head-to-tail) fashion. Electron microscopy has shown that

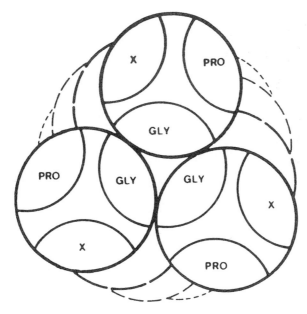

Figure 8.1 Cross section of a tropocollagen molecule showing the internal position of glycine residues and the external location of X and Y molecules. Proline is shown in position Y. (Reproduced by permission from Walton AG. Polypeptide and Protein Structure. New York: Elsevier, 1981, p. 309.)

collagen microfibrils are bonded, the bonds being perpendicular to the microfibril axis. The bands observed have a repeat of 670 Å in hydrated collagen. Such bands represent the "staggered" arrangement of tropocollagen molecules in a microfibril and include the gaps discussed above. This is illustrated in Figure 8.2. A summary of the different levels of structure making up a collagen microfibril is shown in Figure 8.3. Several microfibrils can associate into a fibril, and several fibrils form the collagen fiber. A fiber 1 mm in diameter can withstand a load of 10–40 kg before it breaks. Hence, the collagen infrastructure provides a final product with a tremendous amount of strength. When collagen is heated in aqueous solutions, however, much of it becomes denatured and goes into solution. When cooled, collagens in such solutions assume another type of structure, the result of which is gelatin.

Tropocollagen molecules become stabilized by forming hydrogen bonds. However, the special tensile strength of collagen fibers is partly provided by covalent interactions within the tropocollagen molecules themselves. Most important, such strength is provided by hydrogen bonds formed among the tropocollagen molecules within microfibrils and even among microfibrils making up the fibril structure. Cross-links require that aldehydes be synthesized from certain lysine and hydroxylysine residues of extracellularly located immature tropocollagen. These aldehydes are allysine and hydroxyallysine. They are formed at the N- and C-terminal regions of tropocollagen, regions that are called telopeptides. Telopeptides are relatively short; they do not contain the Gly-X-Y sequences and hence are not helical. Such aldehydes can form two types of linkages with uncharged lysine and hydroxylysine residues: Schiff bases and

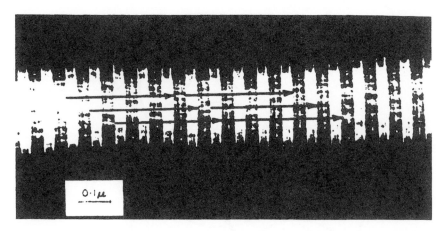

Figure 8.2 Electron microscopic image of a collagen microfibril. Superimposed on this are arrows representing tropocollagen molecules in the N to C direction. The gap between the N-terminus of one molecule and the C-terminus of another is 400 Å. The bands correspond to the gaps. (Reproduced by permission from Walton AG. Polypeptide and Protein Structure. New York: Elsevier, 1981, p. 116.)

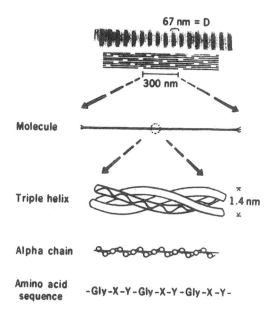

Figure 8.3 Organizational levels of the collagen microfibril showing individual polypeptide chain helices, arrangement of three such helices into the tropocollagen superhelix, and the "staggered" interaction among several tropocollagen molecules to form the microfibril. (Reproduced by permission from Eyre DR. Collagen: molecular diversity in the body's protein scaffold. Science 207:1315–1322, 1980.)

aldols. Aldol condensations (Equation 8.1) occur mostly between two allysine residues at the N-terminal end of a tropocollagen molecule:

$$-\text{Allysine}-\overset{\overset{\displaystyle O}{\|}}{C}-H + HO-C=CH-\text{allysine} \rightarrow -\text{allysine}-\overset{\overset{\displaystyle H}{|}}{C}=\overset{\overset{\displaystyle H}{|}}{C}-\text{allysine}- \quad (8.1)$$

Aldol form   Enol (alcohol) form $H-C=O$

The free carbonyl residue can further condense with a histidyl group of another polypeptide chain to give a more complex cross-link. Schiff base formation, illustrated in Figure 8.4, involves an allysine residue at either the C- or N-terminal telopeptide and an uncharged lysine or hydroxylysine residue of another properly juxtaposed tropocollagen molecule. Such bonds are therefore intermolecular. Several other types of covalent cross-links are possible in collagens. They almost always involve lysine, allysine, hydroxylysine, hydroxyallysine, or histidine.

The oxidation of lysine and hydroxylysine to allysine and hydroxyallysine is achieved with molecular oxygen and the action of lysyl oxidase (hydroxylase), an enzyme that contains copper and acts only on aggregated tropocollagen. Cross-links do not form in sufficient quantity in animals poisoned by β-aminopropionitrile, which is a compound found in Lathyrus odoratus, a sweet pea. Animals so poisoned are said to suffer from lathyrism. This condition affects bones to a greater extent than it affects other tissues. High doses of penicillamine, a metal chelator, will also inhibit cross-linking and cause the weakening of connective tissue. However, its action seems to involve a combination with the aldehyde residues, generated by lysyl oxidase, and not any metal. Increased levels of collagen cross-linking have been associated with the aging process.

Hydroxylysine may be glycosylated in addition to providing the means for cross-linking tropocollagen molecules. It may contain D-galactose that is beta-

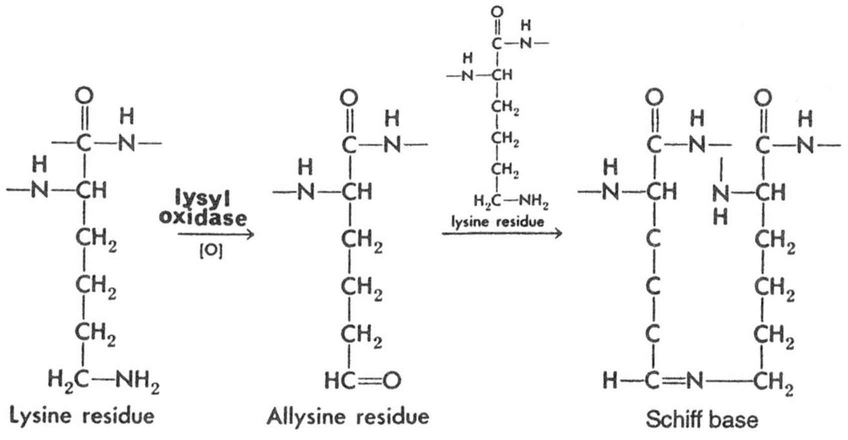

Figure 8.4 Formation of an intermolecular cross-link in collagen. This type of cross-link involves an allysine residue of a telopeptide of one tropocollagen molecule and an amino group of a lysine residue located on the helical portion of another tropocollagen molecule.

Table 8.1 Collagens Tissues in Which They Occur[a]

Collagen type	Designation	Occurrence	Characteristics relative to collagen type I
I	$[\alpha1(I)]_2\alpha2\,(I)$	Skin, bone, teeth, tendons	Two types of polypeptide chains; contains least carbohydrate of known collagens
II	$[\alpha1(II)]_3$	Cartilage, vitreous humor	More highly cross-linked; high carbohydrate; high hydroxylysine
III	$[\alpha1(III)]_3$	Skin, muscle, arterial wall, uterus	High hydroxyproline but low in hydroxylysine; –S–S– bonds present
IV	$[\alpha1(IV)]_2\alpha2(\,IV)$ or a mixture of $[\alpha1(IV)]_3$ and $[\alpha2(IV)]_3$	All basement membranes	Nonfibrillar; highest carbohydrate and hydroxylysine content of known collagens; linked to a globular protein
X	$[\alpha1(X)]_3$	Cartilage developing into bone	May associate with a membrane; gene contains only one intron

[a]This table lists only five of the 11 or more collagen types known.

glycosidically linked to the –OH group of hydroxylysine, or there may be a disaccharide, α-D-glucopyranosyl-1,2-β-D-galactosylhydroxylysine. UDP-glucose and UDP-galactose are used as substrates in the glycosylation reactions catalyzed by Mn^{2+}-containing transferases. Collagen is thus a glycoprotein.

Collagens of different organs possess different types of polypeptide chains. These differ from each other on the basis of their amino acid compositions and other properties. There are over 10 types of collagens known, some more prevalent in a given tissue than others, each containing a different type of polypeptide chain. All, however, have retained the same Gly-X-Y sequence motif as well as the triple-helix structure. A given tropocollagen type may contain three identical polypeptide chains, but another may contain three different polypeptide chains. Thus, type II collagen is a trimer of the same chain. It is designated as $[\alpha1(II)]_3$. But type XI collagen has three different polypeptide chains, all specific for that particular collagen type, and the designation then would be $[\alpha1(XI)\alpha2(XI)\alpha3(XI)]$. Type I collagen is most abundant in the human organism. It accounts for about 90% of all collagen present. Table 8.1 summarizes the properties and occurrences of several types of collagen.

8.1.3   Biosynthesis and Degradation of Collagen

Collagen is synthesized intracellularly in the form of procollagen, which is tropocollagen with additional peptidic material at both the C- and N-terminal ends of the molecule. Procollagen is secreted into the extracellular space, where such additional peptidic material is removed by proteolysis to yield tropocollagen. In the extracellular space, tropocollagen is collected into microfibrils, which involves intermolecular cross-linking as described above and, eventually, the formation of collagen fibers. A number of events occur intracellularly before procollagen is exported into the extracellular space. Individual polypeptide chains are synthesized in the rough endoplasmic reticulum. Next, certain proline and lysine residues are hydroxylated to give hydroxyproline and hydroxylysine. Then sugars are attached to certain hydroxylysine residues (see above). Finally, individual hydroxylated and glycosylated chains assemble to give the triple helix of the procollagen molecule.

Following the export of procollagen into the extracellular space, peptidic material is removed proteolytically from both ends of the molecule. This material is not helical. The N-terminal peptide amounts to about 153 residues in type V collagen. The remaining N-terminal nonhelical telopeptide (part of the resulting tropocollagen molecule) has only 17 amino acid residues. The propeptide material at the C-terminal end of each procollagen type V polypeptide chain has 244 amino acid residues and is extensively cross-linked by both intra- and interchain disulfide bonds. The three C-terminal peptides of procollagen, which contain 3 $\times$ 244 = 732 amino acids, are thus removed as a single unit. The remaining telopeptide has 23 amino acid residues for each polypeptide chain.

Hydroxylation of certain proline and lysine residues occurs post-translationally, that is, there are no codons for hydroxyproline and hydroxy-lysine. The hydroxylation reactions are carried out by two enzymes: proline hydroxylase and lysine hydroxylase. Proline hydroxylase has been studied more extensively than lysine hydroxylase. It is a ferrous iron–containing enzyme that requires oxygen, α-ketoglutarate, and ascorbate, as shown in Figure 8.5. The product is 4-hydroxyproline. There is also an enzyme that can hydroxylate proline in the 3-position. Both the latter and lysine hydroxylase require ferrous iron as well as oxygen α-ketoglutarate, and ascorbate. Ascorbate deficiency severely affects collagen biosynthesis. Clinical findings in scurvy-impaired wound

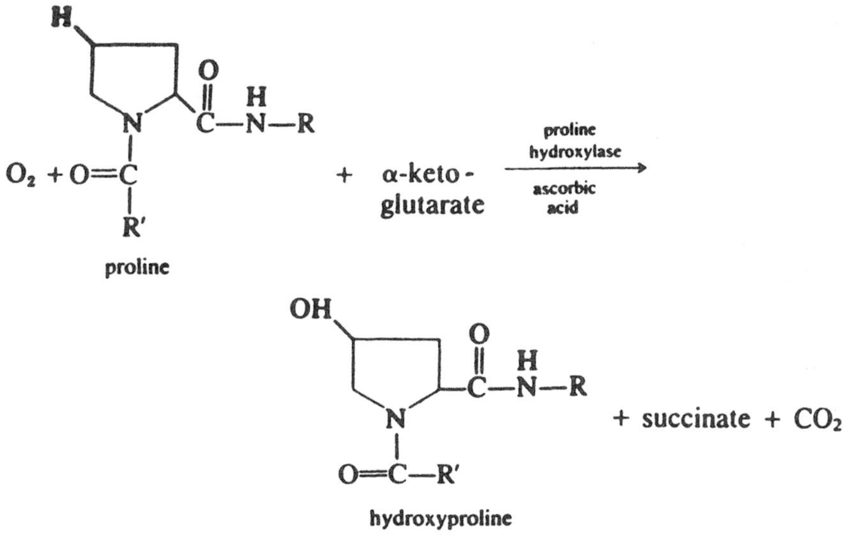

Figure 8.5 Hydroxylation of proline by proline hydroxylase to produce 4-hydroxyproline residues. (Reproduced by permission from Bezkorovainy A. Biochemistry of Nonheme Iron. New York: Plenum, 1980, p. 409.)

healing and incomplete tooth and bone formation are due to incomplete hydroxylation of collagen and hence the inability to stabilize collagen via intrachain hydrogen bond formation.

Degradation of collagen takes place via collagenases, enzymes that initiate the degradation process by splitting a single Gly-Ile bond in each of the three tropocollagen strands. Other proteolytic enzymes do not hydrolyze collagen. However, following the initial action of collagenase, the protein becomes susceptible to attack by intracellular proteases (e.g., cathepsins), and degradation proceeds in a multifaceted way. As a rule, collagens have a very low turnover rate; their half-lives may be as long as a year or more.

Collagen may become damaged as a secondary manifestation in certain disease processes such as homocystinuria, alcaptonuria, and scurvy. However, there can also be a number of inherited errors of collagen biosynthesis, the result of which is damaged and defective collagen with attendant clinical symptoms. There are several diseases commonly called the Ehlers–Danlos syndromes. In most of these, the exact molecular lesions are not known. Exceptions are Ehlers–Danlos type IV, where type III collagen is defective, and Ehlers–Danlos types V and VI, where lysyl oxidase is defective, which results in the incomplete cross-linking of collagen microfibrils. In osteogenesis imperfecta, which is characterized by fragile bones, the biosynthesis of type I collagen is defective. And in Marfan's syndrome, one finds aneurisms, heart problems, and joint dislocation. It is believed that Marfan's syndrome is caused by improper development of collagen cross-links. Chronic copper deficiency will produce similar symptoms.

Deficient collagen degradation occurs in such diseases as scleroderma, excessive scar tissue deposition, and cirrhosis of the liver. Scar tissue is mostly collagen. Collagenase defects have been suggested as a possible reason. Excessive collagen degradation is seen in Paget's disease, rheumatoid arthritis, periodontal disease, and other disorders. Hydroxyproline is often excreted in large amounts in the urine under such circumstances. Increased collagenase activity has been suggested as a reason, but definitive proof to that effect is lacking.

8.2 ELASTIN

Elastin is another important connective tissue protein. It is present in "yellow" connective tissue: large blood vessels, nuchal ligament, lungs, and skin. Whereas the function of collagen is to resist tension, that of elastin is to act as a rubberlike structure: to stretch and relax. Its basic structure is therefore different from that of collagen. It does not have the Gly-X-Y sequence motif, nor does it have the triple helix. Its major amino acids are glycine, alanine, valine, leucine, and proline. There is some hydroxyproline and no hydroxylysine. Its high hydrophobic amino acid content and extensive cross-linking make elastin one of the most insoluble proteins known.

The basic unit of elastin structure is tropoelastin, which has a molecular weight of about 72,000 and contains 800–850 amino acid residues. It has been proposed that tropoelastin units are present in the random coil conformation and are extensively cross-linked. This makes such a network kinetically free: free to stretch and to recoil. It is the entropy effects that permit the stretched elastin to recoil: elastin contains extensive hydrophobic interactions. As the elastin net-work is stretched, these bonds are broken, resulting in a highly ordered water structure (negative entropy change). Recoiling is then driven by water random-ization through the reintroduction of hydrophobic bonding (positive entropy change). Though most of the elastin appears to be amorphous, fibrillar material has also been detected. Its exact conformation is a matter of controversy.

Biosynthesis of elastin is similar to that of collagen in several respects. Elastin is formed in cells in the form of proelastin, which, after entering the extracellular space, is freed of certain peptides through proteolysis. Cross-linking is also an extracellular process involving the action of lysyl oxidase to form allysine. Cross-linking involves four allysine/lysine residues to form new amino acids, desmosine and isodesmosine. Both contain a pyridinium nucleus. The pathway leading to the formation of these two amino acids and cross-linking elastin is illustrated in Figure 8.6. It may be noted that nonspecific inhibitors of collagen cross-linking, such as copper deficiency or lathyrism, will also inhibit cross-linking of elastin. It is well known, for instance, that copper deficiency produces dissecting aneurisms in the blood vessels of animals through incom-plete elastin cross-linking. It appears, however, that elastin abnormalities ob-served in some inherited collagen diseases such as Marfan's syndrome may be secondary to aberrations in collagen structure and deposition because, more often than not, collagen and elastin coexist in the same locus.

8.3 FIBRONECTIN AND LAMININ

Connective tissue matrix contains, in addition to collagen, elastin, and the proteoglycans, certain glycoproteins that have an important function in its physi-ology. Of major importance are fibronectin and laminin. Fibronectin is also found on cell surfaces and in blood plasma, and most studies of this protein have been performed on the plasma material rather than the much more inaccessible connective tissue protein. Fibronectins have two subunits termed the α and β subunits, which are joined by disulfide linkages. The differences between them are due to alternate mRNA splicing, leading to deletion of a part of the β subunit. There are several domains with different functions in fibronectin: two bind to fibrin, one to gelatin (collagen), three to heparin, and one to *Staphylococ-cus aureus*. Most of the carbohydrate is attached to the collagen-binding domain in the form of several oligosaccharide chains. They are asparagine-bound and contain both L-fucose and *N*-acetylneuraminic acid (see Chapter 9). The overall appearance of fibronectin is that of a V, the hinge region being the disulfide bond. Fibronectin structure is illustrated in Figure 8.7. This structure, which is dimeric, allows fibronectin to bridge two cells, or to bridge a ligand and to a cell such as a monocyte, simultaneously.

The binding properties of plasma fibronectin are also a reflection of its biologic function, which is largely opsonic. *Opsonins* are plasma substances that combine with foreign materials or circulating debris to make them susceptible to removal by reticuloendothelial cells such as monocytes and macrophages. Fibronectin also binds to fibrin, becoming cross-linked with it through the action of transglutaminase. The presence of fibronectin in the clot serves, in a later event, to bind to white cells to cause clot dissolution. The collagen-binding

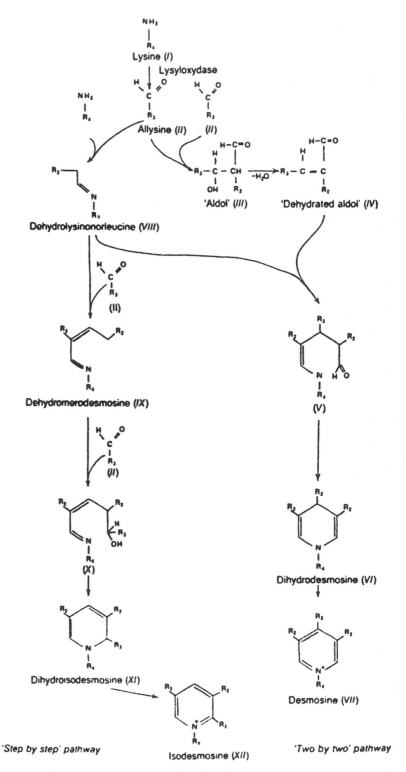

Figure 8.6 Cross-links in elastin involving desmosine and isodesmosine with suggested biosynthetic pathways. Both amino acids contain pyridinium rings, and both contain the elements of four allysine/lysine residues. (Reproduced by permission from Guay M, Lamy F. The troublesome cross-links of elastin 1979. Trends Biochem Sci July, 1979, p. 161.)

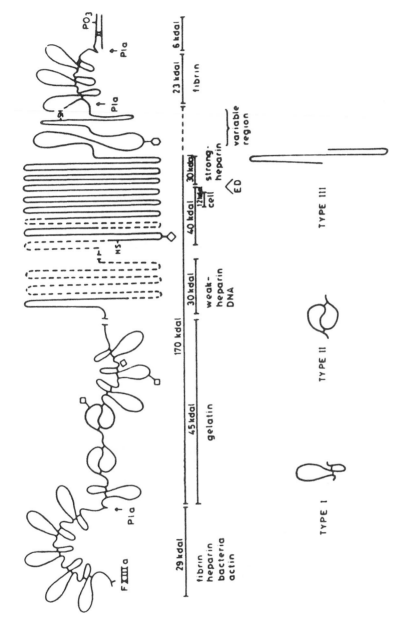

Figure 8.7 Schematic diagram of a human fibronectin subunit. The domains binding to various substances are so indicated. Pla indicates sites of digestion with plasmin. Carbohydrate chains are indicated as follows: square, glucosamine-containing; hexagon, galactosamine. F XIII indicates transglutaminase site. There are extensive internal homology regions, classified as types I, II, and III. (Reproduced by permission from Petersen TE, Skorstengaard K. Primary structure. In McDonagh J (ed). Plasma Fibronectin. New York: Marcel Dekker, 1985, p. 25.)

activity of fibronectin is useful when it binds to newly exposed collagen fibrils at wound sites. This also serves to attract monocytes to dissolve the clot.

In the extracellular matix, fibronectin serves as the matrix organizer. This is still poorly understood, but it is known that fibronectin can interact with proteoglycans, collagens, and cells enmeshed in the matrix, where it binds cells together and anchors them to the matrix. This function also follows fibronectin to act as a mediator of cell growth and differentiation. In some cell systems such as the epithelial cells, this function is replaced by another tissue glycoprotein, laminin.

Laminin is associated with the action of basement membranes. It promotes the attachment of epithelial cells to type IV collagen but not to collagens of the other types. Laminin also binds to certain glycosaminoglycans such as heparin and is believed to be involved in cell–cell interactions, regulation of cellular growth, and differentiation. Its overall molecular weight is around 10^6, and it consists of three small (α) subunits of about 200,000 daltons each and one large (β) subunit with a molecular weight of about 400,000. Its shape, determined by electron microscopic examination, is that of an X, with its shape and subunits being maintained through disulfide bonds. Laminin apparently interacts with tumor cells prone to metastasis but not with nonmetastasizing cells. Laminin levels have been shown to be correlated with metastatic activities of tumor cells.

8.4 KERATINS

Keratins are insoluble proteins that make up such structures as hair, skin, nails, wool, and feathers and form the cytoskeleton structures in all cells of epithelial origin. Along with other fibrous proteins of the same dimensions (e.g., neurofilaments), keratin has been referred to as intermediary filament (IF). In the human being, keratin is one of the more abundant proteins. The basic keratin unit is a relatively small protein with a molecular weight of 40,000–70,000. About 20 different keratin polypeptides have been identified in human hair follicles, various epithelial cells, and tumor cells. They have been assigned numbers 1–20 and have been divided into two classes: acidic (type 1) and neutral/base (type 2). A given tissue or cell line will have a characteristic keratin polypeptide distribution, as shown in Table 8.2. However, both types of peptides are always present in a given cell.

Hair keratin has historically been associated with the α-helical structure. For that reason, it is termed α-keratin. And indeed the basic keratin polypeptides are α-helical except for their N- and C-terminal domains. These are believed to be involved in head-to-tail condensation to form keratin polymers. When hair keratin is stretched, the resulting secondary structure is the parallel pleated sheet (see Chapter 4). Stretched keratin is referred to as β-keratin to emphasize its secondary structure.

The α-helical polypeptide chains, presumably polymerized head-to-tail, interact laterally to form dimers. This is made possible by each polypeptide chain assuming a slightly distorted shape referred to as a "coiled coil." The dimer is referred to as a 2-nm protofilament, because it has a diameter of about 2 nm. It is believed that the dimer consists of one type 1 and one type 2 polypeptide chain. There are a couple of possibilities for the next level of organization: either two 2-

Table 8.2 Major Keratin Polypeptides of Various Tissues and Cell Lines

Polypep- tide[a]	Mol wt (in 1000s)	pI	Epidermis (skin)	Hair follicle	Tissue Cornea	Tracheal epithelium	He La cells[b]	Hepatocellular carcinoma[c]
1	68	7.8	+					
3	63	7.5			+			
5	58	7.4	+	+	+	+		
6	56	7.8	+					
7	54	6.0					+	
8	53	6.1				+	+	+
10	57	5.3	+					
11	56	5.3	+					
12	55	4.9			+			
13	54	5.1				+		
14	50	5.3	+					
15	50	4.9		+		+		
16	48	5.1		+				
17	46	5.1		+		+		+
18	45	5.7						+
19	40	5.2				+		

[a]Other keratin polypeptides may occur in minor amounts in the tissues presented.
[b]Originally isolated from cervical adenocarcinoma.
[c]Keratin pattern is identical to that of normal hepatocytes.
Source: Data from Moll R, Franke WW, Schiller DL, Geiges B, Krepler R. The catalog of human cytokeratins: patterns of expression in normal epithelia, tumors, and cultured cells. Cell 31:11–24, 1982.

nm protofilaments interact laterally to form a 3-nm protofilament, or three 2-nm protofilaments combine to form a 4.5-nm protofibril. The 4.5-nm protofibril can also be generated from two 3-nm protofilaments. Next, the 4.5-nm protofibrils can interact with each other to form either three- or four-membered cables termed 10-nm filaments. A summary of these organizational levels in keratins is provided in Figure 8.8. Interactions between individual polypeptide chains of keratin are apparently brought about by electrostatic effects, though in the final product, extensive –S–S– cross-linking is also present.

8.5 CONTRACTILE PROTEINS

8.5.1 The Skeletal Muscle

Contractile proteins are another group of fibrous proteins that form cyto-skeletons of cells. Muscle proteins, collagen, and the keratins are among the most abundant body proteins because muscle makes up about 40% of total body weight. Anatomically, the smallest unit of the contractile system is the myofibril. Its diameter is 1–2 μm (1000–2000 nm). Myofibrils are gathered into muscle fibers with diameters of 50–100 μm. Muscle fibers are actually very long cells with multiple nuclei and mitochondria encased by a membrane called the sarcolemma. The cytoplasm of muscle cells, the sarcoplasm, contains soluble proteins such as enzymes. The sarcoplasmic reticulum, a cytoskeletal structure, holds the myofibrils together and also forms an internal vesical communications

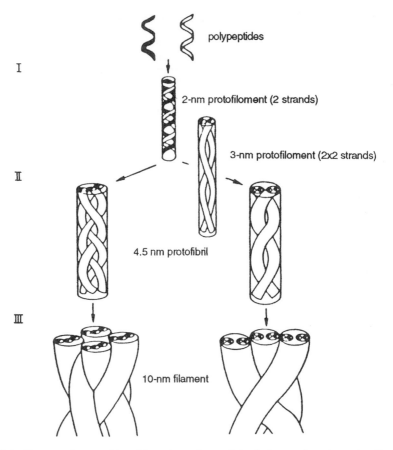

Figure 8.8 Proposed assembly of keratin polypeptide chains to form keratin filaments. (Reproduced by permission from Eichner R, Rew P, Engel A, Aebi U. Human epidermal keratin filaments: studies on their structure and assembly. Ann NY Acad Sci 455:381–401, 1985.)

system. A myofibril consists of two types of fibrils or filaments, the thick (10–15 nm diameter) and the thin (5–7 nm) fibrils or filaments. Lateral microscopic examination of myofibrils further shows a banded structure (Figure 8.9). The repeating unit (Z line to Z line) of a myofibril is called a sarcomere. It is about 2300 nm long. As the muscle contracts, the sarcomere becomes smaller, largely at the expense of the I bands (isotropic bands).

The major component of the thick filaments and the A bands (anisotropic bands) is the protein myosin. It may be rapidly extracted from muscle cells by slightly alkaline 0.6 M KCl. Prolonged extraction produces other proteins such as actin. Myosin has a molecular weight of nearly 460,000 and consists of two very large (heavy) subunits with a molecular weight of 200,000 each and four light chains with molecular weights of 15,000–27,000 each. The light chains are associated with the N-terminal (also called the globular) region of myosin. The bulk of the heavy subunits are in an α-helical conformation intertwined in a supercoil. The total length of the myosin molecule is about 1500 Å (150 nm). The structure of

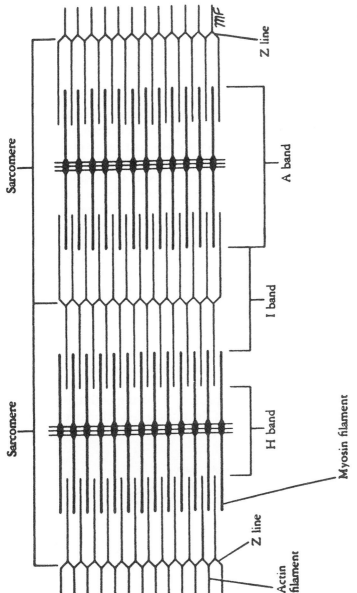

Figure 8.9 Ultrastructure of the myofibril indicating the various bands observed microscopically. The I bands are largely the thin filaments, whereas the A bands are the thick filaments with partially overlapping thin filaments. The thick filaments are about 1600 nm in length, whereas the thin filaments are about 1000 nm in length. The Z line is a transverse tubule that serves to bind the thin filaments together. Thick filaments are bound together by a protein seen as a dark line (M line) in the middle of the H zone. (Reproduced by permission from Snell RS. Clinical and Functional Histology for Medical Students. Boston: Little, Brown, 1984, p. 200.)

myosin has been elucidated with the help of proteolytic enzyme action, as shown in Figure 8.10. Trypsin splits the molecule into the heavy meromyosin, which contains the globular section of myosin, and the light meromyosin. The latter is largely a supercoiled α-helix. Papain, an enzyme, in effect separates the globular portions of the myosin molecule from its fibrous portion. The arrangement of myosin molecules in the thick filaments (1500 nm long) is very peculiar. Within each sarcomere, the myosin molecules interact tail to tail. The interaction is staggered. The globular "heads" of each myosin molecule project outward above the plane of the sarcomere so that each thick filament has a number of knobs appearing at about 14-nm intervals. Each thick filament has 18 myosin molecules.

The thin filaments consist of basically three proteins: actin, tropomyosin, and troponin. Actin has a molecular weight of about 43,000 and is globular (G-actin). It accounts for about 25% of all muscle protein. In the presence of Mg^{2+} and ATP, actin polymerizes to form a beaded string of actin monomers called F-actin (fibrous actin). Two such beaded strings interact to form actin double helices. Associated with the F-actin polymers are the tropomyosin and troponin molecules. The former is a fibrous protein, molecular weight about 66,000, with two subunits of identical molecular weight and both in the α-helical conformation forming a coiled coil. It is situated in the F-actin groove, and in the relaxed state it inhibits the actin–myosin interaction. Troponin is a globular protein, molecular weight about 76,000, with three subunits: TnT, TnI, and TnC. TnT binds to tropomysin, whereas TnC binds Ca^{2+}. TnI also inhibits the interaction between actin and myosin, a normal situation in the resting muscle. The interrelationships among the three proteins to form a thin filament are illustrated in Figure 8.11.

Muscle contraction is a complex process involving both the thin and thick filaments as well as other structures of the muscle cell. Moreover, myosin possesses the ability to hydrolyze ATP (ATPase) at its globular domain, to bind ADP

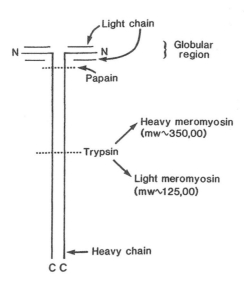

Figure 8.10 Schematic drawing of the myosin molecule. Note that trypsin produces two fragments, light and heavy meromyosins.

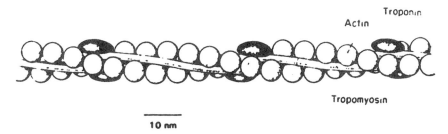

Figure 8.11 Aggregation of F-actin, tropomyosin and troponin to form the thin filaments of myofibrils. (Reproduced by permission from Ohtsuki I, Maruyama K, Ebashi S. Regulatory and cytoskeletal protein of vertebrate skeletal muscle. Adv Prot Chem 38:1–60, 1986.)

and P_i, and to bind to actin. These activities too are involved in the contraction process. The process is initiated by a signal that is propagated along the transverse tubule (Z line). This causes the release of Ca^{2+} from the sarcoplasmic reticulum, whereby $[Ca^{2+}]$ in the sarcoplasm is increased from about 10^{-7} or 10^{-8} M to 10^{-5} M. TnC binds Ca^{2+} and, through a conformation change, moves TnT so that the latter shifts the position of tropomysin in such a way that it can no longer inhibit the myosin–F-actin interaction. At the same time as the myosin head interacts with F-actin (Figure 8.12), the ADP and P_i bound by the globular region of myosin are released, and the myosin ATPase is activated. This makes it possible for ATP to interact with the myosin globular region and for the activated ATPase to hydrolyze the ATP. With ADP and P_i bound to the myosin head, an interaction with F-actin is again indicated. The movement of the thin filaments comes about as the angle of interaction between the myosin head and F-actin changes from 90° to the thermodynamically more stable 45°. The movement of the thin filaments over thick filaments is therefore a ratchet-like action, each "click" moving the thin filament a distance of 10–15 nm. On the supramolecular level, contraction represents the sliding of the thin filaments over the thick filaments with a contraction of the I band. The thin filaments from opposite sides can meet or even overlap each other.

An enhancement of ATPase action comes through the phosphorylation of myosin light chains (MW 18,000). The phosphorylation is achieved because the high cellular $[Ca^{2+}]$ activates myosin kinase, an enzyme that contains calmodulin, a Ca^{2+}-binding subunit. Phosphorylation of myosin is absolutely required for smooth muscle contraction, though not for the contraction of skeletal or cardiac muscle, because smooth muscle has no troponin. Thus, whereas contraction and relaxation in skeletal and cardiac muscle are achieved principally via the action of Ca^{2+} on troponin, in smooth muscle they must depend solely on the Ca^{2+}-dependent phosphorylation of myosin. In skeletal and cardiac muscle, once the stimulus to the sarcolemma is removed, $[Ca^{2+}]$ in sarcoplasm drops rapidly back to 10^{-7} or 10^{-8} M via various Ca^{2+} pump mechanisms present in the sarcoplasmic reticulum, and tropomyosin can once again interfere with the myosin–actin interaction.

It is thus the ATP that drives muscle contraction, given the appropriate stimulus that results in the release of Ca^{2+} from the sarcoplasmic reticulum. ATP

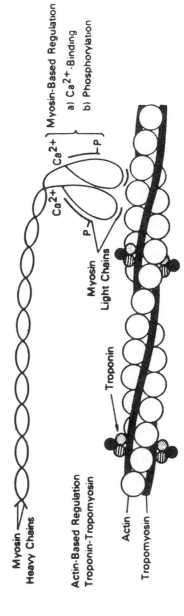

Figure 8.12 Interaction between myosin and actin (thin and thick filaments) during muscle contraction. (Reproduced by permission from Adelstein RS, Eisenberg E. Regulation and kinetics of the actin–myosin– ATP interaction. Annu Rev Biochem 49:921–956, 1980.)

concentration in muscle is very low—about 1×10^{-3} M. This concentration of ATP would support only a second or so of strenuous work. Creatine phosphate, a compound containing a high-energy phosphate bond equivalent to, or of higher energy than, that of ATP (see Chapter 2), is present at a concentration of 3–4 times that of ATP and serves as an ATP backup. It generates ATP through the action of creatine kinase (see Chapter 5) as indicated in the equation

$$
\begin{array}{ccc}
& & \text{H} \\
& & \text{N—P—O}_3\text{H}_2 \\
\text{HN=C} & & \\
& & \text{N—CH}_2\text{—COOH} \\
& & \text{CH}_3 \\
& \text{Creatine phosphate} &
\end{array}
\qquad
\begin{array}{ccc}
& & \text{NH}_2 \\
& \text{NH=C} & \\
& & \text{N—CH}_2\text{COOH} \\
& & \text{CH}_3 \\
& & \text{Creatine}
\end{array}
\qquad (8.2)
$$

ADP → ATP

Nevertheless, there is enough creatine phosphate to sustain only a few seconds of intensive work. Another system available for ATP generation is the myokinase reaction:

$$2\ \text{ADP} \rightleftharpoons \text{ATP} + \text{AMP} \qquad (8.3)$$

But again, only limited amounts of ATP can be produced in this manner, and AMP cannot be further utilized. And so, in order to maintain sustained muscular activity, ATP must be produced rapidly from the oxidation of glucose, and it is the pathway of glycolysis that generates ATP for prolonged muscular work. The AMP and ADP generated by the myokinase reaction or ATP hydrolysis serve to stimulate glycolysis (see Chapter 19). Unfortunately, muscular work cannot be sustained indefinitely, because the lactic acid produced in the glycolysis pathway lowers the pH of the muscle cells and creates a feeling of fatigue. Though lactic acid is exported to the liver through the bloodstream, where it may be reconverted to glucose via the gluconeogenesis pathway, such export is not sufficiently rapid to remove the lactic acid as soon as it is produced in an exercising muscle. The oxidation of glucose via the Krebs cycle is not sufficiently rapid to meet the needs of an active muscle. Other aspects of muscle metabolism will be handled in pertinent metabolism chapters.

8.5.2 Microtubules and Microfilaments

Microtubules and microfilaments are ubiquitous components of almost all cells (red blood cells excluded). Microfilaments are polymers of actin, which in the non-muscle cell can exist in two forms: β-actin and τ-actin. Microfilaments have a diameter of about 6 nm. In certain structures such as the microvilli of intestinal mucosal cells, microfilaments are associated with myosin, so that movement is possible given an appropriate stimulus. Endocytosis and exocytosis events are apparently mediated via microfilaments. Microfilaments are disrupted by the drug cytochalasin.

Microtubules have a diameter of about 25 nm and consist of 13 protofilaments arranged side by side to form a hollow cylinder. Each protofilament is a linear polymer of tubulin molecules in a head-to-tail arrangement. Each tubulin molecule consists of two subunits termed α and β subunits. Both have a molecular weight of 55,000, but their primary structures are different. Microtubules play an important role in cell division, constituting a significant portion of the mitotic spindle. Microtubules are being constantly arranged and rearranged; that is, tubulin molecules are being constantly added to and subtracted from the microtubule. Two molecules of GTP must be used to place one tubulin molecule into a microtubule. The assembly of microtubules is inhibited by colchicine, an anti-inflammatory drug, and by *Vinca* alkaloids vincristine, vinblastine, and vindesine. These have been used as antitumor agents.

It is interesting to note at this point that the keratins and other cytoskeletal proteins such as neurofilaments (from neurons) and vimentin (mesenchymal cells) are referred to as intermediate filaments because their diameter (10 nm) are intermediate between those of the microfilaments and microtubles.

QUESTIONS

8.1. Which of the following statements is incorrect?
   a. Cartilage contains largely type I collagen.
   b. Type I collagen contains approximately 33% glycine.
   c. Link proteins play an important role in the stabilization of the proteoglycan aggregate in cartilage.
   d. Cells in connective tissues are usually separated from one another by extracellular matrix.
   e. Collagen molecules have half-lives of 1–3 years.

8.2. Which of the following statements about the Gly-X-Y triplet of type I collagen is incorrect?
   a. Proline is often found in the X position.
   b. Hydroxyproline is sometimes found in the X position.
   c. Hydroxylysine is sometimes found in the Y position.
   d. The helical portion of the collagen molecule is made up of repeating Gly-X-Y triplets.
   e. Sequences in the telopeptides do not necessarily contain the Gly-X-Y triplet.

8.3. Which of the following statements about the synthesis of the type I collagen molecule is incorrect?
   a. Hydroxylation of proline residues in the chains ceases once the triplet helix is formed.
   b. Disulfide bonds cross-link the triple helix.
   c. Glycosylation of the chains precedes the formation of the triple helix.
   d. Propeptides are removed extracellularly.
   e. Hydroxylysine residues may be glycosylated.

8.4. Which of the following statements about the formation and cross-linking of type I collagen fibrils is incorrect?
   a. Cross-linking is defective in iron deficiency.
   b. Lysine and hydroxylysine are oxidatively deaminated to allysine and hydroxy-allysine, respectively.
   c. Oxidative deamination is mediated by lysyl hydroxylase.
   d. There are two types of cross-linkages: aldol condensation products and Schiff bases.
   e. Aldol condensation products are formed by the interaction of allysine and hydroxyallysine residues.

8.5. Which of the following statements about the different types of collagen is incorrect?
   a. Bone contains predominantly type I collagen.

    b. Cartilage collagen contains three identical polypeptide chains in its triple helix.

    c. Basement membranes contain predominantly type III collagen.

    d. The type II collagen molecule does not contain an α_2-polypeptide chain.

    e. The type I collagen molecule contains two α_1-polypeptide chains and one α_2-polypeptide chain.

8.6. Which of the following statements about elastin is incorrect?

    a. Elastin is the name given to the protein that makes up the amorphous portion of the elastic fiber.

    b. Elastin contains hydroxyproline.

    c. Cross-links in elastin are called desmosine and isodesmosine.

    d. Copper deficiency results in the biosynthesis of insufficiently cross-linked elastin.

    e. Elastin is rich in hydroxylysine.

8.7. Which of the following statements about noncollagenous proteins of connective tissues is incorrect?

    a. The fibronectin molecule contains at least one domain with an affinity for heparin.

    b. The fibronectin molecule consists of a single polypeptide chain of very high molecular weight.

    c. Laminin is found in basement membranes.

    d. The laminin molecule contains a domain with an affinity for type IV collagen.

    e. The laminin molecule contains three α chains and one β chain held together by disulfide bonds.

8.8. Which is *not* true about keratins?

    a. They form the cytoskeleton of both epithelial and mesenchymal cells.

    b. Their basic unit consists of three α-helical chains forming a "coiled coil."

    c. The basic filament has a diameter of 10 nm.

    d. Keratin polypeptide chains may be divided into two classes on the basis of their isoelectric points.

    e. Stretched keratin assumes a pleated sheet structure.

8.9. Which *best* describes the tropocollagen secondary structure?

    a. It is a triple helix with three α-helical polypeptide chains intertwined to form a left-handed superhelix.

    b. Three polypeptide chains form an antiparallel pleated sheet system.

    c. The entire molecule is a cable consisting of three left-handed polypeptide helices containing 3.3 amino acids per turn.

    d. The molecule is largely a cable consisting of three left-handed polypeptide helices with a linear distance of 9.6 Å per turn. At the N- and C-terminal portions, nonhelical segments are present.

    e. None of the above.

8.10. A myofibril is best described by which?

    a. A component of a polynucleated muscle cell containing the thick and thin filaments

    b. An elongated muscle cell, surrounded by sarcolemma and in contact with nerve fiber end plates

    c. An aggregate of globular protein molecules arranged in a cylindrical fashion

    d. Head-to-tail polymer of myosin molecules

    e. A cytoskeletal structure consisting of microfilaments and microtubules

In Questions 8.11–8.13, mark as follows:

    a. Collagen   c. Both

    b. Elastin   d. Neither

8.11. Designed to be stretched and relaxed
8.12. Designed to provide tensile strength
8.13. May act as "intermediate fiber" type of cytoskeleton

In Questions 8.14–8.17, choose answers from the following.
     a. Lathyrism   c. Scleroderma   e. Paget's disease
     b. Scurvy   d. Osteogenesis imperfecta

8.14. Defective collagen degradation
8.15. Defective collagen cross-linking
8.16. Increased collagen degradation
8.17. Destabilization of the triple helix due to inadequate hydrogen bond formation
8.18. Which is not part of the skeletal muscle contraction event?
     a. The binding of Ca^{2+} by troponin
     b. Phosphorylation of myosin light chains
     c. Interaction of myosin globular region with F-actin
     d. Flow of Ca^{2+} into the sarcoplasmic reticulum to increase $[Ca^{2+}]$ to $10^{-5}\,M$.
     e. Hydrolysis of ATP
8.19. In a relaxed state, which best represents the status of skeletal muscle?
     a. Tropomyosin inhibits myosin–F-actin interaction.
     b. $[Ca^{2+}]$ in sarcoplasm is about $10^{-5}\,M$.
     c. Myosin light chains are phosphorylated, thus preventing its interaction with F-actin.
     d. Actin is present in the G-actin form.
     e. Troponin binds Ca^{2+} and thus inhibits actin–myosin interaction.
8.20. Which structure is practically absent from the myofibril when it is in the contracted state?
     a. Z line   c. I band   e. The H zone
     b. A band   d. The sarcomere
8.21. Which cannot provide energy for the contraction of muscle?
     a. ADP   c. Creatine phosphate   e. Glucose
     b. AMP   d. Process of glycolysis
8.22. Which protein molecule *does not* aggregate into oligomers or polymers?
     a. Tubulin   d. β-Actin
     b. G-Actin   e. Tropomyosin
     c. Myosin

Answers

8.1. (a)   Cartilage has largely type II collagen.
8.2. (b)   Hydroxyproline is always found in position Y.
8.3. (b)   Disulfide bonds are not present in the triple helix. They are present in the C-terminal propeptides of procollagen.
8.4. (a)   Copper deficiency, not iron deficiency, produces inadequate cross-linking in collagen.
8.5. (c)   Basement membranes contain predominantly type IV collagen.
8.6. (e)   Elastin does not contain hydroxylysine.
8.7. (b)   Fibronectin is a glycoprotein with two –S–S-linked subunits.
8.8. (a)   Keratin constitutes the cytoskeleton of epithelial cells only.
8.9. (d)   Collagen is a cable consisting of three left-handed helices that have about 3.3 amino acids per turn, with each amino acid accounting for about 2.91 Å. The superhelix of the cable has a right-handed sense.

8.10. (a) A myofibril consists of the thick filaments (myosin) and thin filaments (F-actin with tropomyosin and troponin). The muscle cell, extending the length of the muscle, is termed a muscle fiber and contains a number of myofibrils.

8.11. (b) Elastin is present in large blood vessels and tendons, and its function is to be elastic.

8.12. (a) Collagen is designed to provide tensile strength to tissues.

8.13. (d) Both elastin and collagen are extracellular fibers and do not constitute cytoskeletons.

8.14. (c) In scleroderma, collagen is not degraded normally, perhaps due to a collagenase deficiency.

8.15. (a) In lathyrism, the β-aminopropionitrile inhibits cross-linking generated by lysyl oxidase.

8.16. (e) In Paget's disease, one observes an increased level of collagen degradation and appearance of hydroxyproline in the urine.

8.17. (b) In scurvy, vitamin C deficiency disease, hydroxylation of proline is defective, and the smaller hydroxyproline content of the collagen helix results in weaker hydrogen bonding.

8.18. (d) Muscle contraction is initiated by the *release* of Ca from sarcoplasmic reticulum, whereby sarcoplasmic $[Ca^{2+}]$ increases from 10^{-7}–$10^{-8}\ M$ to 10^{-5}.

8.19. (a) When muscle is relaxed, troponin does not bind Ca because sarcoplasmic $[Ca^{2+}]$ is very low. This permits the tropomyosin to return to the relaxed state in the groove of the thin filaments and interfere with myosin–actin interaction.

8.20. (c) Since the thin filaments slide across (over) the thick filaments during contraction, the I zone, which represents the thin filaments, will decrease greatly in size.

8.21. (b) Muscle contraction depends on the availability of ATP. ATP can be generated from two ADP molecules (myokinase), from creatine phosphate (high-energy phosphate bond), and from glucose via glycolysis.

8.22. (e) All except tropomyosin form larger molecules. Tubulin, under the influence of GTP, aggregates into microtubules; G-actin polymerizes to F-actin; myosin forms thick filaments by tail-to-tail interaction; and β-actin polymerizes to microfilaments. β-Actin is similar but not identical to G-actin. Tropomyosin is a fibrous protein associated with the F-actin polymer. It controls myosin–actin interaction under the influence of troponin.

PROBLEMS

8.1 A 6-month-old infant has been fed unmodified cow's milk supplemented with corn flour. He was healthy except that he was severely anemic, and an X-ray of his wrist showed retarded bone development. His hemoglobin was only 4.5 g/dL, and he had an elevated serum alkaline phosphatase. He was treated with iron supplements, folate, and ascorbic acid to no avail. Then serum copper analysis was done, and it showed a level of 9 μg/dL (normal is 85–163 μg/dL). Thereupon his diet was supplemented with copper sulfate, and he showed dramatic improvement. Address the following questions:

    a. What is the connection between copper and iron metabolisms? Why did iron supplements not cure his anemia?

    b. Was there an indication of a connective tissue disorder? If so, what was it?

    c. What is the connection between copper metabolism and normal functioning of connective tissue?

8.2   A 77-year-old man could no longer walk and complained of pain in his legs and joints. His serum alkaline phosphatase was about 20 times the normal level, and bone scans showed extensive areas of bone turnover (degradation and resynthesis). He was diagnosed as having Paget's disease and was treated with mithramycin and calcitonin with some success. Address the following issues:

    a.   Is Paget's disease hereditary? What are some of the theories on why Paget's disease develops?

    b.   What is excreted in the urine in Paget's disease and similar disorders? Where does it come from?

    c.   Why was the patient treated with mithramycin (look up what mithramycin does) and calcitonin (Chapter 16)? What is the rationale of such treatment?

8.3   Ehlers-Dunlos and osteogenesis imperfecta syndromes are hereditary collagen diseases that are characterized by the biosynthesis of defective collagens. Propose some collagen structural abnormalities that could result in pathology. One type of Ehlers-Dunlos syndrome is characterized by a "paper thin" skin and tendency of blood vessels to burst. Which collagen is abnormal, and why?

BIBLIOGRAPHY

Kreis T, Vale R. Guidebook to the Cytoskeletal and Motor Proteins. Oxford: Oxford University Press, 1993.

Mayne R, Burgeson RE. Structure and Function of Collagen Types. Orlando: Academic Press, 1987.

Nimni ME. Collagen, Vols I, II, and III. Boca Raton: CRC Press, 1989.

Piez KA, Reddi AH. Extracellular Matrix Biochemistry. New York: Elsevier, 1984.

Raxworthy MJ. Microtubules, tubulins and associated proteins. Biochem Ed 16:2–9, 1988.

Ruoslahti E. Fibronectin and its receptors. Ann Rev Biochem 57:375–413, 1988.

Walton AG. Polypeptides and Protein Structure. New York: Elsevier, 1981, chapters 13 and 14.

9

Carbohydrates, Lipids, and Related Structures

After completing this chapter, the student should

1. Be familiar with the general properties and chemistry of carbohydrates: mono-, di-, oligo-, and polysaccharides. Be familiar with their stereochemical properties, reducing properties, terminology used to designate similar sugars (e.g., anomers and epimers), and the nature of the glycoside linkage. Convert Fischer into Haworth structures. Know linkages involved in disaccharides, glycogen, amylopectin, and amylose and the enzymes that serve to hydrolyze them.

2. Know the structures of typical methylpentoses, hexosamine, uronic acids, and sialic acids. Be familiar with the substances in which they occur, and know the differences among the various blood group substances. Be familiar with proteoglycans of connective tissue and how they are assembled into large aggregates. Be familiar with the various mucopolysaccharidoses.

3. Be familiar with the basic properties and classification of lipids, and recognize the various types of lipid structures and their hydrolysis products. Know how lipases work. Recognize amphipathic lipids, and know where they occur. Know the general scheme of sphingolipid degradation and the etiology of lipid storage diseases.

4. Be familiar with the composition and structure of biologic membranes. Be able to place the various phospholipids in the membrane bilayer. Know the function and position of membrane proteins and their possible movements. Know how membrane fluidity is controlled. Know the nature of various mechanisms to transport substances across membranes, receptor-mediated endocytosis, active and facilitated transport, ionophores, and the various types of channels. Be able to solve simple mathematical problems by creating solute gradients across membranes. Know the names of substances that inhibit the various modes of transport across membranes.

9.1 CARBOHYDRATES

9.1.1 General Features of Carbohydrates

The term *carbohydrate* was coined in the midnineteenth century by Karl Schmidt of Dorpat University. He determined that carbohydrates (using modern atomic weights) had the general formula $(C_6H_{10}O_5)_n$. Today it is known that the composition of these constituents of living matter can be represented by $(CH_2O)_n$, that they may contain elements other than C, H, and O (e.g., N, S, and P), that they contain either free or substituted vicinal –OH residues, and that they have reducing carbonyl groups that may be free or present in nonreducing form in *glycoside linkages*.

The number of carbons in a monosaccharide (i.e., simple reducing sugar) may be designated by the prefixes tri- (3), tetr- (4), pent- (5), hex- (6), and hept- (7) and the suffix -ose (e.g., pentose). The simplest carbohydrates are the *trioses*, compounds that contain three carbons. There are two trioses known, D- and L-glyceraldehydes, whose structures are shown in Figure 9.1. They are *optical isomers* (mirror images), also termed enantiomers, because carbon 2 is of the chiral type (see Chapter 3). They have opposite optical rotations. Otherwise, their chemical properties are identical: both have the reducing aldehyde residues and vicinal –OH groups and their composition can be expressed by $(CH_2O)_3$. The glyceraldehydes also serve as a means of classifying all monosaccharides into the D- and L-series. If the *penultimate* (next to last) carbon of a sugar has the configuration of D-glyceraldehyde, then it belongs to the D series. If its configuration is that of L-glyceraldehyde, it then belongs to the L series. With a few exceptions, sugars found in living matter are of the D type. Of greatest biologic importance are the pentoses, which constitute a part of the nucleic acid group of substances (ribose and deoxyribose), and the hexoses.

The reducing group in monosaccharides, the *anomeric carbon*, may be either of the aldehyde type, as shown in Figure 9.1, or of the ketone type, as shown in Figure 9.2 for fructose. The former are *aldoses* and the latter are *ketoses*. Figure 9.2 also shows the structures of D-glucose and D-mannose. The only difference between the two sugars is the configuration of carbon 2. Such sugars are called *epimers*. Another important epimer of D-glucose is D-galactose, which differs from glucose on the basis of carbon 4 configuration. Also note that D-glucose and L-glucose are mirror images of each other. Their physical and

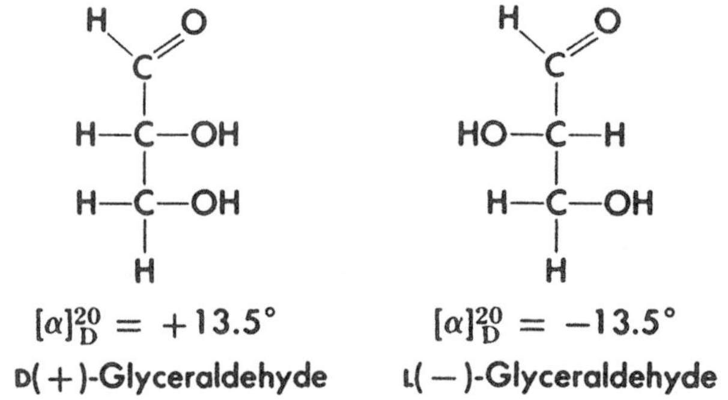

$$[\alpha]_D^{20} = +13.5°$$
D(+)-Glyceraldehyde

$$[\alpha]_D^{20} = -13.5°$$
L(−)-Glyceraldehyde

Figure 9.1 Structures of D- and L- glyceraldehydes.

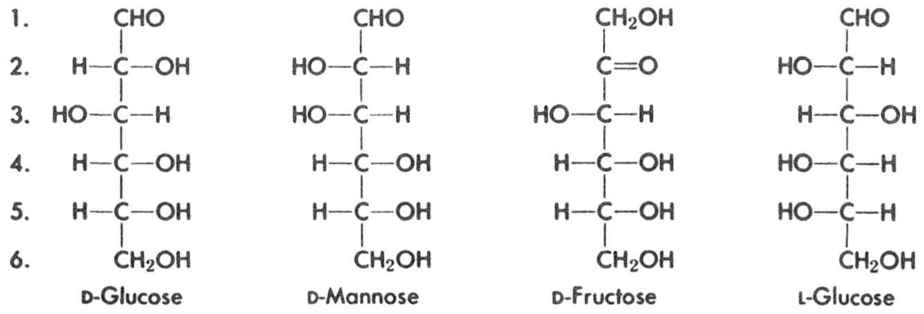

1.	CHO	CHO	CH$_2$OH	CHO
2.	H—C—OH	HO—C—H	C=O	HO—C—H
3.	HO—C—H	HO—C—H	HO—C—H	H—C—OH
4.	H—C—OH	H—C—OH	H—C—OH	HO—C—H
5.	H—C—OH	H—C—OH	H—C—OH	HO—C—H
6.	CH$_2$OH	CH$_2$OH	CH$_2$OH	CH$_2$OH
	D-Glucose	D-Mannose	D-Fructose	L-Glucose

Figure 9.2 Structures of some hexoses. D-Glucose and L-glucose are enantiomers (mirror images), whereas D-glucose and D-mannose are epimers.

chemical properties are identical, except their optical rotations: 113° for D- and −113° for L-glucose.

Glyceraldehyde contains a single chiral carbon, located in position 2. All carbohydrates contain chiral carbons. The number of possible isomers is given by 2^n. For glyceraldehyde, only two isomers are possible, D and L. For a hexose, on the other hand, which in its open form (Figure 9.2) contains four chiral atoms, the number of isomers is $2^4 = 16$, half of them in the D and half in the L series. The first and last carbons in a carbohydrate molecule, if the open structure (e.g., Figure 9.2) is viewed, are nonchiral.

Aldehydes and ketones in solution tend to form hemiacetals or hemiketals with alcohols:

$$R_1\text{-C-H} + \text{HO-}R_2 \rightarrow R_1\text{-C-O-}R_2 \quad \text{Hemiacetal} \tag{9.1}$$

$$R_1\text{-C-}R_2 + \text{HO-}R_3 \rightarrow R_1\text{-C-O-}R_3 \quad \text{Hemiketal} \tag{9.2}$$

Similarly, both aldoses and ketoses can form *internal* hemiacetals and hemiketals with their constituent reducing groups and –OH residues. When this happens, the reducing power of the sugar is not lost. The result is the formation of either five- or six-membered ring structures, *pyranoses* and *furanoses*. Another result is the generation of an additional chiral carbon atom involving the anomeric group. For hexoses, therefore, the number of isomers increases to $2^5 = 32$. Isomerism as a result of the anomeric carbon is illustrated for glucose in Figure 9.3, where the glucose molecule containing a six-membered ring, D-glucopyranose, may assume either the α or the β configuration about the anomeric carbon. In solution, both forms are present in equilibrium with the open structure, but the β-D-glucopyranose is thermodynamically more stable. If we look at the three-dimensional (more realistic) structure of glucose shown in Figure 9.4, we observe the follow-

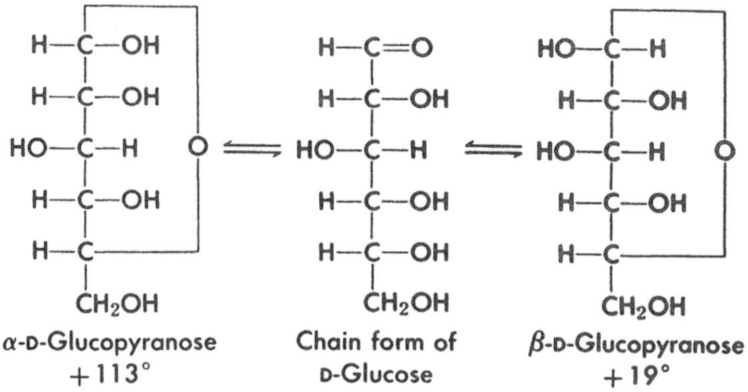

Figure 9.3 Hemiacetal (pyranose) and open structures of glucose showing the phenomenon of mutarotation.

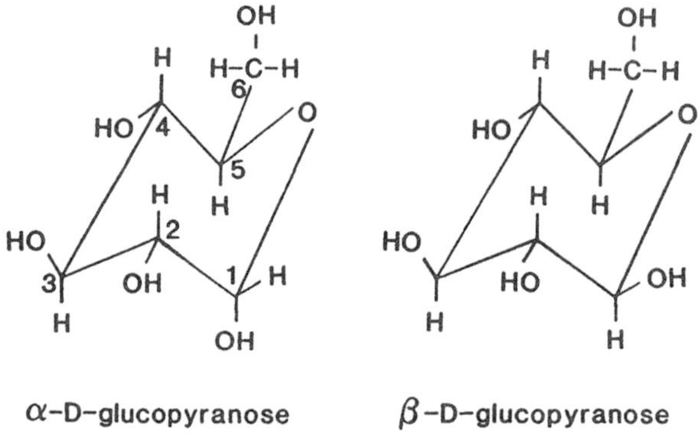

Figure 9.4 Chair forms of glucose anomers. Note that the –OH group on the anomeric carbon (carbon 1) is axial (less stable) in α-D-glucopyranose, whereas it is equatorial in β-D-glucopyranose. Mutarotation therefore favors the latter.

ing: all –OH groups to the right of the carbon chain in Figure 9.3 are down in the three-dimensional (chair) structure. All are of the *equatorial* type (they lie in the plane of the ring), except for the anomeric carbon. In the α-D-glucopyranose, the anomeric –OH is *axial* (down); they are perpendicular to the plane of the ring), and in the β-D-glucopyranose, the anomeric –OH is equatorial (up). It is well known that, from a thermodynamic point of view, bulky groups in the axial position are less stable than they are in the equatorial position, and in this case, equilibrium favors the β form (66%) over the α form (33%). The conversion of α to β glucopyranoses and vice versa is termed *mutarotation*. The α and β forms are anomers, and they make up well over 99% of the total sugar present, the rest being in the open form.

If one takes a look at the structures in Figure 9.3 (these are often referred to as Fischer structures), it is clear that some bonds are short but others are excessively long. This cannot be the case in nature. On the other hand, the more correct chair structures (Figure 9.4) are too cumbersome to use routinely. Carbohydrate chemists most often use the so-called Haworth structures, which are both easy to use and fairly representative of reality. Two such structures are shown in Figure 9.5. Note that those groups that are to the right in the Fischer structures appear down in the Haworth structures (just as in the chair forms), and those appearing to the left in the Fischer formulas point up in the Haworth structure. Fructose, a ketohexose, is usually found in the furanose form, whereas glucose is most stable in the pyranose form. All Haworth structures imply that the ring is perfectly planar. This is not entirely true. Pyranose structures most often assume the chair form, as shown in Figure 9.4. Furanose ring structures, however, are indeed planar.

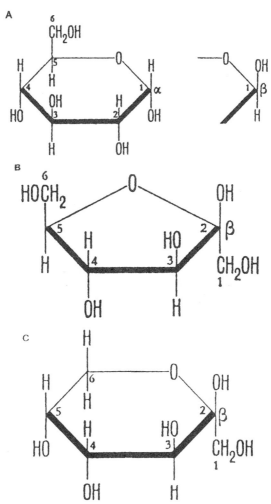

Figure 9.5 Haworth representation of glucose and fructose. (A) Both the α and β anomers of glucose. (B) For fructose, the β anomer of fructofuranose. In the α anomer, the –OH on carbon 2 of fructose would be pointing down and the –CH$_2$OH would be up. (C) The β anomer of D-fructopyranose. (Reproduced by permission from Diem K, Lentner C. Scientific Tables. Basel: Ciba-Geigy, 1971.)

Recall from organic chemistry studies that in addition to forming hemi-acetals and hemiketals, aldehydes and ketones can go a step further and form acetals and ketals:

$$\begin{array}{ccc} \text{OH} & & \text{O--R}_3 \\ | & & | \\ \text{R}_1\text{--C--O--R}_2 + \text{HO--R}_3 \rightarrow \text{R}_1\text{--C--O--R}_2 + \text{H}_2\text{O Acetal} & & \\ | & & | \\ \text{H} & & \text{H} \end{array} \qquad (9.3)$$

$$\begin{array}{ccc} \text{OH} & & \text{O--R}_4 \\ | & & | \\ \text{R}_1\text{--C--O--R}_3 + \text{HO--R}_4 \rightarrow \text{R}_1\text{--C--O--R}_3 + \text{H}_2\text{O Ketal} & & \\ | & & | \\ \text{R}_2 & & \text{R}_2 \end{array} \qquad (9.4)$$

The same is true of monosaccharides that are either pyranoses or furanoses. The bonds generated in forming either acetals or ketals are *glycoside bonds*. They are relatively stable to alkaline hydrolysis but are quite sensitive to acids. The most important glycoside bonds in biology are those between the anomeric group of one monosaccharide and the –OH group of another. Nevertheless, glycosides can be formed between anomeric groups of carbohydrates, on the one hand, and simple alcohols, on the other (e.g., methanol or phenol). The reducing power of the anomeric carbon is lost when it forms a glycoside, and glycosides do not mutarotate, because they cannot generate the open forms of sugars. The formation of a glycoside bond is shown in Figure 9.6. Note also, as indicated in Figure 9.6, that the glycoside bond retains the configuration of the component anomeric carbon atom. When naming a glycoside, the α or β nature of the bond must therefore be specified, as shown in Figure 9.6. The product of the reaction here is a disaccharide, a more complex sugar, consisting of two monosaccharides in a glycoside linkage. There is a nonreducing end (galactose) and a reducing end (glucose). To the reducing or nonreducing end, other sugars may be added via glycoside bond formation to give tri-, tetra-, penta-, and higher sugars, termed oligosaccharides or polysaccharides. The glycoside bond may be broken by a group of hydrolases called *glycosidases*. These are specific to the type of sugars present in an oligosaccharide, the size of the oligosaccharides, and the configuration of the glycoside linkage (α or β).

9.1.2 Hexoses and Related Disaccharides and Oligosaccharides

The most important hexoses in the human organism are glucose (Figures 9.2 through 9.6), fructose (Figure 9.5), galactose (Figure 9.6), and mannose (Figure 9.2). Glucose is important because it is a component of starches and glycogen (mammalian storage sugar); the "blood sugar" often mentioned is glucose, whose levels in plasma are around 100 mg/dL in the fasting state. Red blood cells and the brain utilize glucose exclusively for their energy needs, although the brain in prolonged starvation also utilizes ketone bodies (see Chapter 19). Galactose is a part of milk sugar (lactose, Figure 9.6) and a component of gly-coproteins, complex lipids, blood group substances, and connective tissue

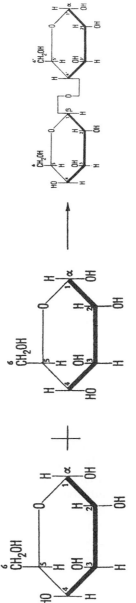

Figure 9.6 Reaction of galactose with glucose to form a disaccharide called lactose via the glycoside bond. Both monosaccharides are shown as their α anomers. The enzyme catalyzing this reaction, however, forms a β-glycoside bond in the product (lactose). (Reproduced by permission from Diem K, Lentner C. Scientific Tables. Basel: Ciba-Geigy, 1971.)

proteoglycans. Mannose is a component of glycoproteins. Glucose is the only sugar that occurs in significant amounts in the free form in the human organism.

A number of disaccharides contain glucose, fructose, and galactose. *Lactose*, present in all milks, including galactose and glucose and is shown in Figure 9.6. Malt sugar, *maltose*, is a glycoside of two glucose molecules linked in an $\alpha(1\rightarrow4)$glycosidic bond. Its isomer, *cellobiose*, which can be derived from *cellulose*, a plant polysaccharide, involves the $\beta(1\rightarrow4)$linkage. *Sucrose*, table sugar, includes glucose and fructose in an $\alpha,\beta(1\rightarrow2)$linkage. In this sugar, both anomeric carbon atoms are involved in the glycoside linkage, and the molecule, in contrast to lactose, maltose, and cellobiose, is not reducing. The structures of these disaccharides are shown in Figure 9.7. Because these disaccharides, with the exception of cellobiose, are food substances for the human being, the intestinal tract contains specific glycosidases that can cause the hydrolysis of these sugars into their constituent monosaccharides. Monosaccharides, but not disaccharides, are absorbed. α-Glucosidase (*maltase*) catalyzes the hydrolysis of maltose to glucose but is inactive with cellobiose. *Sucrase* causes the hydrolysis of sucrose to glucose and fructose, and β-galactosidase (*lactase*) converts lactose to galactose and glucose. *Lactose intolerance*, caused by the absence of lactase, results in an inability to digest lactose. Lactose, when ingested, causes diarrhea and bloating in such patients. This may be the result of a genetic trait, in which case it is absent in infants, who must be given a nonmilk artifical formula, or more commonly in adults, in whom lactase disappears after adolescence.

Glucose is a component of several important *homopolysaccharides*, sugar polymers containing a single monosaccharide species. Starch, a very common plant food source, consists of two kinds of glucose polymers, amylose and amylopectin. Amylose is a straight polymer of α-1,4 glycosidically bound glucose with one nonreducing and one reducing end. Amylopectin is a branched homopolymer of glucose. There are α-1,4 linkages, but there are also α-1,6 linkages that constitute branch points. Amylopectin thus has a single reducing end and numerous nonreducing ends. *Glycogen*, a mammalian homopolysaccharide, is very much like amylopectin except that it has more branch points and its α-1,4-linked oligomers are shorter. It has more nonreducing ends than amylopectin of comparable size. Glycogen can be found in both muscle and liver. The molecular weight of amylopectin is in the hundreds of thousands, whereas that of glycogen is in the millions. Another plant homopolymer of glucose is cellulose, which constitutes plant cell walls. It is equivalent to amylose except that the glucose residues are linked in a β-1,4 linkage. Partial hydrolysis yields cellobiose in addition to other products.

A very important digestive enzyme, which generates maltose and maltotriose from amylose and linear sections of amylopectin and glycogen, is α-*amylase*. It is specific for α-1,4 linkages in large glucose homopolymers and has no action on maltose or maltotriose. It is an *endoglycosidase* because it cleaves internal glycoside bonds. It has no effect on the α-1,6 linkages, and for this reason, its action on amylopectin produces, in addition to maltose, a branched homopolymer called *limit dextrin*. Complete digestion of amylopectin requires a *debranching enzyme*, an α-1,6 glucosidase. Such an enzyme is indeed present in intestinal cell secretions. Complete digestion of amylopectin to glucose thus requires α-amylase, α-1,6 glucosidase, and maltase. There are two types of α-amylases in the human being: one produced by salivary glands and the other by

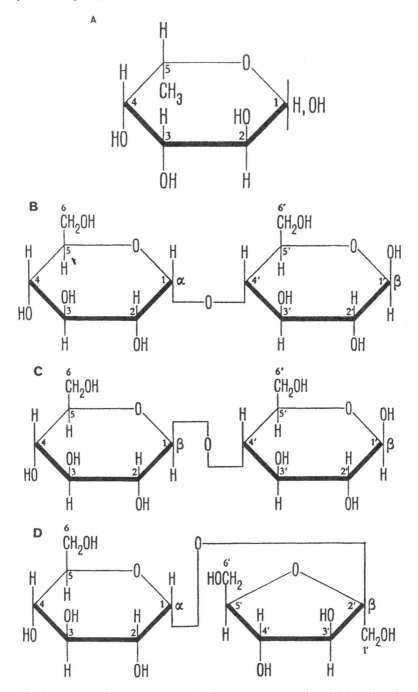

Figure 9.7 Structures of some sugars. (A) L-Fucose (pyranose form). Note that the –CH₃ group points downward; this indicates L series in the Haworth structural convention. (B) Maltose (α-D-glucopyranosyl-1,4-D-glucopyranose); (C) cellobiose (β-D-glucopyranosyl-1,4-D-glycopyranose); and (D) sucrose (α-D-glucopyranosyl-1,2-β-D-fructofuranoside). (Reproduced by permission from Diem K, Lentner C. Scientific Tables. Basel: Ciba-Geigy, 1971.)

pancreas. There is only a 1% difference in amino acid composition between the two enzymes. Pancreatic α-amylase is the more important from a quantitative point of view, because food does not generally remain long enough in the mouth to be thoroughly digested by salivary α-amylase. In acute pancreatitis, pancreatic α-amylase levels in serum are highly elevated, and this serves as a convenient tool in the diagnosis of this disorder.

9.1.3 Derived Sugars

The term *derived sugars* is applied to monosaccharides that do not fit the $(CH_2O)_n$ definition or have some unusual features. Among these sugars are the deoxy sugars, in which a hydrogen residue replaces the normal –OH group on a carbon atom. One such sugar is *L-fucose*, sometimes called methylpentose, which appears in glycoproteins, blood group substances, and complex lipids. Its structure is shown in Figure 9.7. Another deoxy sugar is *deoxyribose*, component of deoxyribonucleic acid (DNA). The reduced carbon here appears in position 2. Deoxyribose and ribose, a standard pentose and a component of ribonucleic acid (RNA), are shown in Figure 9.8.

The first and last carbon residues of glucose, as well as other aldoses, may be oxidized to carboxyl groups. If the first carbon is oxidized, the product is an *aldonic acid* (gluconic acid in glucose). These are not of any biologic importance. If the last carbon atom of a hexose is oxidized, the product is a *uronic acid*. Glucose gives *glucuronic acid* (Figure 9.9), and galactose gives *galacturonic acid*. *Iduronic acid*, an L sugar (L-idose)-derived uronic acid, is also shown in Figure 9.9. Uronic acids are important components of connective tissue proteoglycans. When both the first and sixth carbons of glucose are oxidized to carboxyl groups, the product is *saccharic acid*. The first carbon atom of glucose, or the anomeric carbon of fructose, can be reduced to an alcohol in several tissues, the product being *sorbitol*, a polyalcohol. The reversible reduction is carried out by an enzyme called *sorbitol dehydrogenase*. In diabetes, sorbitol accumulates in those tissues that do not require insulin for glucose transport (see Chapter 16). One such tissue is the eye lens, and sorbitol is believed to be involved in the etiology of cataract formation in individuals with poorly controlled diabetes.

A large group of derived monosaccharides are the amino sugars. An amino group replaces the –OH residue on carbon 2 of such hexoses as glucose, galactose, and mannose. The corresponding compounds are glucosamine, galactosamine,

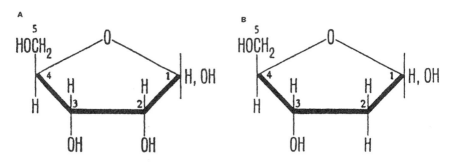

Figure 9.8 Structures of D-ribose (A) and D-deoxyribose (B). (Reproduced by permission from Diem K, Lentner C. Scientific Tables. Basel: Ciba-Geigy, 1971.)

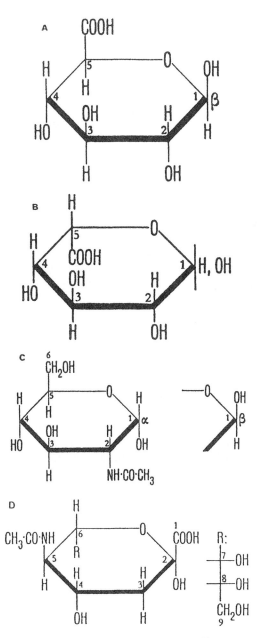

Figure 9.9 Structures of some derived sugars. (A) β-D-Glucuronic acid; (B) L-iduronic acid; (C) α-D-N-acetylglucosamine; (D) α-D-N-acetylneuraminic acid.

and mannosamine. The amino group is normally acetylated, as shown for N-acetylglucosamine in Figure 9.9. N-acetylglucosamine and N-acetylgalactosamine are components of connective tissue proteoglycans, glycoproteins, and complex lipids. An unusual amino sugar is N-acetylneuraminic acid (see Figure 9.9), sometimes called sialic acid, although the term "sialic" should be reserved for a group of

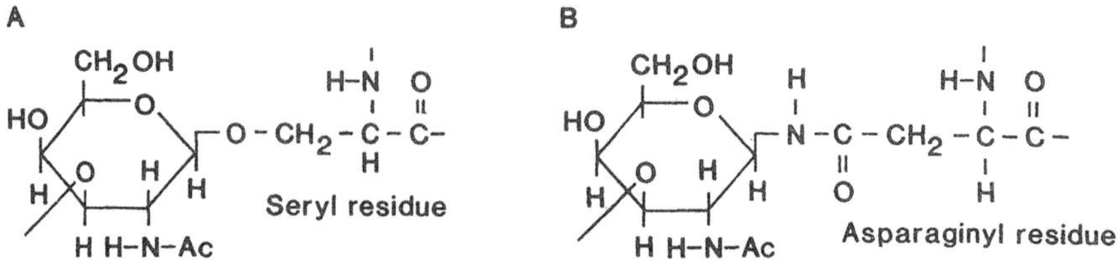

A

CH$_2$OH
HO
O
H H
H H–N–Ac

—O – CH$_2$ – C – C–

H–N   O

Seryl residue

B

CH$_2$OH
HO
O
H H
H H–N–Ac

– N – C – CH$_2$ – C – C –

H
H–N   O

Asparaginyl residue

Figure 9.10 Oligosaccharide-polypeptide linkages found in glycoproteins and pro-teoglycans. (A) *N*-acetylgalactosamine in a β linkage with serine; (B) same in β linkage with asparagine. Ac is acetate.

N-acetylneuraminic acid-like substances. *N*-acetylneuraminic acid is derived from pyruvic acid and *N*-acetyl-D-mannosamine. It therefore contains a carboxyl group and a deoxy carbon. It occurs in glycoproteins and complex lipids.

Most of the derived sugars just described do not occur to any great extent in the free form in the human organism. They are a part of various *heterooligo-saccharides* or *heteropolysaccharides*, sugar polymers consisting of at least two types of monosaccharides and at least two types of glycoside linkages. Glyocoproteins are an example. This group of complex proteins contains various quantities of carbohydrates in the form of one or more heterooligosaccharide units in addition to amino acids. There are two types of carbohydrate-polypeptide linkages in human tissues: O-glycoside bonds and N-asparaginyl linkages, illustrated in Figure 9.10. In the former, the reducing end of the oligosaccharide unit is linked in a glycoside bond with the –OH residue of a serine, a threonine, or a hydroxylysine group. In the latter, the reducing group, usually *N*-acetylglucosamine, is linked in a glycoside-like bond (termed N-glycoside linkage) with the amide residue of asparagine. Figure 9.11 illustrates the structure of one of the two oligosaccharide units of human serum transferrin. The sequence Man(Man)$_n$-Man-GlcNAc-GlcNAc-Asp is common to most, if not all, asparaginyl-linked oligosaccharides.

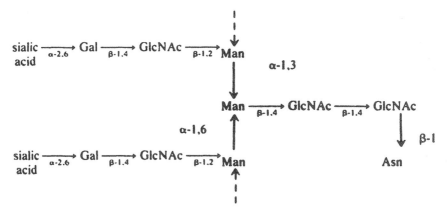

Figure 9.11 Structure of an oligosaccharide unit of human transferrin. The linkage between the oligosaccharide and polypeptide chains is of the N-asparaginyl type. Dotted arrows indicate positions in which one sometimes finds NeuNAc-Gal-GlcNAc units. Gal is galactose, GlcNAc is *N*-acetylglucosamine, NeuNAc is *N*-acetylneuraminic acid (sialic acid), and Man is mannose. (Reproduced with permission from Bezkorovainy A. Biochemistry of Nonheme Iron. New York: Plenum Press, 1980, p. 175.)

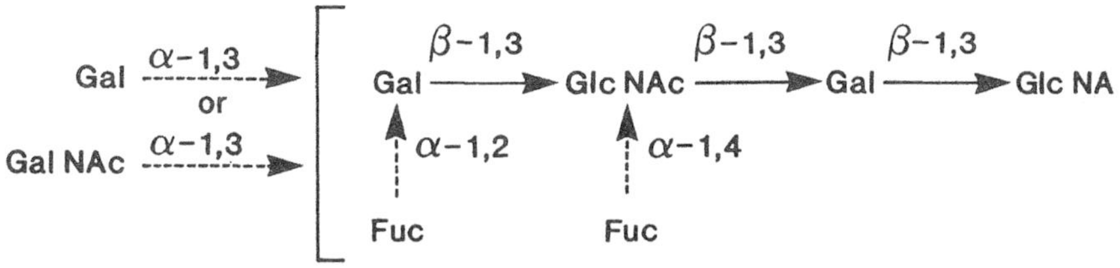

$$\left[\begin{array}{c} \text{Gal} \xrightarrow[\text{or}]{\alpha-1,3} \\ \text{Gal NAc} \xrightarrow{\alpha-1,3} \end{array}\right. \left.\begin{array}{c} \text{Gal} \xrightarrow{\beta-1,3} \text{Glc NAc} \xrightarrow{\beta-1,3} \text{Gal} \xrightarrow{\beta-1,3} \text{Glc NA} \\ \uparrow \alpha-1,2 \qquad\qquad \uparrow \alpha-1,4 \\ \text{Fuc} \qquad\qquad\qquad \text{Fuc} \end{array}\right]$$

Figure 9.12 Antigenic sections of some blood group substances. The structure in brackets is the parent compound of all ABH and Lewis substances. In substance H a Fuc residue is attached to residue 1 (Gal) as indicated by the broken arrow. In Lewis a the Fuc residue is attached to residue 2 (GlcNAc). In Lewis b Fuc groups are attached to residues 1 and 2. In blood group substance A GalNAc and a Fuc group are attached to residue 1; and in group B, a Gal and a Fuc groups are attached to residue 1. Fuc is fucose, GalNAc is *N*-acetylgalactosamine, and other abbreviations are the same as in Figure 9.11.

A clinically important series of oligosaccharides are the *blood group substances*. The major ones are the A, B, and H. They are glycoproteins embedded in red blood cell membranes. All persons have the H blood group substance and no antibodies to it. Individuals with type A red blood cells have substance A and have antibodies to substance B in their serum. Individuals with type B red cells have the B substance and antibodies to the A substance. Individuals with AB group red cells have both A and B substances and no antibodies to either. Individuals with the O red cell type have only the H substance and antibodies to both A and B substances. Thus, a person with type O blood may be transfused with type O blood only, whereas a person with the AB group may receive blood from any individual. Blood types are hereditary characteristics. The nonreducing (antigenic) ends of the major blood group substances are shown in Figure 9.12. Other blood group substances, such as the Lewis types (Le^a and Le^b, Figure 9.12), the MN types, and the Rh (rhesus) types are also oligosaccharide in nature. Blood group substances are also found in the soluble (nonmembrane) form in saliva and milk, and in membranes they may also be attached to complex lipids.

Associated with the discovery of and research on blood group substances are certain plant proteins called *lectins*. Lectins are capable of combining with the blood group substances and aggregating susceptible red blood cells. Thus, the agglutinin from lima beans (*Phaseolus limensis*) recognizes the *N*-acetylgalactosamine residue of substance A and agglutinates red blood cells of that type. Lectin from winged peas (*Lotus tetragonolubus*) reacts with the L-fucose residues of substance H to agglutinate the O type of red cells. Lectins are also known to transform neutrophils and to agglutinate malignant cells. The best known lectins in this area are wheat germ lectin and concanavalin A, which has been crystallized from jack bean meal. It reacts with mannose and glucose residues and can also agglutinate red blood cells from various animal species, as well as yeasts.

9.1.4 Connective Tissue Proteoglycans and Their Function

Oligosaccharide units, discussed in the previous section, are relatively small. The molecular weight of the transferrin oligosaccharide group, for example, is around 2200. Heteropolysaccharides found in connective tissue, however, may be very large: hyaluronic acid, for instance, has a molecular weight of 1–80 million. These large heteropolysaccharides contain hexosamines (GlcNAc and GalNAc) and for this reason are termed *glycosaminoglycans*. Because they are also associated with proteins, they are often referred to as *proteoglycans*. In addition to hexosamines, most glycosaminoglycans also contain uronic acids and sulfate residues. The sulfate groups are most often found as esters of the –OH residues on position 4 or 6 of the hexosamine components, although N-sulfated groups are also encountered.

Major glycosaminoglycans are hyaluronic acid, dermatan sulfate, the chondroitin sulfates, and the heparins. Keratan sulfate differs from the others in that galactose replaces the uronic acid in its structure. Hyaluronic acid is distributed both in mammals and in bacteria. It is the only glycosaminoglycan that is usually not found in the sulfated form. It contains glucuronic acid and *N*-acetylglucosamine. Its structure and that of other proteoglycans are indicated in Figure 9.13. Chondroitin sulfates consist of glucuronic acid and *N*-acetylgalactosamine. There are two types, one sulfated on the 4 position of the *N*-acetylgalactosamine residue and the other at the 6 position. The molecular weight of chondroitin sulfate may be as high as 50,000. Dermatan sulfate is similar to chondroitin sulfate (it was once called chondroitin sulfate B), except that it has L-iduronic acid as the major uronic acid. Nevertheless, glucuronic acid is also present to the extent of about 10–20% of the total uronic acid. The molecular weight of dermatan sulfate is approximately the same as that of chondroitin sulfate. Sulfate residues are present in the 4 position of the *N*-acetylgalactosamine residues and at the 2-O position of iduronic acid.

Keratan sulfate differs from the other heteropolysaccharides in that it contains no uronic acid. Its repeating unit consists of galactose and *N*-acetylglucosamine. Depending on tissue or animal source, it may also contain *N*-acetylneuraminic acid, mannose, L-fucose, and galactosamine. It is extensively sulfated on both the galactose and *N*-acetylglucosamine residues. Its molecular weight is smaller than that of chondroitin sulfate, in the range of 20,000 or less. Heparin and heparan sulfate are related glycosaminoglycans. The former is an intracellular substance present in granules of mast cells, whereas the latter is extracellular and may be anchored to cell surfaces. Both contain L-iduronic and D-glucronic acids. L-Iduronic acid predominates in heparin, whereas D-glucornic acid predominates in heparan sulfate. In heparin, most of the –NH$_2$ groups of glucosamine are sulfated and therefore de-acetylated, whereas in heparan sulfate most of them are acetylated. Heparin has a molecular weight of up to 10^6, whereas that of heparan sulfate is closer to 10^5. Heparin is an effective anticoagulant, because it binds certain coagulation factors (IX and XI) and antithrombin, a plasma protein. The latter interaction increases the ability of antithrombin to inactivate thrombin. Heparin is also used to clear lipids from serum in patients with lipid clearance disorders (see Chapter 19).

All glycosaminoglycans and keratan sulfate, except hyaluronic acid, are covalently linked to protein. Such linkages, shown in Figure 9.13, may be of the O- or the N-glycoside type. Also, at the link region, all glycosaminoglycans contain the -Gal-Gal-Xyl-sequence, in which the xylose molecule, a pentose, is

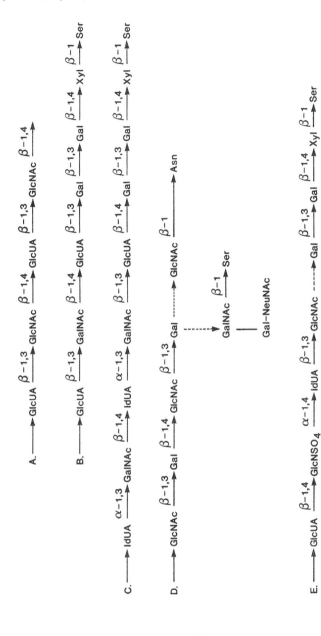

Figure 9.13 Structures of repeating units of glycosaminoglycans: (A) hyaluronic acid; (B) chondroitin sulfate; (C) dermatan sulfate; (D) two types of keratan sulfate; type I is N linked and type II is O linked; (E) heparan sulfate. Sulfate residues have been omitted in all cases.

linked to a serine via the O-glycoside linkage. Keratan sulfate is an exception: it may be linked to the protein via a GlcNAc-N-asparaginyl linkage or via the GalNAc-O-seryl bond, as in glycoproteins.

It is now possible to look at an assembled (complete) proteoglycan unit, and we take the cartilage variety as an example. There is the extended hyaluronic acid molecule to which are attached, in a noncovalent manner, numerous "bottlebrush proteoglycan" units, illustrated in Figure 9.14. The proteoglycan consists of a *core protein*, molecular weight about 400,000, to which are attached numerous units of chondroitin sulfate and keratan sulfate. Each proteoglycan unit is anchored unto hyaluronic acid via the N-terminal domain of the core protein as well as through the action of *link protein*. Hyaluronic acid aggregates

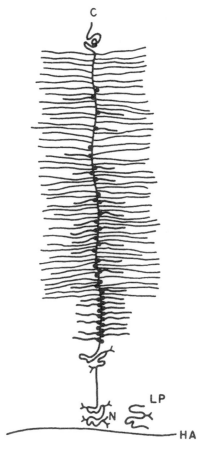

Figure 9.14 Proteoglycan aggregate found in cartilage. C and N are C and N termini of the core protein. Long wavy lines represent chondroitin sulfate, whereas the short lines represent keratan sulfate. All are linkied to the core protein via the O-serine linkage, except for a few oligosaccharide chains near the N terminus of the core protein. LP is link protein, and HA is hyaluronic acid. (Reproduced by permission from Hascall V. Introduction. Functions of the Proteoglycans, Ciba Foundation Symposium 124. New York: Wiley & Sons, 1986, p. 2.)

are very large: the molecular weight may be $2–3 \times 10^8$. This is accounted for by the fact that some 100 proteoglycan units may be associated with a single hyaluronic acid molecule, and furthermore, there may be 100–140 chondroitin sulfate (MW 15,000–25,000 each) and 30–60 keratan sulfate (MW 5000–10,000) chains associated with each molecule of core protein.

Cartilage proteoglycans function in many capacities. They act as polyelectrolytes, drawing water into their compartment and thus making cartilage stiff and resilient. The rather thick network of proteoglycans also restricts the volume available for other substances to dissolve and thus may, in fact, induce the precipitation of certain substances within such a matrix. The formation of collagen fibers and the mineralization of bone have been mentioned in this context. Proteoglycans also provide a barrier to water flow and large molecules. It is believed that the smaller nutrient molecules have no trouble diffusing through the matrix for the purpose of feeding chondrocytes, cells embedded in the cartilage matrix.

Proteoglycans are degraded by lysosomal hydrolases. There are numerous such enzymes, most of them of the exoglycosidase type (hydrolysis from the nonreducing end). These enzymes are of clinical interest in inherited lysosomal enzyme deficiency syndromes, in which an impeded degradation of one of the proteoglycans may be observed. Of the known *mucopolysaccharidoses*, as these disorders are known, the most common involve the degradation of dermatan and heparan sulfates and, to a lesser extent, keratan sulfate. This results in proteoglycan accumulation in the tissues and excretion of undegraded glycosaminoglycan fragments. Because the degradation process is stepwise, involving exoglycosidases or sulfatases, the inability to affect the removal of a sulfate residue from iduronic acid, for example, stops the progress of glycosaminoglycan degradation. The Sanfilippo disorders affect heparan sulfate degradation only, whereas the other diseases may affect the other glycosaminoglycans. The most common disorders of glycosaminoglycan degradation are listed in Table 9.1.

Table 9.1 Lysosomal Glycosaminoglycan Degradation Disorders[a]

Common name	Enzyme deficiency	Glycosaminoglycan affected
MPIIIA, Sanfilippo A	GlcN sulfate sulfatase	HS
MPIIIB, Sanfilippo B	α-N-acetylglucosaminidase	HS
MPIIIC, Sanfilippo C	Acetyltransferase[b]	HS
MPII, Hunter	Iduronic acid-O-2 sulfate sulfatase	HS, DS
MPIH/IS Hurler-Scheie	α-Iduronidase	HS, DS
MPVII	β-Glucuronidase	HS, DS
MPVIII	GlcNac-6-sulfate sulfatase	HS, KS
MPVI Maroteaux-Lamy	GalNAc-4-O-sulfate sulfatase	DS
MPIV Morquio	Gal/GalNAc-6-O-sulfate sulfatase	KS
MPVII	β-Glucuronidase	HS, DS

[a]MP, mucopolysaccharidoses; HS, heparan sulfate; DS, dermatan sulfate; KS, keratan sulfate.
[b]This enzyme catalyzes the transfer of an acetyl group from acetyl-CoA to the desulfated NH_2 group of glucosamine. This is necessary for the α-N-acetylglucosaminidase to work.

9.2 LIPIDS

9.2.1 Fatty Acids and Glycerol-Containing Lipids

Lipids (fats) are generally insoluble in water but are soluble in organic solvents. Solubility characteristics depend on structural features: those fats that have no polar residues are least water soluble, and they exist away from the aqueous environments of the organism (e.g., cholesterol esters and triglycerides). Others have hydrophilic along with hydrophobic residues. These are called *amphipathic* substances (also *amphiphiles*), and they may exist at the interface between aqueous and nonaqueous environments (e.g., phosphoglycerides).

Fatty acids are the simplest amphipathic lipids. They are organic acids with long hydrophobic (hydrocarbon) tails. They are present in the free form to a very limited extent and are mostly esterified with various alcohols. Some fatty acids have double bonds (they are termed unsaturated), but others do not (they are termed saturated). The most abundant fatty acid in the human organism is oleic acid. Naturally occurring unsaturated fatty acids have the cis configuration about each double bond. Several fatty acids have two or more double bonds, two of these (linoleic and linolenic) being *essential fatty acids*. They are required in our diets because they are precursors of prostaglandins, leukotrienes, and thromboxanes (Chapter 16). Table 9.2 lists the most important human fatty acids. Note that as the chain length increases, the melting point increases, and as the number of double bonds increases, the melting point decreases. The double bonds are capable of adding halogens, the result of which are dihalogen fatty acids. This property is often used to assess the extent of "unsaturation" in fats and oils via reaction with iodine (I_2) to obtain the so-called iodine number. The higher the iodine number, the more unsaturated the oil.

The most abundant fatty acid-containing compounds in the human organism are the *triglycerides*. These are esters of three fatty acids and one glycerol molecule, and they most commonly occur in fat storage areas—the *adipose tissue*. Triglycerides are nonamphipathic. Because about two-thirds of all fatty acids in

Table 9.2 Fatty Acids That Occur Most Commonly in the Human Organism

Fatty acid	No. of carbons including the carboxyl group	Melting point (°C)	Position of double bonds[a]	Occurrence (% of total)
Myristic	14	53	None	3
Palmitic	16	63	None	23
Stearic	18	70	None	6
Palmitoleic	16	−1	Δ^9	5
Oleic	18	13	Δ^9	50
Linoleic[b]	18	−9	$\Delta^{9,12}$	10
Linolenic[b]	18	−11	$\Delta^{9,12,15}$	<1
Arachidonic[c]	20	−50	$\Delta^{5,8,11,14}$	<1

[a]The Δ indicates a double bond; Δ^9 means a double bond between carbons 9 and 10; $\Delta^{9,12}$ means double bonds between carbons 9 and 10 and carbons 12 and 13.
[b]Essential fatty acids.
[c]Generated from linoleic acid in vivo; a more immediate precursor of prostaglandins.

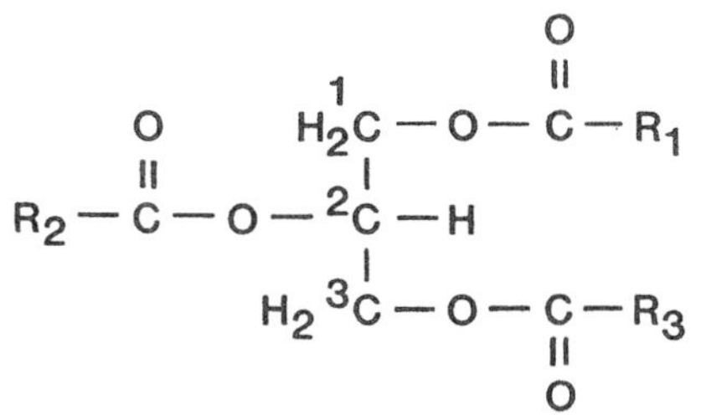

$$\begin{array}{c}
\qquad\qquad\qquad\qquad O \\
\qquad\qquad\qquad\qquad \| \\
\qquad\qquad 1 \\
\qquad\qquad H_2C - O - C - R_1 \\
O \qquad\qquad | \\
\| \qquad\qquad 2 \\
R_2 - C - O - C - H \\
\qquad\qquad | \\
\qquad\qquad 3 \\
\qquad\qquad H_2 C - O - C - R_3 \\
\qquad\qquad\qquad\qquad \| \\
\qquad\qquad\qquad\qquad O
\end{array}$$

Figure 9.15 Structure of a triglyceride. R_2-COOH and R_3-COOH are usually unsaturated fatty acids, whereas R_1-COOH is a saturated fatty acid.

the human organism are unsaturated, triglycerides reflect this usually by containing two molecules of unsaturated and one molecule of a saturated fatty acid. At body temperature, such triglycerides are liquids. A typical triglyceride is shown in Figure 9.15, where the β carbon (carbon 2) is chiral. Naturally occurring triglycerides carry the L conformation. Fatty acids may be esterified with other alcohols as well. A *wax* is an ester containing a fatty acid and a long-chain monohydroxy alcohol.

Triglycerides are hydrolyzable into their component fatty acids and glycerol. They are especially susceptible to alkaline hydrolysis. If KOH or NaOH is used, the process is *saponification* and the products, sodium and potassium salts of fatty acids, are called *soaps*. In the human organism, triglycerides are hydrolyzed by various esterases called *lipases*. These enzymes are quite specific, and they do not necessarily remove all three fatty acid molecules from a triglyceride molecule. Thus, pancreatic lipase, the main lipid digestive enzyme of the small intestine, catalyzes the removal of fatty acids from positions 1 and 3 only.

A very important group of glycerol derivatives are the phospholipids or phosphoglycerides. These amphipathic compounds are components of all membranes, in which they form the well-known lipid bilayers. They are also excellent biologic detergents. Complete hydrolysis of phosphoglycerides yields, per molecule of lipid, two molecules of fatty acid, one glycerol molecule, one phosphate ion, and one molecule of choline, ethanolamine, serine, or myoinositol. Choline-containing phosphoglycerides (*phosphatidylcholines*) are often referred to as *lecithins*. The others are collectively called *cephalins*. The parent compound of phosphoglycerides from a chemical point of view is *phosphatidic acid*, which occurs only sparingly in the free form. Its structure, as well as those of its lecithin and cephalin derivatives, are shown in Figure 9.16, which also shows a compound called phytic acid, a derivative of myoinositol, whose –OH residues are esterified by phosphate. Phytate is a potent metal binder, present in grains, and its excess ingestion leads to metal (especially Ca^{2+}) deficiency. The principal enzymes hydrolyzing phosphoglycerides are phospholipase A_1 and phospholipase A_2. The former removes the fatty acyl residue from position 1 of phosphoglycerides, whereas A_2 removes the fatty acyl residue from position 2. In the latter case, if the substrate of A_2 is lecithin, the product is *lysolecithin*, and it, too, is an excellent biologic detergent. Such detergent action is especially important in the small intestine, where lipids must be emulsified for digestion purposes.

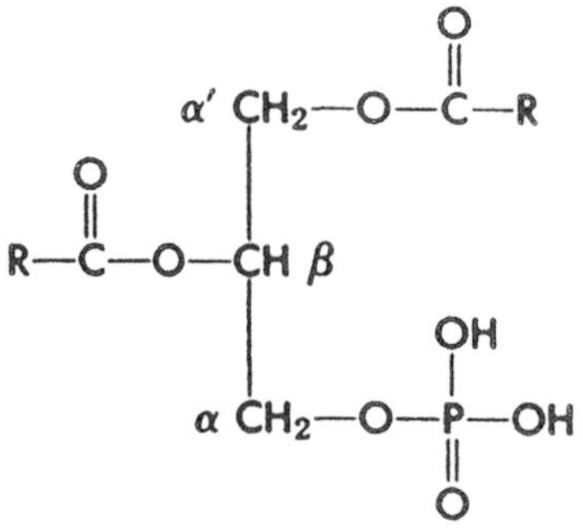

L-α-Phosphatidic acid

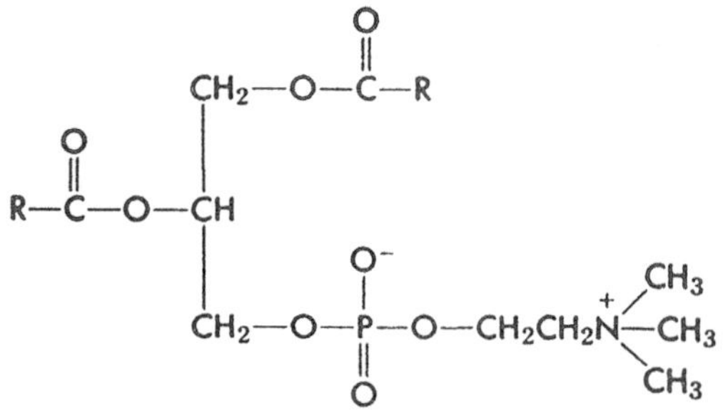

L-α-Phosphatidyl choline
α-Lecithin (zwitterion form)

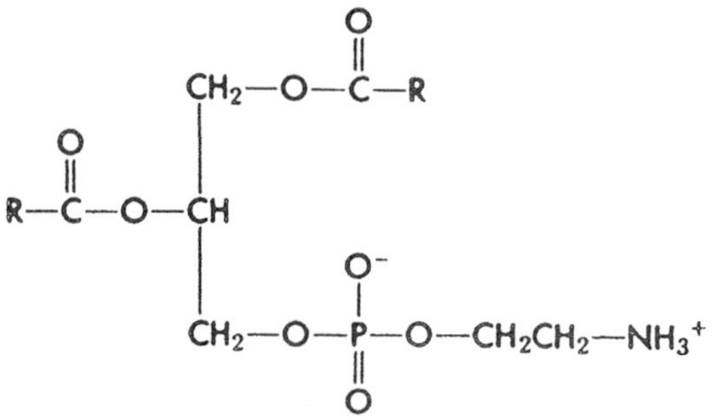

Phosphatidyl ethanolamine

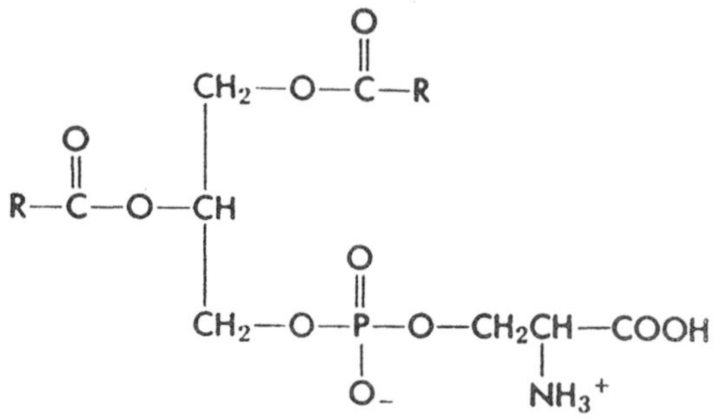

Phosphatidyl serine

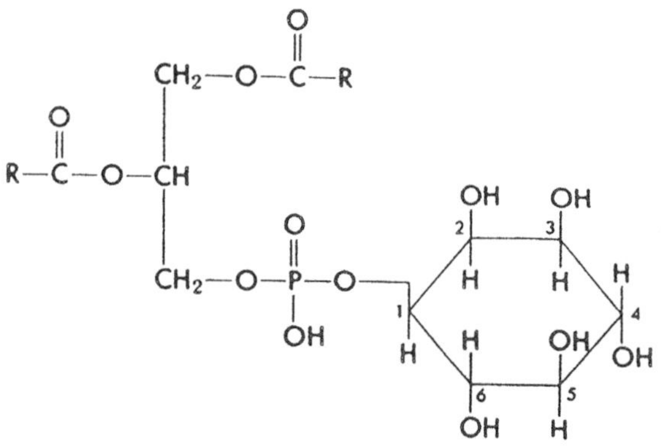

Phosphatidyl inositol

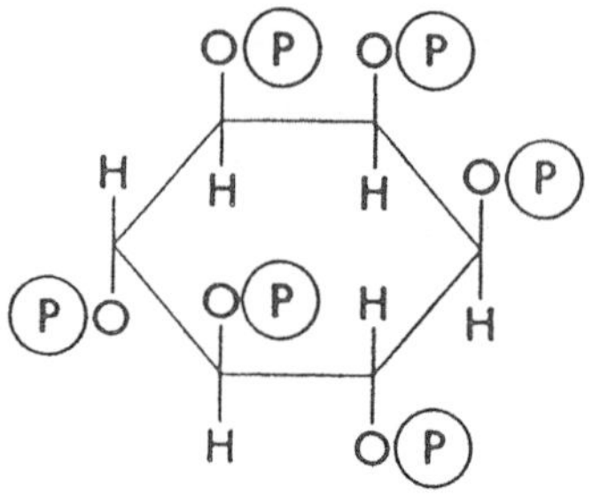

Phytic acid

Figure 9.16 Structures of phosphoglycerides and related substances. The –OH groups of phosphate residues (also indicated by P in phytic acid) are deprotonated at neutral pH.

Other phosphoglycerides include cardiolipins and plasmalogens. Cardiolipins (diphosphatidylglycerols) are present in abundance in inner mitochondrial membranes, and their complete hydrolysis yields four molecules of fatty acid, three glycerol molecules, and two phosphate ions. Plasmalogens (phosphatidal ethanolamines) are present in brain and muscle cell membranes. Complete hydrolysis yields one fatty acid, one glycerol, one phosphate ion, one

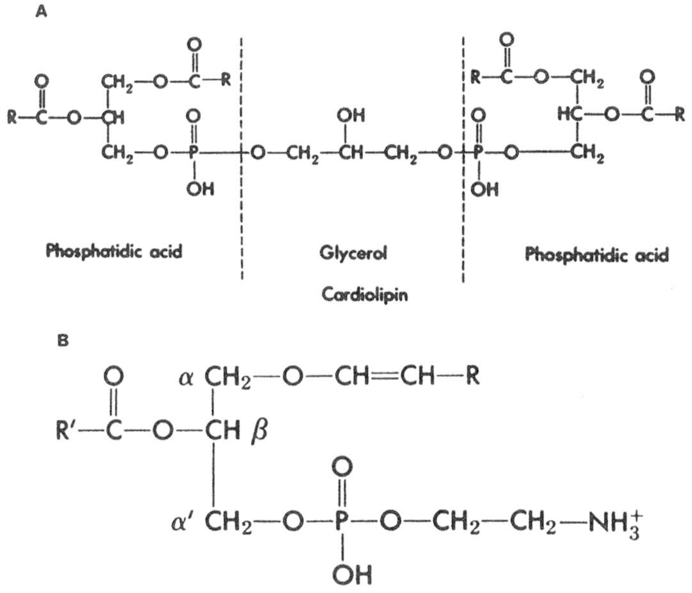

Figure 9.17   Structures of cardiolipin (A) and plasmalogen (B).

ethanolamine molecule, and a fatty acid aldehyde. The structures of a cardio-lipin and plasmalogen are shown in Figure 9.17.

9.2.2   Sphingolipids and Lipid Storage Disorders

Sphingolipids are those lipids that contain *sphingosine,* a complex substance that is synthesized from palmitic acid and serine with the loss of CO_2. They, too, are amphipathic, as shown in Figure 9.18. The amino group of sphingosine is substituted in a peptide-like bond by a fatty acid that may be as long as 24 carbons (e.g., nervonic acid, a $\Delta 15$, C_{24} fatty acid). Such derivatives of sphingosine are called *ceramides.* Both sphingosine and ceramide occur in nature in the free form in negligible amounts. When the terminal –OH group is substituted by another substance, the result is a sphingolipid: phosphocholine gives a sphingomyelin, galactose or glucose (glycoside linkage!) gives a cerebroside, a hexosamine-containing oligosaccharide gives a globoside, and a sialic acid-containing oligosaccharide gives a ganglioside. The structures of these types of compounds are shown in Figure 9.18.

Gangliosides (abbreviated G) can be classified on the basis of the number of component *N*-acetylneuraminic acid molecules and by the length of their oligosaccharide units. If we label the various components of gangliosides as shown in Figure 9.19, then the following classification can be devised, where T is trisialyl, D, disialyl, and M, nonosialyl: the structure in Figure 9.19 is a GT_1 ganglioside. It has three NeuNAc residues and four other sugars (I, II, III, and IV). A GD_{1b} ganglioside has only two NeuNAc residues, labeled A and C, whereas the GD_{1a} ganglioside has NeuNac residues, labeled A and B. A GM_1

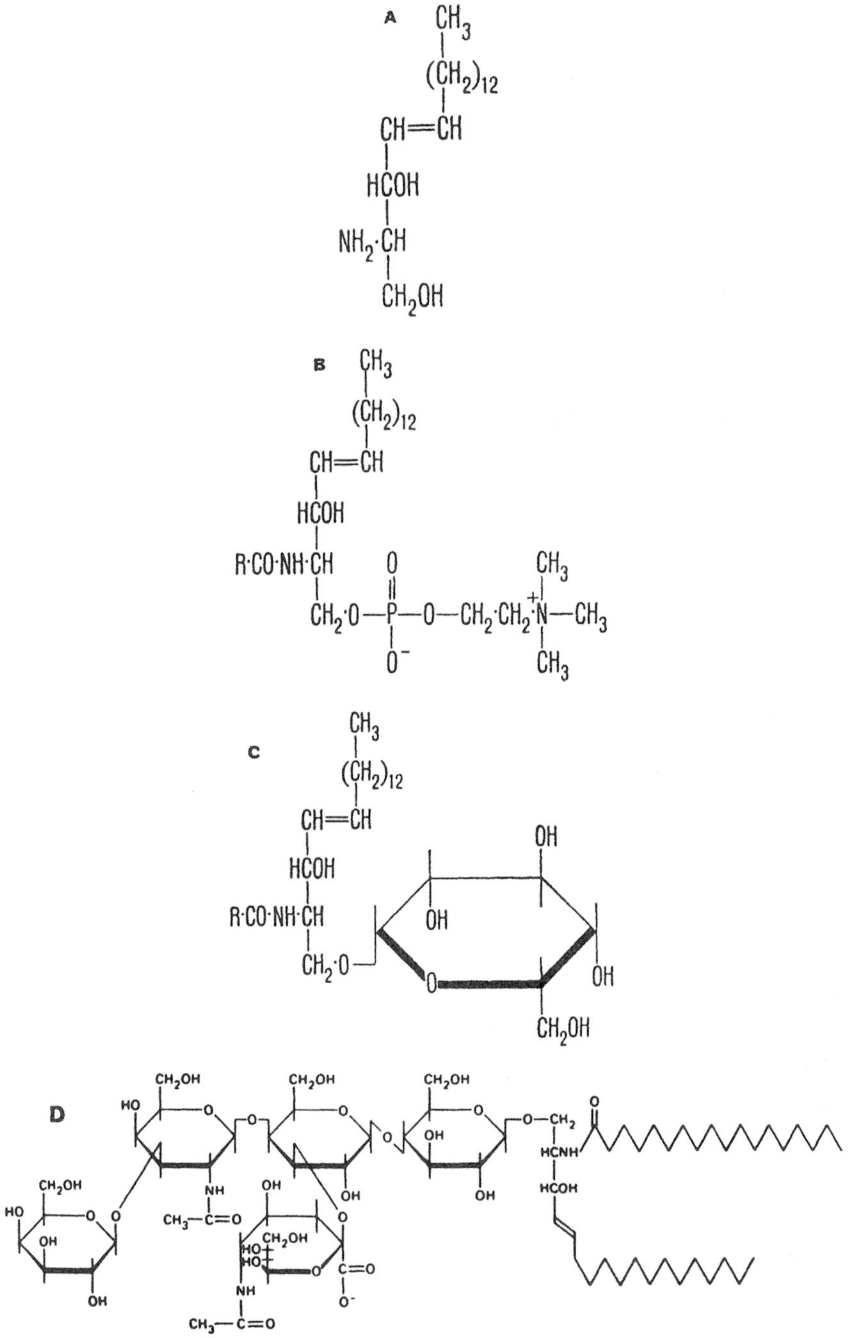

Figure 9.18 Structures of sphinogosine (A), a sphingomyelin (B), a glucocerebroside (C), and a ganglioside (D). In the last, stearic acid is attached to the –NH₂ residue of sphingosine. The structure shown represents a GM₁ ganglioside. (Parts A, B, C reproduced by permission from Diem K, Lentner C. Scientific Tables. Basel: Ciba-Geigy, 1971, p. 376; part D reproduced with permission from Fishman PH, Brady RO. Biosynthesis and function of gangliosides. Science 194:906–915, 1976.

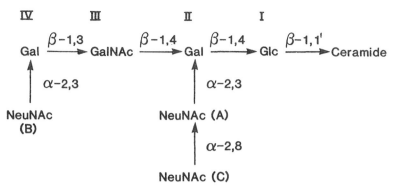

Figure 9.19 Structure of a GT_1 ganglioside.

ganglioside (Figure 9.18D) has a single NeuNAc, labeled A. The GM series may have all four sugars, labeled I, II, III, and IV, or any number less than this. A GM_2 ganglioside does not have galactose in the IV position, and GM_3 gangliosides are without sugars IV and III.

With this classification in mind, it is possible to look at a normal sphingolipid degradative procedure and its disorders. Sphingolipids are degraded by lysosomal hydrolases (see preceding discussion of glycosaminoglycan degradation). A number of hereditary (autosomal recessive) disorders are characterized by the deficiency of one of the hydrolases, and this results in sphingolipid accumulation in the nerve tissue. These are *lipid storage diseases* or *cerebral lipidoses*. The degradation of sphingolipids is shown in Figure 9.20, where various lipid storage diseases are also identified. The most common are Tay-Sachs, Gaucher's, and Niemann-Pick diseases. In Tay-Sachs disease, large quantities of the GM_2 ganglioside accumulate. In Niemann-Pick disease, sphingomyelin accumulates, and in Gaucher's disease glucocerebroside is the material in excess.

Genetic lesions in some lysosomal storage disorders have been elucidated. Thus, in the adult form of *metachromatic leukodystrophy*, the proline residue in position 426 of aryl sulfatase A is substituted by leucine. Amino acid substitutions (point mutations) are also responsible for Gaucher's disease: serine substitutes for asparagine in position 370 of glucocerebrosidase in one form, and proline replaces leucine in position 444 in another. In the French-Canadian form of infantile Tay-Sachs disease, exon 1 (a portion of DNA) is deleted from the gene coding for the α subunit of hexosaminidase A. In the Sandhoff variety of the Tay-Sachs disease, exons 1–5 of the β subunit gene of hexosaminidase A are deleted.

There are other lysosomal disorders in addition to those shown in Figure 9.20 and Table 9.1. For instance, several types of fucosidoses exist, which affect such structures as glycoproteins and blood group substances. Sialidoses also exist. However, lysosomal fucosidase and sialidase (neuraminidase) deficiencies do not affect the degradation of gangliosides.

It has already been stated that phosphoglycerides are good biologic detergents. This property is especially important in the function of lungs, where lecithin, through its action as a surfactant, prevents the collapse of the air sacs.

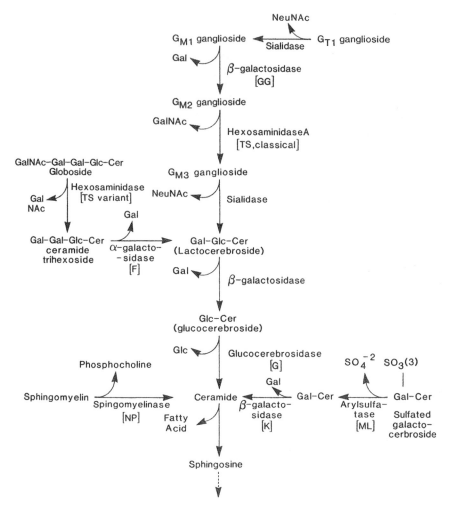

Figure 9.20 Degradation of sphingolipids. Lipid storage diseases are indicated by brackets as follows: TS, Tay-Sachs; ML, metachromatic leukodystrophy; GG, generalized gangliosidosis; G, Gaucher's disease; NP, Niemann-Pick disease; K, Krabbe's disease; F, Fabry's disease. The sulfate residue on galactocerebroside is located on position 3 of the galactose residue. Note the sequential nature of the process: if one step cannot take place, all subsequent steps cannot take place, either.

The infant is occasionally born with immature lungs that do not have the appropriate quantity of lecithin. The clinical result is the *respiratory distress syndrome* (RDS). It is possible to predict lung maturity in a newborn by measuring the lecithin/sphingomyelin (L/S) ratio in the amniotic fluid. Normal amniotic fluid, after 34–36 weeks of gestation, gives an L/S ratio of 2:1. The lecithin measured is the saturated type (saturated phosphatidylcholine, SPC). Mature lungs are characterized by an SPC value of about 500 μg/dL or above. It should be noted that sphingomyelin exerts no detergent activity in the lungs. It is measured only as a convenient reference point for the lecithin.

A better predictor of RDS, especially in complicated cases, such as diabetes, is phosphatidylglyceride (PG); phosphatidic acid esterified with glycerol at its phosphate residue. An amniotic fluid PG level of less than 0.5 μg/mL predicts RDS after birth.

9.2.3 Cholesterol and Other Steroids

Cholesterol is an amphipathic substance present in various biologic membranes, in the bloodstream, and in tissue storage sites. Cholesterol and substances derived from it are called *steroids*, and their most prominent feature is the four-ring structure shown in Figure 9.21. Cholesterol is synthesized in the human organism from acetyl coenzyme A (acetyl-CoA), and all other steroid substances in the human organism are biosynthesized from it. These substances are the bile salts, the detergents of the gastrointestinal tract that emulsify lipids for digestion purposes (Chapter 20), and steroid hormones, such as cortisol, whose chemistry and metabolism are covered in Chapter 16. Cholesterol may be present in the form of cholesterol esters, in which its –OH group is esterified by a fatty acid. Cholesterol esters are not amphipathic. Serum cholesterol amounts to 150–300 mg/dL, two-thirds of which is esterified cholesterol.

Cholesterol may exist in two forms with respect to the configuration of its carbon 3, which is chiral: in the β form, the –OH residue is cis with respect to the methyl group (carbon 19), whereas in the α form they are trans to each other. The cis relationship is indicated by a solid line, the trans by a broken line (see Figure 9.21). Naturally occurring cholesterol is of the β configuration, and because the ring system is practically planar, it is possible to state that the –OH group, the two methyl groups (C-18 and C-19), and the eight-carbon side chain are all located above the plane of the ring (all cis).

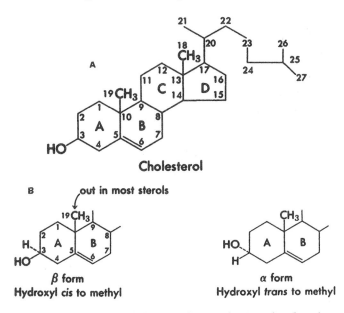

Figure 9.21 Structure of cholesterol showing the numbering of each carbon, ring nomenclature, and the configuration about C-3.

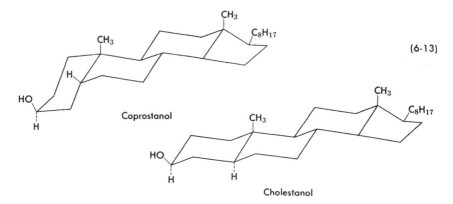

(6-13)

Figure 9.22 Coprastanol and cholestanol, products of cholesterol reduction. Dotted lines indicate positions below the plane of the ring (trans with respect to –CH₃ on position 10); solid lines indicate positions above the plane of the ring (cis with respect to –CH₃ on position 10). Both structures are of the β type.

It should be realized that the various cholesterol ring structures have three-dimensional shapes, the chair forms predominating. This is best illustrated by looking at the two isomers of reduced cholesterol, *coprostanol* and *cholestanol*. In these isomers, the H in position 5 may be either cis or trans with respect to –CH₃ attached to position 10 of the steroid ring structure. This is illustrated in Figure 9.22. Both coprostanol and cholestanol may, of course, exist as the α or β isomers when the –OH group in position 3 is related to the –CH₃ in position 10. The two compounds in Figure 9.22 are both β isomers. Most naturally occurring steroids are related to either coprostanol or cholestanol, with the latter predominating.

9.3   MEMBRANES

9.3.1   Composition and Structure of Membranes

Membranes serve to delineate cellular entities, in which case they are termed *plasma membranes*, and various subcellular particles, such as mitochondria, nuclei, and lysosomes. Such subcellular structures as endoplasmic reticulum and the Golgi apparatus also consist, in large part, of membranous materials. The basic structure of membranes is lipid in nature, and it is the amphipathic nature of such lipid that permits them to aggregate into bilayers. Lipid is not the only component of membranes, however; there are protein and carbohydrate components as well. It is these components that function as the means by which hydrophilic substances can cross membranes or that serve as recognition beacons that permit various substances to affect the metabolic activities of cellular and subcellular particles.

If an amphiphile, such as lysolecithin, is suspended in water, it forms *micelles*, whose three-dimensional shape is that of an inverted cone. The basis for this type of assembly is that the hydrophobic fatty acid tails will interact with each other and exclude water from their environment, whereas the hydrophilic phosphocholine section remains in contact with the aqueous environment. If lecithins, cephalins, or cardiolipins are suspended in water, they aggregate into

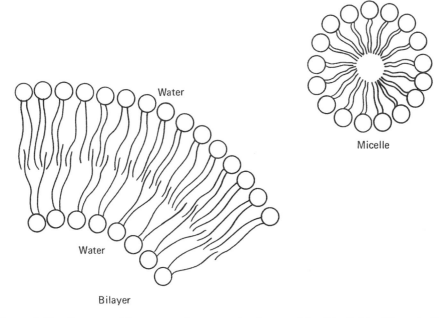

Bilayer

Figure 9.23 Two possible means of aggregation by amphipathic lipids. The micelle is formed by lysolecithin, for example, whereas the bilayer may be formed by lecithins, sphingomyelins, or cephalins.

bilayers, whose three-dimensional shape is that of a cylinder. Other aggregation patterns are also possible. These structures are illustrated in Figure 9.23. Thus, it is the lecithins, cephalins, sphingolipids, and cardiolipins that are the major components of biologic membranes. The membrane composition from various sources is illustrated in Table 9.3, which shows that the ratio of protein to lipid can vary substantially from one membrane to another and that cholesterol is also an important component of mammalian (but not of prokaryotic) membranes. As seen later, cholesterol is a mediator of membrane fluidity. Note also that cardiolipin is found largely in the inner mitochondrial membranes, whereas glycolipids (cerebrosides and gangliosides) are largely found in myelin.

Figure 9.24 illustrates the current concept of a typical membrane. The phospholipid framework is shown in the form of a bilayer, in which one finds embedded various types of proteins. Some proteins are *glycoproteins*—they contain carbohydrate, which is always on the outer surface of the membrane. Some proteins span the entire length of the bilayer. They cannot be separated from the membrane, unless the entire membrane structure is disrupted by detergents. They interact with the hydrophobic portion of the lipid bilayer through their hydrophobic amino acid side chains. These are termed *intrinsic* proteins. Other proteins may exist in loose combination with either the outside (plasma) or the inside (cytosol) surface of the membrane. These are removable with relative ease, by washing with water or aqueous buffers containing salt or metal chelating agents. These are termed extrinsic proteins (peripheral proteins), and they generally interact electrostatically with the hydrophilic residues of bilayer lipids. A

Table 9.3 Composition of Membranes[a]

Component	Myelin (human)	Erythrocyte (human)	Mitochondria (rat) Inner	Mitochondria (rat) Outer	ER (rat) Rough	ER (rat) Smooth	Hepatocyte plasma (rat)	Nuclear (rat)
Protein, %	20	49	70–80	60–70	60–80	40	50–70	60–80
Carbohydrate, %	5	8	2	4	—	—	—	—
Total lipid, %	75	43	20–25	30–40	15–30	60	30–50	15–40
Cholesterol[b]	22	23	<3	<5	6	10	20	10
PC	10	17	45	50	55	55	64	55
PE	15	18	25	23	16	21	17	20
PI			6	13	8	7	11	7
PS	9	7	1	2	—	—	—	3
SM	8	18	3	5	3	12	—	3
Glycolipid	28	3	—	—	—	—	—	
Cardiolipin	—	—	18	4	—	2	—	—
Other	8	13	—	—	—	—	2	—

[a]PC, phosphatidylcholine; PE, phosphatidylethanolamine; PI, phosphatidylinositol; PS, phosphatidylserine; SM, sphingomyelin; ER, endoplasmic reticulum.
[b]All lipids are listed as % of total lipid.
Source: From Jain MK, Wagner RC. Introduction to Biological Membranes. New York: Wiley-Interscience, 1980, Table 3-5.

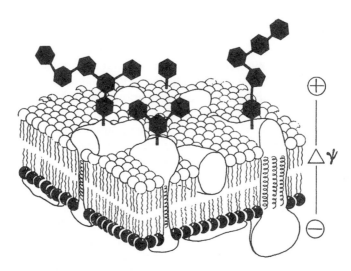

Figure 9.24 The fluid-mosaic model of plasma membrane. Phospholipids with darkened heads are on the cytosol side of the bilayer, and the lipids with unfilled heads are on the outer surface. In intrinsic proteins one or more α-helical segments are in contact with the hydrophobic environment of the bilayer. They usually have hydrophobic amino acid side chains. Carbohydrate is indicated by hexagons. The membrane potential (negative inside) is indicated by $\Delta\Psi$. (Reproduced by permission from Vance DE, Vance JE. Biochemistry of Lipids and Membranes. Menlo Park: Benjamin/Cummings, 1985, p. 26.)

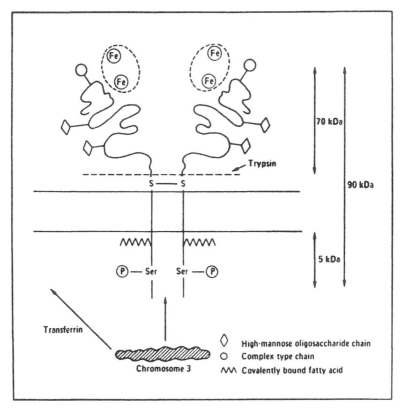

Figure 9.25 The transferrin receptor, an intrinsic membrane protein. (Reproduced by permission from Newman R, Schneider C, Sutherland R, et al. The transferrin receptor. Trends Biochem Sci November: 397–400, 1982.)

typical intrinsic protein is the transferrin receptor, shown in Figure 9.25 (see also Chapter 7), which combines with iron-saturated serum transferrin before the latter is internalized by the cell via the endocytic process. Other intrinsic proteins are the red blood cell membrane proteins glycophorin and "band 3," the latter having been implicated in Cl^- and HCO_3^- transport, and bacterial rhodopsin. The latter functions to generate a H^+ gradient across the membrane of *Halobacterium halobium* by capturing light energy. It is a single-chain protein that loops in and out of the cell membrane. Seven α-helical regions are present in this protein, each embedded in the lipid bilayer. These helices contain largely hydrophobic amino acid side chains. Such *transmembrane proteins*, which contain hydrophobic helices and hydrophilic components that are in contact with either the extracellular or intracellular aqueous environments, are also termed *amphipathic*. Of the extrinsic (peripheral) proteins, the best known are spectrin and ankyrin, which occur on the cytosol side of the red blood cell membrane; and β_2-microglobulin, which occurs on the plasma side of various cell membranes.

Figure 9.24 also distinguishes between the phospholipids on the plasma and cytosol surfaces of the bilayer. Most membranes are *asymmetric* in this respect: phosphoglycerides on the cytosol side are largely anionic—phosphatidylserine, phosphatidylinositol, and phosphatidylethanolamine (the latter is very weakly cationic). Phosphoglycerides on the outer surface of the bilayers are largely cationic—sphingomyelins and phosphatidylcholines. Figure 9.26 illustrates lipid asymmetry for the erythrocyte and *B. megaterium* membranes. Note also that phosphatidylglycerol occurs in quantity in bacterial but not in mammalian cell membranes.

Physically, the membrane may exist in two states: the "solid" gel crystalline and the "liquid" fluid crystalline states. For each type of membrane, there is a specific temperature at which one changes into the other. This is the *transition temperature* (T_c). The T_c is relatively high for membranes containing saturated fatty acids and low for those with unsaturated fatty acids. Thus, bilayers of phosphatidylcholine with two palmitate residues have a $T_c = 41°C$ but that with two oleic acid residues has a $T_c = -20°C$. The hybrid has a $T_c = -5°C$. Sphingomyelin bilayer, on the other hand, may have a T_C of close to body temperature. In the gel crystalline state, the hydrophobic tails of phospholipids are ordered, whereas in the fluid crystalline state they are disordered. At body temperature, all eukaryotic membranes appear to be in the liquid crystalline state, and this is caused, in part, by the presence of unsaturated fatty acids and in part by cholesterol. The latter maintains the fatty acid side chains in the disordered state, even below the normal T_c. There is thus no evidence that membranes regulate cellular metabolic activity by changing their physical status from the gel to the fluid state,

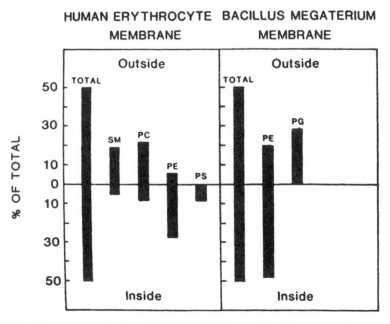

Figure 9.26 Asymmetry of phospholipids in the human erythrocyte and *B. megaterium* plasma membranes. "Total lipid" indicates 50% of lipid on each of the two sides of the bilayer. SM, PC, PE, PS, and PG are sphingomyelin, phosphatidylcholine, phosphatidylethanolamine, phosphatidylserine, and phosphatidylglycerol, respectively. (Reproduced by permission from Vance DE, Vance JE. Biochemistry of Lipids and Membranes. Menlo Park: Benjamin/Cummings, 1985, p. 477.)

or vice versa. The fluid crystalline state of membranes thus permits various movements by constituent lipids and proteins to take place inside the lipid bilayer: rotational diffusion, lateral diffusion, and flexing of fatty acid tails. The presence of cholesterol does not hinder these movements. The transverse (*flip-flop*) movement of membrane components, however, does not take place. Thus, it is not easy to exchange a phosphatidylcholine residue on the plasma surface for a phosphatidylserine residue from the cytosol surface. It has been proposed that the extrinsic membrane proteins (e.g., the filamentous spectrin) may have a function in maintaining membrane integrity and asymmetry.

9.3.2 Transport Functions of Membranes

It is well established that membranes form a barrier to the free passage of various ions in and out of cells. On the other hand, lipid-like substances, such as steroid hormones, can pass through membranes with ease. Gaseous substances, dissolved in the aqueous phase, also cross the membranes with ease, for example CO_2, O_2, and NH_3. Mechanisms must exist for the transport of charged particles across membranes, however. In addition, many substances affect cellular metabolism without entering the cell. The cell surface therefore contains various receptors and transport proteins, which are intrinsic membrane proteins. Some receptors interact with hormones or other metabolic mediators; others serve to transport larger substances into cells by the process of *receptor-mediated endocytosis*. In the latter case, the process is believed to proceed as indicated in Figure 9.27: transferrin receptors (see Figure 9.25) are assembled into a "pit," which is coated on the cytosolic side by the protein *clathrin* (not shown), which aids in the separation of the pit from the cell membrane in the form of a clathrin-coated vesicle. This is eventually changed to the CURL particle (compartment for the uncoupling of receptor and ligand), in which the pH drops to around 5. This serves to dissociate iron from transferrin; iron leaves CURL and is utilized by the cell, and transferrin with its receptor is recycled to the cell surface. The latter process is *exocytosis*. A similar system operates in the internalization of low-density lipoprotein and discussed in Chapter 19. A similar, although non–receptor-mediated process, *fluid pinocytosis*, in which a pocket on the membrane surface is pinched off nonspecifically and is internalized, carrying into the cell a portion of the extracellular fluid. Some cell lines acquire nutrients in this fashion, and macrophages may internalize foreign materials, such as carbon particles, via this process.

Many substances can be transported into the cell (and vice versa) against a concentration gradient. This is an *active transport process*, and it requires energy in the form of ATP. It is to be distinguished from a *passive transport process*, which is simple diffusion across membranes. One of the better understood systems of this type is the *sodium-potassium ATPase* (or Na/K) *pump*, which maintains high potassium and low sodium levels in the cell. These are up to 160 meq/L for K^+ and about 10 meq/L of Na^+ inside the cell. Extracellular fluid contains about 145 meq/L of Na^+ and 4 meq/L of K^+. The simultaneous movement of one substance out of the cell and another into the cell is an *antiport*. A substantial percentage of the basal metabolic rate (see Chapter 21) is accounted for by the activity of the Na/K pump. ATPase (Na/K pump) is lo-

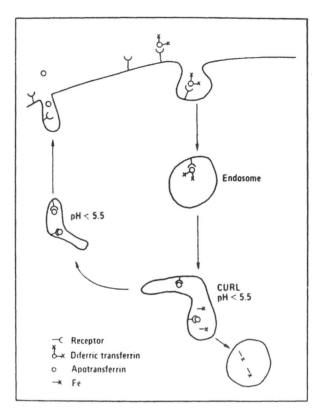

Figure 9.27 Receptor-mediated endocytosis of diferric transferrin in erythroid tissue and certain other cell lines. (Reproduced by permission from Dantry-Varsat A, Ciechanover A, Lodish HF. pH and the recycling of transferrin during receptor-mediated endocytosis. Proc Natl Acad Sci USA 80:2258–2262, 1983.)

cated in the plasma membranes of cells and pumps three Na^+ ions out of the cell for every two K^+ ions pumped in. The action of the pump is illustrated in Figure 9.28. The enzyme itself has two pairs of identical subunits, one of which (MW 95,000) binds ATP and has Na^+ and K^+ binding sites. The other (MW 40,000) is a glycopeptide facing the surface of the cell. The larger subunit combines with cardiac glycosides, such as digoxin and ouabain, which inhibit the Na/K pump.

The unequal distribution of K^+ and Na^+ across plasma membranes gives rise to an electrical potential difference ΔE. It can be calculated by the Nernst equation (see Chapter 2):

$$\Delta E = -\frac{RT}{F} \ln \frac{K^+_{in}}{K^+_{out}} \tag{9.5}$$

If we assume that $R = 1.98$ cal/°-mol, $T = 37°C$ or 310K, $F = 23,000$ cal/V-mol, and $K^+_{in}/K^+_{out} = 150/4$, then

$$\Delta E = -\frac{1.98 \times 310 \times 2.3}{23,000} \times \log \frac{150}{4} = -0.61 \times 1.57 = -96 \text{ mV} \tag{9.6}$$

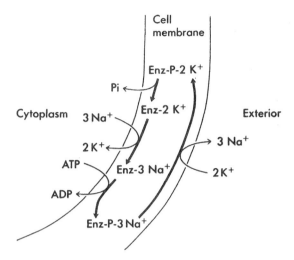

Figure 9.28 Operation of the sodium-potassium ATPase. The process involves phosphorylation of the enzyme and binding of Na^+ on the cytosol side of the membrane and K^+ on the plasma (outer) side.

The charge inside the cell is negative relative to the outside. The actual membrane potential $\Delta\Psi$ is somewhat smaller than ΔE because of nonspecific cation leakage across membranes. In bacteria, an ATPase generates a potent proton gradient across plasma membranes, the pH outside being lower than that inside the cell. In some bacterial cultures, pH difference may be as high as 2 (alkaline inside).

One of the purposes of creating concentration gradients across cell membranes is to transport nutrients into the cell. Thus, the sodium gradient generated across eukaryotic cell membranes serves to transport glucose and galactose into various cells in *symport* with sodium ions. The sodium ions, their concentration being higher outside the cell, tend to move back into the cell through the operation of the second law of thermodynamics. By coupling such a movement of Na^+ with that of glucose, using specific membrane-bound protein carriers, the nutritional requirement of the cell can be satisfied. Mammalian glucose carriers transport one glucose molecule for two Na^+ ions. Glucose absorption operates via this mechanism in both intestinal mucosal cells and kidney tubules. A glycoside named phlorhizin inhibits glucose transport across cell membranes. Glucose may be transported across membranes against a gradient, and hence this has been referred to as an active transport process. Glucose/Na^+ transport per se does not depend on energy expenditure, however; it depends on the operation of the Na/K pump. If the latter is inhibited, glucose transport stops. Symport mechanisms using Na^+ gradients also exist for amino acid transport. Glucose and amino acid transport may be referred to as secondary active processes, as opposed to the primary Na-K pump.

Sodium concentration gradients may serve other purposes as well. Thus, in nerve cells, the outflow and inflow of Na^+ cause the propagation of currents along the axons. We had occasion to observe this in the case of the visual impulse (Chapter 6). Additionally, Na^+ drives a H^+ exchange antiport whose function is to control intracellular pH. As various metabolic reactions produce protons, these are removed from the cell while sodium enters the cell. Such pumps may be activated by low pH (e.g., 7.2–7.4) and become inactive at around pH 7.7. Like the transport of glucose, the Na^+/H^+ pump is a secondary active transport mechanism.

In bacteria, Na^+ is often replaced by H^+ as the carrier of nutrients. The best known mechanisms of this sort are the various galactoside (e.g., lactose) transporters, because lactose is an important carbon source for many bacteria. The work that can be performed (e.g., in transporting a nutrient) by generating a proton gradient across membranes may be expressed by the following, which encompasses both the chemical component (concentration gradient) and the electrical component in the form of the membrane potential $\Delta\Psi$:

$$\Delta G' = RT \ln\frac{H_{in}^+}{H_{out}^+} + F\Delta\Psi = F\Delta\Psi - 2.3RT\,\Delta pH \tag{9.7}$$

If the pH gradient in a bacterial culture is 2 (i.e., H_{in}^+/H_{out}^+) and if the measured $\Delta\Psi$ is -100 mV, then we calculate the $\Delta G'$ at 310 K as

$$\Delta G' = 2.3 \times 1.98 \times 310 \times \log 10^{-2} + 23{,}000\,(-0.1) = -5123 \text{ cal} \tag{9.8}$$

This energy can be used to transport lactose, creating a lactose gradient that can be calculated as

$$\Delta G' = 2.3RT \log\frac{L_i}{L_o} = 5123 \text{ cal} \qquad \text{and} \qquad \frac{L_i}{L_o} = 4273 \tag{9.9}$$

where L is lactose and $\Delta G'$ is positive, because work is being used rather than generated. Theoretically, a pH difference of 2 generates enough work to be able to concentrate lactose 4273-fold inside the cell.

The proton gradient across microbial plasma membranes is created through energy expenditure. A proton pump, associated with an ATPase, pumps protons from the microorganism to the outside. ATP is hydrolyzed to ADP and P_i in the process. Several types of ATPases carrying out this type of reaction are known to exist.

Membrane transport particles also allow the uptake of nutrients by the so-called facilitative transport systems. These involve specific carriers, although no energy is expended. It is therefore impossible to transport a substance against a concentration gradient by this system, and net uptake stops once the substance concentration is equal on both sides of the membrane. Fructose and mannose are transported into cells by a facilitative process. As with active transport particles, it is possible to saturate this transport system in the Michaelis-Menten sense (see Chapter 5). By increasing the substrate concentration outside the cell, a transport V_{max} can be achieved in either case. If a simple diffusion (passive transport) is the means of transport, no saturation phenomenon is observed and transport is proportional to the nutrient concentration outside the cell. L Sugars and pentoses are transported into cells by a simple diffusion process. The active transport process (e.g., glucose and galactose) is usually the fastest, followed by facilitated process, and diffusion is the slowest, given the same types of nutrients. Microbial and mammalian transport systems are summarized in Figure 9.29.

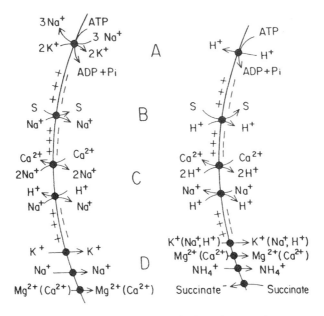

Figure 9.29 Some mammalian (left) and microbial (right) membrane transport systems. (A) Primary electrogenic mechanisms (pumps) creating either a Na^+ or a H^+ gradient. (B) Secondary active transport systems of the symport type, in which the entry of a nutrient S into the cell is coupled with the entry of either the sodium ions or protons. (D) Various passive ion movements, possibly via channels or uniports. (Reproduced by permission from Serrano R. Plasma Membrane ATPase of Plants and Fungi. Boca Raton: CRC Press, 1985, p. 59.)

The transport of small charged ions, especially Na^+, K^+, Ca^{2+}, and Cl^-, may be affected by *ion channels*. Such channels are created by specific integral proteins that span the entire thickness of the membrane. They are very specific for the size and charge of the ion transported. There is no energy input, and the movement of ions through the channels is "downhill." Such movements are extremely rapid, however, much more so than those seen with active and facilitative transport processes. Ion channels are not constantly open; they have "gates," which open in response to specific stimuli. Such a stimulus may be a voltage charge across the membrane, interaction with the ion to be transported, a neurotransmitter, or another substance or process.

Na^+ channels usually respond to voltage changes. They are said to be *voltage gated*, and they are responsible for the propagation of action potentials. The Na^+ channels open locally if the membrane is partially depolarized by electrical stimulation, for example. The influx of Na^+ into the cell further depolarizes the membrane patch, which causes depolarization of neighboring membrane areas, thus passing along the signal. The electrical excitability of cells (nerve muscle cells) thus depends on the opening of Na^+ channels. Another example of channel function is associated with the action of acetylcholine, a neurotransmitter, and the neuromuscular junction. As the nerve cell ending releases acetylcholine and the latter strikes its muscle target cell receptor, the receptor molecule, also a gated channel, opens in response to such stimulation.

The channel admits largely Na^+ into the cell, although K^+ and Ca^{2+} also enter. Depolarization of the membrane patch, where the neurotransmitter receptor is located, causes the opening of neighboring voltage-gated Na^+ channels, causing further depolarization and movement of the action potential along the membrane. The latter affects the membranous sarcoplasmic reticulum and the release of Ca^{2+} from there into the cytosol. Contraction of the muscle follows Ca^{2+} release.

Channels may be created artificially by substances called *ionophores*. Many ionophores are antibiotics and are specific for small ions. Thus, gramicidin (see Chapter 4) creates channels that permit the flow of K^+, Na^+, and H^+ across membranes. Gramicidin is a small α-helical peptide, but when two molecules are lined up end to end, the complex becomes about 3 nm in length and can span the lipid bilayer. The ions pass through its central pore.

Other ionophores act as shuttle systems, often conceptualized as antiports or *uniports*, the latter term indicating the transport of a single ion at a time in a given direction. Valinomycin, for example, a cyclic peptide, is a rather specific carrier of K^+, whereas nigericin is an antiport that exchanges K^+ for H^+ in the cell. Monensin does the same with Na^+ and Li^+, and calcium ionophore (A23187) exchanges Ca^{2+} or Mg^{2+} for H^+. There are several *proton ionophores*, that is, substances that can collapse proton gradients across membranes. The most commonly used proton ionophore is 2,4-dinitrophenol, which acts as a symport of H^+ and as an anion. Thus, a 2,4-dinitrophenol-treated bacterial cell is not able to transport lactose. Another important proton ionophore is carbonylcyanide trifluoromethoxyphenylhydrazone. Proton concentrations in cells can also be disturbed by such agents as NH_3 and CH_3-NH_3. These unprotonated substances cross the cell membrane and bind protons inside the cells, thus increasing cellular pH.

QUESTIONS

9.1.   Clathrin is most likely
    a.   An intrinsic membrane protein
    b.   An extrinsic membrane protein
    c.   A hormone receptor
    d.   An ionophore
    e.   A glycoprotein

9.2.   Which carbohydrate molecule is expected to have the largest number of *nonreducing* ends per mole?
    a.   Amylose
    b.   Amylopectin
    c.   Chondroitin sulfate
    d.   Carbohydrate portion of a GT_1 ganglioside
    e.   Glycogen

9.3.   Suppose a patient had a sialidase (*N*-acetylneuraminidase) deficiency. Which substance do you *not* expect to accumulate in the patient's cells?
    a.   Oligosaccharides from serum glycoproteins
    b. GT_1 gangliosides
    c. GM_1 gangliosides
    d.   Cerebrosides
    e. GM_2 gangliosides

9.4. The best treatment for a patient with Niemann-Pick disease is
   a. Infuse hexosaminidase A intravenously
   b. Administer choline orally
   c. Administer sphingomyelinase intravenously
   d. Give aspirin and plenty of fluids
   e. Administer essential fatty acids

9.5. Which is *not* true about the transport of lactose into *E. coli*?
   a. Dependent on the Na/K pump
   b. Dependent on hydrolysis of ATP
   c. A result of pH gradient across membrane
   d. Inhibited by 2,4-dinitrophenol
   e. Active process

9.6. A new enzyme is specific for β-1,4 linkages and is an endoglycosidase. Which substance does it hydrolyze?
   a. Amylose
   b. Cellulose
   c. Lactose
   d. Cellobiose
   e. Amylopectin

9.7. Which is *not* a hydrolysis product of GM_1 gangliosides?
   a. 1 mole sialic acid per mole lipid
   b. 1 mole fatty acid per mole lipid
   c. 1 mole sphingosine per mole lipid
   d. 2 moles acetate per mole lipid
   e. 1 mole glycerol per mole lipid

9.8. A microorganism creates a pH gradient of 2 across its membrane (alkaline inside). Contrary to mammalian cells, bacterial membrane potentials are caused largely by proton gradients. What is the ΔE across the bacterial membrane at 37°C?
   a. 30 mV
   b. 60 mV
   c. 90 mV
   d. 120 mV
   e. 240 mV

9.9. When pancreatic amylase acts on amylopectin, the products are
   a. Maltose and limit dextrin
   b. Amylose and glucose
   c. Glucose and maltose
   d. Lactose and amylose
   e. Limit dextrin and glucose

In Questions 9.10–9.12, indicate as follows:
   a. Lactose   c. Both
   b. Sucrose   d. Neither

9.10. Nonreducing
9.11. β Linkage present
9.12. α Linkage present

In Questions 9.13–9.22, indicate as follows:
   a. 1, 2, and 3 are correct.
   b. 1 and 3 are correct.
   c. 2 and 4 are correct.

d.   4 only is correct.
e.   All are correct.

9.13. Mammalian cell membranes typically
1.   Contain triglycerides
2.   Control their function by switching from the gel crystalline to the fluid crystalline forms
3.   Undergo transverse movement of component lipids from the cytosol to plasma side
4.   Allow lateral movement of intrinsic proteins

9.14. Membrane surface on the cell exterior
1.   May contain carbohydrate
2.   Contains hydrophilic portions of phosphatidylcholine and sphingomyelin
3.   May have bound extrinsic proteins
4.   Major lipid component is phosphatidylserine

9.15. L Sugars are components of
1.   Blood group substances
2.   Gangliosides and cerebrosides
3.   Dermatan sulfate
4.   Hyalouronic acid

9.16. Transport of glucose across the kidney tubule membrane is inhibited by
1.   Stoppage of the Na/K pump
2.   Phlorhizin
3.   Ouabain
4.   Gramicidin

9.17. Cholesterol that occurs naturally:
1.   Nonamphipathic molecule
2.   Virtually flat molecule with the side chain, methyl groups, and the –OH group pointing in the same direction
3.   Present in bacterial plasma membranes
4.   Interferes with the orderly alignment of fatty acid hydrocarbon chains in membranes

9.18. The "link" protein is
1.   Extrinsic protein in red blood cell membranes
2.   Intrinsic protein of red blood cell membranes
3.   Protein that joins carbohydrate to cell membrane surfaces
4.   Protein that stabilizes connective tissue proteoglycans

9.19. A procedure called β elimination removes carbohydrate from protein when there is an O-glycoside linkage with serine or threonine. β Elimination is active in separating carbohydrate from protein in
1.   Some keratan sulfate from "core protein"
2.   Some chondroitin sulfate from "core protein"
3.   Oligosaccharide from transferrin protein
4.   Oligosaccharide from blood group substance protein

9.20. Hyaluronic acid
1.   Polymer of N-acetylglucosamine and glucuronic acid
2.   Covalently linked to "core protein" carrying glycosaminoglycans
3.   May contain up to 100 proteoglycan units
4.   Heteropolysaccharide containing β-1,3 linkages

9.21. A reducing substance(s) is the product of hydrolysis of
1.   A hemiacetal
2.   A plasmalogen

   3. Fructose
   4. A sphingomyelin
22. A gated Na^+ channel
   1. Pumps sodium out of the cell while pumping in protons
   2. Opens up in response to membrane depolarization
   3. Allows Na^+ to flow out of the cell
   4. When active, propagates the action potential

Answers

9.1. (b) Clathrin is most likely an extrinsic membrane protein on the cytosol side. It participates in receptor-mediated endocytosis processes.

9.2. (e) The two most likely candidates are amylopectin and glycogen. Glycogen is more highly branched and therefore has more nonreducing end residues.

9.3. (d) Look for the substance that has no NeuNAc. The only one is cerebroside.

9.4. (c) Niemann-Pick disease is caused by a deficiency in sphingomyelinase. It has been used to treat this disease. The treatment is termed *enzyme replacement therapy*.

9.5. (a) Lactose is transported into bacteria via a proton symport, and this depends on the generation of a proton gradient via ATP hydrolysis. Proton ionophores equalize the pH outside and inside the cell and stop lactose transport.

9.6. (b) Cellulose has β-1,4 linkages; furthermore, an endoglycosidase operates on glycoside bonds other than those at the reducing or nonreducing terminus.

9.7. (e) Glycerol is not a part of gangliosides.

9.8. (d)
$$\Delta E = \frac{-2.3RT}{F} \Delta pH = \frac{-1.98 \times 310 \times 2.3}{23,000} \times 2 = -123 \text{ mV}$$

9.9. (a) Pancreatic (α) amylase is an endoglycosidase, which removes maltose units from amylose or amylopectin. It splits the α-1,4 glycoside bond. In the absence of an α-1,6 glycosidase, limit dextrin is a product in addition to maltose.

9.10. (b) Sucrose is nonreducing; lactose is reducing.

9.11. (c) Lactose is a β-D-galactopyranosyl-1,4-D-glucopyranoside, and fructose is α-D-glucopyranosyl-1,2-β-D-fructofuranoside.

9.12. (b) See the answer to Question 9.11 for an explanation.

9.13. (d) Cell membranes do not contain triglycerides; their "fluidity" is maintained by cholesterol (there is no gel $\rightarrow$ liquid transition) and there is no transverse (flip-flop) movement of components, but lateral movement (side to side) is permissible.

9.14. (a) Phosphatidylserine is the major membrane component on the cytosol side.

9.15. (b) Blood group substances contain L-fucose, and dermatan sulfate contains L-iduronic acid.

9.16. (e) Transport is inhibited by phlorhizin directly and indirectly by stopping the Na/K pump. Ouabain is an inhibitor of the latter. Because gramicidin is a Na^+/K^+ ionophore, it short-circuits the Na^+ gradient and may thus inhibit glucose uptake by cells.

9.17. (c) Because cholesterol contains an –OH group, it is amphipathic. It controls membrane fluidity in mammals by inhibiting the ordering of fatty acid side chains, but it is absent from bacterial plasma membranes.

9.18. (d) Link protein strengthens the noncovalent interaction between the core protein and hyaluronic acid in proteoglycan aggregates.

9.19. (b) The O-glycoside linkage between protein and carbohydrate exists in blood group substances and chondroitin sulfate. The others are N-asparaginyl linked.

9.20. (b) Hyaluronic acid is linked physically to the core protein, and linkages are β-1,3 between GlcUA and GlcNAc and β-1,4 between GlcNAc and GlcUA.

9.21. (a) Hemiacetal produces an aldehyde and an alcohol upon hydrolysis; plasmalogen produces a fatty acid aldehyde, plus other substances; and fructose, a nonreducing sugar, produces reducing glucose and fructose. Sphingomyelin produces no aldehyde, ketone, or sugar upon hydrolysis.

9.22. (c) The gated Na^+ channel is not a conventional antiport. It responds to changes in membrane potential by allowing Na^+ to flow into the cell, as a result of which the membrane is further depolarized and action potential propagated.

PROBLEMS

9.1. Periodate is often used for carbohydrate structural studies. It oxidizes 1,2-glycols to dialdehydes and hydroxyaldehydes to formate and a new aldehyde. Suppose you treated 100 mg of a glycogen sample (molecular weight 5×10^6) with periodate and generated 1.6×10^{-3} μMol formic acid. Detemine the percentage of glucose residues located at the nonreducing ends of glycogen and the number of branch points (α-1,6 linkages). Determine the average number of glucose residues between each branch point.

9.2. Iodine and saponification numbers are often determined in industries concerned with lipid products. The iodine number is defined as the number of grams of iodine (I_2) that reacts with 100 g fat. The saponification number is mg KOH required to hydrolyze 1 g triglyceride. Now suppose that you have 5 g triglyceride and it required 980 mg KOH for hydrolysis and 4.45 g I_2 to react with the unsaturated fatty acids therein. Calculate or determine the following:
   a. Saponification and iodine numbers of the triglyceride.
   b. Molecular weight of the triglyceride.
   c. Number of double bonds per molecule of the triglyceride.
   d. If one of the fatty acids in the triglyceride is palmitate, what are the other two?

9.3. A newborn child developed normally until the age of 8 months, when a deterioration in various motor functions was observed. At 12 months, she could no longer sit up or swallow. At 22 months, she did not respond to stimuli and could no longer see. She expired at the age of 24 months. Use these data to answer the following questions:

	Normal	Patient
Total brain gangliosides, μg/mg lipid	130	166
GM$_3$, %	0.2	2.5
GM$_2$, %	1.6	86
GM$_1$, %	24.8	5.5
Serum hexosaminidase, specific activity	500	25
Liver globoside, % of total lipid	0.01	1.9

   a. What known disease pattern do these results resemble most?
   b. What are the GM$_1$, GM$_2$, and GM$_3$ gangliosides? Why is the GM$_2$ so high in the patient?

c. What is hexosaminidase? Are there more than one kind, and if so, what are they and what are their specificities?

d. Why should the accumulation of a ganglioside in the brain have such a profound effect on the patient's life expectancy?

e. Is there a way to treat the patient?

BIBLIOGRAPHY

Callahan JW, Lowden JA. Lysosomes and Lysosomal Storage Diseases. New York: Raven Press, 1981.

Goldberg DM, Riordan JR. Role of membranes in disease. Clin Physiol Biochem 4:305–336, 1986.

Harold FM. The Vital Force: A Study of Bioenergetics. New York: WH Freeman, 1986.

Vance DE, Vance JE. Biochemistry of Lipids and Membranes. Menlo Park: Benjamin-Cummings, 1985.

II

NUCLEIC ACIDS AND GENETIC
CONTROL OF BIOCHEMICAL EVENTS

10

Nucleic Acid Chemistry and Nucleotide Metabolism

After completing this chapter, the student should

1. Understand the properties of purine and pyrimidine bases and nucleosides, and nucleotides with varying amounts of phosphate. Recognize the structures of the various xanthines, cyclic nucleotides, uric acid, and bases found in nucleic acids.
2. Understand the purine and pyrmidine *de novo* biosynthetic pathways, with special attention to enzymes controlling pathway rates and the properties of such enzymes; the positive and negative effectors; steps inhibited by the various antitumor agents and their mechanisms; final products of the *de novo* pathways and how the various nucleotides are generated from them; and the biosynthesis of deoxyribonucleotides and the attendant mechanisms.
3. Understand the biosynthesis of FMN, FAD, NAD$^+$, NADP$^+$, and coenzyme A.
4. Know the various salvage pathways using ribose-1-phosphate and phosphoribosylpyrophosphate. Know the action of the various kinases. Know the etiology of Lesch-Nyhan syndrome.
5. Know the purine and pyrimidine degradation pathways and the attendant pathologies.
6. Understand how polynucleotides are assembled and some of their characteristic properties, including hydrolytic enzyme specificities. Understand the properties of various DNAs and how they differ from each other. Understand the differences between DNA and RNA. Know the base relationships in DNA.
7. Understand the process of DNA denaturation and annealing and the information that can be gleaned from such parameters as T_m and C_0t. Know how the physical parameters of DNA change as it is denatured.
8. Know the properties of chromatin components and its organization: nucleosomes, histones, link DNA, and solenoids. Know the dimensions of the various chromatin components. Under-

stand the concept of supercoiling and when it occurs in circular DNA and during DNA replication and transcription.

9. Know the properties of each RNA type. Be familiar with the anatomy of transfer RNA.

10.1 INTRODUCTION

Nucleic acids are nitrogen- and phosphorus-containing components of all living organisms and encode the genetic information necessary for the propagation of specific life forms. It is said that nucleic acids were discovered by the Swiss chemist Friedrich Miescher, who was especially active in this area in 1860s and 1870s. It took many years thereafter to determine the exact nucleic acid composition, to identify unambiguously the role as genetic material, and to elucidate the three-dimensional structure and mode of replication.

Nucleic acids contain purine and pyrimidine bases, phosphate, and carbohydrate. The carbohydrate is either ribose or 2-deoxyribose, and nucleic acids may be divided into two groups on the basis of which of the two sugars they contain. Deoxyribonucleic acid (DNA) is found in eukaryotic nuclei and mitochondria, and represents the genetic material. Its molecular weight is very large—in the hundreds of millions. In prokaryotes, DNA is found in the "chromosome" and smaller structures called *plasmids*. Nucleic acids containing ribose are called ribonucleic acids (RNA). Their molecular weight may be very large or relatively small. They are found in eukaryotic nuclei, endoplasmic reticulum, and cytosol, and they function in the mechanics of protein biosynthesis. The blueprints for protein biosynthesis are contained within the DNA structure, from which RNA receives its instructions.

10.2 CHEMISTRY OF PURINE AND PYRIMIDINE BASES

The major bases found in nucleic acids are *adenine* and *guanine* (purines) and *uracil, cytosine,* and *thymine* (pyrimidines). Thymine is found primarily in DNA, uracil in RNA, and the others in both DNA and RNA. Their structures, along with their chemical parent compounds, purine and pyrimidine, are shown in Figure 10.1, which also indicates other biologically important purines that are not components of nucleic acids. Hypoxanthine, orotic acid, and xanthine are biosynthetic and/or degradation intermediates of purine and pyrimidine bases, whereas xanthine derivatives—caffeine, theophylline, and theobromine—are alkaloids from plant sources. Caffeine is a component of coffee beans and tea, and its effects on metabolism are mentioned in Chapter 16. Theophylline is found in tea and is used therapeutically in asthma, because it is a smooth muscle relaxant. Theobromine is found in chocolate. It is a diuretic, heart stimulant, and vasodilator.

DNA and RNA also contain minor amounts of other bases. Among the minor purines are 1-methylguanine, 6-methylaminopurine (primarily amino group of adenine is methylated), 6-dimethylaminopurine, and 7-methylguanine. Among the minor pyrimidines are 3- or 5-methylcytosine and 5-hydroxymethylcytosine.

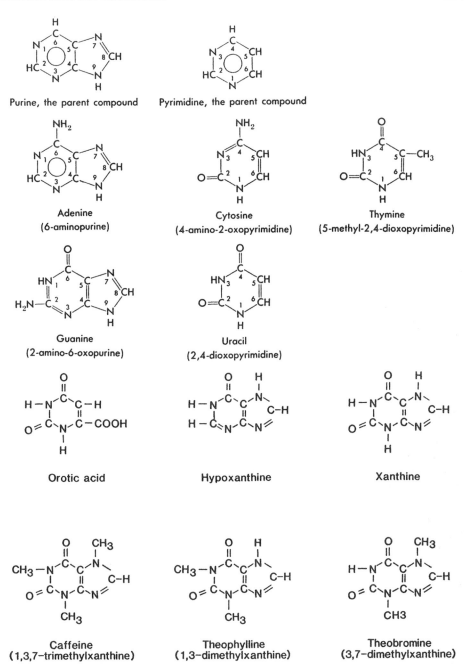

Figure 10.1 Structures of some naturally occurring purine and pyrimidine bases and their structural parent compounds, purine and pyrimidine.

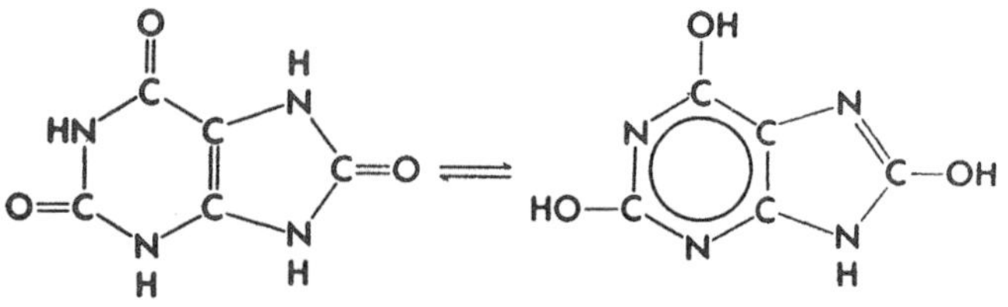

Figure 10.2 Tautomeric forms of uric acid. Although uric acid does not occur in nucleic acids (it is a degradation product of adenine and guanine), the tautomeric structures observed here are typical of all purine bases of this type. At pH 7, the keto forms predominate.

The chemical properties of the purine and pyrimidine bases include highly conjugated double bond systems within the ring structures. For this reason, nucleic acids have a very strong absorption maximum at about 260 nm, which is used for nucleic acid quantitation. Moreover, the bases can exist in two tautomeric forms, the keto and enol forms (Figure 10.2). In DNA and RNA, the keto forms are by far the more predominant, and this property makes it possible for the bases to form intermolecular hydrogen bonds (see Figure 10.18).

10.3 NUCLEOSIDES AND NUCLEOTIDES

10.3.1 Chemistry of Ribo- and Deoxyribonucleosides and Nucleotides

In nucleic acids, purine and pyrimidine bases are associated with a pentose molecule: ribose or deoxyribose. The bond linking the two entities is an N-glycoside bond, it involves the anomeric carbon of the sugar (carbon 1′, β configuration) and either N-3 of purines or N-1 of pyrimidines. An exception occurs with uracil in pseudoridine, in which C-5 instead of N-1 of uracil is involved. Compounds consisting of a purine or pyrimidine base and a sugar are *nucleosides*. The most commonly occurring nucleoside structures are shown in Figure 10.3. *Nucleotides* are nucleosides containing one or more phosphate residues esterified to position 5′ of either the ribose or deoxyribose residue of nucleoside. It is also possible to have the 3′ position of the sugar esterified. Nucleotides containing a single phosphate residue are termed mononucleotides, those with two phosphate residues are dinucleotides, and trinucleotides are those with three phosphate groups. The last two, of course, are carriers of high-energy phosphate bonds. The structures of AMP, ADP, and ATP, nucleotides of adenine, are given in Figure 2.1. Nucleotides may also be called nucleoside phosphates. Table 10.1 lists nucleoside and nucleotide nomenclature.

Trinucleotides, because they are high-energy compounds, are important participants in various metabolic processes. It has already been mentioned that ATP is the principal chemical energy source in the organism and is required for such physiologic processes as muscle contraction and maintenance of electrolyte balances in the organism. UTP is required in the biosynthesis of complex carbo-

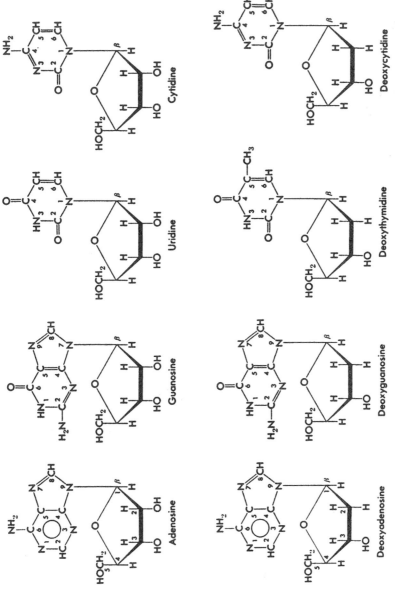

Figure 10.3 Structures of some common ribo- and deoxyribonucleosides.

Table 10.1 Commonly Occurring Nucleosides and Nucleotides

Base	Sugar	Nucleoside	5'-Mononucleotide	5'-Dinucleotide	5'-Trinucleotide
Adenine	Ribose	Adenosine	Adenylic acid; adenosine monophosphate (AMP)	Adenosine diphosphate (ADP)	Adenosine triphosphate (ATP)
	Deoxyribose	Deoxyadenosine	Deoxyadenylic acid; deoxy-adenosine monophosphate (dAMP)	Deoxyadenosine diphosphate (dADP)	Deoxyadenosine triphosphate (dATP)
Guanine	Ribose	Guanosine	Guanylic acid; guanosine monophosphate (GMP)	Guanosine diphosphate (dADP)	Guanosine triphosphate (GTP)
	Deoxyribose	Deoxyguanosine	Deoxyguanylic acid; deoxyguanosine monophosphate (dGMP)	Deoxyguanosine diphosphate (dGDP)	Deoxyguanosine triphosphate (dGTP)
Hypoxanthine	Ribose	Inosine	Inosinic acid; inosine monophosphate (IMP)	Inosine diphosphate (IDP)	Inosine triphosphate (ITP)
Xanthine	Ribose	Xanthosine	Xanthosine monophosphate (XMP); xanthinylic acid	Xanthosine diphosphate	Xanthosine triphosphate
Uracil	Ribose	Uridine	Uridylic acid; uridine monophosphate (UMP)	Uridine diphosphate (UDP)	Uridine triphosphate (UTP)
	Deoxyribose	Deoxyuridine	Deoxyuridylic acid; deoxyuridine monophosphate (dUMP)	Deoxyuridine diphosphate (dUDP)	Deoxyuridine triphosphate (dUTP)
Thymine	Deoxyribose	Thymidine	Thymidylic acid; thymidine monophosphate (dTMP)	Thymidine diphosphate (dTDP)	Thymidine triphosphate (dTTP)
Cytosine	Ribose	Cytidine	Cytidylic acid; cytidine monophosphate (CMP)	Cytidine diphosphate (CDP)	Cytidine triphosphate (CTP)
	Deoxyribose	Deoxycytidine	Deoxycytidylic acid; deoxycytidine monophosphate (dCMP)	Deoxycytidine diphosphate (dCDP)	Deoxycytidine triphosphate (dCTP)
Orotic acid	Ribose	Orotidine	Orotidine monophosphate (OMP)	Orotidine diphosphate (ODP)	Orotidine triphosphate (OTP)

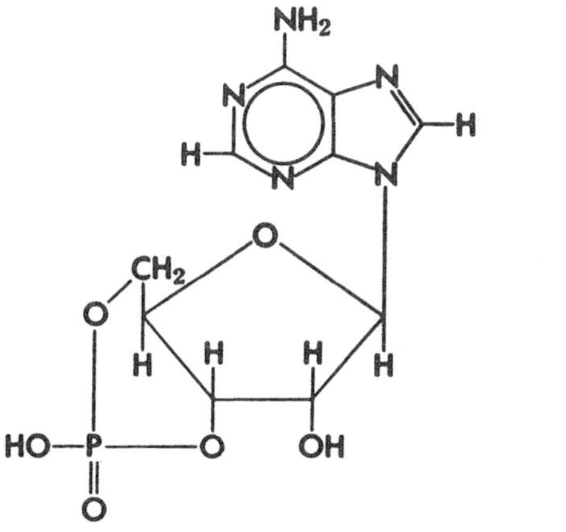

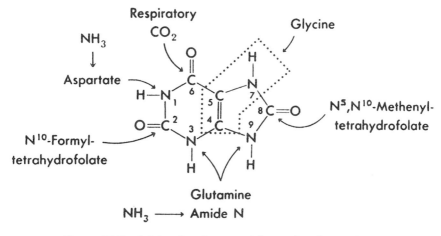

Cyclic-3′,5′-adenosine monophosphate (cAMP)

Figure 10.4 Structure of cyclic AMP (cAMP, cyclic 3′,5′-adenosine monophosphate).

Figure 10.5 Origin of each atom of the purine ring system.

hydrates, CTP in the biosynthesis of complex lipids, and GTP in the second messenger system (see Chapter 16). ATP and GTP are also precursors of their respective cyclic diesters, cyclic AMP (cAMP) and cyclic GMP (cGMP). These are also actors in the second messenger system. The structure of cAMP is shown in Figure 10.4. The enzyme that produces cAMP from ATP is *adenylate cyclase*. Pyrophosphate is the other product of this reaction.

10.3.2 Biosynthesis of Nucleotides

De Novo Purine Biosynthesis

Purine nucleotides can be synthesized in the organism from relatively simple building blocks: ribose, phosphate, glycine, formate, aspartate, glutamine, and CO_2. The origin of each purine base component is summarized in Figure 10.5,

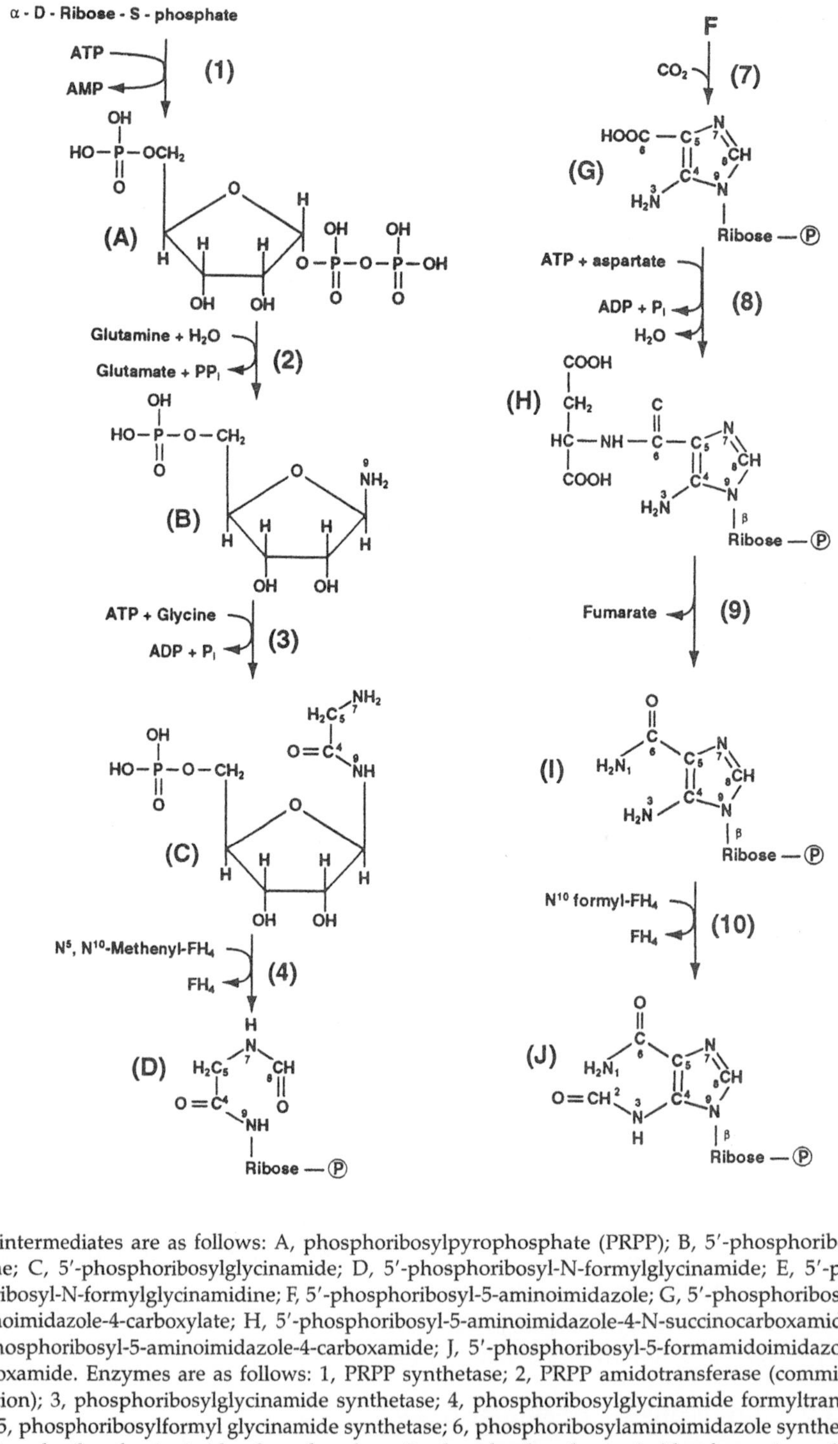

The intermediates are as follows: A, phosphoribosylpyrophosphate (PRPP); B, 5′-phosphoribosyl-amine; C, 5′-phosphoribosylglycinamide; D, 5′-phosphoribosyl-N-formylglycinamide; E, 5′-phos-phoribosyl-N-formylglycinamidine; F, 5′-phosphoribosyl-5-aminoimidazole; G, 5′-phosphoribosyl-5-aminoimidazole-4-carboxylate; H, 5′-phosphoribosyl-5-aminoimidazole-4-N-succinocarboxamide; I, 5′-phosphoribosyl-5-aminoimidazole-4-carboxamide; J, 5′-phosphoribosyl-5-formamidoimidazole-4-carboxamide. Enzymes are as follows: 1, PRPP synthetase; 2, PRPP amidotransferase (committing reaction); 3, phosphoribosylglycinamide synthetase; 4, phosphoribosylglycinamide formyltransfer-ase; 5, phosphoribosylformyl glycinamide synthetase; 6, phosphoribosylaminoimidazole synthetase; 7, phosphoribosylaminoimidazole carboxylase; 8, phosphoribosylaminoimidazole-succinocarboxa-mide synthetase; 9, adenylosuccinate lyase; 10, phosphoribosylaminoimidazolecarboxamide formyl-transferase; 11, IMP cyclohydrolase. Note that azaserine, an analog of glutamine, inhibits reactions 2 and 5. Reactions 4 and 10 are especially susceptible to antifolate agents such as methotrexate. ATP is required in at least 5 reactions shown.

Figure 10.6 *De novo* biosynthetic pathway for inosine monophosphate.

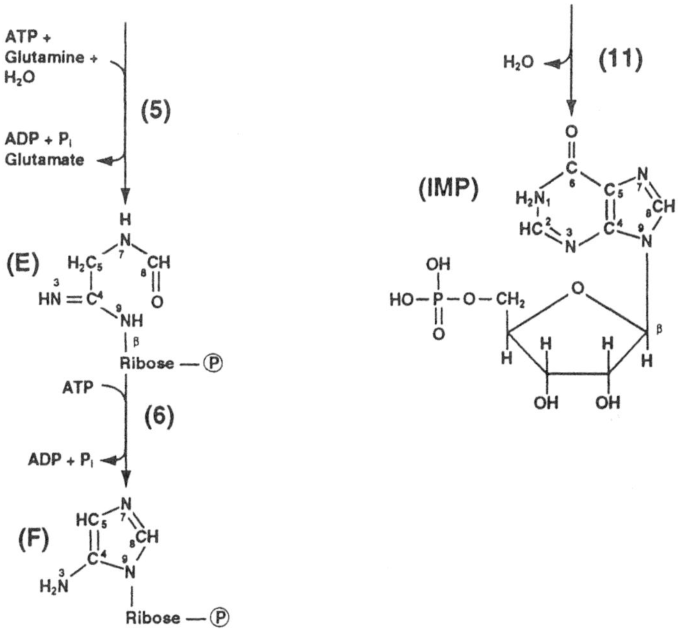

Figure 10.6 Continued

although the process leading to the final product is arduous. The final product is IMP (see Table 10.1), from which other nucleotides are derived. The process is entirely cytosolic, and it requires energy. According to Figure 10.6, which summarizes the enzymatic pathway for IMP biosynthesis, six high-energy phosphate bond equivalents are required for the biosynthesis of a single IMP molecule, not including additional ATPs required for the biosynthesis of ribose-5-phosphate, glutamine, or formyltetrahydrofolate.

Purine biosynthesis is initiated by the phosphorylation of ribose-5-phosphate, which is generated through carbohydrate metabolism pathways (Chapter 18) to give phosphoribosylpyrophosphate [PRPP; reaction (1) in Figure 10.6]. PRPP is an important intermediate in a number of reactions involving nucleotides. The enzyme in reaction (1) is called *PRPP synthetase*. The next step (reaction (2) in Figure 10.6) is the committing and rate-controlling reaction. The enzyme catalyzing this reaction is called PRPP-aminotransferase. Note that there is an inversion in the configuration of the anomeric carbon atom. The enzyme PRPP-aminotransferase is apparently inactive in the dimeric form (molecular weight, MW, 270,000). Increased amounts of PRPP stimulate its dissociation into two subunits (MW 135,000 each), which acquire catalytic activity. Deactivation (dimerization) is promoted by the products of the pathway—IMP, GMP, and AMP. These, as well as ADP and GDP, also inhibit PRPP biosynthesis. The *de novo* purine biosynthetic pathway is therefore controlled by the classic feedback inhibitory mechanisms (see Chapter 5).

Several steps in the *de novo* purine biosynthetic pathway may be inhibited by antitumor agents. Steps requiring glutamine (2 and 5) are sensitive to *azaserine*, a glutamine analog. Its structure is shown in Figure 10.7. Steps requir-

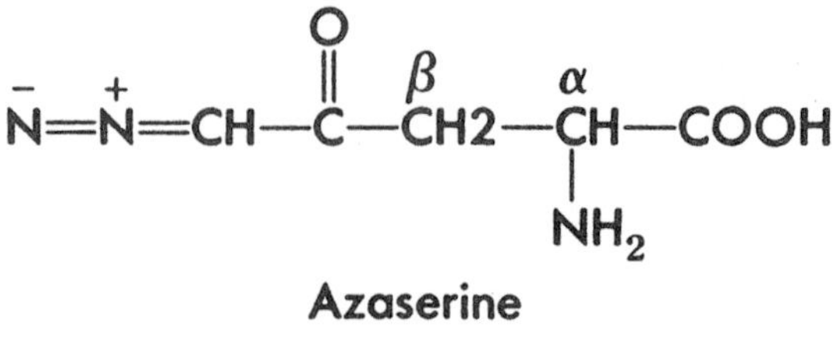

$$\overset{-}{N}=\overset{+}{N}=CH-\overset{\overset{\displaystyle O}{\|}}{C}-\overset{\beta}{CH2}-\overset{\overset{\displaystyle \alpha}{}}{\underset{\underset{\displaystyle NH_2}{|}}{CH}}-COOH$$

Azaserine

Figure 10.7 Structure of azaserine, a glutamine analog and inhibitor of purine biosynthesis.

ing formyl-level tetrahydrofolate-bound one-carbon units (steps 4 and 10; see Chapter 6) are very sensitive to dihydrofolate reductase inhibitors, aminopterin and methotrexate (see Figure 6.3). In bacteria, these reactions are also inhibited by sulfa drugs, when 5'-phosphoribosyl-4-carboxamide-5-aminoimidazole accumulates in the medium. Remember that neither the sulfa drugs nor the folate analogs specifically inhibit the enzymes in the *de novo* purine biosynthetic pathway. They merely make the necessary substrates unavailable, thus reducing nucleic acid biosynthesis and causing an arrest of either bacterial or tumor growth.

The conversion of IMP to AMP and GMP is shown in Figure 10.8. Note that GTP is required for the biosynthesis of AMP and ATP for GMP biosynthesis, and high-ATP levels channel the conversion of IMP to GMP. In addition, IMP dehydrogenase is inhibited by GMP. We therefore have additional loci for controlling cellular concentrations of purine nucleotides by regulating the fate of IMP. The conversion of nucleoside monophosphates to di- and triphosphates is discussed later.

De Novo Pyrimidine Biosynthesis

The design for pyrimidine synthesis differs somewhat from that of purine biosynthesis in that the sugar is attached to the pyrimidine ring at the end of the pathway. In addition, pyrimidine biosynthesis occurs in part in the cytosol and in part in the mitochondria and involves the participation of two multifunctional enzymes. The pathway is summarized in Figure 10.9. One of the initial reactants is the compound carbamoyl phosphate (carbamoyl phosphoric acid). This compound is also formed in the urea biosynthetic pathway, but this takes place in the mitochondria and requires NH_3 (Chapter 20). The cytosolic biosynthesis of carbamoyl phosphate for the purpose of pyrimidine biosynthesis requires glutamine as the nitrogen donor:

$$HCO_3^- + glutamine + 2ATP \rightarrow carbamoyl\ phosphate + 2ADP$$
$$+ P_i + glutamate \tag{10.1}$$

The reaction is catalyzed by carbamoyl phosphate synthetase II (also called carbamoyl phosphate synthetase, glutamine).

The reaction of carbamoyl phosphate with aspartate [Figure 10.9, reaction (1)] is rate controlling and committing in microorganisms, whereas in mammals carbamoyl phosphate synthetase II seems to the major rate-controlling enzyme. The latter is stimulated by PRPP and purine nucleotides (especially ATP) and

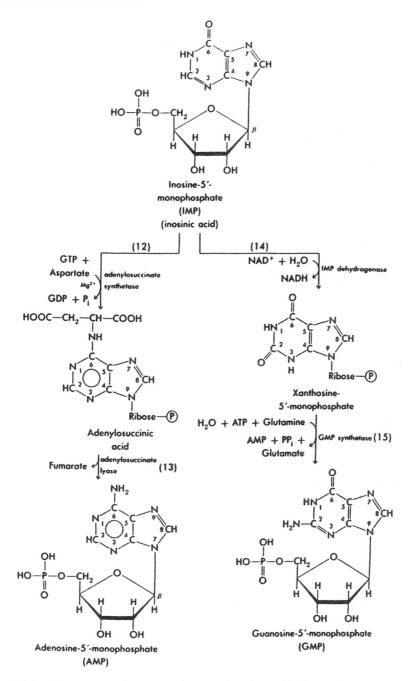

Figure 10.8 Conversion of inosine-5'-monophosphate (IMP) to the corresponding adenosine and guanosine monophosphates (AMP and GMP, respectively). Note that increased levels of GMP inhibit reaction (14) and stimulate reaction (12). Conversely, increased levels of AMP inhibit reaction (12) and stimulate reaction (14).

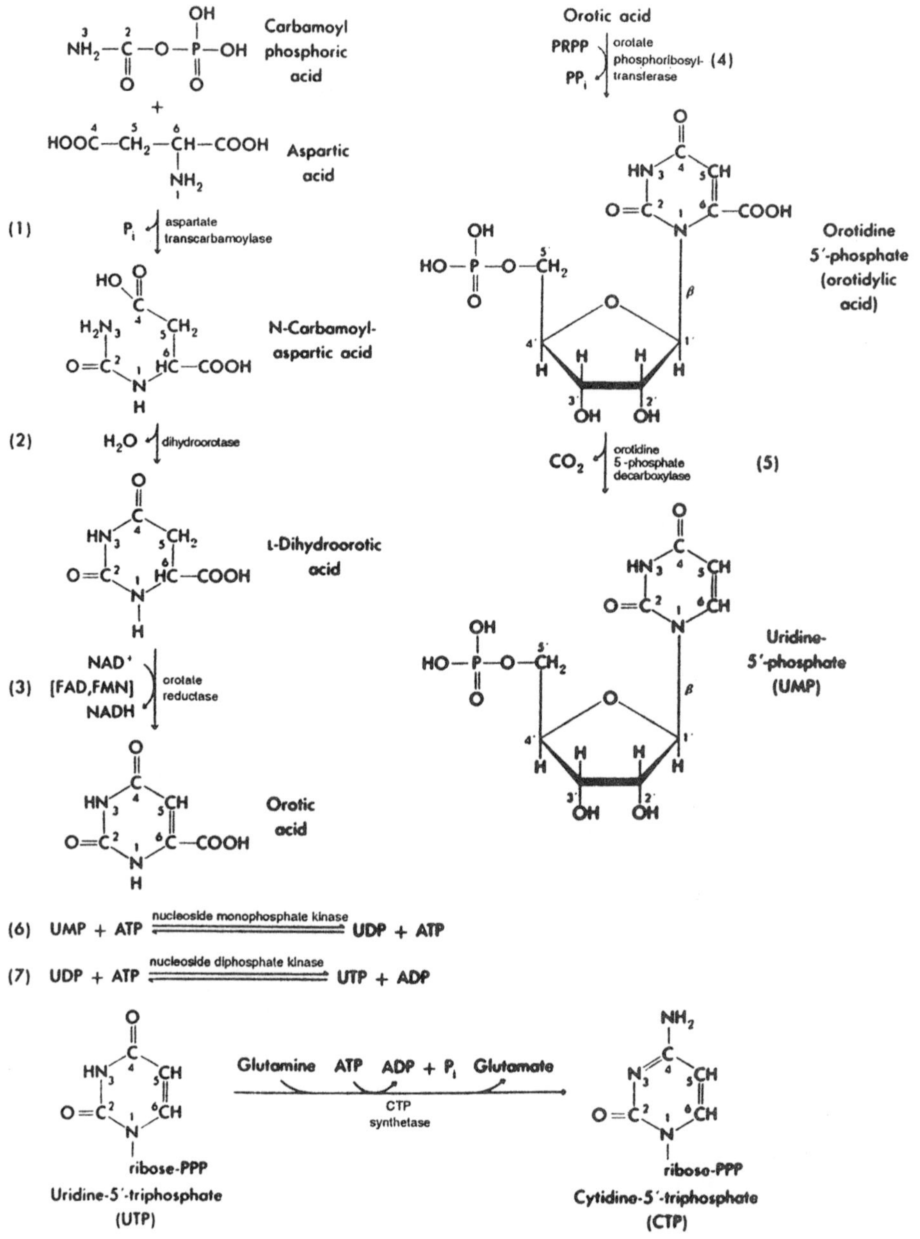

Figure 10.9 *De novo* pyrimidine nucleotide biosynthesis pathway. Note the numbering of the pyrimidine ring in UMP: atoms 2 and 3 come from carbamoyl phosphate and atoms 1, 4, 5, and 6 from aspartate.

inhibited by pyrimidine nucleotides (especially UTP). Aspartate transcarbamoylase in microorganisms is inhibited effectively by CTP and activated by ATP. UMP inhibits microbial carbamoyl phosphate synthetase II, although this is a minor regulatory site. Bacterial aspartate transcarbamoylase is of historical interest, because much of our understanding of the workings of allosteric enzymes comes from studies on this enzyme. ATP is a classic positive effector, whereas CTP is a negative effector.

Although the bacterial set of enzymes leading to the biosynthesis of UMP consists of six separate gene products (proteins), in mammals this represents only three gene products. A single cytoplasmic enzyme with a molecular weight of about 240,000 catalyzes the carbamoyl phosphate II synthetase reaction, plus reactions (1) and (2) in Figure 10.9. A mitochondrial enzyme, dihydroortate dehydrogenase [orotate reductase, reaction (3)], catalyzes the conversion of dihydroorotic acid to orotic acid. It uses stoichiometric amounts of NAD and requires catalytic amounts of FAD. The next two steps, reactions (4) and (5), are catalyzed by another cytosolic multifunction enzyme, which may be called UMP synthase (MW about 51,000). UMP can then be converted to UTP by the expenditure of two ATP equivalents, and finally, CTP is synthesized from UTP via the action of CTP synthetase (Figure 10.9). CTP inhibits the latter via a feedback inhibitory mechanism. In summary, CO_2 contributes carbon 2 of the pyrimidine ring (see Figure 10.1 for numbering of atoms), glutamine contributes nitrogen 3, and the other four ring components are contributed by aspartate.

In an inborn error of metabolism called orotic aciduria, UMP synthase is defective and the urine contains large amounts of orotate. This disorder may be treated by feeding cytidine and uridine. Large amounts of orotate may also be excreted in the urine in the various hyperammonemia syndromes. Carbamoyl phosphate, formed in the mitochondria by the action of carbamoyl phosphate synthetase I, is present in such large amounts that it spills over into the cytosol. There, the carbamoyl phosphate is rapidly converted to orotic acid and the latter is cleared by the kidneys.

Deoxyribonucleotide Biosynthesis

Deoxyribonucleotides are components of DNA, and they are synthesized from ribonucleoside diphosphates: ADP, GDP, CDP, and UDP. This is a reductive process in which the ultimate reducing agent is NADPH. The rate of DNA biosynthesis is largely dependent on the rate of deoxyribonucleotide formation. The focal point of this process is the enzyme ribonucleotide reductase, MW about 240,000, which contains two ferric iron atoms. In some lactobacilli, the Fe may be substituted by Mn or vitamin B_{12}. The immediate electron donor and substrate for ribonucleotide reductase is a small SH-containing protein (MW 12,000) called thioredoxin. The –SH residues are oxidized to –S–S– groups but the reduced protein can be regenerated by NADPH in the presence of the FAD-containing enzyme thioredoxin reductase. In some microorganisms, thioredoxin is replaced by glutaredoxin, another small, heat-stable protein with –SH residues. It, too, becomes oxidized, but it is regenerated by reduced glutathione (G–SH) in the presence of the enzyme glutaredoxin reductase. Oxidized glutathione (GSSG) is reduced through the action of NADPH and glutathione reductase, another FAD-containing enzyme. These reactions are summarized in Figure 10.10.

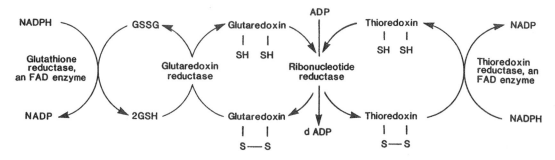

Figure 10.10 Summary of reactions involved in the conversion of ribo- to deoxyribonucleotides.

The control of ribonucleotide reductase activity is affected in the classic feedback fashion by cellular nucleotide concentrations. dATP inhibits the reduction of all four ribonucleoside diphosphates. dTTP inhibits the reduction of only CDP and UDP. ATP is the positive effector for the reduction of these two nucleotides, and both dTTP and dGTP stimulate the reduction of GDP and ADP. Hydroxyurea, an antitumor agent, inhibits ribonucleotide reductase, and this depletes the deoxyribonucleotide supply required for tumor DNA biosynthesis.

The biosynthesis of thymine deoxyribonucleotides is affected by dUDP. The latter may lose a P_i to give dUMP, or dUDP may be phosphorylated by a *kinase* (an enzyme that transfers a phosphate residue from ATP to an acceptor) to give dUTP and then lose a pyrophosphate group to yield dUMP. At any rate, dUMP is subject to the action of thymidylate synthase, which uses 5,10-methylenetetrahydrofolate as both the methyl group donor and reducing agent, as shown in Figure 10.11, to give dTMP. The dihydrofolate produced may regenerate tetrahydrofolate (THF) via dihydrofolate reductase (Chapter 6). Thymidylate kinases can then phosphorylate dTMP to dTDP and dTTP, the latter being utilized for DNA biosynthesis.

Thymidylate synthase is inhibited by several antitumor agents. Because it requires THF-bound one-carbon units, it is susceptible to the folate analogs methotrexate and aminopterin. In addition, 5-fluorouracil inhibits the enzyme, first by being converted to its deoxyribonucleoside and then by combining permanently with thymidylate synthase instead of dUMP to make the enzyme unavailable.

Salvage Pathways

The so-called salvage pathways are available in many cells to scavenge free purine and pyrimidine bases, nucleosides, and mononucleotides and to convert these to metabolically useful di- and trinucleotides. The function of these pathways is to avoid the costly (energy) and lengthy *de novo* purine and pyrimidine biosynthetic processes. In some cells, in fact, the salvage pathways yield a greater quantity of nucleotides than the *de novo* pathways. The substrates for salvage reactions may come from dietary sources or from normal nucleic acid turnover processes.

Free bases can be salvaged using either PRPP or ribose-1-phosphate. The products are nucleoside monophosphates in the former case and nucleosides

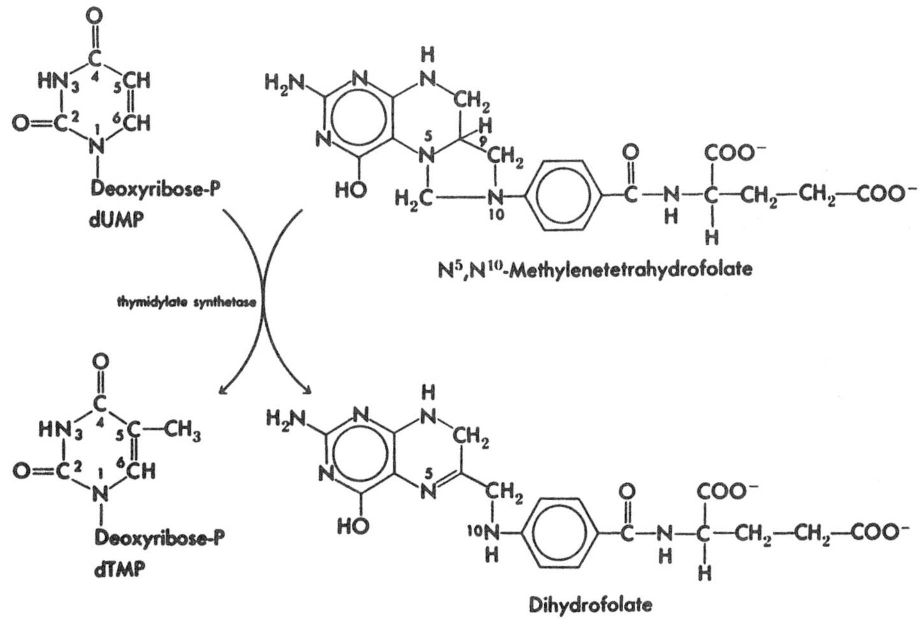

Figure 10.11 Biosynthesis of thymidylic acid from deoxyuridylic acid.

in the latter. For purines, two enzymes are available: hypoxanthine-guanine phosphoribosyltransferase (HGPRTase) and adenine phosphoribosyltransferase (APRTase). The reactions are as follows:

$$\text{Guanine} + \text{PRPP} \underset{\text{HGPRTase}}{\overset{\text{Mg}^{2+}}{\rightleftharpoons}} \text{GMP} + \text{PP}_i \qquad (10.2)$$

$$\text{Hypoxanthine} + \text{PRPP} \underset{\text{HGPRTase}}{\overset{\text{Mg}^{2+}}{\rightleftharpoons}} \text{IMP} + \text{PP}_i \qquad (10.3)$$

$$\text{Adenine} + \text{PRPP} \underset{\text{APRTase}}{\overset{\text{Mg}^{2+}}{\rightleftharpoons}} \text{AMP} + \text{PP}_i \qquad (10.4)$$

In the pyrimidines, a mammalian erythrocyte enzyme, pyrimidine phosphoribosyltransferase, converts uracil, orotic acid, and thymine into nucleotides as follows:

$$\text{Pyrimidine} + \text{PRPP} \rightleftharpoons \text{pyrimidine nucleotide} + \text{PP}_i \qquad (10.5)$$

Such conversions in mammals are not very efficient, however, with the exception of, perhaps, the orotate phosphoribosyltransferase, which is a component of the pyrimidine nucleotide biosynthetic pathway (Figure 10.9). A very active uracil phosphoribosyltransferase has been isolated from microorganisms. It converts uracil to UMP using PRPP.

Nucleosides are formed by the reaction of a purine or pyrimidine base with ribose-1-phosphate, and in mammals, this provides the most effective salvage pathway for pyrimidines:

$$\text{Purine or pyrimidine} + \text{ribose-1-phosphate} \rightleftharpoons \text{nucleoside} + P_i \qquad (10.6)$$

A close look at this reaction reveals that in the opposite direction, the reaction is of the phosphorolysis type. For this reason, the enzymes catalyzing the reaction with ribose-1-phosphate are called *phosphorylases*, and they also participate in nucleic acid degradation pathways. Purine nucleoside phosphorylases thus convert hypoxanthine and guanine to either inosine and guanosine if ribose-1-phosphate is the substrate or to deoxyinosine and deoxyguanosine if deoxyribose-1-phosphate is the substrate. Uridine phosphorylase converts uracil to uridine in the presence of ribose-1-phosphate, and thymidine is formed from thymine and deoxyribose-1-phosphate through the action of thymidine phosphorylase.

The various nucleotides can be generated from nucleosides and monophosphonucleosides by a group of enzymes called *kinases*, which use ATP as the phosphate group donor, as shown in Equations (10.7) and (10.8):

$$\text{Nucleoside} + \text{ATP} \rightarrow \text{monophosphonucleoside} + \text{ADP} \qquad (10.7)$$

$$\text{Monophosphonucleoside} + \text{ATP} \rightarrow \text{diphosphonucleoside} + \text{ADP} \qquad (10.8)$$

Thus, uridine-cytidine kinase converts uridine and cytidine to UMP and CMP, respectively; thymidine kinase converts thymidine to dTMP; and adenosine kinase converts adenosine to AMP. Specific kinases convert monophosphonucleotides to dinucleotides using ATP as a phosphate donor. The conversion of diphosphonucleotides to triphosphonucleotides is carried out by a nonspecific nucleoside diphosphate kinase. This includes both the ribo- and deoxyribonucleotides. Cytosine and its nucleoside and nucleotide transformations are often associated with the metabolism of uracil and its nucleosides and nucleotides. Note that UTP can give rise to CTP (Figure 10.9), and also that, in the presence of cytidine deaminase, cytidine can be converted to uridine.

A serious genetic disorder is associated with the salvage pathways, the Lesch-Nyhan syndrome. It is believed that it is caused by a failure to control the *de novo* purine biosynthetic pathway. In the Lesch-Nyhan syndrome, the enzyme HGPRTase is severely depressed. Because the *de novo* pathway is controlled largely via feedback effects of purine nucleotides, the pathway is derepressed and excessive quantities of purine nucleotides and their degradation product, uric acid, are accumulated. This results is neurologic effects, self-mutilation, and mental retardation.

Biosynthesis of Coenzyme Nucleotides

Coenzymes of riboflavin, niacin, and pantothenic acid are nucleotides of adenine (see Chapter 6). The activation of riboflavin is most straightforward:

$$\text{Riboflavin} + \text{ATP} \rightarrow \text{flavin mononucleotide (FMN)} + \text{ADP} \qquad (10.9)$$

$$\text{FMN} + \text{ATP} \rightarrow \text{FAD} + PP_i \qquad (10.10)$$

Reactions (10.9) and (10.10) are catalyzed by flavokinase and FMN pyrophosphorylase, respectively. For the structures of FMN and FAD, see Chapter 6. The biosynthesis of NAD^+ from nicotinamide is shown in Figure 10.12. An additional phosphorylation step with ATP is required to form $NADP^+$. If one

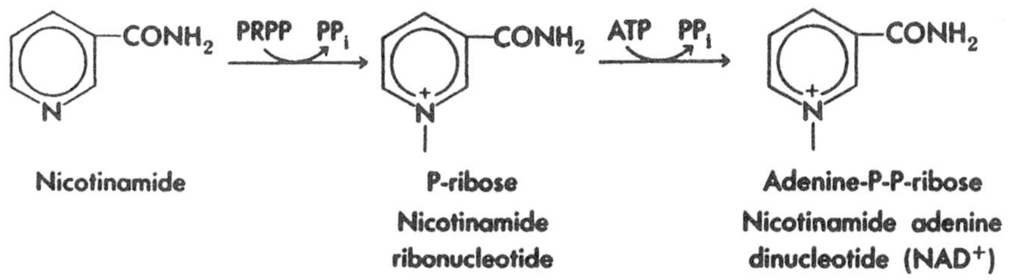

Figure 10.12 Biosynthesis of NAD$^+$ from nicotinamide.

starts with nicotinic acid rather than nicotinamide, the process is the same except that the final product, deamido-NAD$^+$, must be converted to NAD$^+$ by amination:

$$\text{Deamido NAD}^+ \xrightarrow[\substack{\text{ATP, Glutamine} \qquad \text{AMP, PP}_i, \text{Glutamate}}]{\text{NAD}^+ \text{ Synthetase}} \text{NAD}^+ \tag{10.11}$$

In the biosynthesis of coenzyme A from pantothenate, a five-step process is required, which results in the attachment to pantothenate of the active –SH group and an adenine dinucleotide group. This set of reactions is summarized in Figure 10.13. For structures not shown, see Chapter 6.

10.3.3 Degradation of Nucleotides

Nucleic acids undergo the process of turnover just like all other substances. Nucleic acids, because they are polymers of monophosphonucleotides, undergo hydrolysis by a group of enzymes collectively called *nucleases*. There are many types of nucleases, some producing fragments of nucleic acids, others removing single nucleotides or nucleosides from such fragments. Some of these are discussed later. However, their end products are always monophosphonucleotides and, to a smaller extent, nucleosides. These may be degraded further to compounds that are ultimately excreted from the organism. Figure 10.14 shows the purine degradation pathway. One of the first steps is the hydrolytic removal of phosphate via enzymes called *nucleotidases* to give nucleosides. AMP may be first deaminated to IMP (especially in the mammals) and then lose its phosphate. The guanosine and inosine are then converted to xanthine and then to uric acid, the excretion product of purine metabolism in the human. Most of the hypoxanthine and guanine produced, however, are salvaged via HGPRTase. In some animals, uric acid may be degraded further to more water-soluble compounds, such as allantoin and urea. The deoxyribonucleotides are handled exactly as the ribonucleotides.

A very important enzyme is *xanthine oxidase*, which catalyzes two reactions in the purine degradation process. It contains a number of subunits, and Fe, Mo, and FAD are its prosthetic groups. It acts, in this case, as an oxidase using O_2 as an electron sink. In other reactions, however, this enzyme can act as a dehydrogenase using NAD$^+$ as an oxidizing agent. A xanthine oxidase

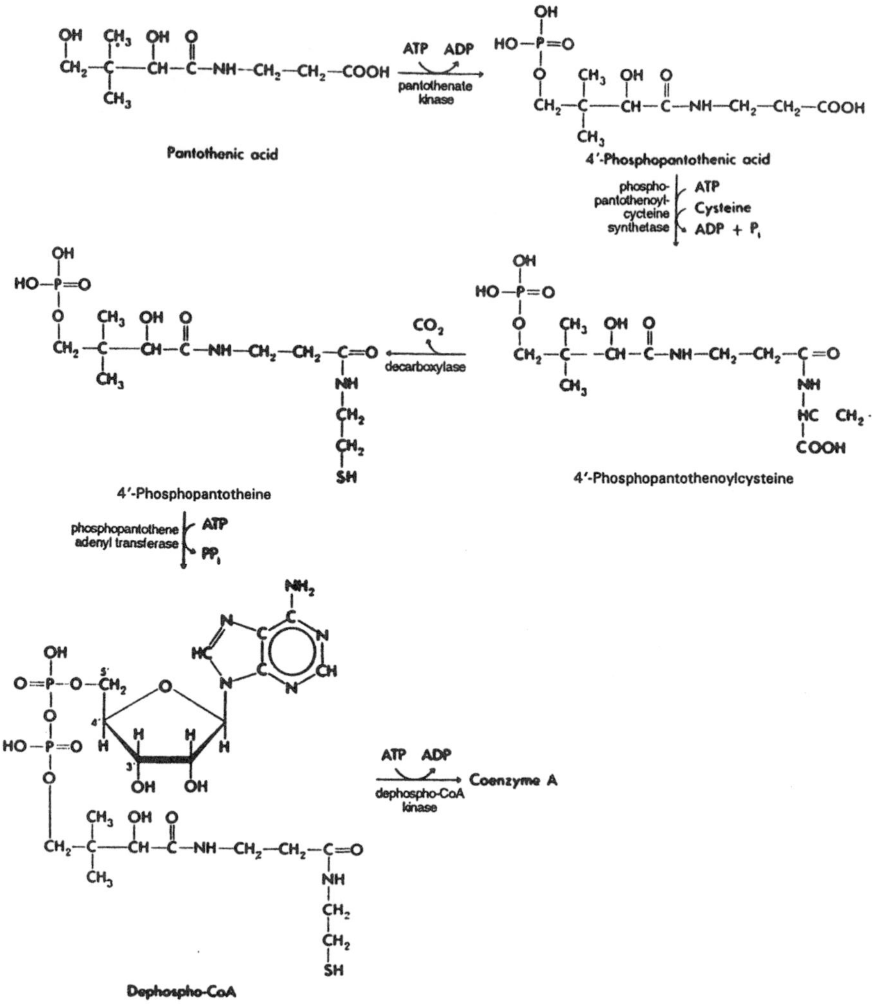

Figure 10.13   Biosynthesis of coenzyme A from pantothenate.

inhibitor and an analog of xanthine, *allopurinol*, is used as a drug in *gout*. In this disease, for largely unknown reasons, the production of uric acid in the patient is either above normal or excretion is below normal and uric acid accumulates in the organism. Uric acid is relatively insoluble in water and may precipitate in the joints, causing inflammation, or in genitourinary tract, producing stones. Gout patients given allopurinol do not convert the xanthine to uric acid and excrete the much more soluble hypoxanthine and xanthine. Normal blood uric levels are 3.5–7.2 mg/dL in males and 2.6–6.0 mg/dL in females. Gout is suspected if these values are exceeded. Daily uric acid excretion ranges from 250 to 750 mg in people on a normal diet. As much as 5 g purine bases is produced per day, although most of this amount is reutilized through the salvage pathways. Another disease associated with the purine nucleotide degradation process is *adenosine deaminase deficiency*. This enzyme converts adenosine and

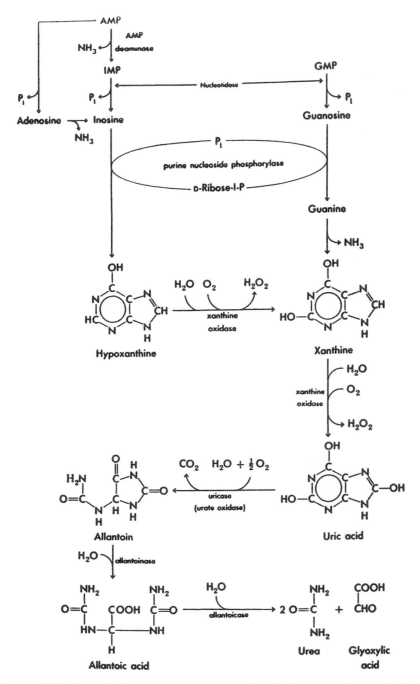

Figure 10.14 Degradation of purines to uric acid and other excretion products. In human beings, uric acid is the end product of purine base catabolism.

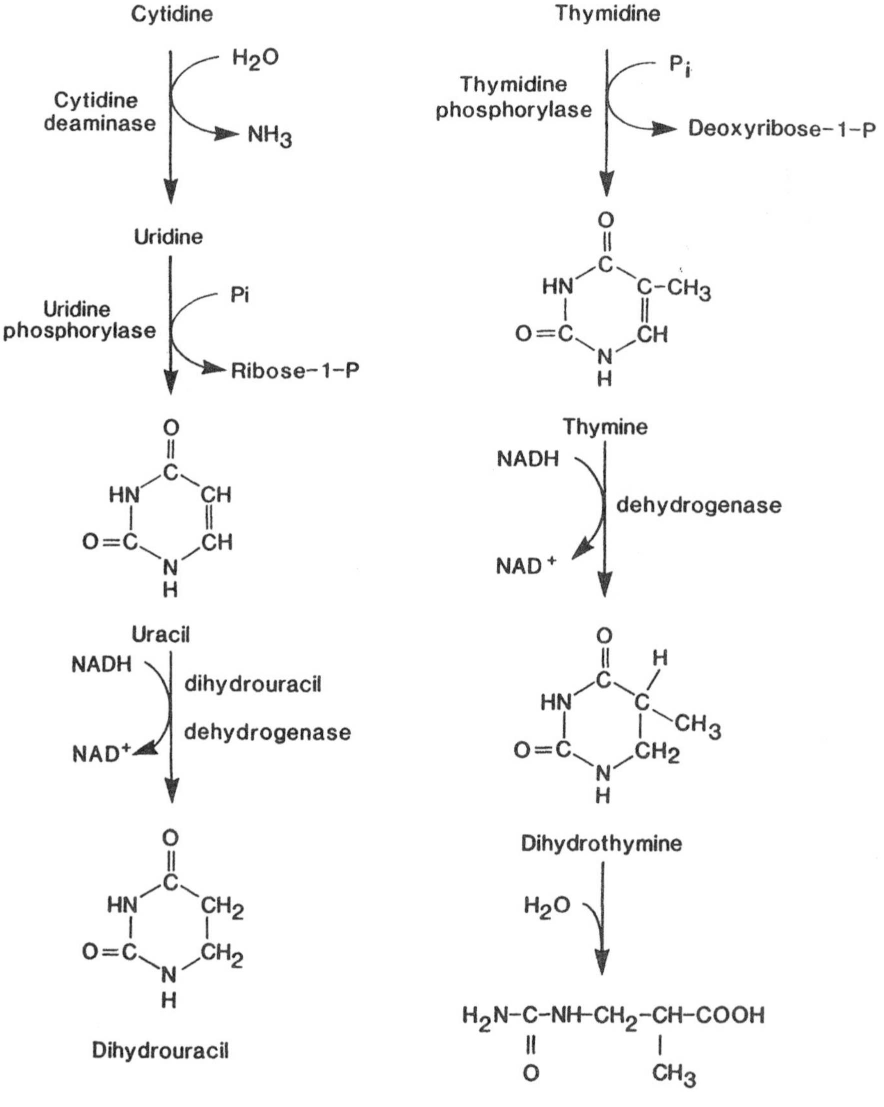

Figure 10.15 Degradation of pyrimidines to their excretion products.

deoxyadenosine to inosine or deoxyinosine (see Figure 10.14). If this enzyme is deficient because of a genetic lesion, the activity of lymphocytes is severely limited and the affected children die of infections. It is believed that the buildup of dATP and other precursors of inosine and deoxyinosine is poisonous to the lymphocytes.

Pyrimidines are metabolized largely as shown in Figure 10.15. β-Aminoisobutyric acid, the product of thymine catabolism, is excreted in the urine in some individuals. In others it is further catabolized to CO_2 and H_2O.

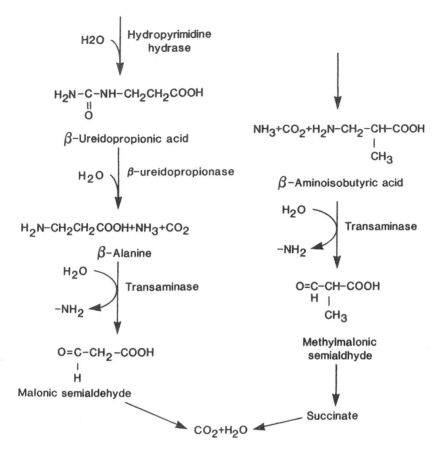

Figure 10.15 Continued

10.4 POLYNUCLEOTIDES

10.4.1 Basic Chemistry

In the previous sections of this chapter we saw that inorganic phosphate could become esterified with the 5'-OH group of a nucleoside to form a nucleoside monophosphate. Because inorganic phosphate has three potential esterification sites (–OH residues), it could conceivably form an ester linkage with, say, the 3'-OH of another nucleoside monophosphate to form a phosphodiester dinucleotide. A trinucleotide could be formed by a third monophosphate forming a diester bond with the free 3'-OH group of the dinucleotide, and so on. It is thus possible to build very large polymers of nucleotides containing ribose (RNA) or deoxyribose (DNA). Such polymers have a terminus with a phosphate monoester, called the 5' end, and another terminus that has a free 3'-OH group. This is analogous to looking at proteins with the N and C termini. Figure 10.16 shows sections of DNA and RNA, with the 5' end at the top and the 3' end at the bottom. A shorthand method of representing polynucleotides is also illustrated in Figure 10.16.

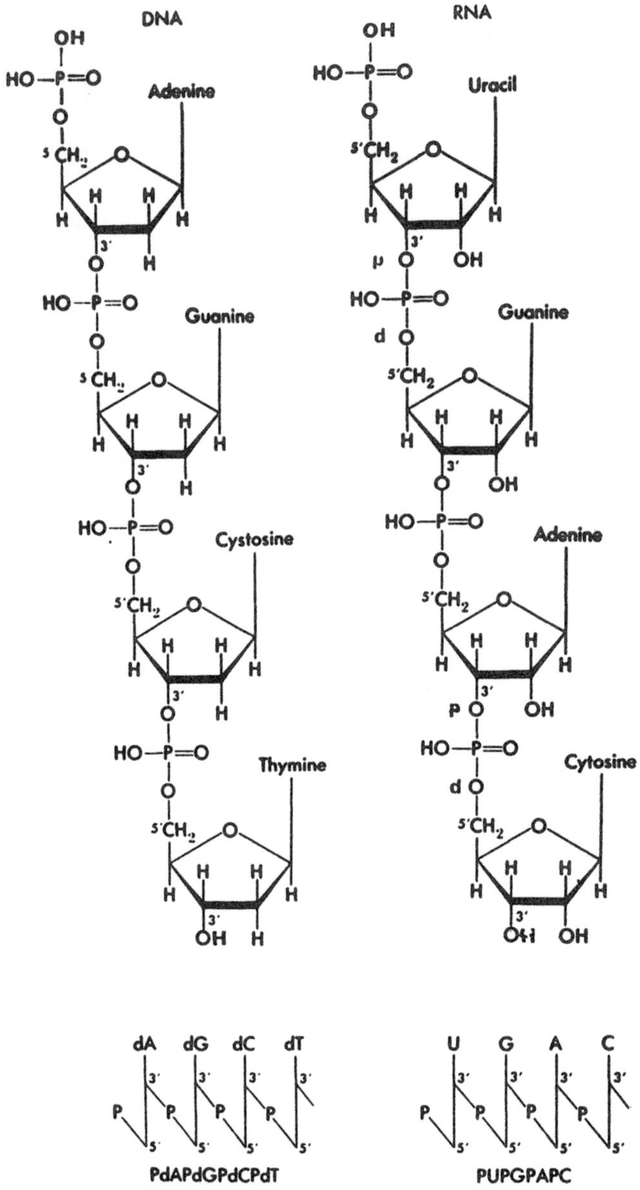

Figure 10.16 Structures of tetranucleotides representing DNA and RNA. p indicates proximal bond with respect to 3'-OH and d indicates the distal bond.

In a given phosphodiester bond, hydrolytic enzymatic cleavage can occur at two locations, indicated by p and d in Figure 10.16. The former is *proximal* with respect to the 3'-OH group; the latter is *distal* with respect to the 3'-OH. Enzymes that catalyze the hydrolysis of nucleic acids are *nucleases* (see Table 10.2). *Exonucleases* remove nucleotides (or nucleosides) from either the 5' or the 3' end of the polynucleotide. These are specific for either the p or the d bond. Thus, an exo-

Table 10.2 Some Typical Nucleases and Their Specificities

Nuclease	Source	Specificity
Ribonuclease T_1	*Aspergillus oryzae*	RNA endonuclease; splits d bonds where guanine nucleotides are in 3' position
Ribonuclease I	Bovine pancreas	RNA endonuclease; splits d bonds where pyrimidine nucleotides are in 3' position
Deoxyribonuclease I	Bovine pancreas	DNA endonuclease; splits simple or double-stranded DNA; specific for p bonds where pyrimidine nucleotides are in 3' position, producing largely tetranucleotides
Deoxyribonuclease II	Porcine spleen	Same as DNA as I, except that d bonds are broken and average product is a hexanucleotide
Micrococcal nuclease	*Staphylococcus aureus*	RNA and DNA endonuclease; splits d bonds in areas rich in adenosine, uracil, and thymine
Phosphodiesterase I	Snake venom	RNA and DNA exonuclease; splits p bonds from 3' ends, releasing 5'-phosphonucleosides
Phosphodiesterase II	Bovine spleen	RNA and DNA (single-stranded) exonuclease; splits d linkages at 5' end, releasing 3'-phosphonucleosides

nuclease working on the p bond at the 5' end of RNA (see Figure 10.16) will remove uridine-5'-monophosphate. An exonuclease specific for the d bond will remove uridine-3', 5'-diphosphate. An exonuclease specific for the p bond at the 3' end of RNA will remove cytidine-5'-monophosphate, but one specific for the d bond will remove cytidine. Endonucleases cause the hydrolysis of phosphodiester bonds anywhere in the polynucleotide chain. They, too, are specific for either p or d bonds. Both exo- and endonucleases may also have specificity with respect to bases and the single- or double-stranded DNA or RNA of the polynucleotide.

RNA but not DNA is susceptible to alkaline hydrolysis. This is because for such hydrolysis to occur, the susceptible phosphodiester must form a triester with the 2'-OH residue adjacent to the 3' residue, as shown in Figure 10.17. The resulting cyclic phosphate triester may be hydrolyzed in any two positions indicated by the broken lines. Because DNA lacks the reaction −OH residues at 2' positions, no intermediate cyclic triester can be formed and DNA is resistant to alkaline hydrolysis. This confers a greater stability upon DNA. Teleologically speaking, DNA is supposed to be permanent, whereas RNA is transient and hence less stable.

10.4.2 Secondary Structure of DNA

Properties of the DNA Double Helix

Both RNA and DNA can exist in various helical conformations, although much of the RNA is globular. DNA, on the other hand, is mostly helical, and this

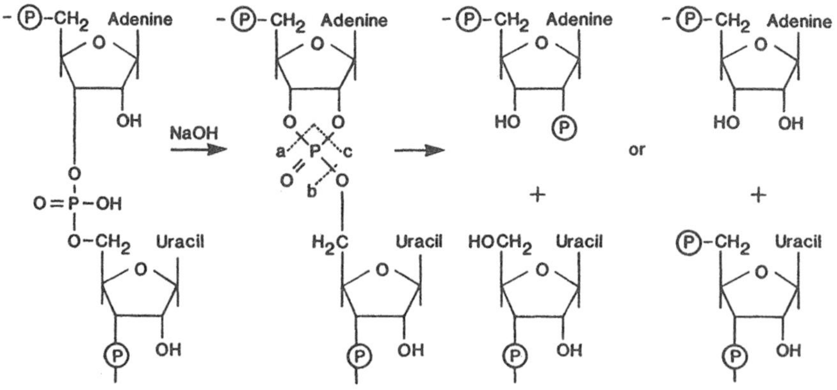

Figure 10.17 Alkaline hydrolysis of RNA, showing only a single diester bond. The intermediate cyclic triester can be hydrolyzed at any two of the three locations indicated by dotted lines and labeled a, b, and c. If cleavage occurs at positions a and b, the first set of products is obtained. Cleavage at a and c produces the second set. A third set may be obtained by cleaving at b and c. P designates esterified phosphate.

section deals with DNA with the understanding that the principles enunciated are applicable to RNA as well. As with proteins, native DNA is not a random coil, but instead assumes a helical conformation because of the interactions among its constituent bases. Such interactions are of hydrophobic, van der Waals, and base-stacking nature. The resulting helix has a spiral staircase appearance, the deoxyribose phosphate acting as the backbone and the bases (which are planar) acting as the steps. The bases are thus partially *stacked* on top of each other, each base being turned about 35° with respect to the next. The distances between stacked bases is about 3.6 Å.

Although some DNA exists in nature as a single helical strand, most DNA is double-stranded, originally described by Watson and Crick in 1953. In this structure, two DNA strands are intertwined to form two-strand cables. As an analogy from the field of protein chemistry, one may mention the keratins and the collagens, which also form superhelices. The double helix cannot be formed with any two DNA strands; to interact, the two strands must be *complementary*. This means that strong hydrogen bonding must be present to maintain the double-stranded structure, and such bonding can be achieved only if an adenine (A) base of one strand can pair with thymine of (T) of another (or with uracil in RNA) and a guanine (G) base with a cytosine (C) base. To form hydrogen bonds, the tautomeric forms of the bases must be of the keto type (see Figure 10.2). Chargaff and his associates discovered, before the double helix was described in the literature, that in any DNA, the quantity of purines is the same as that of pyrimidines (A + G = C + T), the quantity of adenine was always equal to that of thymine, and the quantity of guanine was equal to that of cytosine (A = T; G = C). This precisely fits the double-helix concept of Watson and Crick. Hydrogen bond formation between the two pairs of nucleotides is shown in Figure 10.18. Note that two hydrogen bonds are present in the A-T interaction, whereas three are formed between G and C. It should be remembered that despite these base relationships, the base compositions of the two complementary DNA strands are

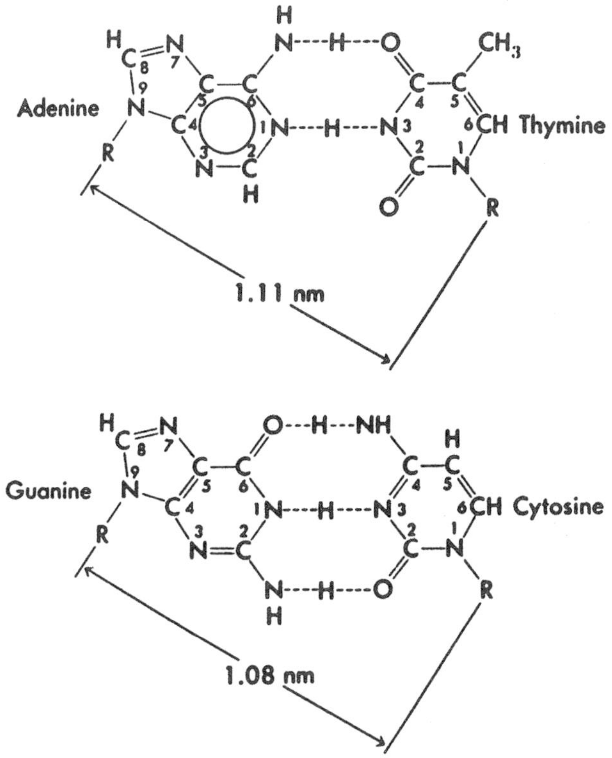

Figure 10.18 Hydrogen bonds formed between purine or pyrimidine pairs in double-stranded DNA.

not equal. Furthermore, DNA compositions from all cells of the same organism are the same.

A section of a typical double-stranded DNA molecule showing both helices as well as the superhelix twisted around a central axis is shown in Figure 10.19. Note that the planar bases (shaded), which are perpendicular to the superhelix axis, are located in the superhelix interior, where the environment is hydrophobic. Thus, hydrogen bond formation between base pairs is favored, as are interactions resulting from base stacking. The more hydrophilic deoxyribose and phosphate residues are on the superhelix exterior, in contact with the aqueous environment. Note also that the two complementary strands of DNA run in opposite directions that is, $5' \rightarrow 3'$ in one case and $3' \rightarrow 5'$ in another. Note the analogy to antiparallel pleated sheet structures in proteins (Chapter 4).

It is easy to imagine that the double helix may assume a number of shapes in three dimensions. Three major forms of DNA are recognized: A-DNA, B-DNA, and Z-DNA. B-DNA is the most common physiologic form. It is right-handed, with 10 base pairs per turn and a 3.4 Å rise per base pair. In the laboratory, it is observed at low salt concentrations and a maximum degree of hydration. When the salt concentration is increased and degree of hydration lowered, DNA may assume the A conformation. It is also right-handed, but there are 10.7–11 base pairs per helical turn with a rise of only 2.3 Å per base

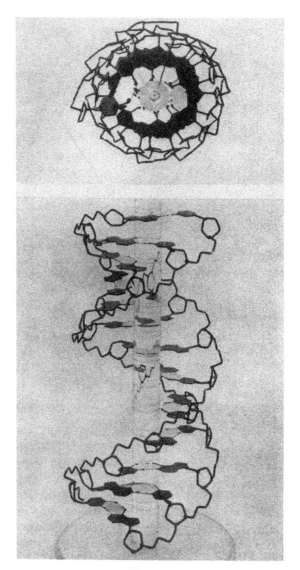

Figure 10.19 Model of a double-stranded DNA molecule. Upper frame is top view; lower frame is side view. Outlined pentagons are deoxyribose molecules. Shaded structures perpendicular to the sugars are the bases. (Reproduced by permission from Crick FHC. The structure of the hereditary material. Sci Am October:2–8, 1954.)

pair. It is thus thicker than B-DNA. Sections of A-DNA are found in the conventional B-DNA strands. Double-stranded RNA and DNA–RNA hybrids assume the shape of A-DNA, because the –OH groups in the 2′ positions prevent the B conformation. Both A- and B-DNAs are illustrated in Figure 10.20.

A recently discovered form of DNA is Z-DNA, which may be universally present as a component or section of other DNA types. It, too, is shown in Figure 10.20. Z-DNA is left-handed, with 12 pairs per turn and a 3.8 Å rise per

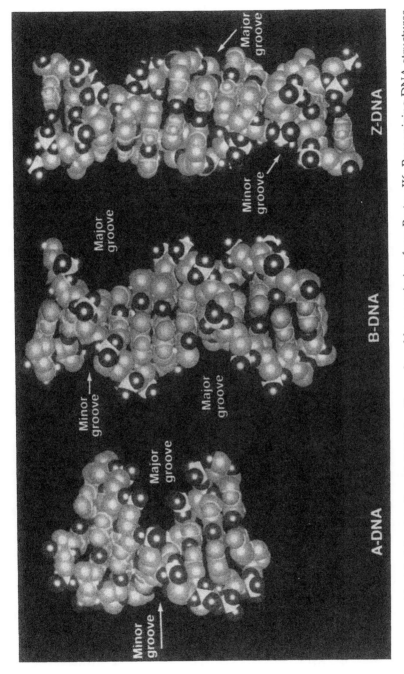

Figure 10.20 Models of A, B, and Z DNAs. (Reproduced by permission from Barton JK. Recognizing DNA structures. Chem Eng News September:30–42, 1988.)

base pair. It is thinner than either A- or B-DNA. Z-DNA is formed in DNA segments in which purine and pyrimidine bases alternate, especially where G and C follow each other and C is methylated in the 5 position. Another important feature that distinguishes Z-DNA from A- and B-DNA is that the relationship between G and deoxyribose is *anti* (across from each other) as shown in Figure 10.21, whereas in Z-DNA their relationship is *syn* (on the same side). The conformation of deoxycytidine is anti as in B-DNA. The Z in Z-DNA means zigzag: the location of the phosphodiester groups on the outer surface of Z-DNA can be connected by a broken (zigzag) line rather than a smooth spiral as in B-DNA (Figure 10.22). All DNAs have grooves, which can interact with proteins, such as histones (see Figure 10.20 and 10.22). Such grooves have different dimensions in the various types of DNA, and it is possible that the formation of Z-DNA within the normal B-DNA strand is a means of regulating its biologic activity through changes in protein binding. Dimensions of the three types of DNA are summarized in Table 10.3.

The DNA double helix is not necessarily the continuous smooth structure shown in Figure 10.20. There may be bulges of various sorts, loops, and palindromic hairpin turns. A *palindrome* is a section of DNA in which the two DNA strands have an identical base sequence running in opposite directions. Figure 10.23 shows a double-stranded DNA with some such features. Of most interest are the cruciform bulges and palindromic structures. Note that in the *cruciform* structure, there are two pairs of palindromic sequences on the vertical

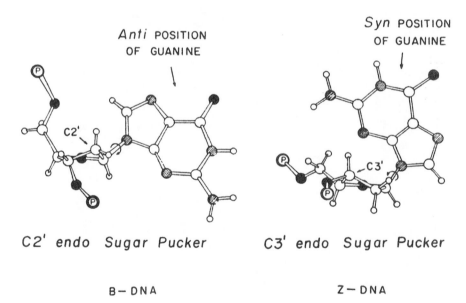

Figure 10.21 Relationship of deoxyribose and the guanine base in B- and Z-DNA. Rotation to affect either the syn or the anti conformations is done about the N-glycoside bond, as shown by the curved arrow. Also note that in Z-DNA, the 3' carbon is above the plane of the sugar, whereas in B-DNA, the 2' carbon is. This is the endo conformation. (Reproduced by permission from Rich A, Nordheim A, Wang AHJ. The chemistry and biology of left-handed Z-DNA. Annu Rev Biochem 53:701–846, 1984.)

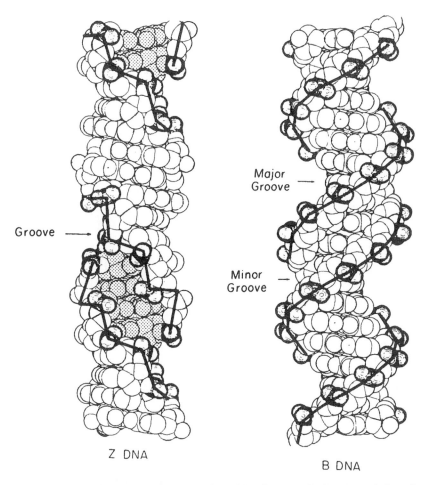

Groove →

Major Groove →

Minor Groove →

Z DNA

B DNA

Figure 10.22 Space-filling models of B- and Z-DNA showing the location of phosphodiester groupings. Note the zigzag distribution of phosphates in Z-DNA and the smooth distribution in B-DNA. (Reproduced by permission as from Rich A, Nordheim A, Wang AHJ. The chemistry and biology of left-handed Z-DNA. Annu Rev Biochem 53:701–846, 1984.)

Table 10.3 Dimensions of the Most Commonly Occurring Forms of DNA

	DNA form		
	A	B	Z
Helical handedness	Right	Right	Left
Base pairs per turn of helix	10.7	10	12
Rise per base pair, Å	2.3	3.4	3.8
Pitch per turn of helix, Å	25	34	46
Diameter, Å	25	24	18
Rotation per base pair, degrees	33	35	30

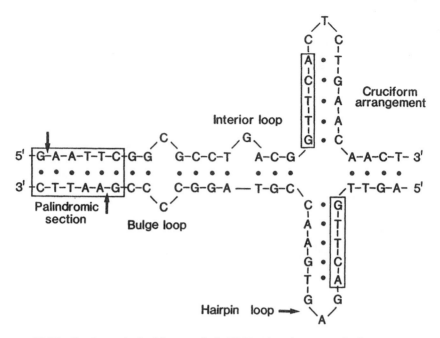

Figure 10.23 Section of double-stranded DNA showing a palindrome section, a cruciform hairpin loop structure, a bulge loop, and an interior loop. Palindromic sequences are boxed. A black dot between bases indicates hydrogen bonding. The interior loop is common in RNA and relatively uncommon in DNA.

portions of the cross on opposite sides (one pair is boxed). A more common palindromic structure is shown on the left side of Figure 10.23. Palindromic structures of this sort are important because they serve as recognition sites for a group of DNA endonucleases called restriction endonucleases. These enzymes recognize identical sequences on the two DNA strands (even if they run in opposite directions) and proceed to hydrolyze specific diester bonds, as shown by arrows in Figure 10.23. The restriction endonuclease that recognizes the sequence shown in Figure 10.23 is called EcoRI, from *Escherichia coli*.

Denaturation of DNA

The DNA double helix is exceptionally stable. However, methods exist that *denature* DNA, that is, seperate DNA into its individual randomly coiled strands. For the most part this involves the breakage of hydrogen bonds linking the two strands. It is believed that, locally, hydrogen bonds are constantly broken, forming "bubbles," and then reformed to regenerate native DNA. Factors that cause the denaturation of DNA include high and low ionic strength solvents, acids and bases, various chemicals, such as ethyl urea and urea, and increases in temperature. The last has been especially useful in studying DNA structures.

For any type of DNA, as the heat is applied, the transition between the double helix and random coil is sudden and occurs at a typical temperature called the melting temperature T_m. The T_m of a DNA depends on its G and C content: the higher G + C, the higher the T_m because it takes more energy to break the three hydrogen bonds linking G and C than the two hydrogen bonds between A and T. One also often expresses the relationship among the bases in terms of the ratio A + T/G + C. Such ratios vary from one organism to another and have been used in microorganism classification schemes. A plot of G + C versus T_m is shown in Figure 10.24. It is obvious that the T_m depends on the ionic strength of the DNA solution: higher T_m are observed at higher ionic strengths. Note that the lowest T_m is obtained with an A-T double helix, the highest with the G-C double helix. The DNAs of the various organisms shown fall between these two extremes.

Denatured DNA can be renatured: the separated DNA strands can be *annealed* under proper circumstances, and the rate of annealing has provided valuable information on DNA structure. Annealing of native DNA strands is often incomplete, and for this reason, the denatured DNA may be broken into smaller fragments by *shearing*. Sheared DNA anneals completely. Annealing is a

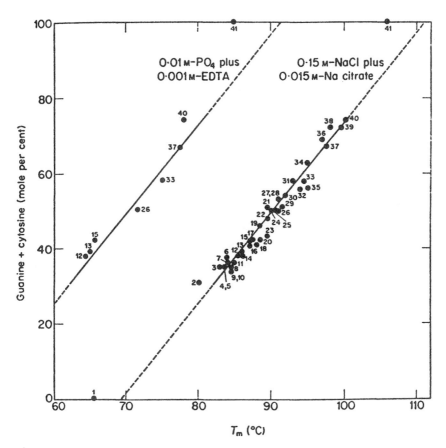

Figure 10.24 Relationship between the G + C content of DNA and its melting temperature. Experiments were done at two different ionic strengths. Numbers indicate DNA sources: 1 is an A-T copolymer, whereas 41 is a G-C copolymer; 2 is *Clostridia perfringens*, and 40 is *Streptococcus viridochromogenes*. (Reproduced by permission from Marmur J, Doty P. Determination of the base composition of deoxyribonucleic acid from thermal denaturation temperature. J Mol Biol 5:109–118, 1962.)

second-order process, that is, the rate of annealing depends on the concentrations of the two complementary strands. The integrated form of the rate equation is

$$\frac{C}{C_0} = \frac{1}{1 + KC_0 t} \tag{10.12}$$

where C is single-stranded DNA, C_0 is total DNA, t is time, and K is the rate constant. Characteristic sigmoid (nonstraightline) curves are obtained if C/C_0 is plotted against log $C_0 t$ (Figure 10.25). When $C/C_0 = 0.5$, or 50%, log $C_0 t$ at this point is related to the number of base pairs and therefore the molecular weight of the DNA. Thus, for *E. coli* DNA, there are about 4.5 million base pairs per genome, which translates to a molecular weight of about 3×10^9 (1500 base pairs accounts for about 10^6 daltons). For the MS2 viral DNA, there are only 5000–6000 base pairs and the molecular weight is between 3×10^6 and 4×10^6. The rate of DNA renaturation depends on its "complexity." The more repetition in base pairs, the faster the DNA anneals. Thus, poly (A) and poly (U) anneal the fastest. Mouse satellite DNA is composed of repetitive nucleotide sequences, so it, too, anneals rather rapidly. MS2, T4, and *E. coli* DNAs are all unique, and they anneal rather slowly, rates of annealing depending on their molecular weights. Rat liver and total calf thymus DNAs are composed of repeating and unique types of DNA, and their annealing rates show a complex nature (Figure 10.25).

When DNA is denatured, a number of physical parameters change. For instance, the absorption of ultraviolet light at 260 nm rises, especially in DNAs with a high A content. This is the *hyperchromic shift*. The viscosity of denatured DNA falls, because native DNA is rigid, whereas denatured DNA is flexible. The buoyant density of denatured DNA increases. It is greater in DNAs rich in G and C. Native and denatured DNAs can be separated by *density gradient centrifugation* using $CsCl_2$ to form the density gradient.

10.4.3 Supramolecular Organization of DNA

DNA molecules are very large. Viral DNA has a MW of $2–100 \times 10^6$, bacterial DNA around 3×10^9, and eukaryotic DNA close to 10^{11}. For each 10^6 daltons, there are 1500 base pairs. Mammalian DNA codes for some 50,000 proteins, and it may be as long as 1 m. Yet all this DNA must be packed into a relatively small volume, for example, into a nucleus with the dimensions of 6×9 μm. DNA has thus responded to this challenge over the course of evolution by assuming various compact shapes and forms. In bacteria and vertebrate mitochondria, the DNA is circular. The 5′ and 3′ ends are joined by phosphodiester linkages. It is not clear whether mammalian chromosomal DNA is also circular. It is known that each chromosome consists of a single, very long double-stranded DNA molecule and that, for packing purposes, it is associated with a group of basic proteins called histones. Such DNA-protein complexes are called *chromatin* when the nucleus is lysed and chromosomes disrupted to reveal the extended genetic material. Chromatin from the interphase is usually studied.

There are five histones associated with DNA, neutralizing the acidic DNA (DNA is acidic largely a result of the phosphate residues). Table 10.4 lists the histones and their properties. Clusters of histones consisting of two molecules each of H2A, H2B, H3, and H4 (octamers) serve as the framework around which

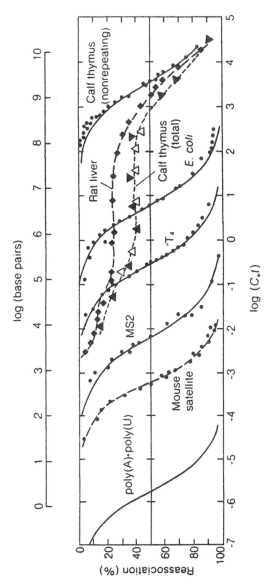

Figure 10.25 Reassociation of denatured sheared DNA expressed as a plot of % annealed DNA versus log C_0t. (Reproduced by permission from Guschlbauer W. Nucleic Acid Structure. New York: Springer-Verlag, 1976, p. 61; Britten RJ, Kohn DE. Repeated sequences in DNA. Science 161:529–540, 1968.)

the double-stranded DNA is wrapped. Histones fit into the major groove of the DNA. The histone octamer with its DNA is a *nucleosome*. There are two types of nucleosomes: one containing a DNA section with 146 base pairs corresponding to about 1.75 DNA turns (incomplete nucleosome) and the complete nucleosome with 166 base pairs corresponding to 2 full DNA turns. The latter is associated with the H1 histone and is sometimes termed the chromatosome. The nucleosomes are shown in Figure 10.26. The diameter of each nucleosome is about 100 Å, and the pitch is 27 Å. A string of nucleosomes and chromatosomes, called the 100 Å fiber, is linked by a *bridge* or *linker* DNA, which is between 10 and 100 base pairs long. Thus, there is a nucleosome for every 200 base pairs in the 100 Å fiber.

The 100 Å fiber can arrange itself into a solenoid or a 300 Å fiber. The solenoid has a diameter of 300 Å and a pitch of about 110 Å. It is held together by H1 histone interactions; without the H1 histone, the 100 Å fibers are unable to form solenoids. Chromatin observed in the laboratory is largely an array of the 300 Å fibers. The solenoids can be further compacted by twisting about themselves to form "knoblike" structures that are very compact and constitute the chromosomes. The organization of DNA into the 100 and 300 Å (solenoid) fibers is shown in Figure 10.27.

When DNA is wrapped around histone octamers, it is said to be *supercoiled*, that is, another coiling level is superimposed upon the double-helical

Table 10.4 Histones and Their Properties

Designation	Molecular Weight	No. of amino acids	Predominant basic amino acid present
H$_1$	21,500	216	Lysine
H2A	14,000	129	Lysine
H2B	13,800	125	Lysine
H3	15,300	135	Arginine
H4	11,300	102	Arginine

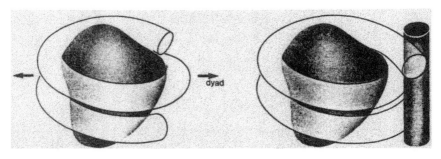

Figure 10.26 Appearance of the two types of nucleosomes. The cores are histone octamers, around which is wound the double-stranded DNA. The cylindrical object in the right frame represents H1 histones. (Reproduced by permission from Saenger W. Principles of Nucleic Acid Structure. New York: Springer-Verlag, 1984, p. 442.)

structure. Another form of DNA supercoiling is observed in the DNA of bacterial chromosomes and plasmids, which most of the time are circular in nature. This type of DNA may of course exist in the so-called relaxed state, that is, if the dimensions of B-DNA are strictly adhered to. Thus, a relaxed circular DNA of the B type with, say, 1050 base pairs, has 10.5 base pairs per turn and a total number of 100 turns. If the number of turns is increased (overwinding) or decreased (underwinding), however, we have a thermodynamically strained condition, which can be relieved by supercoiling. By convention, if DNA is underwound, the supercoil is said to be *negative*, and if it is overwound, the resulting supercoil is *positive*. Suppose we change the number of turns in this example by 10: in a negative supercoil, we now have a total of 90 turns, and

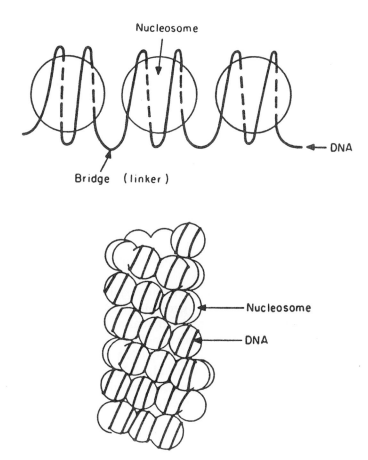

Figure 10.27 Organizations of genetic material in the nucleus. Upper frame represents several nucleosomes (chromatosomes) arrayed in a beaded string fashion (100 Å fibers) Circles represent histone octamers. H1 histones are not shown. Lower frame represents a 100 Å fiber wound in a solenoid fashion. There are six nucleosomes per turn in a solenoid (300 Å fiber). DNA is wound around the histone octamer in a left-handed superhelix. In the solenoid, the winding may be left- or right-handed. (Reproduced by permission from Mainwaring WIP, Parish JH, Pickering JD, Mann NH. Nucleic Acid Biochemistry and Molecular Biology. Oxford: Blackwell Scientific, 1982, pp. 268, 269.)

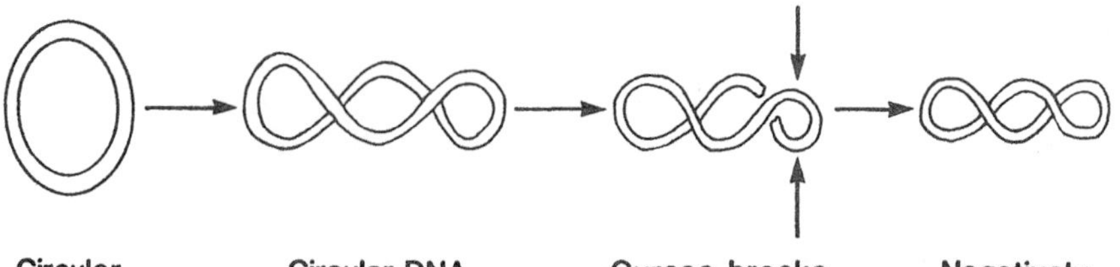

| Circular DNA | Circular DNA folded over | Gyrase breaks double–stranded DNA | Negatively supercoiled DNA with two twists reformed |

Figure 10.28 Formation of negatively supercoiled circular DNA by gyrase. This type of DNA is present in bacterial chromosomes and plasmids. Positively supercoiled DNA has the opposite handedness.

1050/90 = 11.7 base pairs per turn (higher than the 10.5 of B-DNA). On the other hand, if we have a positive supercoil with 110 turns, we have 1050/110 = 9.5 base pairs per turn. In both cases, supercoiling relieves the stress. Note that to show supercoiling, the DNA must be circular or, if it is linear, both ends must be attached to something.

Supercoiling of the type just described aids in the process of DNA packing, and it also is the result of DNA uncoiling during DNA replication and transcription (Chapter 11). Circular DNA of bacteria is usually negatively supercoiled, and this is helpful in the two processes just mentioned, because negative supercoiling counteracts to some extent the positive supercoiling introduced in DNA upstream of the unwinding locus. Negative supercoiling, shown in Figure 10.28, is introduced into circular DNA by an enzyme called gyrase, with the expenditure of ATP energy. Gyrase does not occur in eukaryotic cells, and it is inhibited by the antibiotic nalidixic acid.

Gyrase is a member of a group of enzymes called *topoisomerases*. The function of most topoisomerases is not to generate DNA supercoils, but to relieve them during the processes of DNA replication and transcription. They perform this function by breaking phosphodiester bonds of one or both DNA strands and then resealing the "nick" after rotation of the DNA strand(s) to relieve tension. Topoisomerases I break only one DNA strand, and topoisomerases II break both. Gyrase is a topoisomerase II. Topoisomerases are thus integral components of the DNA replication and transcription mechanisms.

10.4.4 Ribonucleic Acids

Cytosolic RNA occurs mostly in the single-stranded although helical form. Such helices contain six nucleotides per turn and are stabilized by the base-stacking effects described earlier. Double-stranded RNA has A-DNA dimensions, because the –OH groups in position 2′ of ribose interfere with B-RNA formation.

Both pro- and eukaryotic cells have three types of RNA. The largest is *messenger RNA* (mRNA), whose molecular weight can be as high as 10^6. It carries genetic information from DNA to the protein synthesis machinery. It is a product of DNA transcription, and it is *translated* (expressed) into a protein via the action of ribosomes. The flow of information from DNA via mRNA for the purpose of protein expression is referred as the *central dogma* of molecular biology.

By far the most abundant form of RNA in the cell is *ribosomal RNA*. It may account for as much as 80% of total cellular RNA. Its molecular weight is $0.5–1 \times 10^6$, and it is associated with ribosomes, the protein biosynthesis factories.

Transfer RNA (tRNA) has the lowest molecular weight, that is, near 28,000. Its function is to activate amino acids for protein biosynthesis. It has a unique cloverleaf structure (Figure 10.29), and there are sections of double-helix, bulges, and hairpin turns. Of all RNAs, it has the highest number of unusual bases (10–15%). Thus, the hairpin arm pointing east contains pseudouridine Ψ and is

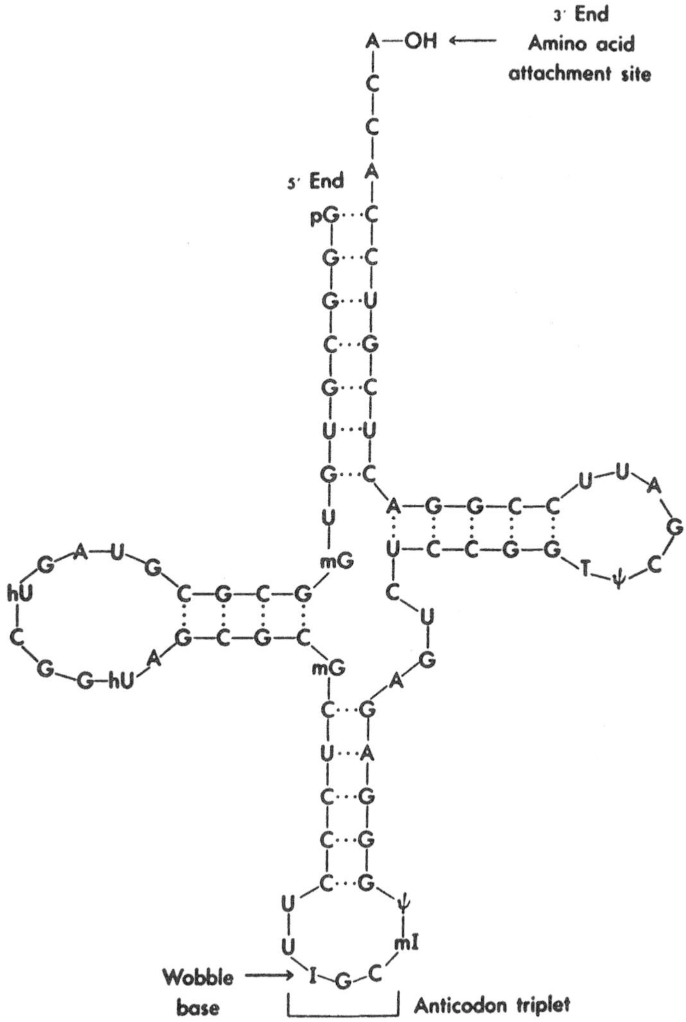

Figure 10.29 Diagram of tRNA from yeast, specific for alanine. I, inosine; Ψ, pseudouridine; mG, methylguanosine; m^{2}G, dimethylguanosine; T, ribothymidine; hU, dihydrouridine; mI, methylinosine.

termed the pseudouridine arm (TΨ arm). The arm pointing west contains dihydrouridine (hU) and is termed the dihydrouridine (DHU) arm or loop. The arm pointing south is called the anticodon arm. The bulge under the TΨ loop is called the variable extra arm. All "arms" have a function in the protein biosynthesis and recognition processes. The open end of tRNA containing the phosphorylated 5' terminus and the 3' end (-C-C-A) is called the *stem*. Amino acids are activated by combining with the 3' end of tRNA, creating an ester linkage between the α-carboxyl group of the amino acid and either the 2'- or 3'-OH group of the 3'-terminal adenylic acid nucleotide. The details of protein biosynthesis are presented in Chapter 12.

QUESTIONS

10.1   Which substance is *not* required for the biosynthesis of deoxyribonucleotides from ribonucleotides?
   a. FAD-containing enzyme
   b. Protein with –SH groups
   c. NADPH
   d. Iron-containing enzyme
   e. ATP in stoichiometric amounts

10.2.   What is the most efficient way to obtain CTP in the mammal?
   a. UMP $\rightarrow$ UDP $\rightarrow$ UTP $\rightarrow$ CTP
   b. Cytosine + PRPP $\rightarrow$ CMP $\rightarrow$ CDP $\rightarrow$ CTP
   c. Cytosine + ribose-1-phosphate $\rightarrow$ cytidine $\xrightarrow{ATP}$ CMP $\xrightarrow{ATP}$ CTP
   d. Uracil + NH_3 $\rightarrow$ cytosine $\xrightarrow{PRPP}$ CMP $\rightarrow$ CDP $\rightarrow$ CTP
   e. Two of these

10.3.   What would be the best pathway to obtain dTTP from CTP? *Note*: Some steps in the following may have been omitted for the sake of brevity.
   a. CTP $\rightarrow$ CDP $\rightarrow$ dCDP $\rightarrow$ dUDP $\rightarrow$ dUMP $\rightarrow$ dTMP $\rightarrow$ dTTP
   b. CTP $\rightarrow$ cytidine $\rightarrow$ uridine $\rightarrow$ thymidine $\rightarrow$ dTMP $\rightarrow$ dTTP
   c. CTP $\rightarrow$ cytidine $\rightarrow$ uridine $\rightarrow$ UMP $\rightarrow$ UDP $\rightarrow$ dUDP $\rightarrow$ dUMP $\rightarrow$ dTMP $\rightarrow$ dTTP
   d. CTP $\rightarrow$ UTP $\rightarrow$ UDP $\rightarrow$ UMP $\rightarrow$ dTMP $\rightarrow$ dTTP
   e. CTP $\rightarrow$ UTP $\rightarrow$ dTTP

10.4.   What would be the easiest way to measure the molecular weight of DNA from *B. breve*?
   a. Gel filtration
   b. Viscosity measurements
   c. Nucleotide composition
   d. Annealing of denatured DNA
   e. Determination of the T_m

10.5.   Which is the one nucleotide that is the end product of purine biosynthetic pathway?
   a. Orotic acid
   b. Hypoxanthine ribonucleoside phosphate
   c. AMP
   d. GMP
   e. Inosine

10.6.   Which substance is absent if 100 Å DNA fibers cannot form solenoids?
   a. Pseudouridine
   b. Double-stranded DNA

     c. Nucleosomes
     d. ATP
     e. Histone H1

10.7. Phosphoribosylpyrophosphate does not react with which compound?
     a. Hypoxanthine
     b. Xanthine
     c. Orotic acid
     d. ATP
     e. Uracil

10.8. You have isolated an exonuclease that is specific for *d* linkages at the 5′ end of a polynucleotide chain. The products will be
     a. A 3′,5′-diphosphonucleotide and an RNA dephosphorylated at the 5′ terminus.
     b. A 5′-nucleoside and a new RNA.
     c. A nucleoside and an RNA phosphorylated at the 3′ position.
     d. The original RNA dephosphorylated at the 5′ end.
     e. A 5′-nucleotide, phosphate, and an RNA dephosphorylated at the 5′ end.

10.9. The salvage pathways in nucleotide metabolism are not capable of which procedure?
     a. Guanine + ribose-1-P → guanosine + P_i.
     b. GDP + ATP → GTP + ADP.
     c. Adenine + phosphodeoxyribosylpyrophosphate → dAMP + PP_i.
     d. Thymine + deoxyribose-1-phosphate → thymidine + P_i.
     e. Adenosine + ATP → AMP + ADP.

In Questions 10.10–10.14, use the following key:
     a. 1, 2, and 3 are correct.
     b. 1 and 3 are correct.
     c. 2 and 4 are correct.
     d. 4 is correct.
     e. All are correct.

10.10. Which are substrates for ribonucleotide reductase?
     1. Thioredoxin
     2. GTP
     3. ADP
     4. NADPH

10.11. Which of the following antitumor agents work by impairing *de novo* purine synthesis?
     1. Azaserine
     2. 5-Fluorouracil
     3. Methotrexate
     4. Hydroxyurea

10.12. In nucleic acid degradation,
     1. There are nucleases that are specific for either DNA or RNA.
     2. Nucleotidases convert nucleotides to nucleosides.
     3. The conversion of a nucleoside to a free base involves the reversal of a salvage reaction.
     4. Hypoxanthine is an intermediate because of the presence of purine deaminases.

10.13. The following is true of uric acid:
     1. It is formed from xanthine in the presence of O_2.
     2. It is oxidized in humans before it is excreted.

   3. It precipitates in joints in gout when its blood levels are above 7.5 mg/dL.
   4. It is a degradation product of cytidine.
10.14. In double-stranded DNA,
   1. A + T = G + C.
   2. Melting temperature depends on G + C content.
   3. Denaturation results in decreased absorption at 260 nm (hypochromic shift).
   4. Strands are held together via hydrogen bonds.

In a–e are listed a number of enzymes. Match these with their physiologic properties enumerated in Questions 10.15–10.20.
   a. Ribonucleotide reductase
   b. Phosphoribosylpyrophosphate amidotransferase
   c. Xanthine oxidase
   d. Carbamoyl phosphate synthetase II
   e. Hypoxanthine-guanine phosphoribosyltransferase

10.15. Active as monomer only.
10.16. Rate-controlling enzyme in the pyrimidine biosynthetic pathway.
10.17. Rate-controlling enzyme in DNA biosynthesis.
10.18. Inhibited by allopurinol.
10.19. Low levels associated with Lesch-Nyhan syndrome.
10.20. Part of a cytoplasmic multifunctional enzyme that has three enzymatic activities.

Use the following data which shows the origins of various atoms found in purine and pyrimidine bases to answer Questions 10.21–10.23.

	a	b	c	d	e
Aspartate	1N, 3C	1N	2N	1N, 3C	1N
Glutamine	2N	3N	2N	1N	1N
Asparagine	0	0	0	0	1N
Glycine	0	1N, 2C	1N, 2C	0	1N, 2C
Tetrahydrofolate-bound 1-carbon unit	0	2C	2C	1C	2C
NH_3/NH_4^+	0	0	0	0	1N
HCO_3^-/CO_2	1C	1C	1C	1C	1C

10.21. Base (guanine) portion of GMP
10.22. Base (thymine) portion of dTMP
10.23. Base (cytosine) portion of CMP
10.24. Which coenzyme does *not* contain adenine?
   a. FAD
   b. FMN
   c. Coenzyme A
   d. NAD^+
   e. $NADP^+$
10.25. Which statement about histones is incorrect?
   a. They form a core for the nucleosomes.
   b. They are highly conserved from an evolutionary standpoint.
   c. They are acidic proteins that neutralize the basic character of DNA.
   d. They fit into the major groove of DNA.
   e. Their molecular weights are relatively low, less than 25,000.
10.26. The following is true of transfer RNA:
   a. A single molecule accommodates all amino acids.

  b. It is circular and twisted, with a negative handedness.

  c. It has about the same molecular weight as messenger RNA.

  d. It transfers information from the nuclear DNA to the protein biosynthesis machinery.

  e. It contains double-helical sections and pseudouridine.

10.27. Which structures of double-stranded DNA are perpendicular to the DNA long axis?

  a. Deoxyribose residues

  b. Phosphate residues

  c. Diester bonds

  d. Purine and pyrimidine bases

  e. Only the purine bases

Answers

10.1. (e) ATP operates only as an effector, not a reactant, in the formation of deoxyribonucleotides.

10.2. (a) UTP is converted to CTP by amination (see Figure 10.9). UMP is the product of *de novo* pyrimidine biosynthesis process.

10.3. (c) Thymine deoxyribonucleotides can be generated from ribonucleotides only via UDP. Hence, one must first convert CTP to UDP, then UDP to dUDP, and then to dTTP (see Figure 10.11).

10.4. (d) By determining the $(C_0t)_{1/2}$ of a simple nonrepetitive DNA, one can determine the number of its base pairs (see Figure 10.25).

10.5. (b) Inosinic acid (hypoxanthine ribonucleoside phosphate) is the end product of purine biosynthesis. It then gives rise to GMP and AMP.

10.6. (e) H1 histone stabilizes and "glues" together segments of the 100 Å fiber to form 300 Å fibers.

10.7. (b) Xanthine does not react with PRPP. ATP reacts in the formation of carbamoyl phosphate, orotic acid in the pyrimidine pathway, and uracil and hypoxanthine in the salvage reactions.

10.8. (a) The *d* linkage in phosphodiester is *distal* to the 3' position. Hence the nucleotide removed will have a phosphate residue from the 5' RNA end and one esterified to the 3' position. The new RNA will *not* have a phosphate residue at the 5' end.

10.9. (c) There is no substantial enzymatic activity to salvage adenine as dAMP in the human organism.

10.10. (b) Thioredoxin is used by ribonucleotide reductase as reducing agent to reduce such diphosphonucleotides as ADP and UDP. NADPH is a substrate for thioredoxin reductase, and GTP is not used at all.

10.11. (b) Azaserine inhibits glutamine-requiring steps, and methotrexate, albeit indirectly, affects formyl-tetrahydrofolate–requiring steps. 5-Fluorouracil inhibits thymidylate synthase, and hydroxyurea inhibits ribonucleotide reductase.

10.12. (e) All are correct.

10.13. (b) Only in certain animals is uric acid further degraded, and it is a purine degradation product, not a pyrimidine.

10.14. (c) In double-stranded DNA, A + G = T + C, and denaturation results in an increase in absorption at 260 nm (hyperchromic shift).

10.15. (b) PRPP amidotransferase is inactive as a dimer. Dimer formation is promoted by IMP, GMP, and ADP, monomer formation by PRPP.

10.16. (d) Carbamoyl phosphate synthetase is a rate-controlling step in the pyrimidine biosynthetic mechanism. It is inhibited by UTP and other pyrimidine nucleotides.

10.17. (a)   Ribonucleotide reductase controls DNA biosynthesis via various feedback effects involving ribo- and deoxyribonucleotides.

10.18. (c)   Allopurinol is an inhibitor of uric acid formation, administered to some gout patients.

10.19. (e)   Lesch-Nyhan syndrome is associated with HGRRP deficiency.

10.20. (d)   Carbamoyl phosphate synthetase is part of a multifunctional enzyme that catalyzes the first three steps in pyrimidine biosynthesis.

10.21. (b)   See Figure 10.5.

10.22. (d)   See Figures 10.9 and 10.11.

10.23. (a)   See Figure 10.9.

10.24. (b)   FMN is simply phosphorylated riboflavin. It forms an adenine diphosphonucleotide (FAD) by reacting with ATP.

10.25. (c)   Histones are basic proteins containing large amounts of either lysine or arginine, and they neutralize the acidic character of DNA.

10.26. (e)   Transfer RNAs are different for each amino acid. They combine with their respective amino acids in the cytosol and carry them to the protein biosynthesis machinery.

10.27. (d)   All bases (stacked) are perpendicular to the long DNA axis. See Figure 10.19.

PROBLEMS

10.1.   Patients with orotic aciduria can be successfully treated with UMP but not with uracil. Explain why.

10.2.   Discuss the causes and consequences of Lesch-Nyhan syndrome. Be sure to address the following issues:

    a. How does the purine biosynthetic pathway activity in Lesch-Nyhan patients differ from that in normal individuals?

    b. Why are such patients treated with allopurinol?

    c. Why do such patients present with megaloblastic anemia?

10.3.   Discuss some metabolic abnormalities that could result in gout. Why would an overconsumption of caviar, meat, and alcohol bring on gout attacks?

10.4.   You have isolated an RNA type of octanucleotide containing A, G, C, and U in a 1:1:1:1 ratio. Treatment with enzymes (consult Table 10.2 if you wish) produces the following compounds, among others:

    a. Phosphodiesterase I: pU

    b. Phosphodiesterase II: pAp

    c. Ribonuclease T_1: pApGp and ApU

    d. A ribonuclease of the d type and no other specificity: UpGpAp

  What is the nucleotide sequence? *Note*: p is phosphate; all nucleotides are written in the 5′ and 3′ direction.

BIBLIOGRAPHY

Alberts B, Bray D, Lewis J, et al. Molecular Biology of the Cell, 2nd ed. New York: Garland, 1989.

Guschlbauer W. Nucleic Acid Structure. New York: Springer-Verlag, 1976.

Mainwaring WIP, Paris JH, Pickering JD, Mann NH. Nucleic Acid Biochemistry and Molecular Biology. Oxford: Blackwell Scientific, 1982.

Saenger W. Principles of Nucleic Acid Structure. New York: Springer-Verlag, 1984.

11

DNA and RNA Information Flow

After completing this chapter, the student should

1. Understand the Messelson-Stahl experiment and its interpretation to verify semiconservative DNA replication.
2. Know the roles of DNA polymerase I, II, III, and eukaryotic DNA polymerases, the roles of primers, helicases, single-stranded binding proteins (SSB), topoisomerases (gyrase), ligases, primase, and RNA polymerases, and the differences between the leading and lagging strands of DNA.
3. Know the main inhibitors of DNA synthesis and their modes of action.
4. Know the chief mechanisms for DNA proofreading.
5. Know the details of the four steps in transcription (binding of polymerase, initiation, elongation, and termination).
6. Be able to discuss the posttranscriptional modification and processing of RNAs (rRNA, mRNA, and tRNA).
7. Know some of the inhibitors of RNA synthesis and how they function.

11.1 INTRODUCTION

DNA is the genetic material in all prokaryotic and eukaryotic organisms. It may be either DNA or RNA in viruses. The genetic material must fulfill certain basic requirements:

1. It must contain the information for cell structure, function, and reproduction.
2. It must have chemical and physical stability, so that significant information is not lost.
3. It must be replicated with a high degree of fidelity.
4. It must be capable of limited variation to provide a basis for the evolutionary process.

Both DNA and RNA meet these requirements, although RNA is not as suitable because it lacks the redundancy associated with a double helix as well as the inherent chemical and physical stability of DNA.

Although DNA was first isolated by Miescher in 1869, it was not until much later that DNA was accepted as the genetic material of all prokaryotic and eukaryotic organisms. Even the persuasive experiments of Avery, Macleod, and McCarty (1944) were not generally accepted as proof that DNA was the genetic material. They determined that DNA extracted from an encapsulated (smooth) strain of *Pneumococcus* transformed an unencapsulated (rough) strain into encapsulated cells. The smooth cells produced by this transformation propagated indefinitely as a smooth strain without further exposure to DNA. The DNA preparations from the smooth strain had induced a specific heritable function and had initiated its own replication, functions usually attributable to genes. The DNA preparations employed were shown to be free of protein and their activity destroyed by treatment with deoxyribonuclease but not destroyed by treatment with ribonuclease.

Additional support for DNA as the bearer of genetic information came from studies by Hershey and Chase (1952) in the replication of DNA-containing bacteriophages. Using virus particles isotopically labeled in either the viral DNA or in the viral protein, it was shown that the viral DNA entered the host cell (*Escherichia coli*), whereas the viral protein did not. Later experiments demonstrated that viral DNA alone was infectious and led to the formation of mature infectious virus particles of the appropriate genotype. The DNA contained *all* the information required for the synthesis of progeny phage particles.

One of the more attractive features of the DNA model proposed by Watson and Crick was the proposal that the replication of DNA occurred by separation of the two complementary chains followed by the formation of a new complementary chain on each of the parental chains to yield two daughter duplex molecules, each containing one parental chain. This mechanism is termed *semiconservative replication*, because one strand of the parental DNA is conserved in each daughter duplex molecule. Other mechanisms were possible, such as conservative, in which new double-stranded DNA molecules are formed directly and the parent molecule is left intact, and dispersive, in which chains fragment and the parental fragments combine with newly formed fragments to form new daughter molecules containing sections of old and sections of new DNA.

That DNA was replicated by the semiconservative mechanism was confirmed in vivo at the molecular level by Messelson and Stahl. They grew the bacterium *E. coli* for several generations in a medium containing ^{15}N-ammonium chloride as the single source of nitrogen. It is possible by density gradient centrifugation in cesium chloride to separate ^{15}N-DNA (heavy) from ^{14}N-DNA (light) and from DNA of intermediate densities. Fully ^{15}N-labeled cells were transferred to a medium containing ^{14}N-ammonium chloride, and the DNA was isolated and examined at various generation times. After one generation, there was single band of DNA halfway between those of ^{14}N-DNA and ^{15}N-DNA. After two generations, there were equal amounts of two bands, one of which was hybrid DNA (^{14}N/^{15}N-DNA) and the other ^{14}N-DNA. For the conservative model to be correct, some heavy DNA must be present at each generation and all new DNA must have normal density with no hybrid DNA ever being formed. The semiconservative model predicts at generation 1 that *all* DNA molecules have one normal and one heavy strand and after two generations equal amounts of hybrid and ^{14}N-DNA and no ^{15}N-DNA (Figure 11.1).

The semiconservative replication of DNA at the chromosomal level was shown by J. H. Taylor and coworkers. Using autoradiography and bean seedling root cells in tissue culture, they showed that, after a part of a cycle of duplication with [^{3}H]thymidine (a selective label for DNA), the two chromosomes, descended from an original unlabeled chromosome, were both labeled. Following an additional duplication in the absence of labeled thymidine, the labeled chromosome yielded one labeled and one unlabeled descendant, as predicted by the semiconservative mechanism.

DNA is not a direct template for protein synthesis. A limited segment of *one* of the DNA strands is first *transcribed* into a complementary strand of messenger RNA (mRNA). The mRNA sequence is then *translated* into the amino acid sequence of the protein by a complex, called a *ribosome*. Each amino acid to be used for protein synthesis is attached by a specific synthetase enzyme to a specific transfer RNA (tRNA; Figure 10.27) to form an aminoacyl-tRNA, which recognizes by base pairing of its *anticodon* to a set of three nucleotides in mRNA, a *codon*. The codons or triplets in mRNA are read from one end to the other according to a virtually universal genetic code; the exceptions are mitochondria and ciliated protozoa. Although there are similarities in the basic mechanism of protein synthesis in eukaryotes and prokaryotes, there are significant differences between them. These include larger ribosomes in eukaryotes, difference in the initiator tRNA, differences in the nature and number of start signals, more initiation factors in eukaryotes, and differences in elongation and termination factors.

The basic DNA replication mechanism is identical for prokaryotes and eukaryotes in that an asymmetric replication fork and a RNA primer are in-

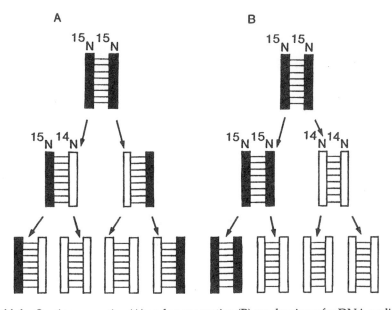

Figure 11.1 Semiconservative (A) and conservative (B) mechanisms for DNA replication.

volved. Because eukaryotic DNA is replicated as chromatin, not as bare DNA, the process and its control are more complicated. It is now clear that only a fraction of the eukaryotic DNA codes for proteins and as much as 90–95% is involved in other functions, such as control of expression of genes in differentiated tissue and the organization of eukaryotic genomes. Whereas genes in prokaryotic DNA are continuous and often overlapping, eukaryotic genes do not overlap and, with few exceptions, the coding sequences (called *exons* for for expressed regions) are interrupted by noncoding intervening sequences called *introns*. These intron sequences are excised from each RNA transcript, and the coding RNA sequences on either side of an intron sequence are joined to form a mRNA molecule that is colinear with its polypeptide product. This is known as *RNA splicing*.

In the discussion to follow, we consider many of the intimate details of these complex processes and some aspects of their regulation.

11.2 DNA REPLICATION AND PROOFREADING

Enzymatic replication of DNA is a complex process and requires the cooperation of some 20 or more proteins. Arthur Kornberg and his colleagues first discovered an enzyme in *E. coli* that catalyzed the polymerization of deoxyribonucleotides under the direction of a DNA template. This enzyme, *DNA polymerase I* (Pol I), is now known to be only one of a group of similar enzymes that can copy DNA or RNA templates or both. Three distinct enzymes (Pol I, Pol II, and Pol III) have been isolated from bacterial cells (Table 11.1). These enzymes catalyze the stepwise addition of deoxyribonucleotide residues to the free 3'-hydroxyl end of a preexisting DNA or RNA primer strand; thus the enzymatic elongation proceeds in the $5' \rightarrow 3'$ direction. The overall reaction is

$$(\text{Deoxyribonucleotide})_n\text{-3'-OH} + \text{dNTP} \xrightarrow{\text{Pol I, Mg}^{2+}}$$
$$(\text{deoxyribonucleotide})_{n+1}\text{-3'-OH} + \text{PP}_i \qquad (11.1)$$

in which dNTP represents any deoxyribonucleotide-5'-triphosphate (dATP, dGTP, dCTP, and dTTP) and PP_i represents pyrophosphate cleaved from the dNTP.

Table 11.1   Properties of *Escherichia coli* DNA Polymerases

Property	Pol I	Pol II[a]	Pol III holoenzyme
Molecules per cell	400	100	15
Turnover number[b]	$\leq$50	30	9000
Molecular weight[c]	110 kD	120 kD	760 kD[d]
$3' \rightarrow 5'$-exonuclease	+	+	+
$5' \rightarrow 3'$-exonuclease	+	−	+

[a]Role unknown; mutant cells lacking this enzyme appear to grow normally.
[b]A $5' \rightarrow 3'$ polymerizing activity; nucleotides polymerized/minute/molecule of enzyme at 37°C.
[c]Kilodaltons.
[d]Dimer.

Hydrolysis of PP_i ensures that the reaction proceeds in the direction of synthesis. The reaction requires for the synthesis of DNA all four deoxyribonucleotide-5'-triphosphates, Mg^{2+}, and a DNA template with a 3'-OH primer, which can be single-stranded or duplex DNA with a single-strand nick or break in the sugar-phosphate backbone. The *template* is the polynucleotide strand that is copied according to the Watson-Crick base pairing rules, and the *primer* is the poly-nucleotide strand containing a 3'-hydroxy terminus from which the DNA chain is covalently extended. Pol I catalyzes some 20 polymerization steps before disso-ciating from the DNA template and is termed a *moderately processive* enzyme. The enzyme contains a single active polymerizing site that can bind any of the four dNTPs, the one selected depending on the base in the template strand.

Pol I is also a 3' → 5'-exonuclease, removing only nucleotides that are not part of double helix and that have a free 3'-hydroxyl terminus. It removes mismatched residues and thus performs a *proofreading* or *editing* function. Af-ter removal of a mismatched base, exonuclease activity ceases and polymeriz-ing activity is restarted. This editing activity enhances the fidelity of DNA replication by rechecking the correctness of base pairing before proceeding with polymerization.

Pol I also has 5' → 3'-exonuclease activity that is different from the 3' → 5'-exonuclease action. It hydrolyzes DNA from the 5' end of a chain, cleaving a bond in the double-helical region at the terminal phosphodiester bond or a bond several residues distant from the 5' terminus. Either deoxy- or ribonucleotides can be removed. In fact, the main function of the 5' → 3' exonuclease activity may be to remove ribonucleotide primers (p. 308). This activity can also excise thymine dimers formed by exposure to ultraviolet (UV) light. The three Pol I enzymatic activities are located at distinct sites (*domains*).

The complementary actions of these mechanisms, as well as others not discussed, ensure the stability of genetic information by continuously scanning the DNA to remove and replace damaged and mismatched nucleotides. Al-though Pol I has essential roles in the replication process and in DNA repair, it is not the enzyme that replicates most of the DNA in *E. coli*. Pol III performs this function. Pol III is a very complex enzyme, and its most active form, the *Pol III holoenzyme*, is composed of at least seven different proteins (Θ, α, and ϵ and the catalytic core β, γ, δ and π) in a dimeric structure. It has high *processivity*, catalyzing the addition of several thousands of nucleotides before dissociating from the template, and a high turnover number, 9000 versus $\leq$ 50 for Pol I. Pol III shares with Pol I requirements for a primer and a template and possesses 3' → 5'-exonuclease activity that plays the major editing function in DNA replica-tion. The role of the 5' → 3'-exonuclease activity is unknown.

All known DNA polymerases (RNA polymerases also) are capable of chain elongation only in the 5' → 3' direction. At low resolution in autoradiographic experiments, the apparent direction of DNA replication was 5' → 3' for one daughter strand and 3' → 5' for the other (Figure 11.2). It was found subse-quently that a significant amount of newly synthesized DNA existed as transient fragments in the vicinity of the replication fork and were later attached to one another to generate a continuous strand. These *precursors* or *Okazaki fragments* are units of about a thousand nucleotides in *E. coli* and about 150 nucleotides long in eukaryotes. The strand formed from Okazaki fragments is the *lagging* strand. It

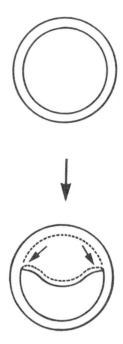

Figure 11.2 Apparent direction of DNA replication at low resolution.

is made overall in the 3′ → 5′ direction, but each fragment is synthesized in the conventional 5′ → 3′ direction (Figure 11.3). As replication proceeds, the fragments are covalently joined by DNA ligase to complete the lagging strand.

The leading strand is synthesized continuously in the direction of unwinding and precedes the lagging strand. Because the modes of synthesis differ for the two strands, the Y-shaped replication fork is *asymmetric*.

DNA replication in *E. coli* starts with the unwinding of the chromosome at a specific *origin site* (oriC) and proceeds sequentially in opposite directions. There are two replication forks, one moving clockwise and the other moving counter-clockwise. Because the bacterial genome is small, two replication forks are sufficient to duplicate the DNA for each cell generation. Eukaryotic DNA, because of its large size, requires thousands of replication forks per DNA molecule. The oriC locus consists of a unique sequence of 245 base pairs that is recognized by an enzyme responsible for the unwinding of the template DNA and the synthesis of a primer to initiate the bidirectional replication. Table 11.2 lists some of the DNA replication proteins in *E. coli* and their functions, when known.

Separation and subsequent unwinding of duplex DNA are required to produce the single-stranded DNA (ssDNA) template required for DNA replication by a DNA polymerase. Separation of the strands is accomplished by a class of specific proteins called *helicases* that disrupt the hydrogen bonds holding the two duplex strands together. Unwinding, in a strict sense, is accomplished by the action of topoisomerases, discussed later. The dissolution of the hydrogen bonds by a helicase is coupled to the hydrolysis of a bound nucleoside-5′-phosphate. How the hydrolysis energy is utilized is unclear, but it seems to propel the unidirectional translocation of the helicase along ssDNA. It is likely

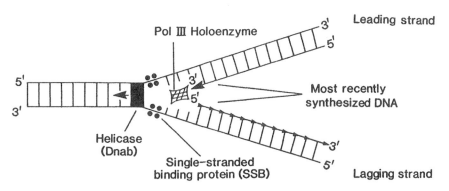

Figure 11.3 Continuous synthesis of leading strand and discontinuous synthesis of lagging strand in the 5′ → 3′ direction. Joining the fragments gives the appearance of overall growth of the lagging strand in the 3′ → 5′ direction.

Table 11.2 *Escherichia coli* DNA Replication Proteins

Protein	Function
DNA A	Recognizes and binds specifically at replication origin for leading strand
Dna B	Primary helicase lagging strand
Dna C	Required for loading Dna B at origin
Primase	RNA primer synthesis
SSB	Single-stranded binding protein (helix destabilizing)
Pol III holoenzyme	Progressive chain elongation
Pol I	Gap filling, primer excision
Topoisomerase I	Removes negative supercoils
Topoisomerase II	Forms negative supercoils, ATP dependent
Ligase	Connects Okazaki pieces, ATP dependent
Rep protein	Helicase on leading strand?

that the hydrolysis of ATP could produce a cyclic change in shape of the helicase and enable it to perform mechanical work. In *E. coli*, the nature of the helicase is complicated by the fact that at least eight DNA helicases are involved in some aspect of DNA metabolism, as well as other enzymes acting on RNA duplexes and DNA-RNA hybrids. It appears, however, that *DNA binding protein* (Dna B, Table 11.2 and Figure 11.3) is the major and perhaps only helicase employed by *E. coli*. It is absolutely required for initiation of replication from the origin of replication and propagates the replication fork in the 5′ → 3′ direction. Dna B is a known component of the *primosome* (see later) that synthesizes primers on the lagging strand. Once the strands have been separated, the single-stranded regions are stabilized by specific single-stranded binding proteins (SSB). The SSB exists as a tetramer, and the binding of one SSB tetramer facilitates the binding of another to an adjacent region of single-stranded DNA. This is called *cooperative binding*. Regions of single-stranded DNA covered with SSB are rigid and semi-extended, an appropriate configuration for its role as a template for the initiation and elongation of a complementary DNA strand. As the helicase moves in ad-vance of the replication fork, the SSBs move on and off the DNA and are recycled for use on another site. The unwinding during replication could lead to positive supercoiling (overwinding) of the circular DNA and cessation of unwinding. This is prevented by the action of *DNA gyrase*, a type II DNA topoisomerase that introduces negative supercoils at the expense of ATP. Type II topoisomerase makes a transient double-strand break in the DNA double helix through which a second DNA double helix can pass before resealing (Figure 10.28).

Despite that the template strands have been transiently separated and unwound by the helicase and topoisomerase and stabilized by SSB proteins, DNA synthesis cannot proceed until a primer with a 3' group is formed (Figure 11.4). This is accomplished on the lagging strand by a specific class of enzymes called *primases*. Primase forms a short stretch (usually three to five ribonucleotides) of RNA complementary to specific sites along the lagging strand DNA template. To function effectively, primase must be complexed with various other proteins (Table 11.2) to form a *primosome*, which moves processively in the 5' → 3' direction on the lagging strand template to prime for the repeated initiation of the Okazaki fragments. The components of the primosome work cooperatively in some manner to bring about movement of this complex along the DNA, displace SSBs, recognize start loci, and synthesize RNA.

The mechanism for the initiation of the leading strand is not clearly understood. An RNA polymerase must transcribe origin DNA sequences into short RNA chains. RNA polymerase, but not primase, is inhibited by the antibiotic

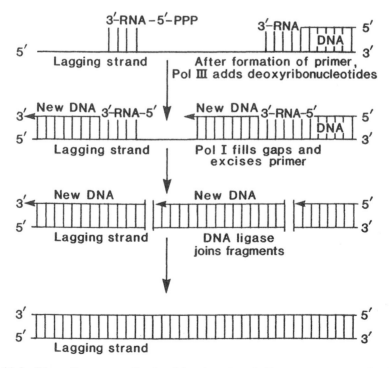

Figure 11.4 Discontinuous synthesis of lagging strand. Fragments are synthesized in the 5' → 3' direction, and overall chain growth is in the 3' → 5' direction.

rifampicin. Because initiation of leading strand synthesis is inhibited by this antibiotic in *E. coli*, RNA polymerase is presumed to be the enzyme involved in priming leading strand synthesis. In some instances, these RNA chains may function as a primer for leading strands after unnecessary regions are removed by the enzyme RNase H that specifically removes the RNA strand of DNA-RNA hybrid molecules. In other cases, the apparent function of the RNA transcript may be to separate the two DNA strands at the origin to allow the binding of a primosome that forms the primer. DnaA protein is absolutely required for the initiation of leading strands.

The leading strand is synthesized continuously in the direction of unwinding by the Pol III holoenzyme. It has been proposed that more or less simultaneous synthesis of both the leading and lagging strands occurs at the replication fork. A dimeric DNA Pol III holoenzyme, a primosome, a helicase, and replication proteins may form a complex termed a *replisome*. Simultaneous synthesis of both strands could occur by the action of a replisome if the DNA of the lagging strand template is looped backward so that it is in the same orientation as the leading strand template during polymerization. The lagging strand template would pass through the polymerase site in one subunit of the dimeric Pol III holoenzyme in the same direction as the leading strand template in the other polymerase subunit. After the addition of about 1000 nucleotides, the polymerase would release the lagging strand template to allow the formation of a new loop. Primase would synthesize a short RNA primer, and the process would repeat. Leading strand synthesis would not be too far ahead of lagging strand synthesis. The gaps between fragments on the lagging strand are filled by Pol I, which also excises with its $5' \rightarrow 3'$-exonuclease action the RNA primer that lies ahead. DNA ligase joins the fragments to produce an intact strand. An energy source, which is NAD^+ in bacteria and ATP in bacteriophages and mammals, is required. This is shown schematically in Figure 11.5.

In *E. coli*, termination of replication occurs when the two replication forks, one moving clockwise and one moving counterclockwise, meet opposite the origin site.

Although DNA replication is basically similar in prokaryotes and eukaryotes, the size and organization of the eukaryotic DNA introduce additional complexities into an already complex process. There is need for multiple origins of replication operating simultaneously for the DNA doubling to take place in a reasonable length of time (Figure 11.6). Nucleosomes must be disassembled in front of the replication and the newly formed DNA reassembled into nucleosomes with the newly formed histone octamers (Chapter 10). There are also some differences in the enzymes involved.

There are four species of DNA polymerases in eukaryotes, designated Polα, Polβ, Polγ, and Polδ. All require a template and a primer with a 3'-OH group. Polα is composed of four distinct subunits and is the only one that can use a RNA primer. One of its subunits constitutes a primase enzyme capable of synthesizing short RNA transcripts that can serve as primers for DNA chain elongation by a catalytic subunit. Polα is a moderately *processive* enzyme (the capacity to remain associated with the template strand), adding about 100 nucleotides per binding event. Its activity correlates with cellular proliferation, being high when there is rapid cell division and dropping to a low level in

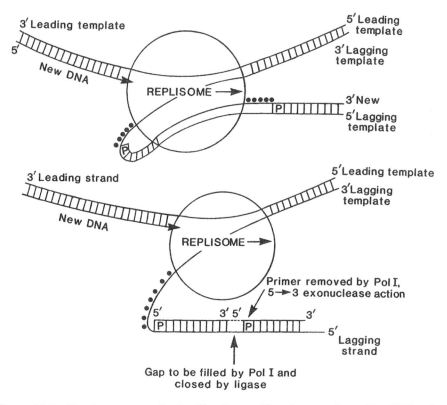

Figure 11.5 Simultaneous synthesis of leading and lagging templates. P = RNA primer; SSB = single-stranded binding protein.

quiescent cells. It is clear that Polα has a direct role in chromosomal DNA synthesis. However, recent experiments with a mammalian cell-free system and the chromosome of simian virus 40 (SV40) suggests that Polδ may be the polymerase for the leading strand, whereas Polα may be the polymerase for the lagging strand. This possibility is attractive because the lagging strand polymerase (Polα) would require moderate processivity and would benefit from the associated primase activity. On the other hand, the leading strand polymerase (Polα) with high processivity would not require an associated primase activity.

Polα has a cryptic 3' → 5'-exonuclease that is revealed only upon dissociation of its four subunits. This proofreading ability probably contributes to the fidelity of DNA replication. Polδ also has proofreading 3' → 5'-exonuclease activity and can carry out editing functions similar to that of the prokaryotic enzymes.

Polβ, like Polα and Polδ is also located in the nucleus and is probably involved in DNA repair. Polγ is localized in mitochondria, and although there is no direct evidence, it is thought to be responsible for the replication of that organelle's DNA. Polδ has 3' → 5' proofreading exonuclease action that is highly selective for base mismatches.

Human mitochondrial DNA (mtDNA), a circular supercoiled DNA of about 16,469 base pairs, codes for 13 proteins, 22 tRNAs, and 2 ribosomal RNAs (rRNAs) using a code slightly different from the virtually universal code (page

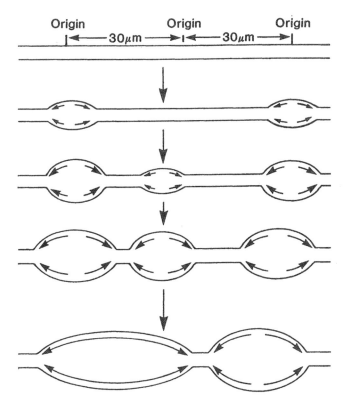

Figure 11.6 Multiple origin of replication forks in eukaryotic DNA replication. Termination of replication occurs where two growth forks come together.

340). In mammals, mtDNA is maternally inherited; this is probably a result of the egg cell contributing much more cytoplasm to the zygote than to the sperm.

There are two known topoisomerases, type II (discussed earlier) and type I. Type I makes a reversible *single-stranded break* that allows the two ends of the DNA double helix to rotate relative to each other and relax negatively supercoiled DNA. Resealing is rapid, and no additional energy is required because the covalent DNA-enzyme linkage retains the energy of the broken phosphodiester bond. Both of these appear to function in SV40 DNA replication. Type I acts as a swivel to remove superhelical tension that could prevent the unwinding of the parental strands as the replication fork advances. Type II acts to separate the multiply intertwined circular daughter molecules into separate unlinked molecules. This is referred to as *decatenation*. Yeast also appears to use the same strategies during replication and segregation of its chromosomes.

Inhibitors of DNA replication can be classified in three general categories:

1. Inhibitors that interact directly with DNA
2. Inhibitors that interact with enzymes involved in DNA synthesis
3. Inhibitors of deoxyribonucleotide synthesis

In the first category are such compounds as actinomycin, acridine, and ethidium that bind between the stacked bases of the DNA duplex, disrupting the normal structure of the DNA and producing some unwinding. This inhibits the DNA from serving as a template for both replication and transcription.

There are several compounds in the second category that act selectively on various DNA polymerases. For example, DNA polymerase γ is much more sensitive to 2′,3′-dideoxythymidine (which lacks a 3′-OH group of the sugar) than is DNA polymerase α, whereas DNA polymerase α is sensitive to N-ethylmaleimide, γ less so, and β is totally resistant. Aphidicolin is a highly specific inhibitor for DNA polymerases α and δ, and arylhydrazinopyrimidines are highly specific for Pol III. The nucleotide analog butyl-phenyl-dGTP is a strong inhibitor of Polα and weakly active against Polδ.

A large number of compounds in category 3 act at different sites in the pathways for purine and pyrimidine biosynthesis. These compounds are very toxic for rapidly growing tumors and bacteria, making them useful in cancer chemotherapy and treatment of bacterial infections. 6-Mercaptopurine is a potent inhibitor of purine biosynthesis, and 5-fluorouracil inhibits thymidylate synthesis. Some compounds, such as hydroxyurea and sulfonamides, inhibit the synthesis of both purine and pyrimidine nucleotides. These are only a few of the many compounds useful in treating cancer and infectious diseases (see Chapter 10).

Most if not all of these compounds are highly toxic to rapidly growing cells, in which continuous nucleic acid synthesis is required, and can severely damage normally replicating cells, such as those in the bone marrow and intestinal tract.

11.3 RNA TRANSCRIPTION

The *central dogma*, proposed by Crick in 1956, summarizes the flow of genetic information in normal cells:

$$\text{Replication } \overset{\frown}{\text{DNA}} \xrightarrow{\text{transcription}} \text{RNA} \xrightarrow{\text{translation}} \text{protein}$$

Proteins never serve as templates for RNA. However, RNA chains can in rare circumstances reverse the flow of information from RNA to DNA. An example of this is the infecting RNA of retroviruses that serves as a template for the synthesis of a single-stranded complementary DNA (cDNA) chain that functions as a template for a complementary DNA chain. The resulting double-stranded DNA then acts as a template for the synthesis of the original viral RNA chain. The virus-specific enzyme, *reverse transcriptase*, catalyzes the synthesis of DNA on the RNA template. Little if any reverse transcriptase activity is present in normal cells, so that very little DNA is formed on RNA templates.

In prokaryotic cells, with the exception of DNA primers, all types of RNA are transcribed by a single enzyme, a DNA-dependent *RNA polymerase*. This RNA polymerase has strict requirements for all four nucleotide-5′-triphosphates, a divalent cation, and a DNA template. Unlike DNA polymerase, there is no requirement for a primer. Initiation and elongation of RNA is in the 5′ → 3′ direction and the product is complementary to one of the two DNA strands, the template strand that runs in the 3′ → 5′ direction. The reaction may be formulated similarly to that catalyzed by DNA polymerases:

$$NTP + (NMP)_n \, RNA \overset{Mg^{2+}}{\rightleftharpoons} (NMP)_{n+1} \, RNA + PP_i \qquad (11.2)$$

As with DNA polymerases, subsequent hydrolysis of PP_i to $2P_i$ ensures that the reaction proceeds in the direction of synthesis.

E. coli RNA polymerase holoenzyme has a molecular weight of about 450,000 and contains *five different* polypeptide chains ($\alpha_2\beta$, $\beta\beta'$, ω, σ) and two zinc atoms, one associated with the β' and the other with σ polypeptides. The β subunit is the catalytic site for RNA polymerization, the β' subunit the site for DNA binding, and the σ subunit the site for promoter recognition and initiation. The functions of the α and ω subunits are not known.

Eukaryotic cells contain at least four different DNA-dependent RNA polymerases. Their localization, cellular transcripts, and susceptibility to the cyclic octapeptide α-amanitin (derived from poisonous mushrooms) are shown in Table 11.3. α-Amanitin blocks the elongation phase of RNA synthesis. Although the structures of these enzymes are much more complex than that of the prokaryotic RNA polymerase, the basic mechanism is very similar to that of the prokaryotic enzyme.

The antibiotic rifamycin and a semisynthetic derivative, rifampicin, specifically inhibit the initiation of RNA synthesis by interfering with the formation of the first phosphodiester bond of the RNA chain. The elongation of chains already being synthesized is unaffected.

The process of transcription involves four steps: binding of polymerase, initiation, elongation, and termination and release. We consider first the simpler and better understood prokaryotic system.

Binding of RNA polymerase occurs at specific sites, *promoters*, which are specific DNA sequences that occur with great regularity, and are called *conserved* or *consensus* sequences. Two consensus sequences of six nucleotides occur about -10 base pairs (Pribnow box) and -35 base pairs upstream of the initiation site (the first nucleotide copied into RNA), which is defined as 1. The consensus sequence at position -10 is $T_{89}A_{81}T_{50}A_{65}A_{65}T_{100}$ and that at position -35 is $T_{85}T_{83}G_{81}A_{61}C_{69}A_{52}$, the subscripts showing the percentage frequency with which each nucleotide was found at that specific position in a large number of promoters. The optimum distance between the two consensus sequences is highly conserved at 17 nucleotides, the exact sequence being unimportant. Strong promoters match the consensus sequences very closely, whereas weaker promoters differ from the consensus sequences. RNA polymerase binds first to the RNA

Table 11.3 Eukaryotic DNA-Dependent RNA polymerases[a]

Type	Location	RNAs transcribed	Inhibition by α-amanitin
I(A)	Nucleolus	Pre-rRNA (18, 5.8, 28 S)	Resistant
II(B)	Nucleoplasm	Pre-mRNA, hnRNA	Sensitive
III(C)	Nucleoplasm	Pre-tRNA, 5 S rRNA	Sensitive to high concentrations
Mitochondrial	Mitochondria	Mitochondrial	Resistant

[a]rRNA = ribosomal RNA; mRNA = messenger RNA; hnRNA = heterogeneous nuclear RNA; tRNA = transfer RNA.

promoter at the -35 region to form a *closed complex,* the DNA remaining double helical or unmelted. This enzyme binding covers about 60 base pairs from -40 to 20 and includes the Pribnow box. The next step involves a conformational change in the polymerase and an unwinding (melting) of about 10 base pairs from positions -9 to 2 to form an *open complex,* a very stable structure. Once the complex has formed, RNA synthesis can be initiated (Figure 11.7).

The initiation site binds only purine nucleoside triphosphates, usually ATP. Thymine is therefore the first DNA base usually transcribed. A second nucleoside triphosphate is selected by virtue of its ability to form hydrogen bonds with the next base in the DNA strand. The two nucleotides are joined into a phosphodiester bond by a nucleophilic attack of the 3'-hydroxyl group of the initiating nucleoside triphosphate on the phosphorus atom of the second NTP with the release of inorganic pyrophosphate. *Elongation* proceeds by the successive binding of the NTP complementary to the next base in the DNA template strand. After some 8–10 nucleotides have added to the elongating chain, the σ-subunit dissociates from the holoenzymes to yield what is termed the core polymerase. The core polymerase continues the elongation until a termination signal is reached. The released σ subunit can bind to free core polymerase to re-form the holoenzyme that is able to bind to the promoter and initiate a new RNA chain.

Termination of RNA synthesis occurs at specific sites along the DNA template. There are two modes of termination events: those that require a termination protein, the ρ factor, and those that depend only on the transcription of regions of DNA containing stop signals.

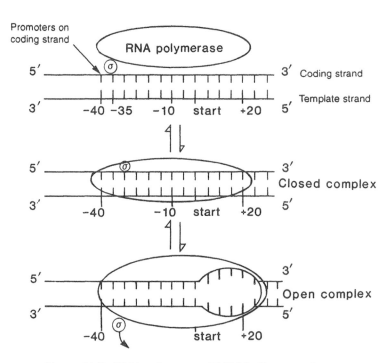

Figure 11.7 RNA polymerase DNA binding complexes.

ρ-Independent terminators are better characterized and involve a consensus type of sequence. This sequence is a GC-rich *palindrome* (inverted repeat) that precedes a sequence of six to eight U residues in the RNA chain. The transcribed RNA chain can form a stem and loop structure (Figure 11.8) preceding the U sequence. Such a structure is believed to stop elongation and expel the RNA and the polymerase.

The second type of terminator lacks the U region and requires the ρ termination factor for RNA chain release. The ρ factor is a hexamer of 45 kD subunits that binds a stretch of 72 nucleotides of single-stranded RNA. The ρ factor hydrolyzes ribonucleoside triphosphates to nucleoside diphosphates in the presence of single-stranded RNA and moves unidirectionally along nascent mRNA toward the transcription bubble and breaks the RNA-DNA hybrid, pulling away the RNA.

Prokaryotic ribosomes attach to the nascent mRNA while it is still being transcribed. Because transcription and translation are coupled, prokaryotic mRNAs undergo little modification and processing before being used as templates for protein synthesis. Prokaryotic tRNA and rRNA are transcribed in units larger than those ultimately used and must be processed to generate the functional molecules. The processing of these and the eukaryotic primary transcripts, almost all of which require modification, is discussed in a later section.

Unlike prokaryotes, eukaryotes have three types of nuclear RNA polymerases (Table 11.3), each of which is responsible for the transcription of different classes of genes.

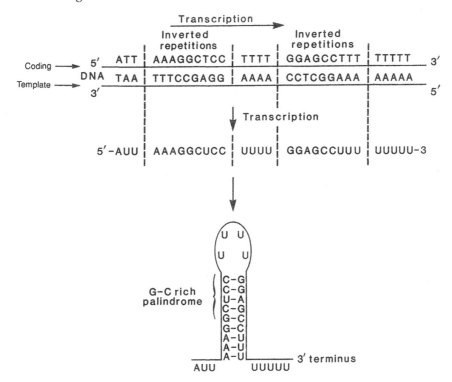

Figure 11.8 Sequence of ρ-independent terminator and terminated RNA.

RNA polymerase I produces a primary RNA transcript (45 S RNA) containing three rRNA sequences in order from the 5′ terminus, a 28, a 5.8, and a 2.8 S ribosomal RNA. The three genes are separated by spacer regions of varying length. Core promoters have been defined about −150 base pairs upstream and between positions −35 and 9. The 45 S primary transcript is subsequently processed to yield the functional RNA species (see later). In mice, there appears to be a termination site some 500 base pairs downstream of the 3′ end of the gene. Initiation and termination appear to be highly variable between different species, so that no clear understanding of the processes is currently available.

RNA polymerase II requires promoters on the 5′ side of the transcription start site. There is a TATA box (Hogness box), like the Pribnow box in prokaryotes, at around −25 with the consensus

$$T_{85}A_{99}T_{93}A_{83}^{T_{31}}A_{63}A_{83}^{T_{33}}A_{50}$$

Additional promoters are located between −40 and −110. Most of these contain a CAAT box [5′GG(C, T)CCA(A, T)CT³′] and some a GC box (⁵′GGGCG³′, or CCGCCC). Very little is known about eukaryotic mRNA termination. It apparently occurs hundreds or even thousands of nucleotides downstream. The 3′ ends of mRNA are produced mainly by processing (see later).

The promoters for RNA polymerase III have been clearly proven to be internal on the template. In one instance the 5 S gene promoter lies between 45 and 83, whereas in tRNA genes it is split into two separate locations, one between 8 and 30 and a second between 51 and 72. Termination in 5 S genes is caused by a sequence of four A residues situated between two GC-rich regions. tRNA precursors are converted into mature tRNAs by a series of alterations (see later).

11.4 POSTTRANSCRIPTIONAL MODIFICATION AND PROCESSING OF RNA

Nearly all eukaryotic and some prokaryotic primary RNA transcripts require a number of modifications before they can carry out their functions. Among others, these include 3′- and 5′-terminal additions, base and sugar modifications, changes in tertiary conformations, and specific exo- and endonucleolytic cleavages, with splicing of pieces. The extent and type of processing are different for each type of RNA. In prokaryotes, most proteins are encoded by a single uninterrupted DNA sequence that is copied without alteration to yield a mRNA. It was found in the late 1970s that in most eukaryotic genes the coding sequences (*exons*) are interrupted by noncoding sequences (*introns*). In this case the entire gene DNA, including introns and exons, is transcribed into a large DNA molecule, the *primary transcript*. Before leaving the nucleus, all of the introns are removed by RNA-processing enzymes, the exons assembled linearly, to produce shortened RNA molecules. The RNA moves to the cytoplasm as a mRNA that specifies the synthesis of a specified protein. Introns range in size from some 80 to 1000 nucleotides. Only the intron nucleotide sequences at the ends of introns are highly conserved and cannot be altered without affecting the splicing process that removes the intron from the primary RNA transcript. This is critical because an error in even one nucleotide would shift the reading frame in the mRNA and disrupt its message (see later).

11.4.1 Ribosomal RNA

In both prokaryotes and eukaryotes, the primary transcript is considerably larger than the ultimate molecule.

In both eukaryotic and prokaryotic cells, large precursors to rRNA are transcribed and processed to produce the mature rRNAs. Processing involves methylation of bases and/or ribose and endolytic cleavage to cut out unwanted sequences. The eukaryotic products are the 18, 5.8, and 28 S rRNAs. In prokaryotes, the final products are the 16 S rRNA, a spacer region that includes one or two tRNAs, the 23 S rRNA, and the 5 S rRNA and, in some instances, one or two additional tRNAs.

11.4.2 Messenger RNA

Prokaryotic mRNAs function in translation with no processing, whereas a very complex process is used by eukaryotes to produce a mature, functional mRNA.

Because of the wide range of sizes, all RNA polymerase II transcripts were called *heterogeneous* nuclear RNA (hnRNA). Some 20% of these molecules leave the nucleus as mRNA molecules. Before their selective transport to the cytoplasm, however, they undergo covalent modification. Shortly after initiation of mRNA synthesis, a guanosine residue is attached at the 5' terminus in an unusual 5',5' $\rightarrow$ triphosphate linkage. The N-7 of the terminal guanine is then methylated by *S*-adenosylmethionine. This unit, 7MeG-5'PPP-5'G or A-3'-P, is called a *cap*. Occasionally the ribose moieties on adjacent nucleotides are also methylated at the 2'-OH positions. These caps remain during subsequent processing. Caps facilitate binding to ribosomes, stabilize mRNAs by protecting their 5' ends from nucleases and phosphatases, and are important for subsequent splicing reactions. rRNA and tRNA are not capped.

Most eukaryotic mRNAs contain a long (up to 250 A residues) polyadenylate [poly(A)] tail at the 3' end. The poly(A) tail is not coded by the RNA template but is added to the mRNA before leaving the nucleus. Because some effective eukaryotic mRNAs do not contain poly(A) (for example, those mRNAs encoding histones), the role of the 3' poly(A) tail is unclear. The primary nuclear transcripts are much larger than the cytoplasmic mRNAs and contain introns (non-coding regions). Intron sequences must be excised and the exons joined to each other to produce a mRNA colinear with its polypeptide product. This is accomplished in general by RNA splicing in which introns are removed by endonucleolytic enzymes and the exons are joined or spliced together. Figure 11.9 is a schematic representation of the formation of the ovalbumin mRNA. Splicing is carried out by *spliceosomes*, which are large (60 S) nucleoprotein complexes containing several kinds of small nuclear ribonuclear particles (snRNPs) and a mRNA precursor. Individual roles have been defined for some of these snRNPs (Table 11.4). The individual snRNPs apparently recognize specific nucleic acid sequences in the mRNA precursor by RNA-RNA base pairing. The sites are specified by sequences at the ends of introns, and the joining of exons is accomplished by two transesterification reac-

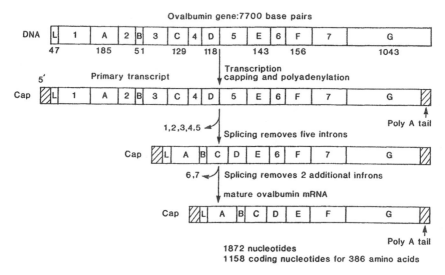

Figure 11.9   Maturation of ovalbumin mRNA. L and A–G = exons; 1–7 = introns.

Table 11.4   Small Nuclear Ribonucleoprotein
Particles (snRNP) in Splicing of mRNA Precursors

snRNP	Size of RNA (nucleotides)	Function
U1	165	Binds 5′ splice site
U2	185	Binds branch site
U5	116	Binds 3′ splice site
U4	145	Required for assembly
U6	106	of spliceosome

tions. Spliceosome-catalyzed splicing may have evolved from RNA self-splicing catalytic RNA (see later).

Abnormal mRNA splicing can be one cause of β^+-thalassemia in which the production of β-hemoglobin chains is greatly reduced. The defect appears to be caused by mutations that interfere with the correct removal of introns from the globin pre-mRNAs.

11.4.3   Transfer RNA

In both prokaryotic and eukaryotic cells, tRNAs are processed from larger precursors. Generally, specific endonucleases that cleave at internal sites and exonucleases that sequentially remove single nucleotides from the 5′ end are employed. CCA is added to the 3′ end of chains that do not have this terminal sequence. Many modifications of bases and ribose occur *posttranscriptionally*. These include the formation of unusual bases (pseudoridylate and ribothymidylate) and methylation of bases and sugar. As noted for *E. coli*, the three rRNA molecules and a tRNA molecule are excised from a single primary transcript that contains spacer regions. Other primary transcripts may contain several different tRNAs or several copies of the same tRNA in addition to the rRNAs. It is advantageous to have the three rRNA sequences in a single transcript. This ensures that appropriate amounts of the three molecules are available for the assembly of ribosomes.

RNA polymerase III transcribes the small genes for the many different tRNAs and the 5 S rRNA of the large ribosomal subunit. The primary tRNA transcripts in eukaryotes are transformed into mature tRNAs by endonuclease removal of a 5'-leader sequence, and replacement of a 3'-terminal UU by CCA.

11.4.4 Self-splicing Catalytic RNA

It was first discovered in 1981 by Thomas Cech and coworkers that a primary transcript for the 26 S rRNA from the protozoan *Tetrarhymena* could cut, splice, and assemble itself into the mature 26 S rRNA. Subsequently it was shown that a specific rRNA could catalyze the assembly of RNAs other than itself and that this could occur in the absence of any protein. Such enzyme-like RNAs were termed *ribozymes*. Self-splicing has been found to occur for RNAs from a variety of species. Two main types of self-splicing mechanisms are known:

> Group I is found in *Tetrahymena*; it requires Mg^{2+} and a guanosine unit, but no ATP.
> Group II requires spermidine and Mg^{2+} but no ATP or guanosine.

For the intimate details of these reactions, the reader is directed to the Bibliography.

11.5   RNA TURNOVER

DNA is metabolically very stable and is replicated only once during the S phase of the cell cycle (Chapter 13). DNA has a finite stability, however, and is subject to various kinds of damage that can change the coding properties of the bases. The various DNA editing and repair mechanisms are essential for maintaining its informational integrity. Repair systems for RNA apparently do not exist, and damaged or unneeded RNAs are degraded to nucleotides that can be reutilized (Chapter 10).

Nuclear rRNA precursors and cytoplasmic rRNA formed by RNA polymerase I account for some 70+% of mammalian cell RNA and 35–40% of total RNA synthesis. The products of RNA polymerase II, hnRNA and mRNA, comprise some 10% of the total RNA and 55–60% of total synthesis. The hnRNA and mRNA transcripts are unstable and have half-lives in higher eukaryotes of about 24 h, compared with an average half-life in bacteria of 90 s. Pre-tRNAs, synthesized along with 5 S rRNA by RNA polymerase III, are relatively stable, with an average half-life of 4–6 days.

A number of exoribonucleases and endoribonucleases with varying specificities degrade RNA in the cytoplasm to nucleotides. Unusual nucleotides derived from rRNA and tRNA are excreted, whereas the four common nucleotides (A, G, C, and U) are readily recycled.

QUESTIONS

11.1. RNA polymerase first binds on a site on DNA called the
   a. Enhancer
   b. Promoter
   c. Repressor
   d. Operator
   e. ρ Factor

11.2. In DNA replication of the lagging strand the following enzymes are used:
   DNA ligase: 1
   Gyrase: 2
   DNA polymerase III: 3
   DNA polymerase I: 4
   Helicase: 5
   Primase: 6

Using the number for the enzymes, select the correct sequence for the DNA replication process.
   a. 1, 2, 3, 4, 5, 6
   b. 4, 3, 5, 2, 1, 6
   c. 6, 5, 4, 3, 2, 1
   d. 5, 6, 2, 3, 4, 1
   e. 1, 3, 5, 6, 2, 4

11.3. The negative supercoiling of DNA requires the action of
   a. Reverse transcriptase
   b. DNA ligase
   c. DNA polymerase
   d. Type II DNA topoisomerase
   e. DNA

11.4. All the following statements are true about DNA replication, *except*
   a. Chain growth on one DNA strand is discontinuous.
   b. Chain growth on new strands is in the $5' \rightarrow 3'$ direction.
   c. A transient covalent linkage is formed between RNA and DNA.
   d. Only deoxyribonucleoside triphosphates are used by DNA polymerases.
   e. The overall process is bidirectional.

In Questions 11.5–11.9, use the following key:
   a. 1, 2, and 3 are correct.
   b. 1 and 3 are correct.
   c. 2 and 4 are correct.
   d. Only 4 is correct.
   e. All are correct.

11.5. Which of the following are required for nuclear DNA replication?
   1. DNA polymerase
   2. Helicase
   3. ATP-dependent DNA ligase
   4. DNase

11.6. Thymine dimers in DNA
   1. Can be excised completely by enzymatic action
   2. Can arise from action of UV light
   3. Distort the double helix
   4. Undergo excision through $5' \rightarrow 3'$ Pol I exonuclease activity

11.7. The DNA of prokaryotes and most viruses
   1. Is supercoiled
   2. Is circular
   3. Has a closed structure with an internal loop during replication
   4. Is replicated in a single direction
11.8. Okazaki fragments are produced by
   1. Primase
   2. DNA ligase
   3. DNA polymerase III (Pol III)
   4. DNA polymerase I (Pol I)
11.9. Prokaryotic RNA polymerase has strict requirements for
   1. All four nucleoside triphosphates
   2. A monovalent cation
   3. A DNA template
   4. A primer

In Questions 11.10–11.14, match the correct term with each statement:
   a. Characteristic of prokaryotes
   b. Characteristic of eukaryotes
   c. Neither
   d. Both

11.10. Binding of RNA polymerases is at specific sites called promoters.
11.11. tRNAs are synthesized via processing of a larger RNA precursor.
11.12. rRNA is synthesized via processing of a larger RNA precursor.
11.13. Most mRNA contains a long polyadenylate tail at the 3′ end.
11.14. Ribosomes attach to nascent mRNA while it is still being synthesized.
11.15. Which of the following statements is *untrue* about caps on RNA molecules?
   a. They are important for subsequent splicing reactions.
   b. They facilitate binding to ribosomes.
   c. They remain during subsequent processing.
   d. They stabilize mRNAs by protecting their 3′ ends from nucleases and phosphatases.
11.16. All of the following statements concerning DNA polymerase III (Pol III) are true, *except*
   a. Pyrophosphate is a product of the reaction.
   b. Pol III is composed of at least seven different proteins.
   c. Pol III has high processivity.
   d. It adds deoxyribonucleotides to the 5′-hydroxyl terminus of preexisting DNA.
   e. It adds deoxyribonucleotides to the 3′-hydroxyl terminus of preexisting DNA.
11.17. Which of the following statements about the ρ termination factor is *false*?
   a. It breaks the RNA-DNA hybrid pulling away the RNA.
   b. It is a hexamer of 46 kD subunits.
   c. It contains six to eight poly (U) regions.
   d. It hydrolyzes ribonucleoside triphosphates to nucleoside diphosphates.
11.18. Which of the following statements about eukaryotic mRNA is *false*?
   a. It contains a poly(A) tail of up to 250 residues.
   b. The poly(A) tail is coded by the DNA template.
   c. The primary nuclear transcripts are much larger than the cytoplasmic mRNAs and contain introns.

    d. A guanosine residue is attached at the 5′ terminus in an unusual 5′-5′-triphosphate linkage.

11.19. Which of the following statements about RNA transcriptase is *false*?
    a. It is involved in DNA synthetase.
    b. It synthesizes DNA from a DNA template.
    c. It utilizes deoxynucleoside triphosphates.
    d. It synthesizes DNA from an RNA template.

11.20. Which of the following statements about DNA polymerase I (PolI) is *false*?
    a. It has $3′ \rightarrow 5′$-exonuclease activity.
    b. It has $5′ \rightarrow 3′$-exonuclease activity.
    c. It has ligase activity.
    d. It removes ribonucleotide primers.

Answers

11.1. (b) Initial binding occurs at specific DNA sites called promoters. These sequences occur with great regularity and are called *conserved* or *consensus* sequences. The optimum distance between two such sequences is highly conserved at 17 nucleotides, the exact sequences being unimportant.

11.2. (d) The order is helicase, primase, gyrase, DNA polymerase III, DNA polymerase I, and DNA ligase.

11.3. (d) Type II DNA topoisomerase prevents positive supercoiling by introducing negative supercoils at the expense of ATP.

11.4. (c) RNA and DNA are held together by the conventional Watson-Crick base pairing hydrogen bonding rules. There is no covalent bond.

11.5. (a) DNase hydrolyzes.

11.6. (e) All statements are true.

11.7. (a) The DNA replication is bidirectional.

11.8. (b) Ligase joins fragments, and Pol I fills in gaps.

11.9. (a) A primer is not required.

11.10. (d) Both require binding to promoters.

11.11. (d) In both, tRNAs are synthesized by processing of a larger RNA precursor.

11.12. (d) In both, rRNAs are processed from larger precursors.

11.13. (b) Prokaryotic mRNAs function in translation with no processing.

11.14. (a) Because prokaryotic mRNAs are not compartmentalized and not processed, translation can begin before the mRNA synthesis is complete.

11.15. (d) Caps are at the 5′ ends.

11.16. (d) Deoxyribonucleotides are added to the 3′-hydroxyl terminus.

11.17. (c) ρ does not contain poly (U) sequence like ρ-independent terminator.

11.18. (b) The poly (A) tail is not coded by DNA but is added to the mRNA before leaving the nucleus.

11.19. (b) RNA transcriptase synthesizes DNA from a RNA template, not from a DNA template.

11.20. (c) Pol I does not have ligase activity.

PROBLEMS

11.1. In *E. coli*, mRNAs comprise some 3–4% of total RNA but represent some 45% of the RNA synthesized at any given time. What is the explanation?

11.2. One strand of a DNA molecule is transcribed into mRNA by RNA polymerase.

This strand, the template strand, has a base composition of A, 15%; T, 40%; C, 25%; and G, 20%. What is the composition of the mRNA molecule synthesized?

11.3. A purified sample of double-stranded DNA contains 16% thymine on a molar basis. What are the percentages of the other bases?

11.4. A 20-year-old male exhibited extreme sensitivity to sunlight that began at an early age and increased as time went on. Following exposure to sunlight, the skin showed erythema, followed by atrophy and dilation of small and terminal blood vessels. The skin was overgrown with a horny layer (keratosis), and the cornea was ulcerated. Malignant skin lesions developed at multiple sites. Cultured skin fibroblasts of the patient had a reduced survival time after ultraviolet irradiation, and the survival of various irradiated viruses grown in these cells was less than that in normal cells. What do these results suggest as the underlying biochemical defect?

BIBLIOGRAPHY

Alberts B, Bray D, Lewis J, Raff M, Roberts K, Watson J. Molecular Biology of the Cell, 3rd edition. New York: Garland, 1994.

Beebe T, Burke J. Gene Structure and Transcription. Oxford: IRL Press, 1988.

Cech T. RNA as an enzyme. Sci Am 182(4):6–14, 1990.

Challberg MD, Kelly TS. Animal virus replication. Annu Rev Biochem 58:682–689, 1989.

Freifelder D. Essentials of Molecular Biology. Boston: Jones and Bartlett, 1985.

Kornberg A. DNA replication. J Biol. Chem. 263:4265–4268, 1989.

McCarty M. The Transforming Principle. New York: W.W. Norton, 1985.

Sharp PA. Splicing of messenger RNA precursors. Science 235:766–771, 1987.

Singer M, Berg P. Genes and Genomes. Mill Valley, CA: University Science Books, 1991.

Watson JD, Hopkins NH, Roberts JW, Steitz JA, Weiner AM. Molecular Biology of the Gene, 4th edition, Vol. I. Menlo Park: Benjamin/Cummings, 1987.

12

Protein Biosynthesis

After completing this chapter, the student should

1. Be able to describe the mechanisms and requirements for activation of amino acids.
2. Be able to describe the mechanism for peptide chain initiation, elongation, and termination in prokaryotes and eukaryotes on the ribosome.
3. Know ribosome general structure (A site, P site, and peptidylsynthetase).
4. Know the common inhibitors of protein synthesis and how they work.
5. Be able to discuss protein targeting and posttranslational modification.
6. Know the principles of the genetic code, the wobble hypothesis, and the concepts of nonsense, missense, and frameshift mutations and how they may be suppressed.

12.1 INTRODUCTION

The biosynthesis of a protein is a complex, integrated process involving the interaction of more than a hundred macromolecules. Involved are ribosomes, mRNAs, tRNAs, aminoacyl-tRNA synthetases, ATP, GTP, and various soluble protein factors for initiation, elongation, and termination (Table 12.1). Although the mechanism and individual steps of protein biosynthesis are similar in prokaryotic and eukaryotic cells, there are substantial differences in ribosomal structure and the soluble factors employed as one proceeds from simpler to more complex organisms. This is perhaps a result of the need for additional features in eukaryotic cells, in which regulation is much more complex. We consider both systems in four stages: activation, initiation, elongation, and termination. The various components currently believed to be required at each stage in protein biosynthesis are presented in Table 12.2. We do not attempt to discuss in detail the roles of all the soluble factors involved.

12.2 ACTIVATION OF AMINO ACIDS AND FORMATION OF AMINOACYL-tRNAs

The enzymes activating the amino acids and forming aminoacyl-tRNAs are called *aminoacyl-tRNA synthetases* and are localized in the cytosol. These enzymes catalyze two distinguishable reactions. In the first reaction, which is analogous to fatty acid activation (Chapter 19), the amino acids are converted to transient enzyme-bound aminoacyl adenylates in which the carboxyl group of the amino acid is linked to the 5'-phosphate group of AMP by an anhydride bond (Figure 12.1). In a second reaction, the aminoacyl moiety is transferred to either the 2'- or 3'-hydroxyl of the ribose unit at the 3' terminus of the tRNA to form aminoacyl-tRNA. Because subsequent acyl migration can readily occur, some equilibrium mixture of the 2' and 3' isomers is found. When the amino acid is transferred to the growing polypeptide chain, however, it must leave the 3'-hydroxyl group. Because the free energy of hydrolysis of the ester bond in tRNA is similar to that of the terminal phosphate group of ATP, the reaction proceeds with little free energy change. The overall reaction is driven by the subsequent hydrolysis of pyrophosphate. Thus, two high-energy phosphate bonds are ultimately used for each aminoacyl-tRNA formed, making the overall reaction highly exergonic and virtually irreversible.

There are at least one specific synthetase and one specific tRNA for each amino acid. The synthetases are highly specific for both the amino acid and its cognate tRNA. Once an amino acid is specifically attached to its cognate tRNA, it no longer controls its own fate. This was shown by taking enzymatically formed cysteinyl-tRNA^{Cys} and reducing the bound cysteine chemically to alanyl-tRNA^{Cys}. The hybrid aminoacyl-tRNA was incubated with a cell-free system capable of synthesizing hemoglobin. It was found that alanine residues were incorporated in polypeptide linkages in positions normally occupied by cysteine. Thus, the amino acid was selected by virtue of the base sequence in the tRNA adaptor. It is the anticodon triplet in tRNAs that interacts by specific base pairing with the codon on the mRNA chain to select the "correct" amino acid (see Chapter 10 and Section 12.9). The amino acid in aminoacyl-tRNA has no role in selecting the appropriate codon.

There is, however, some proofreading or editing function by most of the synthetases that serves to enhance fidelity. Most synthetases contain both a synthetic and a hydrolytic site. These two sites function together as a *double sieve*, the synthetic site rejects amino acids that are too large, the hydrolytic site destroying activated intermediates that are smaller than the correct aminoacyl-tRNA. For example, isoleucine-tRNA^{Ile} is excluded from the hydrolytic site, which is smaller than the synthetic site. Valine-tRNA^{Ile} is accommodated by the hydrolytic site and hydrolyzed to valine and tRNA^{Ile}. This allows a discrete discrimination between valine and isoleucine, which differ in only a single methylene group ($-CH_2-$).

12.3 INITIATION AND ELONGATION IN PROKARYOTES

The direction of protein biosynthesis is from the amino terminus to the carboxyl terminus, the mRNA being translated in the 5' → 3 direction as in DNA synthe-

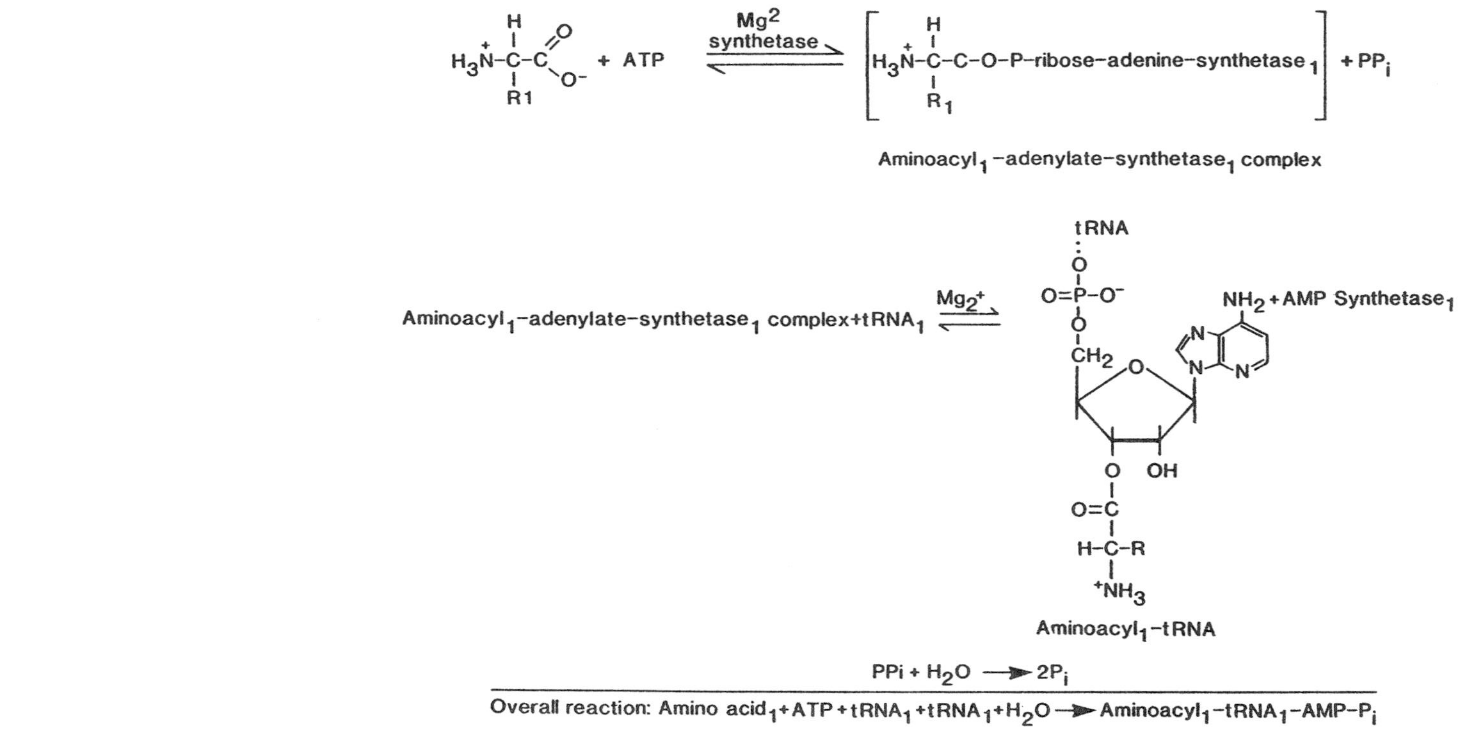

Figure 12.1 Formation of aminoacyl-tRNA involving the intermediate formation of an intermediate aminoacyl-adenylate-synthetase complex.

sis. This establishes a sequence relationship between the nucleotides in DNA (or its mRNA transcripts) and the amino acids in proteins. Protein synthesis in bacteria is initiated by formylmethionyl-tRNA (fMet-tRNAi), which recognizes the AUG initiation code in mRNA (see Table 12.4). This tRNA is different from the one (methionyl-tRNA, Met-tRNA) that inserts methionine at internal positions; methionine cannot be formylated when attached to Met-tRNA.

For initiation, the 30 S ribosomal subunit forms a complex with the three initiation factors [IF; reaction (1) in Figure 12.2]. GTP is then bound to IF-2, allowing mRNA and fMet-tRNAi to join the complex with the release of IF-3 [release (2) in Figure 12.2]. Addition of the 50 S subunit and hydrolysis of GTP causes the release of IF-1 and IF-2 and the formation of the functional 70 S ribosome [reaction (3)]. The fMet-tRNAi occupies the P (peptidyl) site on the ribosome and is positioned so that its anticodon pairs with the initiating AUG of the mRNA. The A (aminoacyl) site is empty. EF-Tu-GTP (an elongation factor) delivers the appropriate aminoacyl-tRNA to the A site [reaction (4)], following which the GTP is hydrolyzed and the EF-Tu-GDP complex dissociates from the ribosome. A second elongation factor, EF-Ts, binds to EF-Tu-GTP, releasing GDP.

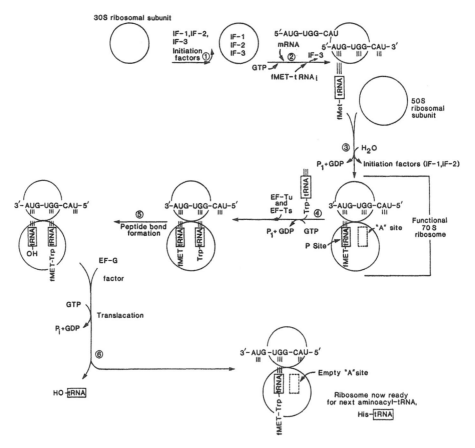

Figure 12.2 Initiation reactions and elongation cycle in prokaryotic protein synthesis.

GTP can again bind to EF-Tu, releasing EF-Ts and re-forming EF-Tu-GTP that can deliver another aminoacyl-tRNA to the A site. A peptide bond [reaction (5)] is then formed by the nucleophilic attack of the amino group of the aminoacyl-tRNA on the esterified carboxyl group of the fMet-tRNA. This reaction step is catalyzed by *peptidyltransferase*, which is an integral component of the 50 S ribosome. The formylmethionine moiety of fMET-tRNA is transferred to the amino group of the aminoacyl-tRNA on the A site, forming a dipeptidyl-tRNA and leaving an uncharged tRNA on the P site. The energy for this reaction derives from the original formation of the aminoacyl-tRNA.

The next phase (step 6) is *translocating*, in which the uncharged tRNA dissociates from the P site, the dipeptidyl-tRNA (shown as formylmethionyltryptophanyl-tRNA) moves to the P site from the A site, and mRNA moves a distance of three nucleotides (one codon). GTP and a third elongation factor, a *translocase* or EF-G, are required. EF-G-GTP drives the translocase reaction. Following hydrolysis of the bound GTP, EF-G is released from the ribosome. The A site is now empty and ready to accept another aminoacyl-tRNA and begin another round of elongation. The same process repeats with the free amino group of the newly bound aminoacyl-tRNA on the A site displacing the tRNA from the peptidyl-tRNA on the P site to form a new peptide bond.

12.4 TERMINATION IN PROKARYOTES

The process of termination involves the release of the completed polypeptide chain from the P site on the ribosome and requires a termination codon (UAA, UAG, and UGA) in the A site, GTP, and release factors (RF-1, RF-2, and RF-3). Normal cells do not contain tRNAs with anti-codons complementary to the termination signals. These stop signals are recognized by the release factors, and the binding of the release factors to a termination codon in some way activates the peptidyltransferase to hydrolyze the ester bond between the last tRNA and the polypeptide on the P site. The polypeptide chain, the tRNA, and the mRNA leave the ribosome. The ribosome then dissociates into its subunits, and futile reassociation in the absence of an initiation complex to the 70 S complex is prevented by the binding of IF-3 to the 30 S subunit. The ribosome must be reassembled before being used for the synthesis of a new polypeptide chain (Figure 12.3). This requires the sequence of events shown in Figure 12.2.

12.5 POLYSOMES

In addition, several ribosomes can independently and simultaneously translate a mRNA molecule and, hence, synthesize several identical polypeptide chains concurrently (Figure 12.3). Such clusters or groups of ribosomes are called *polyribosomes* or *polysomes*. The number of attached ribosomes depends on the size of the mRNA and how frequently ribosomes can initiate at the start of a gene sequence. Because RNA transcription and translation are neither temporally nor spatially separated in prokaryotes, it is possible for translation to begin before transcription is completed. However, we have already noted that prokaryotic mRNAs have short half-lives; this is probably a result of their continuous degra-

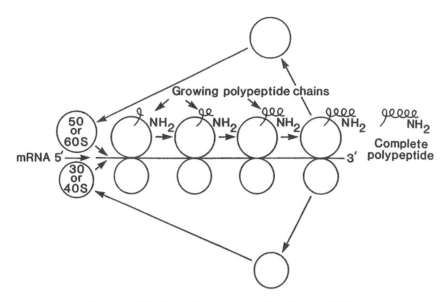

Figure 12.3 Polyribosomes moving along mRNA.

dation, even during translation. If the degradation proceeds beyond the initiation site, this limits the frequency of initiation. Eukaryotic mRNAs have much longer half-lives (hours to days), their degradation being prevented by the 5′ caps.

12.6 INITIATION, ELONGATION, AND TERMINATION IN EUKARYOTES

Although the general mechanism and individual steps of protein biosynthesis are similar in prokaryotes and eukaryotes, there are differences and additional complexities in the eukaryote. The differences in size and composition of eukaryotic and prokaryotic ribosomes are listed in Table 12.1. Differences in the initiator tRNA and in the soluble factors involved with initiation, elongation, and termination are listed in Table 12.2. In eukaryotes, the *initiator* is Met-tRNAi rather than fMet-tRNAi. Nine or more soluble initiation factors are known in eukaryotes that interact in a complicated manner. Eukaryotic elongation factors EF-1α and EF-1β have roles similar to prokaryotic EF-Tu and EF-Ts, and EF-2 acts like prokaryotic EF-G in driving the translocase reaction. Again, a GTP-GDP cycle is involved in the interactions. A single release factor in eukaryotes, eRF, recognizes all three termination codons. eIF-3, like IF-3, prevents the futile reassociation of the ribosomal subunits. Recent experiments with the initiation factor eIF-2 have shown that its level of phosphorylation is one of the mechanisms whereby translation is controlled. Phosphorylation of a subunit of eIF-2 (eIF-2α) on its serine 5′ residue by a specific protein kinase leads to an inhibition of translation. Specific phosphatases have been characterized, and temporal correlations of the levels of phosphorylation and translation activity have been made. A second possible site for the regulation of translation is at the binding of

Table 12.1 Comparison of Prokaryotic and Eukaryotic Ribosomes[a]

	Prokaryotes	Eukaryotes
Ribosome size	70 S, MW 2×10^6	80 S, MW 4.2×10^6
Large subunit size	50 S, MW 1.6×10^6	60 S, MW 2.8×10^6
Size of RNAs	5 S (120 nucleotides) 23 S (2900 nucleotides)	5.8 S (160 nucleotides) 28 S (4700 nucleotides)
Number of proteins	34	49
Small subunit size	30 S, MW 9×10^5	40 S, MW 1.4×10^6
Size of RNAs	16 S (1540 nucleotides)	18 S (1900 nucleotides)
Number of proteins	21	33

[a]Sizes are expressed as Svedberg units determined by ultra centrifugation; they depend upon both size and shape and are not additive. MW, molecular weight.

Table 12.2 Components Required in Stages of Prokaryotic and Eukaryotic Protein Biosynthesis[a]

Stages	Prokaryotes	Eukaryotes
Activation	tRNAs, ATP, Mg^{2+} aminoacyl-tRNA synthetases	tRNAs, ATP, Mg^{2+} aminoacyl-tRNA synthetases
Initiation	mRNAs with AUG initiation code; fMet-tRNAi; IF-1, IF-2, and IF-3 initiation factors, GTP, Mg^{2+}; 30 and 50 S	mRNAs with AUG initiation code; Met-tRNA; eIF_3, eIF_2, eIF_4, eIF_5 initiation factors; GTP, Mg^{2+}, eIF-2 protein kinase; 40 and 60 S ribosomal subunits
Elongation	Functional 70 S ribosomes; aminoacyl-tRNAs; GTP, Mg^{2+}, EF-Tu, EF-Ts, and EF-G elongation factors	Functional 80 S ribosomes; aminoacyl-tRNAs; GTP, Mg^{2+}, EF-1, EF-1, and EF-2 elongation factors
Termination	Termination codons (UAG, UAA, or UGA) recognized by RF-1, RF-2, and RF-3 release factors	Termination codons (UAG, UAA, or UGA) recognized by eRF release factor

[a]fMet-tRNA and Met-tRNA = N-formylmethionyl transfer RNA and methionyl transfer RNA, respectively.

mRNA to the small ribosomal subunit. This involves phosphorylation of a serine residue in one of the IF-4 polypeptides and results in an upregulation of protein synthesis. It seems that the eIF-2 and eIF-4 regulatory mechanisms are probably interlinked rather than operating independently. Whether regulation occurs at other sites is not known at present.

Table 12.3 Antibiotic Inhibitors of Protein or RNA Synthesis

Antibiotic	Mechanism of action
Acting only on prokaryotes	
Chloramphenicol[a]	Binds to 50 S ribosomyl subunit and inhibits peptidyltransferase
Tetracyclines	Binds to 30 S ribosomyl subunit to prevent anticodon binding of aminoacyl-tRNA
Streptomycin	Binds to 30 S ribosomyl subunit and causes misreading of mRNA
Erythromycin	Binds to 50 S ribosomyl subunit and inhibits translocation
Rifamycin	Binds to RNA polymerase blocking initiation of RNA chains
Acting on prokaryotes and eukaryotes	
Puromycin	Acts as an analog of aminoacyl-tRNA, causes premature chain termination
Actinomycin D	Intercalates between two GC base pairs of DNA, blocking the movement of RNA polymerase
Acting only on eukaryotes	
Cycloheximide[b]	Binds to 60 S ribosomyl subunit and inhibits peptidyltransferase
Amanitin	Binds to RNA polymerase blocking mRNA synthesis
Anisomycin	Blocks peptidyltransferase reaction

[a]In eukaryotes, only protein synthesis on ribosomes of mitochondria is inhibited.
[b]Affects only ribosomes in the cytosol.

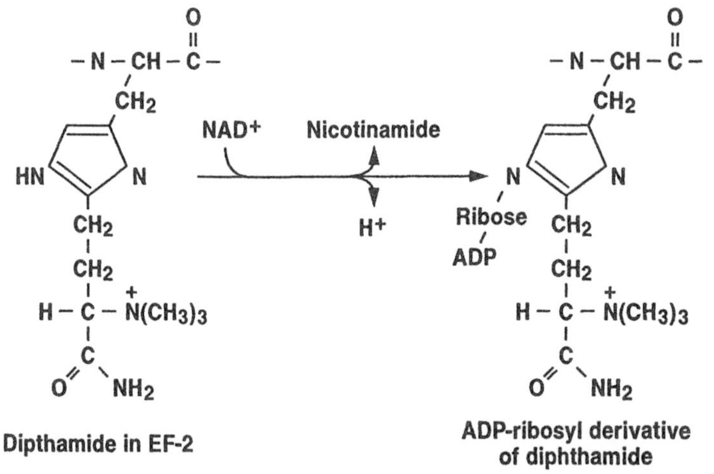

Dipthamide in EF-2   ADP-ribosyl derivative of diphthamide

Figure 12.4 Inhibition of protein synthesis by diphtheria toxin transfer of an ADP-ribose moiety from NAD^+ to a diphthamide residue in the elongation factor EF-2.

12.7 INHIBITORS OF PROTEIN BIOSYNTHESIS

Many antibiotics are inhibitors of protein biosynthesis, and in many instances their mechanisms of action is known (Table 12.3). The clinically useful antibiotics are those that are active against prokaryotes and have little if any effect on eukaryotic protein biosynthesis. Inhibitors other than antibiotics include *diphtheria toxin*, which inhibits protein biosynthesis by modifying the eukaryotic elongation factor EF-2. The toxin interacts with a receptor on the surface of a sensitive cell and is proteolytically cleaved to yield two fragments, an A fragment and a B fragment. The B fragment facilitates the penetration of the A fragment through the cell membrane. The A fragment catalyzes the ADP ribosylation of a single unusual amino residue present in EF-2 (diphthamide), which is formed by posttranslational modification of histidine (Figure 12.4). This ADP ribosylation irreversibly blocks the capacity of EF-2 to carry out the translocation step of protein chain elongation. A single molecule of the A fragment can kill the cell. The function of diphthamide in EF-2 is unknown, but it is clearly critical.

12.8 PROTEIN TARGETING AND PROCESSING

In addition to synthesizing proteins in a controlled manner, cells must also deliver specific proteins to their functional sites. *Escherichia coli* is compartmentalized, with an outer membrane, a periplasmic space, an inner membrane, and a cytosol, each with its own assortment of specific proteins. The situation in eukaryotic cells is even more complex, with their several membrane-enclosed compartments, each again with distinctive protein composition. How is a specific protein directed and conveyed to a specific target site? We shall see that there is a specific signal sequence in the protein being synthesized that determines its destination. The synthesis of proteins begins and continues on free ribosomes in the cytosol unless the nascent protein contains a hydrophobic signal sequence that directs the ribosome to the endoplasmic reticulum (ER). We noted in Chapter 1 the extensive ER membrane system, the *smooth ER*, which is devoid of ribosomes, and the *rough ER*, which has bound ribosomes. There is no structural difference between a free ribosome and a bound ribosome. Ribosomal attachment depends upon the kind of protein it is synthesizing. The nascent proteins synthesized by membrane-bound ribosomes are translocated in an ATP-driven reaction across the ER membrane into an internal space, the ER *lumen* or the ER *cisternal space*. The proteins are modified in various ways and then transferred to the Golgi complex for further modification. They are then targeted for delivery to the plasma membrane, to secretory vesicles, and to lysosomes. Bacterial and eukaryotic signal sequences are functionally similar. In fact, a bacterial signal sequence added to a eukaryotic mRNA converted a cytosolic protein into a secretory protein.

It is the ER that provides the cell with the mechanism for segregating newly synthesized proteins that are to remain in the cytosol and those destined for the plasma membrane, storage in lysosomes, or secretion from the cell.

The signal that directs a ribosome with its nascent protein to the ER membrane is a sequence of amino acids near the amino terminus of its nascent polypeptide chain. In a secretory protein, these signal sequences are present when synthesized *in vitro* by free ribosomes but absent from normally secreted proteins because they are removed by a signal peptidase on the luminal side of the ER membrane. The structure of many of these amino-terminal signal sequences are known; two are shown in Figure 12.5. They all have some common features: (1) a highly hydrophobic sequence of 10–15 residues at the center of the signal sequence, leucine, valine, isoleucine, and phenylalanine being common residues in this region; (2) at least 1 positively charged residue (arginine and lysine in the examples) near the amino terminal end; and (3) 5 residues more polar than the hydrophobic core precede the cleavage site at the carboxyl terminus.

The hydrophobic signal sequence located near the amino terminus of a growing polypeptide chain is recognized as it leaves the ribosome by a cytoplasmic nucleoprotein particle, the *signal recognition particle* (SRP). SRP consists of a 300-nucleotide RNA molecule and six different polypeptide chains. SRP binding blocks further translation. The ribosome-SRP complex then moves to the ER membrane and binds to the *SRP receptor* (docking protein) on the cytosolic face. Two ribosomal binding proteins, *ribophorin I* and *II*, anchor the ribosomal complex, the SRP is released into cytosol for recycling, and elongation continues until the signal peptide moves through the membrane to the cisternal side of the ER. At this point the signal peptide is cleaved by a *signal peptidase* in the ER lumen. Elongation continues, and the remainder of the polypeptide chain is translocated across the membrane. At termination, the ribosome and the mRNA are released to the cytosol (Figure 12.6).

Many secretory and membrane proteins are modified in the lumen of the ER. Protein glycosylation, the addition of covalently bound oligosaccharide chains, is a common reaction in the ER lumen and the Golgi complex. Most proteins in the ER lumen destined for secretion from the cell or for transport to other intracellular sites are glycoproteins. The carbohydrate content of glycoproteins can vary from 0.5 to 80% or more of the glycoprotein mass. Glycoprotein structures were described in Chapter 9, and their biosynthesis are covered in Chapter 20.

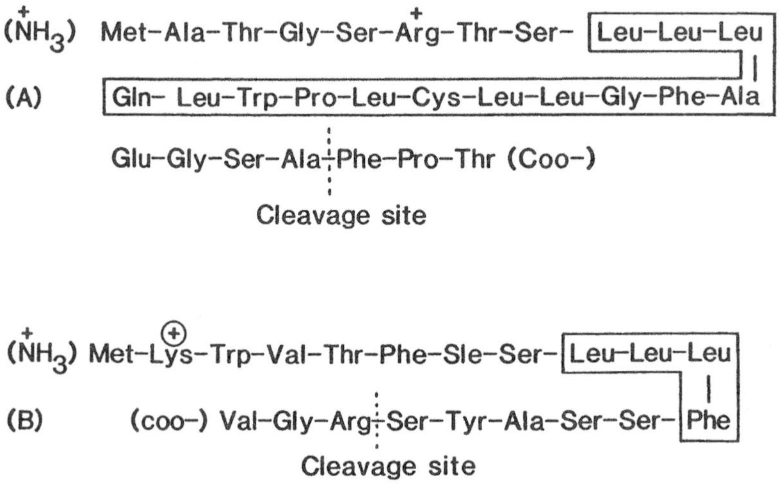

$(\overset{+}{N}H_3)$ Met–Ala–Thr–Gly–Ser–$\overset{+}{A}$rg–Thr–Ser– | Leu–Leu–Leu |
                                                                          | |
(A) | Gln– Leu–Trp–Pro–Leu–Cys–Leu–Leu–Gly–Phe–Ala |

             Glu–Gly–Ser–Ala⋮Phe–Pro–Thr (Coo–)
                           ⋮
                    Cleavage site

$(\overset{+}{N}H_3)$ Met–L$\overset{\oplus}{y}$s–Trp–Val–Thr–Phe–Sle–Ser–| Leu–Leu–Leu |
                                                                                | |
(B)   (coo–) Val–Gly–Arg⋮Ser–Tyr–Ala–Ser–Ser–| Phe |
                         ⋮
                  Cleavage site

Figure 12.5 Amino-terminal signal sequence of (A) human growth hormone and (B) bovine proalbumin. Hydrophobic core is within the box.

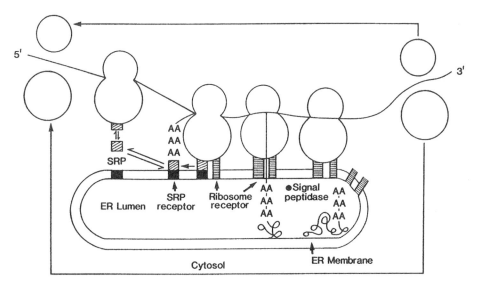

Figure 12.6 Roles of signal recognition particles (SRP), SRP receptor (docking protein), ribosome binding proteins (ribophorin I and II), and signal peptidase in translocation of nascent polypeptide chains across ER membrane. AA, amino acids.

Proteins from the lumen and membranes of the ER are transferred to the cis surface of the Golgi apparatus by coated vesicles (transfer vesicles). The Golgi apparatus in the mammalian cell consists of a stack of some six flattened membranous stacks (cisternae) and is symmetric. There are three compartments: a *cis* compartment, which is closest to the ER; a *medial* compartment; and a *trans* compartment closest to the plasma membrane. These compartments have different enzymes and carry out different processes. Transfer vesicles containing proteins bud off from the ER and fuse with the cis Golgi face. Different vesicles transfer proteins from cis to medial and from the medial to the trans compartment. Vesicles derived from the trans face carry proteins to different target sites, such as the plasma membrane, lysosomes, and secretory vesicles. In the medial Golgi, a N-acetylglucosamine and a fucose residue are added, and two additional mannoses are removed. A galactose and a sialic acid are added sequentially in the trans Golgi. The content of glycosyltransferase enzymes in each of the compartments, as well as the conformation of the glycoprotein, determines the structure of the N-linked oligosaccharide units. Lysosomal enzymes are known to be targeted by the acquisition of a mannose-6-phosphate residue, but plasma membrane proteins and secretory proteins do not appear to be targeted by carbohydrate residues. We do not as yet have a clear understanding of budding and fusion or the specificity of sorting that occurs in the trans Golgi and the vesicles derived from it.

Other kinds of modifications may be necessary to convert a newly synthesized protein to its biologically active form. The N-formyl group of the initiating methionine in prokaryotes is removed by a deformylase. A methionine aminopeptidase removes the initiating residue in many eukaryotic proteins. Other posttranslational modifications may include acetylation, amidation, hydroxylation, methylation, phosphorylation, and sulfation of specific amino acid residues. Enzymatic formation of coenzymes are required in many instances to produce a biochemically functional molecule.

Proteolytic conversion of inactive zymogens to active enzymes was noted in Chapter 5. Other examples of posttranslational proteolytic cleavages include the conversions of proalbumin to albumin (Chapter 7), of preprocollagen to collagen (Chapter 8), and of preproinsulin to insulin (Chapter 16) and the activation of the compounds of the blood-clotting cascade (Chapter 7).

12.9 THE GENETIC CODE

The genetic code is the sequence relationship between the nucleotides in DNA (or its mRNA transcripts) and the amino acids in proteins. Because there are four kinds of bases in DNA (A, T, G, and C) and 20 different amino acids in proteins, a single-base code could specify only four kinds of amino acids. A two-letter code could specify $4^2 = 16$ and a four-letter code $4^4 = 256$ amino acids. A triplet code read three at a time could specify $4^3 = 64$ amino acids, more than enough to specify each of 20 amino acids. Genetic experiments showed that an amino acid was in fact coded by a group of three bases. Allowing for 3 *termination* (stop) codons and 1 *start* codon (AUG) that also specifies internal methionine, all 60 remaining codons correspond to amino acids (Table 12.4). Several codons (*synonyms*) can specify a given amino acid—thus, the genetic code is highly degenerate.

The deciphering of the genetic code was begun by Marshall Nirenberg and coworkers by the use of synthetic polyribonucleotides of known base com-

Table 12.4 The Genetic Code

5′ End First position	Second position				3′ End Third position
	U	C	A	G	
U	Phe	Ser	Tyr	Cys	U
	Phe	Ser	Tyr	Cys	C
	Leu	Ser	Term[a]	Term[a]	A
	Leu	Ser	Term[a]	Trp	G
C	Leu	Pro	His	Aug	U
	Leu	Pro	His	Arg	C
	Leu	Pro	Gln	Arg	A
	Leu	Pro	Gln	Arg	G
A	Ile	Thr	Asn	Ser	U
	Ile	Thr	Asn	Ser	C
	Ile	Thr	Lys	Arg	A
	Met[b]	Thr	Lys	Arg	G
G	Val	Ala	Asp	Gly	U
	Val	Ala	Asp	Gly	C
	Val	Ala	Glu	Gly	A
	Val[c]	Ala	Glu	Gly	G

[a]UAA, UAG, and UGA are termination or "nonsense" codons.
[b]AUG in addition to coding for internal methionine is part of the chain initiation signal.
[c]GUG, in addition to coding for internal valine, is on occasion part of the chain initiation signal.

position as messengers in a cell-free system from *E. coli*. The system consisted of ribosomes and soluble enzymes that had been depleted of mRNA by preincubation and of DNA by treatment with deoxyribonuclease. Such a system has minimal endogenous capacity to synthesize protein. The addition of polyribonucleotides to this system promoted amino acid incorporation, the specific amino acids incorporated depending on the nucleotide content of the added polyribonucleotide. Using a variety of homopolymers and random heteropolymers and assuming a nonoverlapping triplet code, M. Nirenberg and S. Ochoa and their colleagues were able to establish the nucleotide composition, but not sequence, of some 50 triplets coding for amino acids. The sequence of nucleotides within codons was established by two additional techniques: the polyribonucleotide-directed specific binding of aminoacyl-tRNA to ribosomes by nucleotide triplets of known sequence, and the use of long-chain synthetic ribonucleotide polymers, also of known structure, prepared by H. G. Khorana and his associates.

An examination of the "dictionary" in Table 12.4 reveals that the code is degenerate in a semisystematic way. First, for a given amino acid, the first two bases of degenerate codons (synonyms) are the same, whereas the third base (3'-hydroxyl terminal) may be any of four bases (for example, the codons for valine, alanine, and glycine). Second, for a given amino acid, the first two bases of synonyms are the same, whereas the third base may be either of the two purines or either of the two pyrimidines (for example, the codons for lysine, glutamate, phenylalanine, and tyrosine). Third, the first base (5'-hydroxyl terminal) may vary while the second two remain constant (for example, the codons for leucine and arginine). It should be emphasized that although the code is degenerate (redundant), it is not ambiguous: a codon specifies only a single amino acid. Strict Watson-Crick base pairing between codon and anticodon would necessitate 61 different anticodons (tRNAs). Subsequently, it was found in many cases that different codons were recognized by the same tRNA. For example, the anticodon of yeast alanine tRNA is $^{3'}$C-G-I$^{5'}$ and recognizes and binds to 3 codons:

$^{3'}$C G I$^{5'}$	$^{3'}$C G I$^{5'}$	$^{3'}$C G I$^{5'}$	anticodon
$_{5'}$G C U$_{3'}$	$_{5'}$G C C$_{3'}$	$_{5'}$G C A$_{3'}$	codon

Crick proposed the *wobble hypothesis* to explain this stearic freedom. Models of various base pairs [including inosine (I), which appears in several anticodons] were constructed to determine which combinations were plausible with minimum geometric distortions from the normal Watson-Crick base pairs (A-U and G-C). The base pairs listed in Table 12.5 were permissible in the third position (3' of the codon). Thus, for the alanine anticodon ($^{3'}$C G I$^{5'}$), the pairing is as predicted, that is, I with U, C, or A. Phenylalanine-tRNA, which has the anticodon GAA, recognizes codons UUC and UUU but not UUG or UUA, again according to prediction. The wobble hypothesis explains the arrangement of all synonyms in the code. The minimum number of tRNAs needed to translate all 61 codons is 31, or 32 if the initiator tRNA is included. Cells contain more tRNAs than the minimum, some 50–60, the number varying in different cells of differ-

Table 12.5 Permissible Pairings
According to the Wobble Hypothesis

5′ Base of anticodon	3′ Base of codon
C	G
A	U
G	A or G
G	C or U
I	U, C, or A

ent organs and with the state of development. This may be related to changes in the patterns of gene expression.

It has been suggested that the degeneracy of the code minimizes the effects of mutations. Were it not degenerate, 20 codons would specify amino acids and 44 would lead to chain termination, which usually produces inactive proteins. A substitution of one amino acid for another can be benign in many instances, although critical in some instances for normal function (see later).

The direction of translation of mRNA is the same as its direction of synthesis, that is, from the 5′ end to the 3′ end. Ribosomes attach to the 5′ end of the mRNA, and the initiation codon for the N-terminal amino acid is at or near this end. The order of codons in mRNA is colinear with the amino acids in the corresponding polypeptides, as is the information in the DNA genome. The RNA code is non-overlapping, and contiguous triplets are read sequentially and consecutively. This was clearly shown in studies with synthetic polyribonucleotides containing alternate triplets. For example, the alternating copolymer AC, which contains two alternating trinucleotide sequences ApCpA and CpApC, directed the synthesis of a polypeptide containing alternate threonine (codon ACA) and histidine (codon CAC) residues.

Important support for the validity of the cell-free technique for assigning the code has come from the study of known mutations in which a single amino acid in a protein molecule is known to be changed. For example, in sickle cell hemoglobin, glutamate is replaced by valine in position 6 of the β chain. Because glutamate is coded by GAA and GAG and valine in GUA and GUG, a single base change from A to U could account for the substitution. Many other examples could be given (other abnormal hemoglobins, the coat protein of tobacco mosaic virus, or the chain of the tryptophan synthetase of *E. coli*) to show that the substitution of one amino acid for another may be related in a logical way to the change of a single base in a coding triplet.

The code appears to be universal to the extent that synthetic polyribonucleotides seem to code in the same way in mammals, bacteria, and other species, and components of the protein-synthesizing system of various species can operate with components from certain others. Mitochondria and ciliated protozoa have genetic codes slightly different from the standard. For example, in human mitochondria, UGA codes for tryptophan instead of as a termination signal, AUA codes for methionine rather than isoleucine, and AGA and AGG are termination signals rather than coding for arginine.

12.10 MUTATIONS

Mutation refers to any change in the base sequence of DNA that yields a mutant phenotype. Mutations are produced by the replication errors, the deletion and insertion of bases, the covalent modification of bases by physical agents (ionizing radiation and ultraviolet light), and by a variety of chemical agents. Much of this DNA damage can be repaired, because the appropriate genetic information can be recovered from the undamaged DNA strand. We discussed briefly in Chapter 11 the repair roles of the $3' \rightarrow 5'$ and $5' \rightarrow 3'$ activities of the DNA polymerases.

The change in a codon specific for one amino acid to a codon specific for another amino acid is *missense* mutation. A change to a chain termination codon is known as a *nonsense* codon. Because there are 61 codons for amino acids and only 3 codons for termination, it is far more likely that missense rather than nonsense mutations will occur. Nonsense mutations cause a premature release of the peptide chain. The size of the incomplete chain depends on the location of the mutation. Because most incomplete chains have no biologic activity, they are easily detectable. The missense mutations usually have some activity and are more difficult to detect. The effects of a harmful mutation are often reversed by a second mutation. The simplest case is a *reverse* (back) mutation that restores the original nucleotide sequence. A different mutation at the same site might specify another amino acid that partially or fully restores the original activity. More difficult to understand are those mutations that suppress the harmful effect of the original mutation and occur at a different site on the same gene (*intragenic suppression*), or on a different gene (*intergenic suppressor*). Genes that cause suppression of other genes are *suppressor genes,* and they exist for missense, nonsense, and frameshift mutations caused by single-nucleotide insertions or deletions. Suppressors act by altering the reading of mRNA, their actions being mediated by mutant tRNAs. In nonsense suppression, suppressor genes for each of the chain-terminating codons (UAG, UAA, and UGA) act by reading a stop signal as if it were a codon for an amino acid. One suppressor gene inserts tyrosine, a second serine, and a third glutamine. The anticodon of a tRNA species has been altered by a single-base change in each case so that it recognizes one of the stop codons and inserts a specific amino acid that may lead to the synthesis of a functional protein. Normal cells do not contain tRNA with anticodons complementary to the stop signals.

Suppression of missense mutations is, at least in some instances, also mediated by mutant tRNAs. This is probably because a cell processes multiple tRNAs, each with a different anticodon and each capable of recognizing different codons for a given amino acid. One of these tRNAs (I) recognizes only a single codon for a given amino acid. This same codon is also recognized by another tRNA (II), whose anticodon can wobble to pair with other codons for the amino acid; thus, tRNA(I) is not essential for protein synthesis. A change in the anticodon of tRNA(I) to another anti allows it to decode for another amino acid without the cell simultaneously losing its ability to read the codon for the original amino acid. However, the efficiency of suppression is low.

Suppression of frameshift mutations caused by insertion of nucleotides is also mediated by mutant tRNAs. One known frameshift suppressor has an extra base in its anticodon loop (Figure 10.27) and allows this tRNA to pair with a four-base codon. It also allows the translocation of four nucleotides of mRNA from the A to the P site (Figure 12.1), restoring the correct reading frame. There are also frameshift suppressor tRNAs that act on deletions by reading only two bases.

Specific mutations in 30 S ribosomal proteins affect the accuracy of reading and can weakly suppress nonsense as well as missense mutations in the absence of any suppressing tRNAs.

QUESTIONS

12.1. Puromycin inhibits protein synthesis by
   a. Blocking the attachment of methionine to tRNA
   b. Mimicking an aminoacyl-tRNA
   c. Distorting reading of the genetic code
   d. Mimicking a ribosome protein
   e. Inhibiting the binding of mRNA to the 30 S ribosomal subunit

12.2 A codon consists of
   a. Four individual nucleotides
   b. Two complementary base pairs
   c. A ribosome
   d. Three consecutive base pairs
   e. A polysome

12.3. In eukaryotic cells, the first step in the incorporation of amino acids into polypeptide chains requires
   a. Initiation factors
   b. Binding of mRNA to the 40 S ribosomal unit
   c. Participation of aminoacyl-tRNA synthetase
   d. Binding of the 30–50 S ribosomyl subunit
   e. Binding of formylmethionyl-tRNA to ribosome

12.4. In mammalian secretory cells, the synthesis of protein takes mainly in the
   a. Rough endoplasmic reticulum
   b. Smooth endoplasmic reticulum
   c. Nucleolus
   d. Nucleus
   e. Peroxisomes

12.5. Following translation, a protein can undergo all of the following *except*
   a. Formation of disulfide bonds
   b. Hydroxylation, methylation, phosphorylation, acetylation, amidation, or removal of initiating amino acid residue (methionine in eukaryotes)
   c. Removal of N-formyl group of initiating methionine in prokaryotes
   d. Removal of intron segments
   e. Proteolytic cleavage of protein to yield active molecule

12.6. tRNA reacts specifically with
   a. Free amino acids
   b. Specific aminoacyl adenylates
   c. ADP
   d. Nuclear DNA
   e. None of these

In Questions 12.7–12.12, match the correct statement with the antibiotics a–f:
   a. Chloramphenicol
   b. Tetracyclines
   c. Streptomycin

    d.   Puromycin
    e.   Erythromycin
    f.   Cyclohexamide

12.7.   Binds to 50 S ribosomyl subunit of eukaryotes and inhibits peptidyltransferase.

12.8.   Binds to 60 S subunit of eukaryotes and inhibits peptidyltransferase.

12.9.   Binds to the 30 S ribosomyl subunit and causes misreading of mRNA.

12.10. Acts as analog of aminoacyl-tRNA and causes premature chain termination in both prokaryotes and eukaryotes.

12.11. Binds to 30 S ribosomal subunit to prevent the anticodon binding of aminoacyl-tRNA.

12.12. Binds to the 50 S ribosomal subunit and inhibits translocation.

In Questions 12.13–12.21, use the following key:
    a.   1, 2, and 3 are correct.
    b.   1 and 3 are correct.
    c.   2 and 4 are correct.
    d.   Only 4 is correct.
    e.   All are correct.

12.13. Because of "wobble" in the fit of tRNA with its codon, the tRNA may recognize several bases in the
    1.   First and second position of the codon
    2.   First position of the codon
    3.   First and third positions of the codon
    4.   Third position of the codon
    5.   Second and third position of the codon

12.14. Protein biosynthesis requires
    1.   GTP
    2.   Ribosomes
    3.   Peptidyltransferase
    4.   mRNA

12.15. During protein synthesis,
    1.   More than one ribosome can be bound to a mRNA at one time.
    2.   The carboxyl terminus of a polypeptide chain is synthesized before the amino terminus.
    3.   Two high-energy bonds are ultimately used for the synthesis of a aminoacyl-tRNA.
    4.   Formation of peptide bonds is coupled directly to GTP hydrolysis.

12.16. In prokaryotes, the formation of a functional 70 S ribosome requires
    1.   Formation of a complex of the 30 S ribosome with three initiation factors (IF-1, IF-2, and IF-3).
    2.   The binding of GTP to IF-2, which allows mRNA and fMet-tRNA to join the complex with the release of IF-3.
    3.   Addition of the 50 S subunit.
    4.   Hydrolysis of GTP causing release of IF-1 and IF-2.

12.17. Termination of protein synthesis in prokaryotes requires
    1.   A termination codon (UAA, UAG, or UGA) in the A site
    2.   GTP
    3.   Release factors (RF-1, RF-2, and RF-3)
    4.   tRNAs with anticodons complementary to termination signals

12.18. In eukaryotes,
    1.   The initiator tRNA is methionine tRNA.

2. There are several release factors as in prokaryotes.
3. Nine soluble initiation are known.
4. There is no GTP-GDP cycle as with prokaryotes.

12.19. The genetic code is
1. Degenerate (redundant) in a semisystematic way
2. Nonoverlapping
3. Nonambiguous
4. Absolutely universal

12.20. Suppressor genes
1. Act by altering the reading of mRNA
2. Exist for missense, nonsense, and for frameshift mutations caused by single nucleotide insertions and deletions.
3. Have actions that are often mediated by mutant tRNAs.
4. Have low efficiency is low.

12.21. In protein targeting and processing,
1. A hydrophobic signal sequence in the protein being synthesized on a free ribosome directs the ribosome to the endoplasmic reticulum.
2. The nascent protein synthesized by membrane-bound ribosomes is translocated in an ATP-drive reaction across the ER membrane into the ER lumen.
3. Many secretory and membrane proteins are modified in the lumen of the ER.
4. Proteins from the lumen and membrane of the ER are transferred by coated vesicles to the Golgi apparatus, where additional modifications (addition and removal of specific residues) take place.

Answers

12.1. (b) Puromycin causes premature chain termination in both pro- and eukaryotes; chloramphenicol binds to 50 S ribosomal subunit and inhibits peptidyl-synthetase; streptomycin binds to 30 S ribosome, causing misreading of mRNA, and so on. See Table 12.3.

12.2. (d)

12.3. (c) Amino acids must be activated by the formation of aminoacyl-tRNAs by the action of aminoacyl-tRNA synthetases.

12.4. (a)

12.5. (d) Introns are excised at the mRNA level.

12.6. (b)

12.7. (a) See Table 12.3.

12.8. (f) See Table 12.3.

12.9. (c) See Table 12.3.

12.10. (d) See Table 12.3.

12.11. (b) See Table 12.3.

12.12. (e) See Table 12.3.

12.13. (d)

12.14. (e)

12.15. (b) The peptide is synthesized in the amino to carboxyl direction. GTP does not provide the direct energy for peptide bond formation. This is provided by the original formation of the aminoacyl-tRNAs.

12.16. (e) See Figure 12.1.

12.17. (a) Normal cells do not contain tRNAs with anticodons complementary to termination signals. The stop signals are recognized by the release factors.

12.18. (b) There is a single release factor in eukaryotes, and a GTP-GDP is involved.

12.19. (a) It is not absolutely universal, being slightly different in human mitochondria.

12.20. (e)
12.21. (e)

PROBLEMS

12.1. A sequence of DNA is shown here. What are the sequences of all mRNAs that could be synthesized using this DNA as template?
5'-CAGTAAGGCTC-3'
3'-GTCATTCCGAG-5'

12.2. What happens if the following transversion mutations (change of a pyrimidine to a purine or the reverse) occur in the coding strand of a DNA molecule?
   a. From TCG to TAG
   b. From AAT to ATT
   c. From TTC to TTT
   d. From TTT to TGT

12.3. What are the accuracies of DNA synthesis, RNA synthesis, and protein synthesis? What mechanisms are employed, if any, to ensure some degree of fidelity in each case?

12.4. How many high-energy bonds are required to synthesize a protein of 100 amino acid residues? Assume that all components are available (amino acids, tRNA, ATP, and GTP).

BIBLIOGRAPHY

Alberts E, Bray P, Lewis J, Raff M, Roberts K, Watson J. Molecular Biology of the Cell, 3rd edition. New York: Garland, 1994.

Celis JE, Smith JD, editors. Nonsense Mutations and tRNA Suppressors. New York: Academic Press, 1979.

Freifelder D. Molecular Biology, 2nd edition. Boston: Jones and Bartlett, 1987.

Hershey JWB. Protein phosphorylation controls translation rates. J Biol Chem 264:20823–20826, 1989.

Pugsley AP, Protein Targeting. San Diego: Academic Press, 1989.

Rhoads RE. Regulation of eukaryotic protein synthesis by initiation factors. J Biol Chem 268:3017–3020, 1993.

Watson JD, Hopkins NH, Roberts JW, Steitz JA, Weiner AM. Molecular Biology of the Gene, 4th edition. Benjamin/Cummings Menlo Park, 1987.

13

Regulation of Gene Expression

After completing this chapter, the student should

1. Be able to define constitutive enzymes, inducible enzymes, enzyme repression, coordinate repression, and derepression.
2. Understand the function of the operon and its components.
3. Know the roles of a regulator gene, repressor and corepressor, catabolite gene activator protein (CAP), cyclic AMP, and attenuator.
4. Be able to describe the action of transposons.
5. Understand the basis for the lytic and lysogenic pathways for λ bacteriophage and its significance.
6. Be able to discuss the levels at which gene expression is controlled in prokaryotes.
7. Understand the differences in the structural organization of the genomes of prokaryotes and eukaryotes and the consequences for gene control.
8. Understand the role of condensation and decondensation of chromatin in eukaryotes.
9. Know what eukaryotic gene families are and how they are transcribed.
10. Understand gene amplification and its role.
11. Understand the role of enhancers and their general properties.
12. Understand the role of mRNA half-life in the regulation of gene expression.
13. Be able to discuss the various levels at which control of gene expression can be exercised in eukaryotes.
14. Know the stages in the eukaryotic cell cycle and the more important biochemical events in each stage.

13.1 INTRODUCTION

The diverse biochemical processes within a cell must be precisely regulated to ensure the integrated and orderly functioning of the cell. Numerous factors govern whether an enzyme, once present, functions: the availability of sub-strates and cofactors, the local pH, the effects of mass action, the competition of various enzyme systems for specific substrates in specific areas within the cells, and feedback inhibition are some of the factors that regulate biochemical pro-cesses (Chapter 5).

Genetic mechanisms must also exist that regulate when and if a gene is expressed and to what extent.

In this chapter we first discuss the better understood prokaryotic regula-tory mechanisms and follow this with a brief consideration of the less well understood and more complex eukaryotic regulatory mechanisms.

13.2 GENE REGULATION IN PROKARYOTES

It has been known for some time that bacteria can alter their enzyme composi-tion in response to changes in their environment. Early studies demonstrated that certain enzymes in microorganisms were produced in significant amounts only when their substrates were present in the culture medium. Such enzymes were considered a special group and were first called "adaptive" enzymes; now they are called *inducible* enzymes because they are formed *de novo* from amino acids rather than from protein precursors. Opposed to the inducible enzymes were the *constitutive* enzymes, which were formed in constant amounts regard-less of the metabolic state of the organism.

A classic example of an induced enzyme is the formation of β-galactosidase when wild-type *Escherichia coli* cells are grown on lactose as the sole source of carbon. After a brief lag period, large amounts of β-galactosidase are synthe-sized, the increase being from 5 to 10 molecules per cell to several thousand copies per cell. In addition to β-galactosidase, two other functionally related enzymes are formed, β-galactoside permease, and β-thiogalactoside trans-acetylase. The permease is required for the transport of lactose into the cell; the function of the transacetylase is uncertain. The induction of a group of related enzymes by a single inducing agent is *coordinate induction*, which can occur in bacteria because the genes for these three enzymes are contiguous and their products are encoded by a single polycistronic mRNA. This type of regulation does not occur in eukaryotes whose mRNA is monocistronic. A *cistron* is the smallest unit of genetic expression.

An effect opposite to induction is *enzyme repression*. Wild-type *E. coli* cells can be grown on a medium containing an ammonium salt as the sole source of nitrogen. Under these conditions, all nitrogenous compounds must be formed from ammonium ion and a carbon source, and such cells have all the enzymes necessary for the synthesis of the 20 amino acids requisite for protein synthesis. If, for example, the amino acid tryptophan is added to the culture medium, all the enzymes required for the biosynthesis of tryptophan disappear from the cell. In this case, the synthesis of five enzymes catalyzing five consecutive steps in tryptophan biosynthesis is repressed. This is a termed *coordinate repression*. It will become clear that induction and repression are manifestations of the same phenomenon.

The *operon model* was described in 1961 by F. Jacob and J. Monod to account for the molecular and genetic mechanisms involved in bacterial enzyme induction and enzyme repression. The model, slightly modified from that originally proposed and using the lactose (*lac*) operon as a specific example, is shown in Figure 13.1. According to this model, there are two basic types of genes: *structural* genes, whose primary product is mRNA, which carries structural information from cistrons (genes) to the ribosomes, and *control* genes, which regulate the rate at which structural genes function. Control genes were considered to be of two types, *operator* genes and *regulator* genes. The operator gene lies adjacent to the structural genes it controls. The operator locus was visualized as controlling the transcription of an entire group of coordinately induced genes to form a single polycistronic mRNA. The operator and its associated structural genes are called an *operon*. Operators act only on adjacent structural genes and have no action on genes on the other chromosomes of diploid organisms.

The activity of the operator gene is controlled by the *regulator* gene (i), which produces a specific protein, the *repressor*. The repressor protein can com-

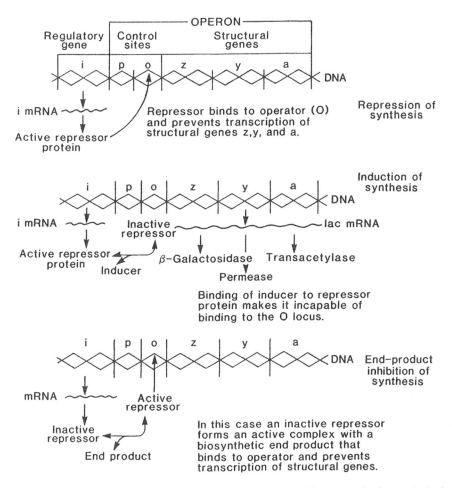

Figure 13.1 Operon model for control of protein synthesis. The example chosen is the lactose (*lac*) operon. I, regulatory gene; p, promoter site; o, operator gene; z, y, and a represent the structural genes for β-galactosidase, permease, and transacetylase, respectively.

bine with the operator, blocking the action of the operator gene and preventing transcription of the operon and, thereby, protein synthesis. The repressor protein acts on the operator genes of both homologous chromosomes. In *enzyme induction*, the inducer combines with the repressor protein to yield an inactive repressor–inducer complex incapable of binding to the operator. This releases the operon from inhibition and allows the initiation of protein synthesis. The inactivation of the repressor by the inducer is *derepression*.

In *end-product repression* (see later), it was postulated that the repressor protein is inactive until it binds the repressing metabolite (*corepressor*) to form an active repressor–corepressor complex that can combine with the operator gene to block synthesis at the operon.

The *lac* repressor protein is a tetramer of 37 kD identical subunits, each having one binding site for the inducer. The isolated repressor has a very high affinity for the operator site. The operator binding site for repressor has been isolated and characterized: the region contains 28 base pairs arranged so that rotation of the double helix by 180° yields the same sequence. This twofold axial symmetry is referred to as *dyad* symmetry. Because the *lac* repressor is composed of an even number (four) of identical subunits, its dyad symmetry matches that of its binding site on DNA so that complementary binding readily takes place.

There is yet another site in the *lac* operon immediately in front of the *lac* operator, the *promoter* (p) site, that is recognized by the RNA polymerase and the catabolite gene activator protein (CAP) that binds cAMP. It was found in bacteria that exogenous cAMP could relieve the catabolite repression of β-galactosidase synthesis and other catabolic enzymes by glucose. Other studies showed that cAMP stimulated the transcription of inducible operons by an interaction with the promoter site. When glucose is present (or its metabolites), the level of cAMP is somehow kept low, and the synthesis of enzymes requisite for using such energy sources as lactose is inhibited. When glucose levels decrease and an alternative carbon source, such as lactose, is available, the level of cAMP increases and is bound to CAP. This cAMP–CAP complex then binds to the promoter next to the site for RNA polymerase and stimulates initiation of transcription. CAP is a dimer of identical 22 kD subunits, each containing a DNA binding domain and a cAMP binding domain. As does the *lac* repressor, CAP exhibits 2-fold symmetry that matches its DNA binding site. The transcription rate of the *lac* operon is enhanced some 20- to 50-fold in the presence of cAMP-CAP. This *positive* transcriptional control is probably a result of an increased affinity of RNA polymerase holoenzyme for the promoter produced by the bound cAMP-CAP.

Because the ratios of the number of copies of the three *lac* operon enzymes are 1.0:0.5:0.2 for the galactosidase, permease, and transacetylase, respectively, some translational regulation must also occur. These differences could be the result of a balance between the detachment of the *lac* mRNA from its ribosome following chain termination and the reinitiation at subsequent start codons. This could produce a gradient from the 5′ terminus to the 3′ terminus of the polycistronic mRNA. Also, at any time, there are more complete copies of the Z gene product than the y gene product and more complete copies of the y gene product than of the A gene. Additionally, degradation of *lac* mRNA may occur more frequently in the A gene than in the Y gene and more frequently in the Y gene than in the Z gene.

Other sugars (galactose, maltose, and sorbitol) are converted to either glucose or some intermediate in glycolysis during their catabolism. These sugars are degraded by inducible operons that cannot be induced in the presence of glucose. These are *catabolite-sensitive operons*.

In *E. coli*, tryptophan is synthesized from an aromatic precursor, chorismic acid, in a five-step sequence involving five enzymes. The five proteins are translated from a single polycistronic trpRNA coordinately, sequentially, and in equimolar amounts. Translation occurs *before* completion of transcription. The *trp* operon (Figure 13.2) contains five structural genes for the enzymes of the biosynthetic pathway: two regions, the *attenuator* (a) and the *leader* (trpL), adjacent to trpE, and an *operator* gene (o) situated entirely within the *promoter*. A *repressor* gene (trpR) is located far from the trp operon.

We noted earlier the coordinate repression of the enzymes for tryptophan synthesis in the presence of tryptophan. When the level of tryptophan is depleted or reduced, trp mRNA is synthesized in 3–4 minutes and rapidly degraded; it has a half-life of some 3 minutes. This allows the bacteria to respond quickly to changing requirements for tryptophan.

The product of the *trpR* gene is an *aporepressor* protein consisting of four identical subunits, which does not bind to the operator unless tryptophan is present. A complex of the aporepressor and tryptophan binds tightly to the operator and prevents the RNA polymerase from binding to the *trp* promoter, so that transcription is prevented. The reactions are as follows:

Aporepressor →   no repressor (transcription occurs)
Aporepressor + tryptophan → active repressor
          operator——┐
               inactive promoter (transcription inhibited)

Binding of tryptophan to the aporepressor apparently produces a conformational change that enhances the binding to the trp o site. The target for the tryptophan–repressor complex is again a DNA sequence with twofold symmetry. Contrary to lactose, which causes the release fo the repressor from the *lac* operator, tryptophan acts as a *corepressor*, stimulating the binding of the repressor to the *trp* operator.

The *trp* operon has no positive control system like cAMP-CAP, but it does have an additional transcriptional control mechanism that depends on the concentration of tryptophan. This involves the *attenuator* site, which resides within the *leader* (L) sequence. It consists of 14 adjacent codons beginning with a methionine codon (AUG) and ending with a termination codon (UGA) and, importantly, codons (UGG) for tryptophan at positions 10 and 11. When tryptophan is plentiful, the complete 14-residue polypeptide (*leader polypeptide*) is synthesized. When tryptophan is scarce, the ribosome stalls at the tandem UGG

60	162			1560	1585	1350	1196	804	
P	o	L	a	L	E	D	C	B	A	Spacer

Figure 13.2 *E. coli* tryptophan (*trp*) operon. o, operator; L, leader; a, attenuator; E, D, C, B, A, structural genes. Numbers are base pairs.

codons because of a lack of tryptophanyl-tRNA. The stalled ribosome alters the mRNA structure so that the tryptophan codons are *not* read as a termination signal for the RNA polymerase and the RNA polymerase continues on into the *trp*E gene. Transcription and translation are closely coupled; the ribosome translating the *trp* leader follows closely behind the RNA polymerase that is transcribing the DNA template. When tryptophan is present and there is no need to synthesize tryptophan, transcription stops after the synthesis of a 140-nucleotide transcript. This provides the RNA polymerase a second chance to stop transcription of unneeded tryptophan enzymes. Attenuation has some 10-fold effect on transcription of tryptophan structural genes, and derepression has a 70-fold effect. *E. coli* thus has the ability to vary the rate of production of tryptophan biosynthetic enzymes over a 700-fold range.

Attenuation of transcription is relatively common in bacterial gene expression and occurs in at least six other amino acid biosynthetic pathways (histidine, threonine, phenylalanine, leucine, isoleucine, and valine). These are also based on the coupling of transcription and translation.

There are some recent data suggesting that attenuation of transcription may occur in eukaryotes. If this is true, however, the mechanism must be completely different, because the compartmentalization in eukaryotes would not allow for the close coupling of transcription (in the nucleus) and translation (in the cytoplasm).

The genes for the more than 50 kinds of ribosomal proteins are located in 20 or more operons. Despite this, their synthesis is strictly balanced. Control is exerted at the level of translation rather than transcription. At least one ribosomal protein encoded by a polycistronic operon acts as a translational repressor and acts when ribosomal protein synthesis exceeds that of ribosomal RNAs or when these proteins are not formed in equimolar quantities.

When there are not sufficient amino acids for the cell to maintain protein synthesis, the synthesis of rRNAs and tRNAs is reduced some 20-fold. This adaption is the *stringent response* and is mediated by guanosine tetraphosphate (ppGpp), which is triggered by the presence of an uncharged tRNA in the A site of the ribosome. Further elongation stops, and a protein called *stringent factor* synthesizes guanosine tetraphosphate from ATP and GDP. The exact mechanism of guanosine tetraphosphate action is unknown, but it appears to inhibit the initiation of transcription of the rRNA and tRNA genes.

Most bacterial genes are fixed in the chromosome and their positions relative to other genes do not change, but there are chromosomal segments that are able to relocate (transpose) to another part of the chromosome, to a plasmid, or to a separate chromosome in eukaryotes. These are known as *transposable elements* or *transposons*. Their movement is infrequent and usually random and produces insertions, deletions, and other complicated rearrangements that can disrupt the reading frame, alter mRNA stability, and insert termination signals. They vary greatly in size, from a few thousand base pairs containing two or three genes to many thousands of base pairs containing several genes. Most if not all transposons encode an enzyme, a *transposase*, that carries out the DNA cutting and ligation reactions requisite for their movement. The first 20–40 nucleotides at one end is repeated but oriented oppositely at the other end—these are *inverted repeats* and are essential for the insertion of a copy into another location.

Often they contain genes that encode for antibiotic resistance that can be found on plasmids (a circular DNA duplex that replicates autonomously). Plasmids can be passed from one bacterial strain to another and produce resistance to antibiotics in the recipient strains. This can increase the number of pathogenic strains that become resistant to antibiotics.

A brief discussion of the role of repressors and activators in regulating the life cycle of λ bacteriophage is useful as an example of how a few reciprocally acting gene regulatory proteins can influence a complex pattern of gene expression. It may help in understanding how large numbers of genes are switched on and off in a multicellular eukaryote. The bacterial virus has two available pathways after infection of its *E. coli* host: multiply in the cytosol and kill the host, or become integrated into the host cell DNA and be automatically replicated each time the bacterium divides. There is a switchlike mechanism, governed by proteins encoded by the bacteriophage genome of some 50 genes, that determines the lytic or lysogenic pathways. In the *lytic pathway*, all viral functions are completely expressed, causing lysis of the host cell and the release of several hundred progeny virus particles. In the *lysogenic pathway*, most phage functions are repressed when its DNA is integrated into the host DNA. The viral DNA in this stage is a *prophage*, and the host cell is a lysogenic bacterium. Two regulatory proteins are synthesized by the virus: the λ *repressor protein* and the *cro protein*. Each of these, when bound to the operator site for the other gene, blocks the synthesis of the other. The λ repressor dominates in the lysogenic state, and the cro protein dominates in the lytic state. The lysogenic stage, which occurs more frequently, is usually adopted when the host bacteria are growing well. If the bacteria are damaged or not growing well because of some environmental restriction, the integrated provirus can leave the host chromosome, multiply in the cytosol, and subsequently escape to find a healthy host cell.

13.3   GENE REGULATION IN EUKARYOTES

Knowledge of gene regulation in eukaryotes is significantly less than that for prokaryotes. The genome of the eukaryotic cell is much larger than that of *E. coli* and much more highly organized. We have already noted the tight packaging of DNA with histones to form chromatin in eukaryotes, the presence of introns in most eukaryotic genes, the extensive posttranscriptional modifications in eukaryotes, the segregation of transcription from the translational process in eukaryotes, and the absence of polycistronic RNAs and operons in eukaryotes. It should also be noted that the cells of a multicellular organism all contain the *same* DNA and differ from each other by virtue of the proteins they synthesize. It follows from this that different cell types transcribe different sets of genes. Although the gene regulatory mechanism of prokaryotes could in principle operate in eukaryotes, more complex as well as additional mechanisms not found in bacteria must operate in eukaryotes. Gene regulation could operate at any or all of the steps from DNA to protein: at transcription (probably the most important), at RNA processing, by selection of which mRNAs are transported from the nucleus to the cytoplasm, at translation, and by selectively stabilizing or degrading specific mRNA molecules in the cytoplasm.

It has been speculated that gene activator proteins, rather than gene repressor proteins, predominate in eukaryotic cells. Because only about 6–7% of eukaryotic DNA is transcribed into RNA, it seems unlikely that blocking of this massive amount of untranscribed DNA is achieved by thousands of different repressor proteins. Rather, some general mechanism for gene repression is employed, and specific gene regulatory proteins serve to turn on specific genes for transcription. Although little is known about the mechanism whereby a large number of eukaryotic genes might be switched on and off in an orderly way, we suggested that the λ repressor protein and cro protein are evolutionary prototypes whereby a few gene regulatory proteins might specify different cell types by interacting in a combinatorial fashion. There is evidence from embryogenesis in *Drosophila* that a single mutation can convert one part of the body to another. The proteins coded by the mutant gene are presumed to be master gene regulatory proteins, possibly acting like the λ repressor and *cro* protein.

The heterochromatin region of a eukaryotic chromosome must be *decondensed* to a bead-on-a-string conformation to be accessible to transcriptional proteins. When tightly bound by chromosomal proteins, the DNA is unavailable for transcription. In actively transcribed genes, the regular packaging of DNA into nucleosomes is altered or absent. Decondensed DNA is more sensitive to DNase I, and cytosine sites in or near the gene(s) being transcribed are usually undermethylated compared with genes not being transcribed. Histone H1, which binds to nucleosomes to augment their packing together, is highly acetylated in many transcriptionally active nucleosomes. It is also known that two nonhistone proteins, HMG14 and HMG16, bind to the nucleosomes of active genes. These, as well as other yet unknown factors, probably function in some cooperative manner to convert the chromatin fibers to a bead-on-a-string conformation in which transcription can be initiated. Subsequent transcription of the exposed chromatin is presumed to be regulated by activator and repressor proteins resembling those in prokaryotes. Recondensation of the chromatin would prevent transcription and provide a basis for controlling the expression of a gene by altering the availability of the DNA to the transcriptional process.

One known example of inactivation of a gene by condensation of euchromatin to heterochromatin is the inactivation of one X chromosome in mammalian females. This occurs early in embryonic development, at the 20-cell stage. It has been suggested that this is achieved by heavy methylation.

Many eukaryotic genes are functionally related and are often organized as a set of genes called a gene cluster or gene family. The activity of members of a set is usually coordinately regulated, possibly by chromatin condensation and decondensation. These gene families range from *simple* multigene families, in which one or a few genes are repeated in tandem array, to *complex* multigene families, in which there is a cluster of functionally related genes. In both cases each gene is separated by a spacer that may be severalfold larger than the gene. Each gene is transcribed as a separate RNA molecule that is processed to generate the final molecule. Each gene may be transcribed in the same direction, that is, from the same DNA strand, or in both directions, that is, from both DNA strands.

Hemoglobin (Chapter 14) is an example of a *developmentally controlled complex gene family* in which the presence of α- and β-like subunits depends on the state of development of the organism. The immunoglobulins also represent a developmental regulatory process, but in this case it is fully active in the adult organism. The genetics of hemoglobin and hemoglobin diseases and immunoglobulin genetics are presented in some detail in the next chapter.

Gene alteration, with a resultant change in primary transcripts, can occur by *gene loss, gene amplification*, and *gene rearrangement*. Gene loss in lower eukaryotes occurs by chromosome loss, which has not been seen in higher eukaryotes. Gene amplification (the duplication of a specific gene within a chromosome two or more times) often occurs when there is large demand for a specific gene product. The most thoroughly investigated example of this is in the development of the eggs of the toad (*Xenopus laevis*) in which genes for rRNA increase in number some 4000-fold. This allows the oocyte to synthesize 10^{12} ribosomes needed for the large amount of protein synthesis required for the rapid cell cleavage stages following fertilization. Because it is no longer needed once the oocyte has matured, this excess rDNA is degraded.

Amplification of a specific gene can be selected and stabilized by environmental pressure. If mammalian cells growing in culture are exposed to methotrexate (an inhibitor of the enzyme dehydrofolate reductase, Chapter 6), most of the cells die. The rare survivors are cells capable of producing large amounts of the essential enzyme. Repeated selection yields cells with a 1000-fold amplification of the normally single haploid copy of the enzyme gene. In this procedure, the drug selects those rare cells that have amplified their target; it does not induce gene amplification.

Gene rearrangement is a very complex process, and a detailed consideration is beyond the scope of this book. We discuss only the turning on of immunoglobulin gene expression in which DNA rearrangement positions a promoter in the vicinity of a B cell-specific enhancer (Chapter 14).

Enhancers are DNA sequences that stimulate the rate of transcription for promoters located several kilobases upstream or downstream. They function in either orientation, that is, on either the coding or the template strand. They have no promoter activity themselves and are not gene specific, acting on any nearby gene as long as it is in the same DNA molecule. They often exhibit tissue and species specificity. Tissue-specific enhancers might provide a basis for the differential expression of genes during development. An example discussed later is the initiation of immunoglobulin gene expression after DNA rearrangement that places a promoter near a B cell-specific enhancer. A particular enhancer is effective only in certain cell types: the immunoglobulin enhancer only in B lymphocytes and the glucocorticoid enhancer only in cells that contain the hormone receptor that activates the enhancer. How these elements regulate transcription is unknown. However, they must somehow render the DNA in the vicinity of a promoter more accessible for the binding of RNA polymerase II and/or its associated factors. However they function, they probably play a major role in the control of gene expression.

If a large amount of protein is required over an extended period of time, this could be achieved by increasing the stability of mRNA. Gene amplification would be unnecessary.

Little is known about what determines mRNA half-life. We do not know whether the stability of certain mRNAs, such as hemoglobin mRNA in reticulocytes, is an intrinsic property of the molecule itself or whether stabilizing proteins are involved. The mechanism of action of steroid hormones probably involves the stabilization of specific mRNAs.

In the eukaryotic cell, the levels of histone mRNA vary with the cell cycle (see later). The levels are low during most phases of the cell cycle but rise 20- to 40-fold when DNA is replicated during the S phase. This is a result of transcriptional regulation and an increase in histone mRNA half-life from 8 to 40 minutes. In the absence of DNA synthesis, any histone mRNA is degraded within minutes. This is apparently caused by the activation of a degradation pathway that specifically selects histone mRNA. The 3' terminus of this mRNA is not polyadenylated: this and a 16-nucleotide looped structure apparently allow the specific recognition. The rate of degradation (3' → 5') is equal for all five histone mRNAs. Another example of posttranscriptional regulation by altering the stability of mRNA is the required presence of the hormone prolactin, which stabilizes the mRNA for casein.

Regulation of eukaryotic translation provides a rapid way to control gene expression and is used frequently. In some cases this is achieved by altering components of the translational complex. This is expected to affect the translation of all mRNAs. Such a mechanism is the phosphorylation of 40 S ribosomal proteins, which results in higher polysome levels in cells stimulated by growth factors.

One example of the control of a specific protein at the translational level is the regulation of hemoglobin synthesis by the availability of heme (Chapter 7). This occurs in mammalian reticulocytes that have lost their nucleus but have high levels of stable mRNAs coding for the hemoglobin. When the concentration of heme decreases, the synthesis of hemoglobin decreases. The decline occurs because heme deficiency activates an inhibitor of protein synthesis initiation. This inhibitor, *heme-controlled inhibitor* (HCI), is an active protein kinase that catalyzes the phosphorylation of the α subunit of eIF_2 (Table 12.2). When the eIF_2 α subunit is phosphorylated by HCI, it is unable to hydrolyze GTP to GDP + P_i, an essential reaction in the formation of the 80 S initiation complex. Initiation of protein chains is blocked. Excess heme binds to HCI and inactivates it. A phosphatase can remove the phosphate.

13.4 CELL CYCLE INFORMATION FLOW: STAGES AND GENERAL BIOCHEMICAL EVENTS

Before a cell can divide, it must essentially double its mass and duplicate all of its contents, so that the two new daughter cells have all the components to initiate their own cycles of cell growth and division. Because the events of nuclear division (mitosis) and cytoplasmic division (*cytokinesis*) produced dramatic morphologic changes readily seen with the light microscope, earlier studies focused on these relatively brief events. In the time between divisions (*interphase*), little seemed to be happening. We now know that most of the biochemical events in preparation for division occur continuously throughout interphase.

A typical eukaryotic cell cycle is shown in Figure 13.3. Following *mitosis* and *cytokinesis*, the daughter cells begin the interphase of a new cycle with the G_1 (gap 1) phase in which biosynthetic activities markedly increase. The G_1 phase is

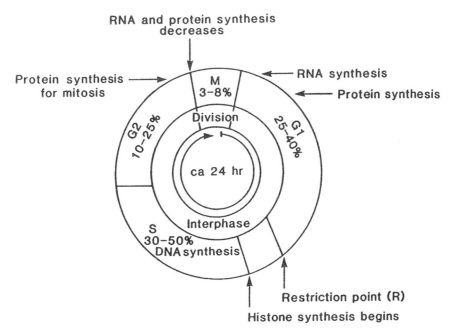

Figure 13.3 Typical eukaryotic cell cycle. *M*, mitotic phase; G_1, gap phase; *S*, synthesis phase; G_2, gap phase 2. The percentage of times shown for each phase are ranges for cells with cell cycle times of approximately 24 h.

much more variable in length than the other three phases, and it is the length of time spent in the G_1 phase that is responsible for differences in cell cycle times. There is some evidence to suggest that the length of this phase is directly related to the cell mass that must be duplicated.

Cells that stop dividing normally arrest in the G_1 phase. Depending on the cell type, cell cycle times can range from 8 to 10 h to 100 days or more. However, the time for a cell to progress from *S* through *M* is unusually constant despite its division rate. It appears that once a cell has passed a point in late G_1, the *restriction point* (*R* point), it is committed to completing the *S*, G_2, and *M* phases. It has been suggested that cells accumulate a threshold level of an unstable protein (*U protein*) that allows the cell to pass through the *R* point and initiate DNA synthesis and subsequent mitosis. Because RNA and protein synthesis are markedly reduced in the *M* phase, the concentration of the putative U protein is reduced and would have to be increased to the threshold level in G_1 to initiate a cycle of cell division.

It has been shown in fission yeast that a gene called *CDC2* is required for the cell to pass through a G_1 control point and continue through the other phases. The gene has been cloned and shown to encode a protein kinase that appears to be a homolog of vertebrate *M*-phase promoting factor (MPF). MPF has two subunits, one of which is a protein kinase that can phosphorylate the other subunit. A similar homologous gene has been found in budding yeast. MPF activity may be regulated by phosphorylation. The MPF kinase phosphorylates several substrates, for example histone H1, and it is possible that a phosphorylation cascade triggers the cell cycle events. There is also an S-phase activator that delays the M phase until DNA synthesis has been completed. A protein, *cyclin*, was first identified in primitive marine organisms and later in more complex organisms. Cyclin concentration was found to rise during interphase to a maximum halfway through M phase, when it abruptly dropped to zero. This suggested that the time between one mitosis and the next could be determined by the time required for the concentration of cyclin to rise from zero to some threshold value, which was supported by the observation that inhibitors of protein synthesis blocked the cell cycle in interphase. Very recently it was found that there are several different types of cyclins (perhaps six to eight in humans) that are produced and destroyed at each step of the cell cycle. Presumably, a different cyclin is active at specific stages of the division cycle, thus requiring the destruction of one type and the creation afresh of a new type. It is thought that a CDC type of protein combines with a specific cyclin to activate the first phase of cell division and each subsequent phase. These CDC-specific cyclin complexes phosphorylate other proteins to alter their form and functions. Such altered proteins could aid in the unwinding of the DNA duplex, activate the genes for the enzymes involved in DNA replication, and promote the separation of duplicated chromosomes before cytokinesis. At this time it appears very likely that a protein phosphorylation cascade has a paramount role in the initiation and control of the cell cycle in yeast and higher organisms.

During the S phase, each strand of parental DNA is replicated only once, and the two new strands combine with both newly synthesized and old histones. Histones are synthesized primarily during the S phase, and once they are assembled in nucleosomes, they remain bound to the DNA strand. It appears that the preexisting histone octamers are transferred to the daughter DNA helix formed on the leading strand at a replication fork (see Chapter 12) while new histones are assembled into nucleosomes on the lagging strand.

Thus, in some cells, parental histones appear to be inherited directly. Simian virus 40 may be an exception. When DNA synthesis ceases at the end of the S phase, any histone mRNA is rapidly degraded. This link between DNA synthesis and histone synthesis may serve as a feedback mechanism to ensure that the amount of new histone formed is consonant with the amount of new DNA synthesized.

Following the S phase is the G_2 phase, in which the cell prepares for mitosis and cytokinesis. Although few of the molecular events that occur in G_2 phase have been identified, it is known that some proteins synthesized during this period are essential for cell division. It is believed that contractile proteins necessary for chromosome separation and cytokinesis accumulate and are accompanied by modifications in the structure of chromosomal proteins. The phosphorylation of histone H1, known to be involved in the packaging of nucleosomes, could cause the initiation of chromosome condensation that directs the cell into mitosis.

G_2 ends as the first of the five stages of cell division, prophase, begins. *Prophase* is defined as the first appearance of condensed chromosomes. This is followed by *metaphase*, in which spindle fibers appear leading from centromeres to opposite sides, or *poles*, of the cells. The sister chromosomes (i.e., the pairs formed by replication of single chromosomes in S) become aligned in one plane in a region called the metaphase plate. During *anaphase*, the chromosomes migrate to the pole region. This serves to segregate the two identical copies of each chromosome to the two poles. In *telophase*, each set of chromosomes acquires a nuclear envelope, the chromosomes disperse, and the nucleolus or nucleoli reforms. In most cases telophase is followed by *cytokinesis*, in which the cell membrane pinches off at the metaphase plate to yield two new cells. Following this, cells commonly enter either the G_1 phase or G_0 phase. In G_0, a stable resting state, phase proliferation ceases, in some cases forever. Cells can return to G_1 after receiving an appropriate biochemical signal. This signal can be the removal of an inhibitor of proliferation.

Although the mechanisms for the control of cell division in tissues are largely unknown, it is clear in normal situations that cells divide only if new cells are needed. A classic example is the liver, which can regenerates its normal mass within a week or so after removal of two-thirds of its mass. Other tissues exhibit a smaller type of limited cell division. Whatever the normal feedback control mechanisms, it is clear that cancer cells have lost the normal growth controls and continue to divide in an uncontrolled manner until the host is destroyed.

QUESTIONS

Answer Questions 13.1–13.5 using the following key:
  a. 1, 2, and 3 are correct.
  b. 1 and 3 are correct.
  c. 2 and 4 are correct.
  d. Only 4 is correct.
  e. All are correct.

13.1   An operon
  1. Codes for a polycistronic mRNA
  2. Has control sequences, such as an operator
  3. Contains promoter(s)
  4. Is a gene that is controlled by a regulatory gene

13.2.   In the tryptophan operon,
  1. Tryptophan is synthesized in five steps, each requiring a specific enzyme
  2. Requires a corepressor
  3. Transcription and translation are closely coupled
  4. There is an attenuator site in a leader sequence

13.3.   In the stringent response,
  1. GTP is involved as a mediator
  2. Synthesis of rRNAs and tRNAs is reduced 20-fold
  3. ATP is required
  4. A protein factor is involved

13.4.   Transposons are chromosomal segments that
  1. Can be relocated to another part of the chromosome
  2. Most encode an enzyme transposase
  3. Often contain genes that encode for antibiotic resistance
  4. Can produce insertions and deletions and disrupt a reading frame

13.5.   All the following statements about λ bacteriophage are true, *except*
  a. Has two pathways available after infection of its *E. coli* host
  b. Produces a λ repressor protein

　　c.　Produces a cro protein
　　d.　The λ repressor dominates in the lytic state
13.6.　All of the following statements about gene regulation in eukaryotes is true, *except*
　　a.　Gene activator proteins rather than gene repressor proteins probably dominate
　　b.　Invites coordinate expression of a polycistronic mRNA
　　c.　Gene regulation could operate at any or all steps from DNA to protein
　　d.　The heterochromatic region of chromosomes must be decondensed to a bead-on-a-string conformation to be transcribed

Answer Questions 13.7–13.9 using the following key:
　　a.　1, 2, and 3 are correct.
　　b.　1 and 3 are correct.
　　c.　2 and 4 are correct.
　　d.　Only 4 is correct.
　　e.　All are correct.

13.7.　Enhancers are DNA sequences that
　　1.　Stimulate the rate of transcription for promoters located several kilobases upstream or downstream
　　2.　Function on either the coding or template strand
　　3.　Have no promoter activity
　　4.　Often exhibit tissue and species specificity
13.8.　In the eukaryotic cell,
　　1.　Levels of histone mRNAs vary with the cell cycle
　　2.　The half-life of histone mRNAs is increased during DNA synthesis
　　3.　In the absence of DNA synthesis, any histone mRNA is degraded within minutes
　　4.　The 3′ terminus of histone is polyadenylated
13.9.　In hemoglobin synthesis,
　　1.　Excess heme binds to an inhibitor (HCI) and inactivates it
　　2.　When the concentration of heme decreases, the synthesis of hemoglobin decreases
　　3.　The HCI inhibitor is a protein kinase that catalyzes the phosphorylation of eIF_2
　　4.　Heme deficiency activates an inhibitor of hemoglobin synthesis

In Questions 13.10–13.17, select the answers from the different phases in the cell cycle listed in a–e.
　　a. M phase　　b. G_0 phase　　c. G_1 phase
　　d. S phase　　e. G_2 phase

13.10.　Replication of parental DNA.
13.11.　The most variable phase with respect to time.
13.12.　Cytokinesis takes place.
13.13.　Microtubules are apparently synthesized.
13.14.　Mitotic spindle forms.
13.15.　Biosynthesis of histones.
13.16.　A phase that does not lead to cell division unless a division command is given.
13.17.　The R point appears at the end of which phase?

Answers

13.1.　(e)　See Figure 13.1.
13.2.　(e)

13.3. (c) GTP is not involved. Guanosine tetraphosphate (ppGpp), which mediates the response, is formed from ATP and GDP by a protein called stringent factor.

13.4. (e)

13.5. (d) The λ repressor dominates in the lysogenic state, the cro protein in the lytic state.

13.6. (b) Polycistronic mRNAs do not occur in eukaryotes.

13.7. (e)

13.8. (a) The 3' terminus.

13.9. (e) Hemoglobin synthesis is controlled at the translational level by the availability of heme. It declines when heme concentration falls and increases when heme concentration rises. Heme deficiency activates an inhibitor.

13.10. (d) DNA is replicated in the S phase.

13.11. (c) Whereas the $S + M + G_2$ phases are quite constant from cell to cell, the G phase may vary considerably.

13.12. (a) Cytokinesis is cytoplasm division, and this occurs during the M phase.

13.13. (e) Proteins necessary for cell division (e.g., contractile).

13.14. (a) The mitotic spindle is part of the cell division process, and this takes place during the M phase.

13.15. (d) Biosynthesis of histones occurs as DNA division occurs. The cell creates exactly the quantity of histones needed, and then the histone mRNA is degraded.

13.16. (b) The cell may be arrested in the G_0 phase after cell division. It proceeds into the G_1 phase. This is a point in the cell cycle beyond which the cell is committed to divide.

13.17. (c) The R point appears at the end of the G_1 phase. This is a point in the cell cycle beyond which the cell is committed to divide.

PROBLEMS

13.1. How does the regulation of transcription in eukaryotes differ from that in bacteria?

13.2. Propose models for the action of enhancers in regulating transcription over large DNA distances.

13.3. Can gene expression be controlled by changes in mRNA stability?

BIBLIOGRAPHY

Alberts B, Bray D, Lewis J, Raff M, Roberts K, Watson JD. Molecular Cell Biology of the Cell, 3rd ed. New York: Garland, 1994.

Darnell J, Lodish H, Baltimore D. Molecular Cell Biology. Scientific American Books, 1986.

Freifelder D. Molecular Biology, 2nd ed. Boston: Jones & Bartlett, 1987.

Levin B. Genes, 3rd ed. New York: Wiley, 1987.

Russel P. Lecture Notes on Genetics. Oxford: Blackwell Scientific, 1980.

Watson JD, Hospkins NH, Roberts JW, Steitz JA, Weiner AM. Molecular Biology of the Gene, 4th ed. Menlo Park: Benjamin/Cummings, 1987.

14

Genetic Control of Synthesis of Immunoglobulins and Hemoglobin

After completing this chapter, the student should

1. Be able to describe the general structure of immunoglobulin molecules.
2. Be able to describe the distribution of the various gene pools and understand how they are rearranged to produce antibody diversity.
3. Understand the clonal selection theory.
4. Be able to describe the distribution of the various hemoglobins' genes.
5. Know the base for hemoglobin variants and why some are harmless and some are not.
6. Understand the etiology of the thalassemias and the hemoglobin profile in each type.

14.1 INTRODUCTION

We discuss in this chapter some specific proteins that not only are important in their own right but also provide in their diversity some insight into the functioning of the complex gene regulatory system that exists in more complex eukaryotic organisms.

14.2 IMMUNOGLOBULINS

The immune system is a highly dynamic system, and its hallmark is its ability to produce an astonishing variety of specific proteins that include both antibodies (immunoglobulin) and T-cell receptor proteins. This is accomplished by molecular and cellular mechanisms that generate a large number of proteins and specifically select a few of these for amplification. This diversity has its origins in genetic rearrangements of relatively few gene segments in the germline DNA, followed by somatic recombination and somatic mutation.

Antibody activity is associated with three major classes of plasma proteins, immunoglobulins that are synthesized in the plasma cells and lymphoid cells, designated IgG, IgA, and IgM. Two additional types of immunoglobulin, designated IgD and IgE, are found in plasma in very small amounts.

IgG, IgA, IgM, IgD, and IgE consist of a pair of identical light chains (that is, they all share the same light chains) designated as κ or λ, with a molecular weight of 25,000 each, and a pair of heavy chains designated γ, α, μ, δ, and ϵ, respectively, with a molecular weight of about 50,000 each. All are joined by disulfide bonds. Thus, an IgG molecule can exist as $\kappa_2\gamma_2$ or $\lambda_2\gamma_2$; an IgA molecule as $\kappa_2\alpha_2$ or $\lambda_2\alpha_2$, and so on. The heavy chains (γ, α, μ, γ, and ϵ) differ in structure from each other and carry the antigenic determinants characteristic of their respective immunoglobulin classes.

IgG molecules can be further subdivided into the IgG_1 through IgG_4 subclasses. The percentages for a normal adult are 70, 20, 8, and 2%, respectively. These subclasses differ with regard to the number of disulfide bonds and amino acids in the hinge region (Figure 14.1) and amino acid sequences in the constant

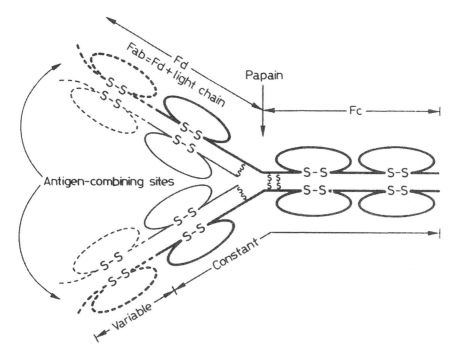

Figure 14.1 The linear polypeptide chain structure of immunoglobulin. Two identical half-molecules are symmetrically arranged; each contains a light chain (the light line) and a heavy chain (the darker line). The light chains may be either κ or λ and the heavy chains γ, α, μ, or ϵ, but hybrid combinations are not observed. The interchain and intrachain disulfide bridges are located in the correct position for human IgG_1 but may differ for other immunoglobulins. The variable region indicated by the dashed line occupies the first half of the light chain but only the first domain of the heavy chain. The Fc and Fab fragments are produced by limited proteolysis with papain or pepsin. Electron micrographs and x-ray crystal structures, as well as other data, suggest a forked structure with a flexible region near the hinge peptide bridging Fc and Fd in the heavy chain. (Reproduced from Clinical Physiology and Biochemistry by permission of S. Karger, A.G., Basel, Switzerland.)

regions of the heavy chains. However, the heavy chains of IgG subclasses carry extensive homologies.

The IgM molecule has a molecular weight of approximately 800,000 and consists of a cluster of five $\lambda_2\mu_2$ or $k_2\mu_2$ units, that is, $(\lambda_2\mu_2)_5$ or $(k_2\mu_2)_5$. Higher IgM polymers are also present in plasma. IgA may exist as a monomer $(\lambda_2\alpha_2$ or $k_2\alpha_2)$ or as a polymer, $(\lambda_2\alpha_2)_n$ or $(\kappa_2\mu_2)_n$, where $n = 2, 4$, and so on. All IgM molecules and polymeric forms of IgA contain an additional subunit, the *J chain*. Its function is to join the monomer units. IgA exists as *secretory* IgA in many external human secretions, such as milk, synovial fluid, tears, and semen. It consists of two IgA units, a J chain, and another subunit, the *secretory piece*. Secretory IgA has a molecular weight near 400,000.

The antigen-combining sites of immunoglobulin are located at the N-terminal ends of their subunits. To accommodate each specific antigen, the N-terminal regions of each specific antibody group of molecules differ from those of other groups of antibodies in amino acid sequences. We thus speak of N-terminal regions of immunoglobulin as *variable*, whereas the C termini are *constant* in amino acid sequences. The constant region carries carbohydrate as well as *complement* (C1q) recognition sites.

Figure 14.1 is a schematic diagram of the linear polypeptide chain structure of immunoglobulin. Both the light (L) and heavy (H) chains of this flexible Y-shaped molecule are divided into a variable, or *V* region, and a constant, or *C* region. The V regions of the H and L chains are the same length, whereas the C region of the H chain is about three times as long as that of the L chain. Both L and H chains are folded into compact domains, the L chain having one V and one C domain and the H chain having one V and three separate C domains, C_H^1, C_H^2, and C_H^3. The μ (IgM) and the ϵ (IgE) heavy chains have one V and four C domains. Note that the immunoglobulins are divalent, having two antigen binding sites at the N-terminal ends of the light- and heavy-chain pairs. This allows the binding of two antigens at a time and the possibility of interconnected matrices of antigens and antibodies, which could promote the removal of antigen molecules by precipitation and agglutination.

For each type of immunoglobulin chain, there exists a separate pool of genes from which a single polypeptide chain is synthesized. V genes in each pool are located far apart from one or more C genes in germline DNA but are closely associated in the DNA of antibody-producing cells. This requires the translocation of genes during the differentiation of lymphocytes.

The gene pools for coding κ, λ, and H chains are located on different chromosomes. The κ pool contains a single C gene and a few hundred V genes. The λ pool contains two V genes, each associated with one or two different C genes. The H gene pool contains some 300 V genes and a sequential cluster of different C genes, each coding for a different class of H chains ($C\mu$, $C\delta$, $C\gamma$, $C\epsilon$, and $C\alpha$).

It was found in embryonic cells that V genes did not encode for the entire variable regions in L and H chains. A short DNA segment, the *joining* or J gene segment, was identified that encoded the last 13 residues of the variable regions. A single J gene is associated with each C gene in the λ gene pool, four in the κ gene pool, and four or five in the H gene pool. The neighboring J gene segments in K and H are separated by an intron.

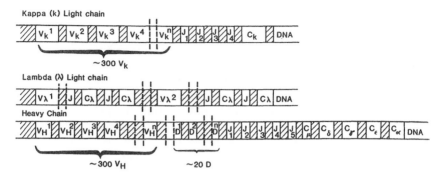

Figure 14.2 Immunoglobulin gene pools found in mammals (not drawn to scale): V, variable-region genes; J, joining segment; C, constant region; hatched areas are introns and leaders.

These relationships are shown schematically in Figure 14.2. Any V gene segment can be joined to any J gene segment in the κ- and H-chain gene pools, thus amplifying the diversity of the germline DNA. Additional diversification in the H chain comes from another gene segment, the D (*diversity*) gene segment. Some 15–20 D segments lie between the hundreds of V_H and J_H segments. A D segment can bind to any J_H segment and V_H gene. The site-specific recombination of D, J, and H genes is mediated by enzymes that recognize specific base sequences to the left and right of three genes. Palindromic sequences and a conserved AT-rich region are involved.

It was noted earlier that there are five classes of immunoglobulin. IgM is first synthesized by an antibody-producing cell, followed by IgG, IgA, IgD, or IgE of the same specificity. In this *class switching*, the L chain is the same and only the constant region of the H chain changes. The genes for the constant region of all heavy chains lie next to each other (Figure 14.2). In addition, there are four subclasses of IgG that differ in the number of disulfide bonds and amino acids in the hinge region. These are not shown in Figure 14.2. Thus, there are eight genes for the constant region of chains. A complete gene for the H chains of IgM consists of joining together V_H, D, J_H, and $C\mu$. This switching takes place in DNA by intrachromosomal recombination but not in RNA.

Figure 14.3 is a schematic representation of the assembly of a κ light chain; the λ chain is formed by a similar mechanism, differing in detail. In the germline DNA, the four J gene segments are separated from each other and the C gene by short introns. The V genes are separated from the J genes by hundreds or thousands of base pairs. During B cell maturation, randomly selected V and J segments are fused by enzymes that delete all intervening DNA (V_κ^3, V_κ^4, and J), bringing together V_κ^2 and J_2. This is followed by transcription of the entire length of DNA from the start of V_κ^2 to the end of C_κ. This is followed by excision of all the RNA from the end of J_2 (J_3 and J_4) to the start of C_κ. The mature mRNA is then translated into protein. The actual mechanism for joining V and J gene segments is unknown but is thought to be achieved by site-specific DNA recombination enzymes that recognize highly conserved DNA sequences downstream from V gene segments and upstream from J gene segments. These DNA recombination enzymes must break and rejoin the DNA double helix at these recogni-

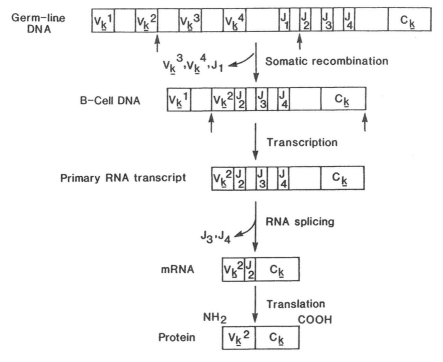

Figure 14.3 Assembly of a κ light chain from randomly selected V and J segments by somatic recombination. Transcription, posttranscriptional modification, and translation follow to yield a specific chain.

tion sites. RNA modifications are probably carried about by standard RNA-splicing enzymes.

It has been shown that the junction with a particular J gene is not absolutely precise. The site of the junction can vary by several base pairs. In some cases additional base pairs are inserted during the combination process. These changes alter the amino acid sequence of the polypeptide and generate more diversity.

Another major source of diversity are *somatic mutations*. These occur in and around V-region genes but not in constant domains. The rate of mutation has been estimated as 1 change in the V region for every 3–30 cell divisions. This is several orders of magnitude greater than the average rate for eukaryotic cells and suggests that there might be some enzymatic process in the B cell for producing mutations in the variable region. Such mutations may increase the number of different antibodies 100-fold.

The combining of different L and H chains, of different V, D, and J segments, of somatic mutant segments, and of other sources of diversity not discussed allow the generation of more than 10^8 different antibody molecules. Note that T cell receptors have α and β chains and contain variable and constant regions that are homologous in sequence and three-dimensional structure to the V and C genes of the immunoglobulin. Their V, D, J, and C genes are rearranged to produce a diversity comparable to that of the immunoglobulin.

The *clonal selection theory*, which is now firmly established, provides a unified explanation of how the immune system produces such a diversity of antibodies. It is based on the proposition that each antibody-producing cell (*lymphocyte*) is committed to synthesize a specific antibody *before* the cell encounters a specific antigen. During maturation, each cell produces small amounts of the specific antibody that appears on the cell surface. If it is a mature cell and encounters the appropriate antigen, it produces more antibody and is stimulated to multiply. Thus, a foreign antigen stimulates those cells that have complementary antigen-specific receptors and are precommitted to respond. The progeny of these cells are *clones*, which have the same genetic content as the original cell. If an immature cell encounters a self antigen corresponding to its antibody, it is destroyed or suppressed during fetal life; the result is an immune system able to respond only to foreign antigens.

Autoimmune reactions, those against self antigens, can occur and are responsible for a number of serious diseases. These *autoimmune diseases* display a spectrum. At one end there are *organ-specific diseases* with organ-specific antibodies, such as Hashimoto's thyroiditis with absolute specificity for certain thyroid components. At the other end of the spectrum are *non–organ-specific diseases*, such as systemic lupus erythematosus (SLE), in which both lesions and antibodies are not confined to a single organ. SLE manifests itself primarily as lesions of connective tissue seen in skin, serous membranes, kidney glomeruli, and blood vessels. At the center of the spectrum are those diseases in which the lesion tends to be confined to a single organ but the antibodies are non–organ specific. Primary biliary cirrhosis is an example: the serum antibodies are mainly mitochondrial but are not liver specific.

There are also *immunodeficiency states* that are primary and can be caused by phagocytic cell defects, deficiencies in the complement system, B- and T-cell deficiency, and other causes. Secondary immunodeficiency disorders can result from malnutrition, cytotoxic drugs, infections with pyrogenic bacteria, and infections with an RNA retrovirus, as in the acquired immunodeficiency syndrome (AIDS).

A group of diseases called *multiple myeloma* is characterized by the extraordinary accumulation of pure (also called *monoclonal*) immunoglobulin molecules in the patient's serum. Such immunoglobulins are termed *paraproteins*, and they may be of the IgG, IgA, IgM, IgD, or IgE type. The cause for the overproduction of the immunoglobulin is a neoplasm of the immunoglobulin-producing cells. In many cases, a multiple myeloma patient excretes protein in the urine. This protein is called *Bence-Jones protein*, and it is nothing but a dimer of κ or λ chains that are also found in the paraprotein. Multiple myelomas is suspected by the finding of a paraprotein upon serum electrophoresis and/or the detection of Bence-Jones protein in the urine of a patient.

14.3 HEMOGLOBIN

The hemoglobin family of macromolecules exhibits virtually all the important features of protein structure, function, and evolution, principles of protein folding, subunit movement and allosteric control in regulating activity, effects of point mutations on molecular behavior, and gene structure and genetic control.

Many of these were discussed in Chapter 7. Gene structure and genetic control are discussed in this section.

The α and β families of hemoglobin genes are located on separate chromosomes in humans. These genes have been mapped and cloned and their sequences determined by the methods of modern molecular biology (Chapter 15). The structures of DNA regions that contain its α and β families of genes are shown in Figure 14.4. On chromosome 11, which contains the β family, an ϵ gene is followed after a long, untranslated intervening sequence by two G_γ and $A\gamma$ genes, a pseudogene β_1, and the δ and β genes. The G_γ and A_γ genes differ in the codon specifying position 136. Chromosome 16 (α family) starts with a ζ gene, followed by two pseudogenes (ψ and ζ) and two α genes (α_2 and α_1). The last four genes are evenly spaced along the chromosome.

Each globin gene is separated from others by long intervening sequences that appear to be important for genetic recombination and gene control, although they are excised during the processing of mRNA.

The pattern of exons and introns (exon-intron-exon-intron-exon) in the α and β families of genes is quite old and apparently developed before the separation of these genes some 500 million years ago. The role of introns is unknown, although their base sequences vary. Because the introns are not transcribed, the protein sequences are unchanged. The introns appear to correspond to structural domains within the folded globulin subunits and are requisite for the posttranscriptional processing of mRNA.

It is interesting that the order of genes (5' $\rightarrow$ 3') along each chromosome is the same order in which the genes are expressed during development from embryo to fetus to adult. The percentage of total globulin synthesis as a function of time is shown for each in Figure 7.4. A similar order is found in most other mammals, although the size of gene clusters may vary. In the chicken, β-globulin genes expressed in the adult are flanked by embryonic genes, indicating that the mammalian arrangement is not obligatory.

Most hemoglobin mutations have little or no effect on hemoglobin function. Most amino acid substitutions on the exterior of the chains are harmless—the notable exception is HbS. Those replacing amino acids in the chain interior or close to the site of heme insertion can produce profound disturbances in the function of the molecule. Some substitutions can distort the tertiary structure and produce unstable hemoglobin. Replacements near the heme can impair oxygen binding, and replacements at subunit contacts can produce changes in oxygen affinity and allosteric properties.

14.4 THE THALASSEMIAS

Forms of anemia prevalent in the Mediterranean region are characterized by the partial or total failure to synthesize either the α or β chains. These can be caused by gene deletions or regulatory failures. For α-thalassemias, there can be the deletion of one, two, three, or all four α-globin genes from chromosome 16. *Hydrops fetalis*, a fatal disease, results when all four genes are deleted. *Hemoglobin H disease* is present when three of the four genes are deleted. It is characterized by anemia and the presence of HbH (β_4^A) and Hb Bart's in the bloodstream of adults and infants, respectively. The two less serious α-thalassemias are the

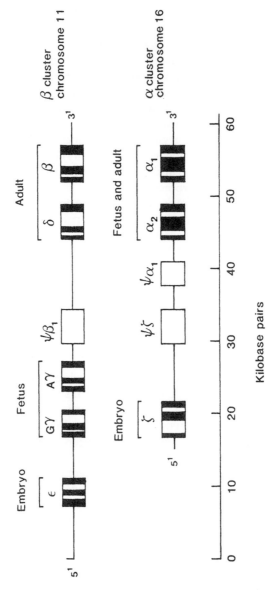

Figure 14.4 Arrangement of hemoglobin genes along human chromosomes 11 and 16. Boxes are transcribed genes, and the horizontal thin lines are intervening, untranscribed spaces. Exons are shaded black, and introns that are removed from mRNA are white. ψ are pseudogenes with sequences resembling genes but are not transcribed. The scheme is roughly to scale.

silent carrier type (one gene deleted) and the α-thalassemia trait in which two genes are deleted. Both show some Hb Bart's at birth. In Asia, one of the most common types of α-thalassemia leading to HbH disease and hydrops fetalis involves the change in termination codon at what should be the end of an α gene to a codon for glutamine. The RNA polymerase continues beyond the normal stop and adds codons for 31 additional amino acids. This extra length does not allow the formation of $\alpha_2\beta_2$ tetramers, the same effect as if the gene had been deleted.

The etiology of β-thalassemias is more complex. One of these is the homozygous β^0-thalassemia, in which only one β-gene may be defective. Some β-thalassemias are caused by gene deletions. An example is the $\delta\beta$ gene deletion syndrome, in which no β or δ chains are produced. Most β^+-thalassemias are caused by mRNA processing disorders. Characteristic symptoms of the β-thalassemias including the persistence of HbF into adulthood, increased levels of HbA$_2$ ($\alpha_2{}^\wedge\delta_2$), and even the presence of Hb Bart's. In β^0-thalassemia, in which there is a total absence of β chains, there is usually an overproduction of α chains, which precipitate in the red blood cells, causing damage to the membrane and low red cell survival time.

Abnormal hemoglobins can be detected by electrophoresis, as shown in Figure 7.4, which includes a pattern observed in β^+-thalassemia and one in a newborn with α-thalassemia (possibly HbH disease). It should also be mentioned that, unless there is a coexisting hemoglobin abnormality resulting from a point mutation or crossover problem, the globin chains of classic α- and β-thalassemia are perfectly normal. It is usually the quantities of either the α or the β chains that are decreased. Some frameshifts have been found near the terminus of the β chain that lead to frameshift mutations in certain areas.

QUESTIONS

For Questions 14.1–14.3, use the following key:
  a. 1, 2, and 3 are correct.
  b. 1 and 3 are correct.
  c. 2 and 4 are correct.
  d. Only 4 is correct.
  e. All are correct.

14.1. The diversity of immunoglobulin is accomplished by
  1. Somatic recombination
  2. Genetic rearrangements of a few gene segments in the germline DNA
  3. Somatic mutation
  4. The imprecise joining of V and J genes
14.2. In the structure of immunoglobulin,
  1. The light (L) and heavy (H) chains are divided into a variable (V) region and a constant C region
  2. The V regions of the H and L chains are the same length
  3. The L and H chains are folded into domains, the H chain having one V and three separate C domains
  4. The C region of the L chain is the same size as the C region of the H chain
14.3. The clonal section theory proposes that

a. Each antibody-producing cell is committed to synthesize a specific antibody before the cell encounters a specific antigen

b. During maturation each cell produces small amounts of the specific antibody that appears on the cell surface

c. If a mature cell encounters the appropriate antigen, it produces additional antibody and is stimulated to multiply

d. If an immature cell encounters a self antigen corresponding to its antibody, it is destroyed or suppressed during fetal life

14.4. All the following statements about the five classes of immunoglobulin are true, *except*

a. An antibody cell first synthesizes IgM

b. IgM synthesis is followed by IgG, IgA, IgD, or IgE

c. In class switching (b), the H chain is the same and the L chain is different

d. There are four subclasses of IgG

e. Class switching takes place in DNA by intrachromosomal recombination

14.5. All the following statements about each type of immunoglobulin are true, *except*

a. There exists a separate pool of genes from which a single polypeptide chain is synthesized

b. V genes are located far apart from one or more C genes in germline DNA

c. V and C genes are closely associated in the DNA of antibody-producing cells

d. No translation of genes is required during the differentiation of lymphocytes

e. Differences in the C regions of the H chain determine the class to which the antibody belongs

14.6. All the following statements about hemoglobin genes are true, *except*

a. The α and β families are located on separate chromosomes

b. Chromosome 11 contains the β family

c. The order of genes $5' \rightarrow 3'$ along each chromosome is inverse to the order in which the gene are expressed during development from embryo to fetus to adult

d. Chromosome 16 starts with a gene, followed by two pseudogenes and two α genes

e. Each globin gene is separated from others by long intervening sequences

14.7. Which of the following statements about hemoglobin mutations is *false*?

a. Some amino and substitutions near the heme can impair oxygen binding.

b. Amino acid replacements at subunit contacts can produce changes in allosteric properties and oxygen affinity.

c. A common type of α-thalassemia is caused by the change in a stop codon to a codon for glutamine.

d. Most amino acid substitutions on the exterior of the chains have severe effects on hemoglobin functions.

For Questions 14.8–14.13, use the following key:

a. Item is associated with 1 only.

b. Item is associated with 2 only.

c. Item is associated with both 1 and 2.

d. Item is associated with neither 1 nor 2.

1. H chains of immunoglobulin

2. L chains of immunoglobulin

14.8. Contains variable regions.

14.9. Contains constant region.

14.10. Contains one V and one C domain.

14.11. Contains one V and three C domains.
14.12. Contains D gene segment.
14.13. Contains J gene segments.
14.14. If a patient has β^0-thalassemia, the most likely red blood cell contents will include (1) increased quantity of HbA_2 ($\alpha_2{}^A\delta_2$); (2) increased quantity of HbH ($\beta_4{}^A$); (3) increased quantity of HbF ($\alpha_2{}^A\tau_2{}^F$); (4) increased quantity of HbL ($\alpha_4{}^A$).
 a. 1, 2, and 3 are correct.
 b. 1 and 3 are correct.
 c. 2 and 4 are correct.
 d. 4 is correct.
 e. All are correct.

Answers

14.1. (e)
14.2. (a) The C region of the H chains is about three times as long as the L chain.
14.3. (e)
14.4. (c) The L chain is the same, and only the constant region of the H chain changes.
14.5. (d) Translation of genes is required during the differentiation of lymphocytes because they are located closely together in the DNA of antibody-producing cells.
14.6. (c) The order of genes is in the same order in which the genes are expressed during development from embryo to fetus to adult.
14.7. (d)
14.8. (c)
14.9. (c)
14.10. (b)
14.11. (a)
14.12. (a)
14.13. (c)
14.14. (b) In β^0-thalassemia, no β chains are produced, and a tetramer of α chains is unknown.

PROBLEMS

14.1. The expression of mammalian hemoglobin genes is regulated only posttranscriptionally. Why?
14.2. What might be the reasons for the switching of α- and β-globin genes during the development from embryo to fetus to adult?
14.3. What types of mutations are found within the hemoglobin β-globin gene cluster?

BIBLIOGRAPHY

Dickerson RE, Geis I. Hemoglobin: Structure, Function, Evolution, and Pathology, Menlo Park: Benjamin/Cummings, 1983.
Ferrus P, Kreppe B, Furley A, et al. Cold Spring Harbor Symp. Quant. Biol 54:191–201, 1989.
Roitt I. Essential Immunology, 7th ed. Boston: Blackwell Scientific, 1991.
Vogel F, Motulsky AG. Human Genetics. New York: Springer Verlag, 1982.

15

Application of Modern Molecular Biology

After completing this chapter, the student should

1. Understand the use and mechanism of action of restriction enzymes.
2. Know how DNA and RNA are characterized by Southern and northern blotting.
3. Know what cloning vectors (plasmid, phage, and cosmids) are and how they are used to insert foreign DNA into a cell.
4. Know the two types of DNA libraries, genomic and complementary.
5. Understand how to isolate a DNA clone of special interest.
6. Be aware of specific applications of recombinant DNA technology, such as the production of useful proteins, the construction of useful organisms, uses in medical diagnosis, for gene therapy, and for basic experimental studies.

15.1 INTRODUCTION

The revolutionary new techniques known collectively as *recombinant DNA technology* or *genetic engineering* have provided the means for analyzing and cloning genes, altering them in precise ways, and introducing them into cells of the same or different species. These abilities depend on the availability of many restriction enzymes that cleave DNA at specific sites: ligase that joins DNA strands, and RNA reverse transcriptase and hybridization techniques for annealing complementary DNA and RNA sequences. Also required are cloning vectors or cloning vehicles that can introduce a DNA fragment into an appropriate host cell for amplification, and the techniques for obtaining the sequence of nucleotides in a cloned DNA segment. These techniques are the product of many years of basic DNA and RNA research.

15.2 RESTRICTION ENZYMES AND CHARACTERIZATION OF PRODUCTS

More than 100 restriction endonucleases (*restriction enzymes*) have been isolated and purified from various bacterial species. All but a few of these enzymes recognize specific palindromic base sequences in double-helical DNA and cleave both strands at specific sites. They do not cleave DNA from their host strain, because their specific cleavage sites are protected by methylation of an A or C residue. Any foreign DNA molecule entering the cell is immediately recognized, however, and both strands are cleaved. There are three major types of restriction enzymes: types I and III recognize a specific sequence but cleave elsewhere, and the more useful type II cleaves only within the recognition sequence. Many restriction endonucleases make staggered cuts at a four- to six-base recognition sequence to produce overlapping *cohesive* or *sticky* ends (Figure 15.1A). These can form complementary base pairs with any other end produced by the *same* enzyme from any other DNA molecule. Once the ends have joined transiently by complementary base pairing, they can be permanently sealed by either *Escherichia coli* DNA ligase or the T_4 ligase. Phosphodiester bond formation is coupled to the cleavage of the pyrophosphate bonds in nicotinamide adenine dinucleotide (NAD) for the bacterial ligase and in ATP for the phage ligase. A circular DNA molecule cuts at a single site by this type of restriction nuclease readily re-forms the circular structure by *annealing* (base pairing).

A second type of cleavage (Figure 15.1B) at the axis of symmetry of the recognition site produces nonoverlapping *blunt-end fragments*. These blunt ends can be joined only by the T_4 ligase. They can be converted to sticky-ended molecules by the enzymatic addition of a double-stranded oligonucleotide (10–12 nucleotides) containing a *restriction site sequence* specific for cleavage by a given endonuclease. By the combined actions of a given restriction endonuclease and a DNA ligase, any segment of DNA on one molecule may be joined to a fragment from another DNA molecule, even those from different species. This is an important means of producing *recombinant DNA molecules* and of cloning genes.

Because a particular restriction enzyme recognizes a unique sequence, the number of cuts made in a DNA molecule is limited. Depending on the size of the

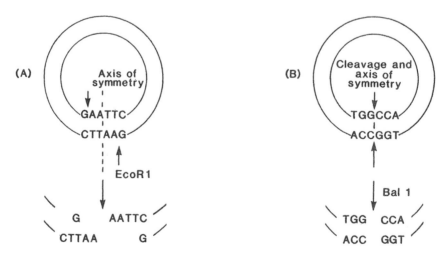

Figure 15.1 Two types of cleavage made by restriction enzymes: (A) cuts symmetrically placed around the line of symmetry to form overlapping cohesive ends; (B) cuts on the line of symmetry to form nonoverlapping blunt ends.

molecule and its sequence, the number of fragments can vary from less than ten in smaller molecules to a few hundred or a few thousands in larger DNA molecules. Each restriction enzyme produces a unique family of fragments from a given DNA molecule. Restriction fragments can be separated by electrophoresis, for example, on polyacrylamide and agarose gels, and visualized by various techniques.

DNA samples can be characterized by a technique called *Southern blotting* (named after its originator, E. M. Southern). In this technique (Figure 15.2), DNA restriction fragments are separated by size by electrophoresis in agarose gel, converted to single-stranded molecules with alkali, and transferred by capillary action to a sheet of cellulose nitrate filter that immobilizes the single-stranded DNA to form a replica of the DNA from the gel. Single-stranded DNA bound to a cellulose nitrate filter is still accessible to hybridization reactions. The filter is dried, and a small volume of ^{32}P-labeled single-stranded DNA (a *probe*) is added and held at a suitable temperature and time period to allow hybridization of complementary sequences. The filter is washed to remove unbound radioactivity, dried, and subjected to autoradiography on x-ray film. The exposed portions of the film indicate the DNA molecules with sequences complementary to the added radioactive molecules. An analogous technique, *northern blotting*, is used for RNA. Bound RNA can hybridize with probes of radioactive RNA or single-stranded DNA.

Base sequences within DNA molecules can be readily determined by the Maxam-Gilbert procedure, which involves *chemical cleavage at particular bases*, and the Sanger dideoxy procedure, which depends upon generating fragments by the *controlled interruption* of enzymatic replication. Both methods are effective, and the fragments generated by both can be separated by gel electrophoresis and visualized by autoradiography or fluorescent tagging. These methods, especially the fluorescent tagging technique, can be readily automated and may make possible the sequencing of the human genome of 3×10^9 base pairs. The student is directed to other sources for details of these procedures.

DNA probes and genes can now be synthesized by automated solid-phase methods. This is accomplished by the sequential addition of activated mono-

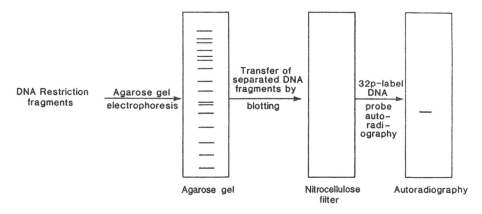

Figure 15.2 Southern blotting. The exposed portion of the film shows the DNA fragment complementary to the radioactive probe.

mers to a growing chain linked to an insoluble resin. The activated monomers are protonated deoxyribonucleoside-3′-phosphoramidites containing blocking groups on the 5′-hydroxyl group and on the bases. The blocking or protection groups are readily removed, leaving the desired product on the insoluble support. The product is removed from the support by hydrolysis and can be purified by electrophoresis on polyacrylamide gels or by high-performance liquid chromatography (HPLC). This automated technique allows the synthesis of specific DNA chains some 100 nucleotides in length that can be used as a probe for complementary sequences in a large DNA molecule. Synthetic new genes can also be made by this process and introduced into a cell for the expression of new proteins with unique properties.

15.3 CLONING VECTORS: PLASMIDS, PHAGES, AND COSMIDS

Plasmid and the λ *phage* have been the primary vehicles whereby a recombinant DNA molecule can be introduced into a bacterium for DNA cloning. Plasmid DNAs exist as free, circular duplex DNA molecules ranging in size from two to several hundred kilobase pairs. They are present as single or multiple copies that replicate independently of the bacterial chromosome. Plasmid DNAs usually encode no essential functions, because bacteria lacking them multiply normally. Instead, they encode for special functions, such as the simultaneous multiple resistance to several antibiotics and factors that allow bacteria to conjugate and transfer genetic material. Plasmids present in a large number of copies per cell (10–20) are usually employed as cloning vectors, because the foreign DNA segments linked to them and the products encoded by them can be amplified many times. The desired foreign DNA can be removed by cleaving the plasmid with the endonuclease specific for the restriction site into which the foreign DNA was originally inserted. Because plasmid DNA is much smaller than the chromosomal DNA and is not membrane bound, it can be readily separated from the latter. Bacteria that have taken up a plasmid are commonly selected by virtue of their antibiotic resistance (Figure 15.3). A commonly used plasmid, pBR322, contains genes that confer resistance to tetracycline and ampicillin and specific cleavage sites for a number of restriction endonucleases (Figure 15.2). If a foreign DNA is inserted into a specific site in the tetracycline gene (for example, at BamH1), this gene is inactivated and the host cell is sensitive to tetracycline but still resistant to ampicillin (Figure 15.4). This effect is *insertional inactivation*. Bacteria containing plasmids with insertions can be selected by their ability to grow in the presence of ampicillin but not tetracycline. Cells that have not taken up the vector are sensitive to both antibiotics. DNA fragments up to some 20 kilobases can be propagated with this vector.

The λ phage is a widely used vector and has the advantages over plasmids of entering the cell more readily and allowing the propagation of DNA fragments as large as 24 kilobases. Phage vectors have been constructed that contain only two cleavage sites for a specific endonuclease (EcoR1). Following cleavage with the endonuclease, the middle segment of the λ DNA molecule can be removed and replaced by an externally derived DNA fragment of about the same

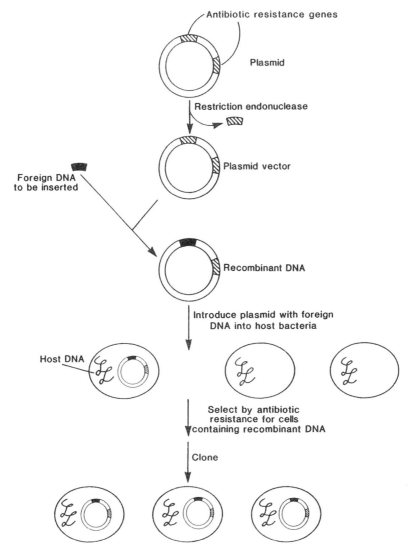

Figure 15.3 Construction and cloning of recombinant DNA, with foreign DNA inserted into plasmid vector. Vector is introduced into cells, and bacteria containing recombinant DNA are selected by antibiotic resistance. The figure is not to scale.

size without influencing phage growth. The chimeric DNA is isolated after the phage has gone through the lytic pathway (page 355), which leads to lysis of the host cell and the production of about 100 mature virus particles. In the lysogenic pathway, the phage DNA is integrated into the host genome, where it can be replicated for many generations. The viral DNA is dormant until activated by certain environmental factors to produce mature virus and lysis of the host cell.

Cosmids are specifically designed cloning vehicles derived from plasmid that contain a plasmid origin of replication and the *cos sites* (cohesive ends) of

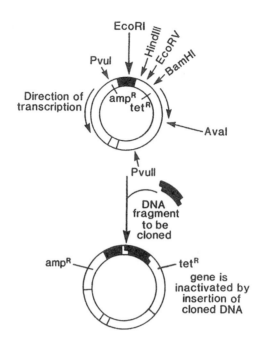

Figure 15.4 pBR322 plasmid vector showing antibiotic resistance genes (tet^R, tetra-cycline resistance; amp^R, ampicillin resistance) and the direction of their transcription. Some restriction sites are also shown, as well as the effect of cloning a new sequence into the HindIII site.

normal λ phage that are required for the packaging of any DNA in λ phage. Cosmid DNA, along with inserted, foreign DNA, can be packaged *in vitro* into λ phage particles from which, with the exception of the cos sites, virtually all of the genome has been deleted. This produces a defective but still infectious phage particle that replicates not as a phage but as a plasmid. These vectors can propagate exogenously derived DNA fragments up to about 48 kilobases in length.

Recently, newly designed vectors have been produced that contain two distinct *origins of replication* derived from two different species, for example *E. coli* and human or *E. coli* and yeast. These are *shuttle vectors*, and they are used to transfer genes between very different cell types.

15.4 GENE LIBRARIES

A *DNA library* is a collection of independently vector-linked DNA fragments corresponding to the entire genome of an organism. There are two types of libraries, a *genomic* DNA library prepared from the total DNA of a cell or an organism, and a *complementary* (cDNA) library that is complementary to the mRNA population present. Each has its advantages and disadvantages for use in specific purposes. The goal is to achieve a complete library that represents all sequences with the least possible number of clones.

For the construction of a genomic library, DNA from a donor organism is degraded by mechanical shearing or endonuclease digestion to produce random fragments that are joined to a vector (plasmid, phage, or cosmid) containing some selective marker so that bacteria containing recombinant DNA can be identified. The minimum number of clones (the size of the library) required to contain the entire genome is a function of the size of the genome and the average size of the cloned fragments. It is necessary to clone 3–10 times the minimum to achieve a high probability that a particular segment is represented. Using DNA fragments of 5×10^3 bases, the minimum number of clones required for a mammalian genome of 3×10^9 bases is approximately 6×10^5 pBR322 plasmid or 2×10^5 λ phage particles. Because most mammalian genes are mosaics of exons and introns, these cannot be cloned and expressed in bacteria that do not have the ability to excise introns from these primary RNA transcripts. This can be avoided by preparing a cDNA library that is a collection of DNA copies of the cell's or organism's mRNA that do not contain introns. This requires the use of reverse transcriptase (page 316), which synthesizes in the $5' \rightarrow 3'$ direction a DNA strand complementary to a RNA template. Required is an oligo (dT) primer containing a free 3'-OH group that can pair with the poly (A) sequence present at the 3' end of most eukaryotic mRNA molecules. DNA polymerase I, in the presence of the four deoxyribonucleoside triphosphates (dNTPs), completes the chain to produce a RNA-DNA hybrid. The RNA strand is removed by alkaline hydrolysis. The 3' end of the new DNA forms a hairpin loop and acts as a primer for the synthesis of the complementary DNA strand. The loop is then excised by a nuclease that recognizes unpaired nucleotides. Following this, the duplex DNA can be inserted into a vector for introduction into a suitable host bacterium. The ability to produce a *foreign* protein can serve as the basis for screening the cDNA clones.

Because a library can contain thousands of different clones, it can be difficult to isolate a clone with DNA of specific interest. This is because the majority of cloned DNAs do not contain a readily selectable genetic marker, such as antibiotic resistance, or lead (as discussed earlier) to the production of a foreign protein. Methods to achieve this have been developed and utilize hybridization, immunochemical, and structural techniques. A specific DNA sequence of only several kilobases can be isolated from a genome containing in excess of 10^6 kilobases. *Hybridization* requires a radioactive DNA or RNA molecule (a *probe*) that is complementary (or partially so) to the sequence of the cloned DNA. *Immunologic* techniques require that the polypeptides coded by the DNAs of interest are available and have specific antigenic properties that allow detection. *Structural* analysis can also be used when the other techniques are inapplicable.

If the amino acid sequence of a peptide is known, the possible nucleotide sequences of the mRNA and the complementary DNA may be deduced from the genetic code (Chapter 12). The number of possible DNA sequences is directly related to the extent of degeneracy of the genetic code. Unique sets of DNA oligonucleotides can be chemically synthesized, labeled at the 5' end with ^{32}P, and used as probes to isolate a clone with DNA of specific interest.

Restriction enzyme analysis (the reverse of the process of insertion and ligation) is suitable, although this requires some knowledge of the size and the restriction pattern of the foreign DNA. (See discussion of *restriction* fragment length polymorphisms in Section 15.6.3.)

15.5 ENZYMATIC AMPLIFICATION OF DNA AND RNA SEGMENTS WITH PCR

Polymerase chain reaction (PCR; Figure 15.5) is a powerful new technique by which a targeted DNA sequence can be exponentially amplified *in vitro* by repeated cycles of enzymatic DNA synthesis. Knowledge of the sequence flanking the targeted region is required to construct two DNA oligonucleotide primers complementary to the DNA on the flanks of the target regions. These primers, 20–30 bases long, can hybridize to opposite strands of the target sequence, are oriented with their 3′ ends pointing toward each other, and define the ends of the DNA that will be replicated. In the first step, the DNA to be copied is heat denatured to separate the two complementary DNA strands. This is followed by annealing (*hybridizing*) the primers to the denatured flanking sequences. The primers are then extended along the single-stranded DNA templates with thermostable DNA polymerase in the presence of the four deoxynucleoside triphosphates that yield double-stranded DNA. At this point there are two copies of the target sequence. The three-step cycle is repeated, producing copies of the original DNA and copies of the primer-defined target DNA. Copies of copies contain only the target sequence, whereas copies of the origi-

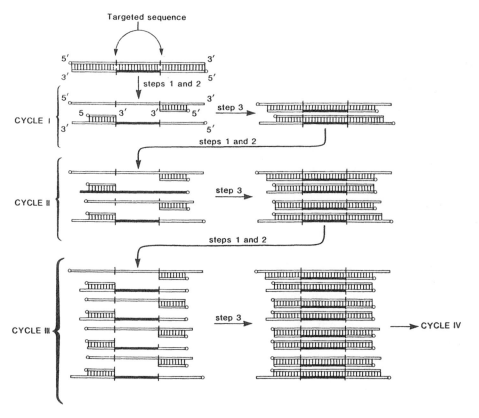

Figure 15.5 Polymerase chain reaction: step 1, separation of strands by heating (98°C); step 2, anneal primers (60°C); step 3, primer extension by polymerase.

nal DNA extend beyond the target sequence. The copies of the copies increase exponentially, whereas the original DNA increases arithmetically, one copy of each strand per cycle. The amount of DNA sequence flanked by the primers is 2^n, where n is the number of amplification cycles. Thus, 20 and 30 cycles produce amplifications of $\sim 10^6$ and $\sim 10^9$, respectively, and can be accomplished in a few hours. It is possible to sequence a PCR product directly, eliminating the need to clone DNA fragments.

PCR is extremely sensitive and allows the DNA in a single cell, hair follicle, sperm, or even a single molecule in a complex mixture to be amplified for analysis. Thus, there are many applications in forensic medicine. Other applications include (1) the detection of specific infectious agents, such as human immunodeficiency virus (HIV) and cytomegalovirus; (2) the study of molecular evolution by going back in time and analyzing archeologic DNA samples that are ancestral to their present-day counterparts; (3) in developmental biology to study gene expression during early embryogenesis and DNA rearrangement during cell differentiation; (4) to enhance prenatal diagnoses of genetic disease, for example cystic fibrosis, Tay-Sachs disease, phenylketonuria, sickle cell anemia, and β-thalassemia; (5) to establish precisely tissue histocompatibility genes for transplantation; and (6) to analyze both normal variations in DNA sequence (allelic polymorphisms) and variations causing diseases, such as point mutations, deletions, insertions, and rearrangements. Note that PCR can also be used for the amplification of RNA. In this case the template RNA is transcribed into DNA by the enzyme reverse transcriptase (page 316), the RNA removed by a ribonuclease, and the DNA amplified by conventional PCR.

A technique called *chromosome walking* or *overlap hybridization* allows the analysis of long stretches of DNA (300 or more kilobases). It involves the use of a series of DNA clones with overlapping DNA complementary to a unique region. A fragment of DNA is used to isolate a second fragment of DNA that overlaps and extends the first fragment. This is repeated to isolate a third piece that overlaps a fourth piece, and so on, until the entire sequence of a gene is obtained. Most recently, the gene for cystic fibrosis was localized in the middle of human chromosome 7 with this technique.

15.6 APPLICATIONS OF RECOMBINANT DNA TECHNOLOGY

Both now and in the future, the uses of this technology for basic research and practical purposes are virtually unlimited. Some current and possible future applications are considered briefly in this section.

15.6.1 Production of Useful Proteins

The human hormones somatostatin, growth hormone, and insulin are examples of proteins synthesized in large amounts by genetically modified *E. coli*.

For *somatostatin* (a 14-residue polypeptide synthesized in the hypothalamus), the appropriate double-stranded DNA was synthesized chemically and coupled to an appropriate plasmid vector for insertion into the bacteria. Because of the small size of somatostatin, the procedure is relatively simple.

The procedure for *insulin* is more complex because insulin is synthesized as preproinsulin and must be processed to yield the A and B chains of insulin (page 415). Bacteria do not have the processing system for converting the precursor to insulin. The appropriate cDNAs for the A and B chains were coupled into individual plasmids and each inserted into separate bacteria for production of the A and B chains. Following purification of the individual chains, the proper disulfide bonds were chemically formed to yield the mature insulin.

Because it contains 191 amino acid residues, although in a single chain, *human growth hormone* presented a more difficult problem than insulin. Two separate segments of cDNA had to be constructed, each inserted and joined in a vector, to obtain the entire coding sequence for the protein.

A group of small proteins called *interferons* are currently produced in *E. coli*. These compounds have antiviral activity and may also be anticancer agents. Before the cloning of several interferon genes, sufficient material was not available to conduct basic studies and clinical trials. *Interleukin-2* (T cell growth factor) has been cloned and is being tested in patients with acquired immunodeficiency syndrome (AIDS) and other viral diseases. Clearly, many other biologically active proteins that are present in nature only in small amounts can be cloned and made available for experimental studies. Examples are erythropoietin, plasminogen activator, and various blood-clotting factors.

15.6.2 Construction of Useful Organisms

Marine bacteria have been constructed that are capable of metabolizing petroleum and are useful in clearing oil spills. Designer bacteria have been exploited to produce increased amounts of industrial chemicals, such as methanol, ethanol, and butanol, from biologic wastes. Attempts are currently being made to introduce the nitrogen fixation system into non–nitrogen-fixing bacteria and plants to reduce the dependence on nitrogen fertilizers. Again, the future possibilities are enormous.

15.6.3 Medical Diagnosis

Cloned genes are currently being used as hybridization probes for the detection of cancer, infectious diseases, and genetic diseases. Antenatal diagnosis of hemoglobinopathies and other diseases is currently being done. Structural variants (point mutations) as well as dysfunctional and absent genes can be detected. Recall (page 373) that α_1-thalassemia can have two different genotypes: one chromosome with two defective α genes in combination with a normal chromosome, or two chromosomes, each of which carries one defective α gene and one normal α gene. The latter case does not lead to hydrops fetalis. Only those couples who have α_1-thalassemia caused by "no-gene" chromosomes can produce a hydropic fetus and can be given the appropriate genetic counseling. Other genetic diseases yielding developmental abnormalities can be detected by changes in the DNA primary structure. Probes are now available for the antenatal diagnosis of such diseases.

The human genome contains about 3×10^9 base pairs of DNA, of which 5% code for some 100,000 genes. The remainder do not code for any particular gene, although they may have some yet unknown function. Variations in DNA sequences in either the coding or noncoding regions produce considerable individual variability. Some of these variations within the coding sequence of a gene may have profound effects on the function of the proteins. Variations in noncoding regions may occur and have no effect on any expressed gene. Nevertheless, variations in noncoding regions may very often be detected by *restriction fragment length polymorphism* (RFLP), a technique that allows the study of genetic individuality at the molecular level and is based on the fact that many changes in DNA sequence can create or destroy a restriction enzyme recognition site, thus changing the restriction fragmentation pattern. Changes in RFLP patterns can be readily detected by Southern blotting and the use of appropriate probes. RFLPs, which are inherited and segregated in a Mendelian manner, are highly conserved in different individuals and therefore applicable to problems of genetic individuality. For example, depending on the combination of probes and restriction enzymes used, complex patterns can be obtained with a probability of 1 in 10^{19} that identical patterns between two randomly selected individuals would be obtained. The value of RFLPs for pedigree analysis, questioned paternity, and forensic medicine is obvious. A recent use of the technique is to map and isolate genes for hereditary diseases in which the responsible gene is unknown.

15.6.4   Gene Therapy

Although not yet a practical technique in humans, the possibility exists for the direct introduction of functional genes into individuals who carry genetic mutations. It has been possible in mice to alter germline cells by the injection of genes into the male pronucleus of a fertilized ovum derived from mice deficient in the production of gonadotropin-releasing hormone. The progeny of these transgenic animals were normal in all respects. A similar transgenic approach involving the microinjection of multiple copies of rat growth hormone (somatotropin) yielded mice of twice the normal weight. These experiments demonstrate both the effective expression of the transgene and its maintenance in germ cells. Somatic cell gene replacement would not be transmitted to offspring. However, bone marrow cells are being used as specific replacement vehicles after the introduction of a specific gene. Following injection, such modified cells can find their way to the bone marrow, replicate, and produce the product of the new gene. This could at least temporarily correct the deficiency in the host cell. Repeated injections would be required with time.

15.6.5   Basic Applications

Basic scientific applications are many and include the ability to explore the molecular basis of development, gene evolution, further elucidation of DNA transcription, and the effects of structural alterations of specific regions of cloned DNA on the function of the gene product. *Site-directed mutagenesis* is a technique whereby specific mutations of DNA at any site can be created *in vitro*. A desired mutation is introduced using an oligonucleotide primer containing the desired mutation flanked by a complementary sequence to the cloned gene. The primer is elongated with DNA polymerase to produce a new copy of the gene containing the mutation. Insertion of the mutant gene into a host cell for expression would yield an altered protein that could be tested for altered function. A known

DNA sequence can be readily modified using a PCR primer differing from the targeted sequence in one or more positions to produce deletions, insertions, or base pair substitutions. The function of the modified PCR products can then be compared to the original, unmodified sequence.

QUESTIONS

In Questions 15.1–15.3, use the following key:
- a.   1, 2, and 3 are correct.
- b.   1 and 3 are correct.
- c.   2 and 4 are correct.
- d.   Only 4 is correct.
- e.   All are correct.

15.1.   The cloning of gene requires, among other procedures,
1.   Ligase
2.   Restriction enzymes
3.   Cloning vectors
4.   Hybridization techniques

15.2.   Restriction endonucleases
1.   Cleave both strands of duplex DNA
2.   Recognize palindromic sequence
3.   Are specific for short symmetric sequences
4.   Attack 5′ ends of DNA strands

15.3.   Southern blotting involves
1.   Separation by size by electrophoresis of DNA restriction fragments
2.   Conversion to single-stranded molecules with alkali
3.   Transfer to cellulose nitrate filler
4.   Hybridization with a ^{32}P-labeled probe

15.4.   Preparation of cDNA copy from mRNA involves (1) hybridization with an oligo(dT) primer; (2) use of reverse transcriptase; (3) DNA olymerase I; (4) alkali treatment; (5) action of nuclease. The correct sequence is
- a.   1, 2, 3, 4, 5.
- b.   2, 3, 4, 5, 1.
- c.   2, 4, 3, 5, 1.
- d.   3, 4, 1, 5, 2.
- e.   5, 4, 3, 2, 1.

15.5.   The Maxam-Gilbert method for DNA sequencing depends upon (one of the following):
- a.   Use of endonuclease
- b.   Chemical cleavage at particular bases
- c.   Use of DNA ligase
- d.   Controlled interruption of enzymatic replication
- e.   Immunoelectrophoresis

15.6.   All the following statements about a genomic DNA library are true, *except*
- a.   It is prepared from the total DNA of the cell
- b.   The DNA is degraded by endonuclease digestion or by mechanical shearing
- c.   The fragments produced are joined to a vector containing some selective marker
- d.   These recombinant DNA molecules (DNA fragment and vector) are readily expressed and cloned in bacteria

e. The size of the library is a function of the size of the genome and the average size of the DNA fragments

15.7. All the following statements about plasmid are true, *except*
   a. They are present as single or multiple copies that replicate independently of the bacterial chromosome
   b. Plasmid DNAs usually encode for no essential functions in bacteria
   c. They exist as free circular DNA molecules from two to several hundred kilobase pairs
   d. They usually code multiple resistance to several antibiotics
   e. They enter the cell more readily than λ phage

15.8. All the following statements about cosmids are true, *except*
   a. Cannot propagate as much exogenously derived DNA as phage
   b. Are designed cloning vehicles
   c. Contain a plasmid origin of replication
   d. Contain *cos sites* (cohesive ends) of normal phage
   e. Replicate not as a phage but as a plasmid

15.9. All the following statements about restriction enzymes are true, *except*
   a. All but a few recognize specific palindromic base sequences
   b. They do not cleave their own DNA, because their specific cleavage sites are protected by methylation of an A or C residue
   c. They cleave only single-stranded DNA
   d. Foreign DNA molecules are recognized and cleaved
   e. There are two types of restriction molecules

Answers

15.1. (e)
15.2. (a)
15.3. (e)
15.4. (c)
15.5. (b)
15.6. (d) Bacteria do not have ability to excise introns, whereas cDNA does not contain introns.
15.7. (e)
15.8. (a)
15.9. (c)

PROBLEMS

15.1. What are the steps involved in cloning a DNA?
15.2. What are the requirements for sequencing DNA with the Sanger dideoxy method?
15.3. Describe another method to obtain a specific probe for a gene other than to prepare a complementary DNA (cDNA) from mRNA. Assume that a portion of the amino acid sequence of the protein encoded by the gene is known.
15.4. What properties must a DNA molecule have to act as a cloning vector?

BIBLIOGRAPHY

Arnheim H, Levenson C. Polymerase chain reaction. Chem Eng News 68 (40):36–47, 1990.

Koshland DE. The new harvest: genetically engineered species. Science 24A:1275–1317, 1989.

Oxendir DL, Fox CF, eds. Protein Engineering. New York: Allan R. Liss, 1987.

White TJ, Arnheim N, Erlich HA. The polymerase chain reaction. Trends Genet (6):185–189, 1989.

Wu R, Grossman L, Moldave K, eds. Recombinant DNA Methodology. New York: Academic Press, 1989.

III

INTERMEDIARY METABOLISM

16

Action of Hormones and Prostaglandins

After completing the chapter, the student should

1. Explain the arrangement of the hypothalamus–pituitary hormone system, including the function of hypothalamic release and release inhibitory factors; tropic and nontropic hormones elaborated by the anterior, intermediary, and posterior pituitary; their chemical natures; and their effects on target tissues. Understand the short- and long-loop control mechanisms for hormone secretion.
2. Know the biosynthesis, functions, and chemical nature of steroid hormones. Be familiar with water and electrolyte metabolism and the control factors involved, and solve problems involving serum electrolytes.
3. Understand how the thyroid gland hormones work, their effect on target tissues, their biosynthesis, and control of their secretion.
4. Be familiar with the biosynthesis and catabolism of catecholamines, their structures, control of their secretion, their effects on target tissues, and diagnostic uses of their catabolic products.
5. Know the effects of parathyroid hormone, calcitonin, and vitamin D in controlling calcium and phosphate metabolism. Know what controls the levels of such hormones in the bloodstream.
6. Know the action of hormones involved in the digestion and metabolism of food substances: insulin, glucagon, secretin, gastrin, and cholecystokinin. Know their chemical and physiologic properties and what controls their blood levels.
7. Know the biochemical basis and signs and symptoms of disease associated with hormone over- or underproduction, such as Addison's, Cushing's and Graves' disease.
8. Have mastered the workings of hormones on the cellular and molecular levels: the concept of membrane and intracellular receptors, nuclear receptors, the various types of second messengers, and the details of their mode of action. Be able to use the Scatchard equation to solve protein–small molecule interaction problems.

9. Recognize the structures of prostaglandins, tromboxanes, and leukotrienes. Understand their classification and origins. Know the action of antiinflammatory drugs at the molecular level. Be familiar with the biosynthetic pathway peculiarities leading to each group of compounds. Be familiar with some major physiologic effects of prostaglandins, thromboxanes, and leukotrienes: platelets, gastrointestinal tract, cardiovascular system, immunity, and reproduction.

16.1 INTRODUCTION

At the end of the nineteenth and beginning of the twentieth century, many physiologists were interested in what controls pancreatic secretions in response to the entry of acidic chyme into the small intestine. One school of thought believed this to be the result of nerve impulses; however, a search for responsible nerve connections proved to be fruitless. In 1902, W. M. Bayliss and E. H. Starling were able to elicit pancreatic secretions into the small intestine by injecting jejunal extracts into the bloodstream of animals. The conclusion was that a chemical substance produced by the small intestine and traveling to the pancreas via the bloodstream was responsible for eliciting the pancreatic response to the entry of chyme into the small intestine. This was the birth of the concept of hormone action.

In 1905, Starling defined a *hormone* as a substance that is produced by a structure, that is, a gland, in one part of the organism and elicits a response in another. Hormones are thus chemical messengers. A chemical or chemicals are produced in the jejunum, which travel via the bloodstream to the pancreas to elicit pancreatic secretions. Many far-reaching discoveries on the nature and action of various hormones have been made since the times of Starling, the most recent activities in this area being the mechanisms of action of *second messengers*, biochemically active substances released intracellularly through the reaction of hormones with specific cell surface receptors. The biomedical area concerned with the properties and action of hormones is known as *endocrinology*, and the structures that secrete hormones into the bloodstream are referred to as *endocrine glands*.

The chemical nature of hormones is varied. A large group of hormones is peptidic in nature and water soluble. Some are relatively large peptides (e.g., insulin); others are very short (e.g., vasopressin in Chapter 4). There are two water-soluble hormones that are derived from amino acids: thyroxine and epinephrine. Another large group of hormones is steroid in nature. They are fat soluble and derived from cholesterol. Finally, the prostaglandin group of hormone-like substances are derived from arachidonic and similar fatty acids and also represent a lipophilic group of substances.

Physiologically, hormones are responsible for maintaining a steady state—*homeostasis*—in the human being, and help the organism to cope with environmental changes that affect it. Hormones control enzymatic activities; this effect is observed in intermediary metabolism, in the digestion of foodstuffs, and in the maintenance of electrolyte and water balance. Such control is accomplished via direct effects on the genetic material responsible for enzyme biosynthesis or through second messengers. In many instances, the exact molecular effect of a hormone is still unclear.

What is clear, however, is that the consequences of hormone imbalance result in profound aberrations in homeostasis. For instance, changes in water, acid-base, and electrolyte balance in the human organism have far-reaching medical implications. The clinical biochemistry laboratory performs numerous acid–base, electrolyte, and osmolarity determinations every day, and the management of the patient depends in a major way on such clinical-chemical data. For this reason, this chapter contains a discourse on water and electrolyte balance, presented from a clinical and biochemical point of view.

16.2   THE HYPOTHALAMUS-PITUITARY SYSTEM

16.2.1   Anterior and Intermediate Pituitary

A significant group of hormones is secreted by peripheral endocrine glands in response to signals from the brain. The brain structures responsible for this are the *hypothalamus* and the *pituitary gland*. The hypothalamus is connected with the pituitary gland by two pathways: a bundle of nerve fibers leading into the posterior pituitary (*neurohypophysis*), and a vascular network, the *hypophyseal portal system*, joining the *anterior* and *intermediate pituitaries* with the hypothalamus, as shown in Figure 16.1.

Various stimuli, such as emotions and stress, result in the secretion by the hypothalamus of peptide hormones termed *release factors*. These travel via the portal system to the anterior pituitary, and possibly the intermediate pituitary, causing these structures to release other peptidic hormones into the general circulation. Some such hormones are called *tropic hormones* because their target tissues are other endocrine glands, which, under the influence of tropic hormones, secrete hormones of their own. The tropic hormones are the *thyroid-stimulating hormone* (TSH), *adrenocorticotropic hormone* (ACTH; see Chapter 4 for structure), *follicle-stimulating hormone* (FSH), and *luteinizing hormone* (LH). In the male, LH is also known as interstitial cell stimulating hormone (ICSH). Other hormones produced by the anterior or intermediate pituitary are not tropic; they act on target peripheral tissues directly. These are *prolactin* (PRL), *melanocyte-stimulating hormone* (MSH), and the *endorphins*. *Growth hormone* (GH) works through intermediary substances (see later).

Endorphins are peptides produced by the intermediate pituitary that react with the brain's opioid receptors and presumably act as endogenous analgesics. The two best known endorphins from bovine brain are the pentapeptides, *met-enkephalin* and *leu-enkephalin*, whose structures are Tyr-Gly-Gly-Phe-Met and Tyr-Gly-Gly-Phe-Leu, respectively. There is evidence that the enkephalins, MSH, and ACTH are produced from the same precursor protein, *pro-opiomelanocortin*, molecular weight (MW) 31,000. This protein is present in both the anterior and intermediate pituitary glands. In the anterior pituitary area, this protein loses the element of ACTH (39 amino acids). In the intermediate pituitary, this protein

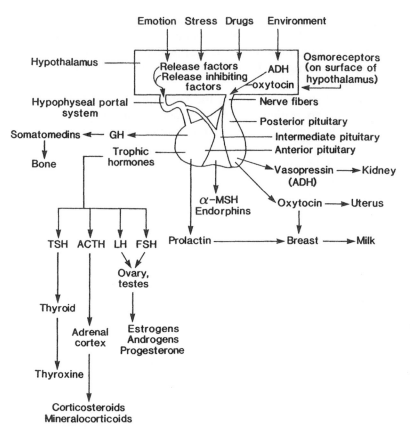

Figure 16.1 Hypothalamic-pituitary system. The hypothalamus receives various types of impulses and responds by secreting appropriate release and release-inhibiting factors. These migrate to the anterior or intermediate pituitary via the hypophyseal portal vein system and elicit the secretion of various tropic or nontropic hormones. For instance, when the organism is exposed to cold, blood TSH levels increase; when under stress, blood ACTH levels rise. In some animals, the absence of light causes the release of α-MSH.

loses MSH, termed α-MSH (see Table 16.1) and another peptide called β-lipotropin (β-LPH). The latter is then degraded to form the met-enkephalin. It should be noted that α-MSH represents the first 13 amino acids of ACTH, the other 26 amino acid peptide being termed "corticotropinlike peptide" (CLIP). It is not known whether in the intermediate pituitary the pro-opiomelanocortin first loses ACTH, the latter then being converted to α-MSH and CLIP, or if α-MSH is directly cleaved from pro-opiomelanocortin. α-MSH stimulates the biosynthesis of the copper-containing enzyme tyrosinase in melanin-producing cells, which catalyzes the rate-controlling step in the biosynthesis of various melanin pigments.

Several anterior pituitary hormones, and possibly α-MSH, are released by the pituitary gland in response to release factors from the hypothalamus. These are summarized in Table 16.1. In addition, the hypothalamus secretes peptidic

Table 16.1 Hormones of the Anterior and Intermediate Pituitary Gland and Their Hypothalamic Release and Release-Inhibiting Factors

Hormone	Chemical nature	Release factor and its chemical nature	Release-inhibiting factor and its chemical nature	Function of the hormone
Growth hormone (somatotropin)	Protein, MW 21,000	Somatocrinin, peptide with 44 amino acids	Somatostatin; peptide with 14 amino acids and an S–S bond	Bone growth; affects carbohydrate, protein metabolism
Prolactin (PRL)	Protein, MW 20,000	Prolactin release factor (PRF); may or may not be identical to thyrotropin-releasing hormone	Prolactin release-inhibiting factor (PIF); most likely dopamine	Supports lactation
Thyrotropin (TSH)	Glycoprotein, MW 28,500, two subunits	Thyrotropin-releasing hormone (TRH); pyro-Glu-His-Pro-NH$_2$[a]	Unknown	Causes release of thyroxine by thyroid gland
Adrenocorticotropic hormone (ACTH)	Polypeptide with 39 amino acids	Corticotropin-releasing hormone (CRH); peptide with 41 amino acids	Unknown	Causes release of steroid hormones from adrenal cortex
Luteinizing hormone (LH)	Glycoprotein, MW 28,500; very similar to TSH	Gonadotropin-releasing hormone (GuRH); pyro-Glu-His-Trp-Ser-Tyr-Gly-Leu-Arg-Pro-Gly-NH$_2$[b]	Unknown	Causes ovulation in female and testosterone secretion in male
Follicle-stimulating hormone (FSH)	Glycoprotein, MW 34,000, two subunits	Same as for LH	Unknown	Egg development (ovary) in female and spermatogenesis in male
Melanocyte-stimulating hormone (α-MSH)	Ac-Ser-Tyr-Ser-Met-Glu-His-Phe-Arg-Trp-Gly-Lys-Pro-Val-NH$_2$[c]	Unknown	MSH release-inhibiting factor (MIF); most likely dopamine	Regulates pigment production by melanocytes

[a]Pyro-Glu (pyroglutamate) is glutamate in which the α-carboxyl group makes an internal peptide linkage with the N-terminal residue. Pro-NH$_2$ is proline amidinated at the C-terminal residue.

[b]Gly-NH$_2$ is amidinated glycine at the C terminus.

[c]The N-terminal residue of α-MSH (Ser) is acetylated; the C-terminal residue (Val) is amidinated.

hormones that *inhibit* the secretion of hormones by the anterior pituitary. These, too, are presented in Table 16.1. Thus, the control of anterior and intermediate pituitary hormone secretion rests, in part, on the elaboration of release- or release-inhibiting factors from the hypothalamus via the portal system. Additional factors that regulate the secretion of anterior pituitary hormones include a very elaborate system of feedback effects called the *long-loop system*. The principle that applies here is that the blood levels of the target tissue hormones (e.g., thyroid gland hormones) have an effect on the secretory activities of either the hypothalamus or anterior pituitary. The better known long-loop effects are illustrated in Figure 16.2. In addition, neural controls also exist. Thus PRL secretion is initiated by suckling, this is accomplished by a nerve impulse that serves to inhibit the secretion of prolactin release-inhibiting factor (PIF). There is also evidence that PRL increases PIF secretion by the hypothalamus via the so-called *short-loop mechanism*. This is a control system in which an increased level of a hormone in the pituitary gland results in its transport into the hypothalamus via a portal venous system to either inhibit the appropriate release factor production or to increase the production of a release-inhibiting factor. This system is summarized in Figure 16.3. GH may act in

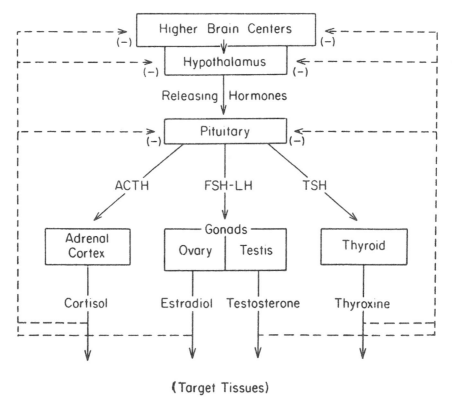

(Target Tissues)

Figure 16.2 Long-loop systems controlling the secretion of various pituitary hormones. A similar effect has been observed with somatomedins, growth factors released by the liver in response to GH. (Reproduced by permission from Hadley ME. Endocrinology, 2nd ed. Englewood Cliffs: Prentice-Hall, 1988, p. 126.)

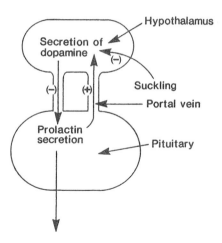

Figure 16.3 Short feedback loop controlling prolactin (PRL) secretion. PRL secretion by the anterior pituitary is normally inhibited by the PRL inhibiting factor (PIF) secreted by hypothalamus. PIF is dopamine. The suckling reflex stops PIF secretion and allows the pituitary to produce and export prolactin. Accumulation of PRL in the pituitary causes its backup through a portal vein into the hypothalamus, eliciting a derepression of PIF production and a subsequent decrease in PRL export.

the same way, either to increase the secretion of somatostatin or to increase the secretion of somatocrinin by the hypothalamus.

The physiologic effects of pituitary hormones are summarized in Table 16.1 and were discussed in more detail earlier (e.g., endorphins, α-MSH, and PRL). The physiologic action of GH is mediated mostly through a group of growth factors called *somatomedins*. These substances are synthesized in the liver under the influence of GH, and their main function is to support growth, for example that of the epiphyseal areas of long bones, and the sulfation of proteoglycans. Structurally, somatomedins are polypeptides very similar to insulin. For this reason they are called *insulin-like growth factors* (IGFs). The best known are IGF-I and IGF-II, both isolated from plasma and both bound to their specific plasma carrier proteins. IGF-I has a long-loop effect on the elaboration of GH by the pituitary gland. *Dwarfism* is the result of GH deficiency; it can be treated in children by GH. Overproduction of GH in children causes *gigantism*, and *acromegaly* is the result in adults.

16.2.2 Posterior Pituitary (Neurohypophysis) and Water Balance Hormones

The posterior pituitary gland is the source of circulating *oxytocin* and *vasopressin* (*antidiuretic hormone*, ADH). These hormones are actually produced in specific nerve cells in the hypothalamus and travel down the axons into the neurohypophysis. The structures of oxytocin and vasopressin are shown in Chapter 4. It may be seen that both are nanopeptides with disulfide bonds and that they differ by two amino acids only. Both hormones originate from larger proteins: vasopressin from prepressophysin and oxytocin from pro-oxyphysin. These are converted to pressophysin and oxyphysin, respectively (collectively, these are termed neurophysins), which then generate vasopressin and oxytocin by proteolysis.

The function of oxytocin is to cause uterine contraction and the release of milk from the mammary glands. As with prolactin, suckling, via the neural pathways, induces oxytocin secretion by the neurohypophysis. Blood oxytocin levels increase greatly just before parturition. Oxytocin is used as a drug to induce labor in pregnant women at term.

The function of vasopressin is to regulate water balance in the human being. A corollary is that vasopressin affects blood volume and blood pressure. There are so-called *osmoreceptors* on the hypothalamus surface, which sense the osmolarity of the blood stream. *Osmolarity* is the sum of all plasma solutes expressed as osmoles per liter. This, in fact, represents the number of particles per liter, where 6×10^{23} (Avogadro's number) particles per liter would depress the freezing point by 1.86°C. A 1 M glucose solution is 1 osmolar, 1 M NaCl would be 2 osm and 1 M CaCl$_2$ would be 3 osm. Normal (calculated) plasma osmolarity is about 0.304 osmol/L; Na$^+$ and Cl$^-$ ions are the major contributors. The actual (effective) osmolarity for plasma is somewhat lower than this because the activities of some solutes are lower than their concentrations. Table 16.2 lists the major solutes that contribute to biologic fluid osmolarity.

Thus, if osmoreceptors sense that osmolarity of the bloodstream is higher than normal, the secretion of vasopressin is increased. In addition, the patient experiences a thirst sensation, although a different set of osmoreceptors is in-

Table 16.2 Constituents of Various Biologic Fluids (mosmol/L)

Component	Plasma	Interstitial fluid	Intracellular fluid
Na$^+$	144	137	10
K$^+$	5	4.7	141
Ca^{2+}	2.5	2.4	0
Mg^{2+}	1.5	1.4	31
Cl$^-$	107	112.7	4
HCO$_3^-$	27	28.3	10
HPO$_4^{2-}$ and H$_2$PO$_4^-$	2	2	11
SO$_4^{2-}$	0.5	0.5	1
Creatine phosphate	—	—	45
Carnosine	—	—	14
Amino acids	2	2	9
Creatine	0.2	0.2	1.5
Lactate	1.2	1.2	1.5
ATP	—	—	5
Hexose phosphates	—	—	3.7
Glucose	5.6	5.6	—
Protein	1.2	0.2	4
Urea	4	4	4
Total	303.7	302.2	302.2
Actual	282.6	281.3	281.3
Osmotic pressure, mm Hg	5454	5430	5430

Source: Taken in part from Guyton AC. Textbook of Medical Physiology, 3d ed. Philadelphia: W. B. Saunders, 1966, p. 426.

volved in this response. The increased blood vasopressin levels increase water absorption by the distal tubules of the kidney. The effect is to dilute the blood by increasing blood volume with water via kidney effects and drinking. This results in an increased blood pressure, although other factors, too, contribute to blood pressure variations. In high osmolarity, the secretion of ADH decreases and water excretion increases. *Diabetes insipidus* is the result of certain pituitary lesions in which ADH secretion is severely limited and water excretion may increase to as high as 10 L/day, the normal being about 1.5 L/day. There is a condition called *inappropriate ADH secretion* (SIDH) in which ADH is secreted continuously (e.g., by a tumor), resulting in excessive water reabsorption and a decreased plasma osmolarity.

Body fluids may be distributed into several compartments that interact with each other. It is possible to speak of the *intracellular fluid*, which is the fluid present inside the approximately 100 trillion cells found in the human organism, including red blood cells; *extracellular fluid*, which includes blood plasma, *interstitial fluid* (fluid found between cells and in lymph), cerebrospinal fluid, synovial fluid, intraocular fluid, and fluids found in the gastrointestinal tract, the peritoneal cavity, the pericardial cavity, and others. The amounts of some such fluids present in normal individuals are summarized in Table 16.3. Overall, water accounts for 55–67% of an individual's weight.

Normally, an individual excretes 1.0–1.5 L of water daily in the urine, about 100 ml each in feces and sweat, and up to 1 L in the expired air and from the skin (the latter quantity is also called insensible water loss). During the course of normal water metabolism, however, some 200 L water passes through the

Table 16.3 Body Fluid Compartments

Compartment	Amount in a 70 kg person	% of Body weight
Total body water weight, kg		
Males	37	52
Females	43	62
Intracellular fluid weight, kg	28	40
Extracellular fluid weight, kg		
Adults	14	20
Infants	—	Up to 40
Interstitial fluid weight, kg		
males	11	16
Blood weight, kg[a]		
Males	5.1	7.3
Females	4.6	6.6
Red cell volume, L		
Males	2.0	—
Females	1.5	—
Plasma volume, L		
Males	2.9	—
Females	2.8	—

[a]Specific gravity of normal blood is approximately 1.

glomerular membrane of the kidneys and 8–10 L is excreted into the gastrointestinal tract. Because a total of only 1.6–2.5 L water is excreted every day via all channels, it is clear that the human has developed very efficient water conservation mechanisms that cause the reabsorption of the bulk of water from the glomerular filtrate and the gastrointestinal tract. Water intake amounts to about 1.2 L from drinking fluids, 1.1 L from solid foods, and 0.3 L from metabolism per day. Sometimes, however, because of disease, one of these reabsorption mechanisms becomes deficient; the individual then proceeds to lose excessive amounts of water either in the urine or through other channels.

Considerable losses of body water may occur rather suddenly via hemorrhage or more slowly via severe diarrhea or vomiting. Excessive losses of blood volume cause *shock*, which may set in when 25–30% of the blood volume is lost. The physiologic mechanism to correct for blood loss involves the rapid movement of interstitial fluid into the circulatory system, into which as much as 50% of the interstitial fluid may thus be transferred within a matter of a few hours. The interstitial fluid is, in turn, partially replaced by intracellular fluid; however, this is a much slower process, and 1 or 2 days is required to reestablish a fluid equilibrium in the organism. The lost fluids and electrolytes must eventually be replaced through diet or intravenous feeding.

In certain instances, fluids may merely shift from one compartment to another without net water loss or gain for the entire organism. This is usually secondary to a pathologic process, such as kidney disease, infection, or malnutrition. If there is an increase in the volume of the interstitial fluid, the condition is called *edema*. Edema may be present in peripheral tissues, in the lungs, or in other tissues, and because this water is otherwise unavailable to the organism, it must be replaced via dietary means.

It is generally impractical to measure body fluid compartment changes as a matter of routine clinical biochemistry procedure, except blood volume shifts. Thus, total red blood cell volume may be estimated via the *isotope dilution* method, using red blood cells tagged with radioactive chromium, and plasma volume may be estimated by the injection of serum albumin labeled with radioactive iodine. An approximation of blood volume changes may also be made by measuring the hematocrit (see Chapter 7) or another blood constituent. Thus if the hematocrit drops from a normal value of 47% to a value of 39% (a 17% drop) in a patient who hemorrhaged but later stabilized the extracellular fluid volume, the patient must have lost 17% of his blood volume in the bleeding episode, and this loss was replaced by the interstitial fluid, which of course has no red blood cells.

16.3   STEROID HORMONE-PRODUCING GLANDS

16.3.1   Biosynthesis of Steroid Hormones

Steroid hormones are produced in the adrenal cortex and the sex glands. All such hormones originate from cholesterol. Figure 16.4 shows the overall scheme for steroid hormone biosynthesis that is applicable to all tissues. The final products may be divided into the following groups: *mineralocorticoids* (e.g., aldosterone), produced by the zona glomerulosa of the adrenal cortex; *glucocorticoids* (e.g., cortisol), produced by the zona fasciculata of the adrenal cortex; and the

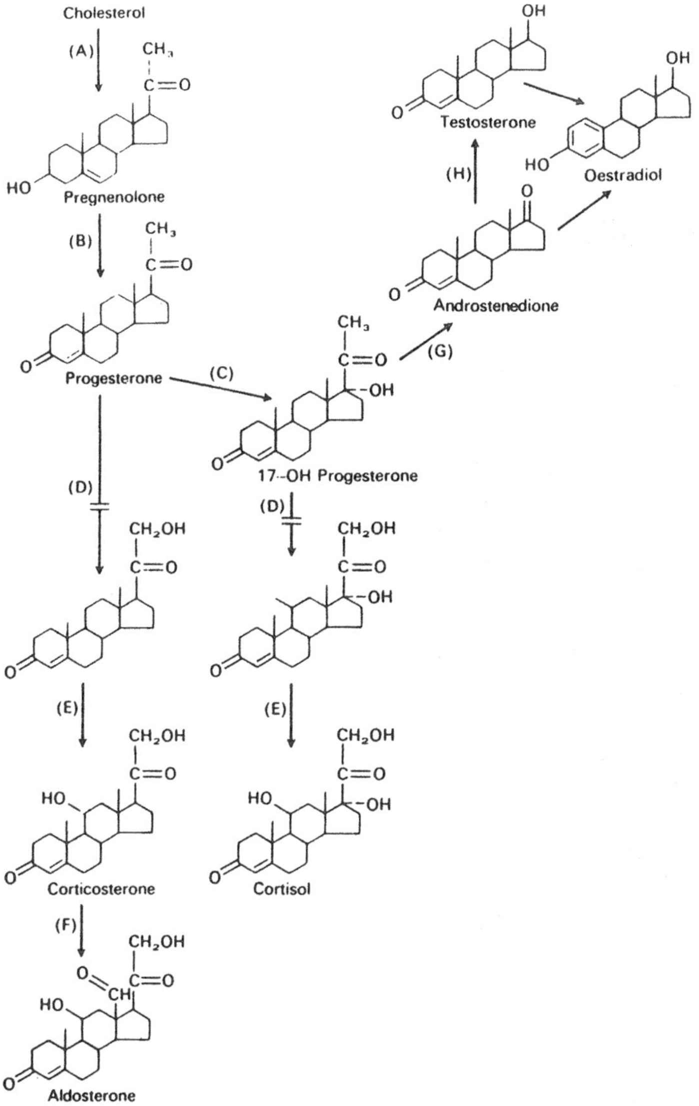

Figure 16.4 Biosynthesis of various classes of steroid hormones. Reaction (A) is cata-lyzed by a cholesterol desmolase, which oxidizes the cholesterol side chain. Reactions (D) are catalyzed by 21-hydroxylases, which are defective in congenital adrenal hyperplasia. (Reproduced by permission from Schwarz V. A Clinical Companion to Biochemical Stud-ies. Reading: Freeman, 1978, p. 94.)

sex hormones, *androgens* (e.g., testosterone), *estrogens* (e.g., estradiol), and *progesterone*, produced by the sex glands. The zona reticularis of the adrenal cortex also produces *androgens*. Progesterone appears to be the intermediate in all steroid hormone biosynthetic processes.

The corticosteroids and to some extent the mineralocorticoids are released from the adrenal cortex under the influence of ACTH. In turn, ACTH secretion by the pituitary is inhibited by high concentrations of plasma glucocorticoids (long loop). Thus, in *Addison's disease*, an adrenal-cortical lesion, blood levels of ACTH are very high. The glucocorticoids affect intermediary metabolism, and this function is discussed in Chapters 18 through 21. Glucocorticoids also have antiinflammatory properties, and these are discussed in connection with prostaglandin biochemistry later in this chapter.

Testicular function is controlled by the anterior pituitary hormones LH and FSH. The former acts on the *Leydig cells* (interstitial cells) to cause the secretion of testosterone, whereas the latter acts on the *Sertoli cells* to promote spermatogenesis. Testosterone, an androgen, is responsible for the development of secondary sex characteristics in the male, and, along with FSH, stimulates spermatogenesis. It is an *anabolic steroid*, which causes an increase in muscle mass. In the female, both LH and FSH act on the ovary. LH presumably causes the *thecal cells* to synthesize androgens, whereas FSH stimulates the *granulosa cells* to produce estrogens from the androgens. Both LH and FSH are required for ovulation. Progesterone is produced largely by the *corpus luteum*. Estrogens are responsible for secondary female sex characteristics, whereas progesterone prepares the organism for pregnancy. There is a cyclic pattern to female sex hormone secretion corresponding to the events during the menstrual cycle. This area is beyond the scope of this volume, however.

Congenital adrenal hyperplasia is a hereditary disorder in which the 21-hydroxylase-catalyzing reaction (D) in Figure 16.4 is inoperative. This lowers plasma cortisol and aldosterone levels, disturbing the long-loop system and thus increasing ACTH production. This further increases adrenal progesterone levels, which respond by synthesizing excessive quantities of testosterone. This, in turn, results in masculinization of the female child. Inborn errors involving 11-hydroxylase deficiency [reaction (E) in Figure 16.4] are also known, and these lead to symptoms similar to those observed in 21-hydroxylase deficiency.

16.3.2 Aldosterone and Its Actions

Aldosterone is produced in the zona glomerulosa of the adrenal cortex. Its function is to regulate sodium ion reabsorption in the distal convoluted tubule of the kidney: under its influence, sodium is retained and K^+, NH_4^+, and H^+ are excreted. Although ACTH exerts some effect on aldosterone secretion, the main control mechanism seems to involve the renin–angiotensin system. This is illustrated in Figure 16.5 and may be described as follows. *Renin* is an enzyme secreted by the juxtaglomerular cells of the kidney, which are situated in the vicinity of the glomeruli. The secretion of renin increases when there is a decrease in blood pressure or blood volume or when the osmolarity of plasma decreases. Its substrate is a circulating α-globulin (also called angiotensinogen, MW 56,000), from which a decapeptide, *angiotensin I*, is removed. The decapeptide is further cleaved by a lung enzyme, *angiotensinase*, into a dipeptide and the biologically active octapeptide, *angiotensin II*. The latter then stimulates the production of aldosterone by the adrenal cortex; it also possesses a vasopressor property.

Aldosterone is expected to work in concert with ADH. Thus, if the appropriate *baroreceptors* (monitors of blood pressure) should detect decreased blood

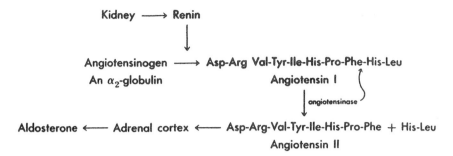

Figure 16.5 The renin–angiotensin system controlling aldosterone secretion by the adrenal cortex cells.

pressure, aldosterone is secreted, causing sodium retention. This increases plasma osmolarity, which is detected by the hypothalamus via its osmoreceptors. The result is the secretion of ADH by the neurohypophysis, resulting in water retention and an increase in blood volume and blood pressure. It is thus clear that increased plasma sodium levels result in increased water retention and an increased blood pressure.

Several relatively common disorders result in aldosterone secretion abnormalities and aberrations of electrolyte status. In *Addison's disease,* the adrenal cortex is often destroyed through autoimmune processes. One of the effects is a lack of aldosterone secretion and decreased Na^+ retention by the patient. In a typical Addison's disease patient, serum $[Na^+]$ and $[Cl^-]$ are 128 and 96 meq/L, respectively (see Table 16.2 for normal values). Potassium levels are elevated, 6 meq/L or higher, because the Na^+ reabsorption system of the kidney, which is under aldosterone control, moves K^+ into the urine just as it moves Na^+ back into plasma. Thus, if more Na^+ is excreted, more K^+ is reabsorbed. Bicarbonate remains relatively normal. The opposite situation prevails in *Cushing's disease,* however, in which an overproduction of adrenocorticosteroids, especially cortisol, is present. Glucocorticoids have mild mineralocorticoid activities, but ACTH also increases aldosterone secretion. This may be caused by an oversecretion of ACTH by a tumor or by adrenal hyperplasia or tumors. Serum sodium in Cushing's disease is slightly elevated, $[K^+]$ is below normal (hypokalemia), and metabolic alkalosis is present. The patient is usually hypertensive. A more severe electrolyte abnormality is seen in Conn's syndrome or *primary aldosteronism,* usually caused by an adrenal tumor. Increased blood aldosterone levels result in the urinary loss of K^+ and H^+, retention of Na^+ (hypernatremia), alkalosis, and profound hypertension.

The kidneys filter about 180 L plasma per day. This contains a total of about $144 \times 180 = 26{,}000$ meq Na^+, which must be reabsorbed into the circulation. Only a small percentage (2%) of this is under aldosterone control: that which is exchanged with K^+. The rest is absorbed by other mechanisms, including that which exchanges protons for reabsorbed Na^+ ions. This is shown in Figure 16.6 and may be explained as follows: both Na^+ and HCO_3^- ions are present in the glomerular filtrate. As they move down the tubular lumen, Na^+ is taken up by the renal tubular cells and is replaced in the tubular lumen by protons, which are actively secreted. The protons combine largely with the luminal HCO_3^-, and

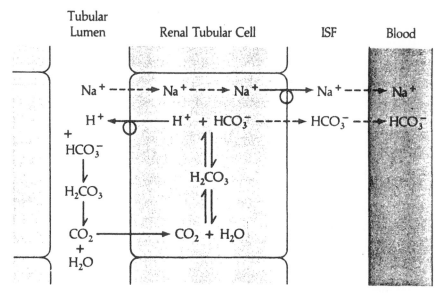

Figure 16.6 Reabsorption of Na^+ into the bloodstream from the kidney tubules. ISF, interstitial fluid. (Reproduced by permission from Keys JL. Fluid, Electrolyte and Acid–Base Regulation. Monterey: Wadsworth Health Science Division, 1985, p. 73.)

the latter then yields CO_2 and H_2O. The CO_2 diffuses into the tubular cell, where under the influence of carbonic anhydrase it regenerates H^+ and HCO_3^-. The H^+ ions are once again transported into the tubular lumen, whereas the HCO_3^- leaves the tubular cell along with the Na^+. One may observe in this scheme of events that the bicarbonate found in the tubular lumen is not the same that is reabsorbed into the bloodstream and that the involvement of H^+ and HCO_3^- in Na^+ transport creates the possibility of acid–base disorders. One form of *renal tubular acidosis* is a reflection of either an impaired secretion of protons into the tubular lumen and/or an impaired movement of HCO_3^- from the tubular cell into the bloodstream. In this disorder, the urine is often alkaline and the bloodstream is hyponatremic (low Na^+), with the presence of metabolic acidosis. Chloride is usually increased in such individuals to compensate for the decrease in HCO_3^-.

It is thus clear that the kidneys are an important means of excreting protons from whatever source and in generating HCO_3^-. This was alluded to in Chapter 3. The kidneys, in fact, generate more HCO_3^- than they receive. The difference is 50–60 meq/day (about 4300 meq/day enters the kidney and is regenerated). This difference is necessary to replenish HCO_3^- lost, when acids produced in the organism are buffered (e.g., lactic acid). Kidneys also acidify urine; that is, they serve to excrete protons as shown in Figure 16.6. In addition to being able to combine with luminal HCO_3^-, the protons can combine with NH_3 and HPO_4^{2-}, which are also present in the tubular lumen. Combination with NH_3 produces NH_4^+, and combination with HPO_4^{2-} generates $H_2PO_4^-$. These are excreted in the urine and represent the so-called titratable acidity of the urine. The excretion of NH_4^+ and $H_2PO_4^-$ also serves to spare an organism's sodium ions.

The determination of serum Na^+, K^+, HCO_3^-, and Cl^- is extremely important in diagnostic work, as well as in the management of surgical patients. A detailed discussion of water, electrolyte, and acid–base relationships in health and disease is beyond the scope of this book; however, certain basic facts and vocabulary are presented here, which should prove useful if further studies in this area are to be undertaken. Table 16.2 lists the normal concentrations of blood electrolytes. It is customary to represent electrolytes in the form of *Gamblegrams* (in honor of J. Gamble), shown in Figure 16.7. An examination of the Gamblegram should indicate that the sum of all cations must equal the sum of all anions. In addition to Na^+, K^+, HCO_3^-, and Cl^-, the "unmeasured" cations and anions (e.g., Ca^{2+} and SO_4^{2-}) are represented by uc and ua, respectively. We can then write the following expressions:

$$[Na^+] + [K^+] + [uc] = [Cl^-] + [HCO_3^-] + [ua] \tag{16.1}$$

and

$$[Na^+] + [K^+] - [Cl^-] - [HCO_3^-] = [ua] - [uc] \tag{16.2}$$

The expression [ua] − [uc] is the *anion gap*. In the normal Gamblegram (Figure 16.7), the anion gap is 17 meq/L (using the values given). In diabetic coma (Figure 16.7), the anion gap is 33 meq/L. It is accounted for largely by "organic acids," otherwise known as *ketone bodies* (see Chapter 19). Calculation of the

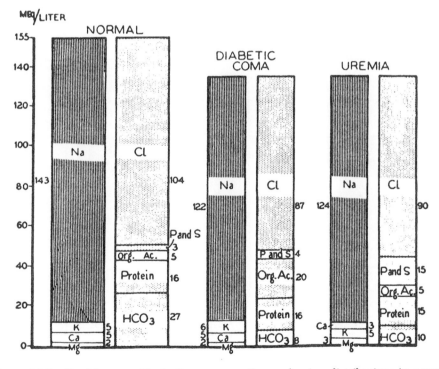

Figure 16.7 Gamblegrams illustrating serum cation and anion distributions in normal, diabetic, and uremic individuals. (Reproduced by permission from Hoffman WS. The Biochemistry of Clinical Medicine, 4th ed. Chicago: Yearbook, 1970, p. 249.)

anion gap may serve both the diagnostic purposes and to verify the accuracy of "measured" electrolyte determinations.

    Because the sum of all cations must equal the sum of all anions per Equation (16.1), it then follows that quantitative changes in one set of electrolytes must be accompanied by those of the other set. Thus, should $[Na^+]$ decrease, the anion content should also decrease. Alternatively, a decrease in one ionic group may lead to its replacement by another ionic form of the same charge. Thus, should serum $[Cl^-]$ decrease, $[HCO_3^-]$ may increase to take its place. Note that whenever $[HCO_3^-]$ changes, aberrations of the acid–base status of the patient follow. For instance, when infants were fed an artificial formula that had a low $[Cl^-]$, serum Cl^- was lowered and was partially replaced by HCO_3^-, leading to metabolic alkalosis and loss of K^+. A similar situation is observed in the uremic patient (Figure 16.7), in whom an increase in phosphate and sulfate (these two ions always change identically) results in a decrease in HCO_3^-, leading to an acidotic condition. In pyloric obstruction (Figure 16.8), in which severe vomiting leads to the loss of HCl, the Cl^- lost is replaced by HCO_3^-, leading to metabolic alkalosis. Vomiting also causes a loss of Na^+ and K^+. In severe diarrhea (Figure 16.8), there is a loss of Na^+, K^+, and HCO_3^-, because the intestinal content is slightly alkaline

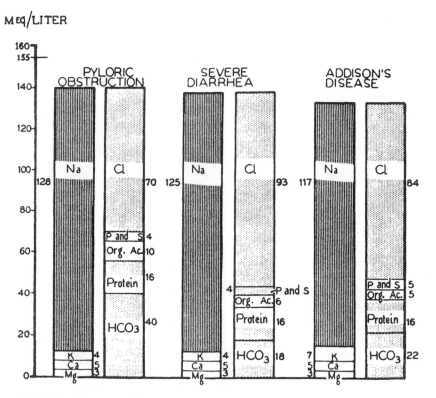

Figure 16.8 Gamblegrams illustrating serum cation and anion distribution in patients with pyloric obstruction, severe diarrhea, and Addison's disease. (Reproduced by permission from Hoffman WS. The Biochemistry of Clinical Medicine, 4th ed. Chicago, Yearbook, 1970, p. 252.)

Table 16.4 Electrolyte Concentration of Selected Biologic Fluids

Fluid	Electrolytes (meq/L)					
	pH	Na^+	K^+	Ca^{2+}	Cl^-	HCO_3^-
Plasma	7.4	144	4.5	5.0	103	24
Sweat	4.5–7.5	30–70[a]	3–6	3–5	30–7	0–10
Gastric juice	1.0–4.0	60[b]	9.2	—	84	0
Large bowel diarrhea	>7	150–360	45	—	—	High
Recent ileostomy	7.6–8.2	100	20	—	110	75
Pancreatic juice	7–8	148	7	6	80	80
Diarrhea in infants	>7	60	30	—	45	—
Small bowel	7.2–7.8	111	5	—	104	30

[a]May be as low as 10 meq/L in heat-acclimated individuals.
[b]May be higher in elderly persons.

(see Table 16.4). This results in lowered serum $[HCO_3^-]$ and an acidotic condition. Figure 16.8 also shows the cation–anion distribution observed in Addison's disease, which was discussed earlier.

The pathologic conditions shown in Figures 16.7 and 16.8 are associated with *hyponatremia*-decreased serum $[Na^+]$. These and other electrolyte disorders may be associated with fluid volume changes in the organism. For instance, in SIADH (increased vasopressin secretion), the hyponatremia observed is a result of an extracellular fluid dilution by the water retained. A similar situation is observed in other fluid retention syndromes, such as *congestive heart failure*. Administration of diuretics also leads to Na^+ (and K^+) depletion and water loss. In fact, water loss occurs because the diuretics interfere with Na^+ reabsorption in the kidney tubules. The loss of water always accompanies increases in the excretion of various solutes, such as glucose and ketone bodies in untreated diabetes. Excessive water losses generally result in losses of K^+ as well. Water may, of course, be lost by avenues other than the kidneys. We have already noted the severe vomiting and diarrhea conditions in which Na^+ losses occur in addition to those of anions, leading to acid-base disorders. In burns, there is a hyposmotic fluid loss but electrolytes are largely retained, leading to hypernatremia. The latter is often associated with metabolic alkalosis, whereas hyponatremia is often associated with metabolic acidosis. There are numerous exceptions to these rules, however, as brought about by many diuretic drugs.

16.3.3 Potassium Metabolism

The maintenance of the appropriate potassium levels in extracellular fluid is extremely important for the normal functioning of cardiac and skeletal muscle. Apparently, the regulation of intracellular potassium is of lesser importance. The control of potassium concentration in the extracellular fluid is affected by its migration in and out of the intracellular fluid and via excretion in the urine. The glomerular filtrate contains the same amount of potassium as plasma; however, practically all of it is reabsorbed in the proximal convoluted tubule. In the distal tubule, however, as the sodium becomes reabsorbed under the influence of aldosterone, some potassium is excreted into the tubules and is lost in the urine.

Abnormal losses of potassium resulting in *hypokalemia* (low serum potassium) occur during diuretic therapy, in which large amounts of sodium pass into the glomerular filtrate and must be reabsorbed, and in diarrhea and vomiting. *Hyperkalemia* (high serum potassium levels), with its possible fatal consequences as a result of cardiac muscle toxicity, is observed in kidney failure and trauma, especially surgical trauma. Although hypokalemia can be treated by potassium infusions, hyperkalemia is usually treated by the infusion of sodium bicarbonate. Alkaline plasma causes potassium to move into the cells, whereas a relatively acidic plasma will bring about its movement out of the cells into the plasma. This occurs because hydrogen ions and potassium ions are antagonistic toward each other; thus, if the hydrogen ion concentration is greater in the intracellular fluid, by the law of mass action the hydrogen ions move into the extracellular fluid, forcing potassium ions to move in the opposite direction to maintain electrical neutrality. Conversely, if acidosis (acid plasma) exists, hydrogen ions move into the cells, causing potassium ions to migrate into the bloodstream. Acidosis is thus associated with hyperkalemia, whereas alkalosis is associated with hypokalemia.

16.4   AMINO ACID-DERIVED HORMONES

16.4.1   Thyroxine and Triiodothyronine

Thyroxine (T_4) and *triidothyronine* (T_3) are produced in the thyroid gland in response to TSH stimulation. Conversely, T_3 and T_4 inhibit TSH release by the anterior pituitary, so that blood serum TSH levels are an excellent indicator of thyroid gland function. The biosynthesis and structures of T_3 and T_4 are shown in Figure 16.9. It is seen that these hormones are derivatives of tyrosine and that they contain iodine. The biosynthesis of thyroid hormones seems to be the only reason human beings require iodide in their diets. The thyroid gland concentrates iodide from the circulation, where it is oxidized by perioxidase to I_2 or possibly I^+. The oxidized form of iodine halogenates certain tryosyl residues of *thyroglobulin*, a thyroid gland protein with a molecular weight of 600,000. Following further posttranslational modification, as indicated in Figure 16.9, T_3 and T_4 are released from thyroglobulin proteolytically and exported into the bloodstream. T_3 and T_4 are bound to carrier proteins in the bloodstream and for this reason are referred to as "protein-bound iodine" (PBI). The proteins in question are the *thyroxine binding globulin* (TBG), thyroxine binding prealbumin (TBPA), and serum albumin. These bind 70–75, 15–20, and 5–10% of circulating T_4, respectively. In tissues, T_4 may be converted by a dehalogenase enzyme to a triiodothyronine that has a different iodine distribution than T_3. The triiodothyronines are biologically more potent than the more abundant T_4.

Several types of effects are ascribed to thyroid hormones. T_3 and T_4 control heat production in the organism by affecting the electron transport pathway (see Chapter 17). Apparently these hormones stimulate electron transport, thereby producing more ATP. The latter is used to increase the activity of Na^+/K^+ pumps throughout the organism, in the process of which ATP is hydrolyzed and heat

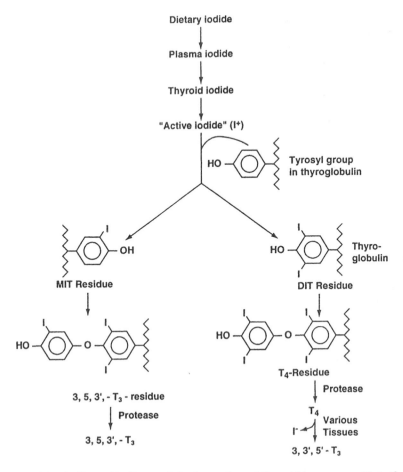

Figure 16.9 Metabolism of iodine and the formation of thyroid hormones. Note that the thyroid gland produces one type of triiodothyronine, whereas peripheral tissue dehalogenases produce another type. (Adapted by permission from Chattoraj SC, Watts NB. Endocrinology. In Tietz NW, ed. Textbook of Clinical Chemistry. Philadelphia: WB Saunders, 1986, p. 1117.)

released. It also induces the biosynthesis of many enzymes, including Na^+/K^+-ATPase, hyalouronidase, and milk synthesis enzymes. It acts in concert with other hormones, such as GH, and it is required for the differentiation of various tissues in the fetus and newborn.

Thyroid disorders may be divided into over- and underproduction of the thyroid hormones. These may be caused by thyroid gland disorders or disorders of the pituitary gland (TSH production) or hypothalamus (thyrotropin-releasing hormone release). Thyroid hormone deficiency in infancy may cause mental retardation if it is not corrected immediately after birth. For this reason, many states require thyroid function tests in all newborns. In adults, thyroid deficiency may be caused by *Hashimoto's thyroiditis,* an immune disorder, or dietary iodine deficiency, in which case it is called *simple goiter.* The term "myxedema" has been used to refer to hypothyroidism of whatever cause. Myxedemas may be treated by thyroxine or iodide administration. Hyperthyroidism, also termed *thyrotoxicosis*, is characterized by excess circulating T_3 and T_4, and it may be caused by a variety of factors: *Graves' disease*, in which there is a constant stimulation of TSH receptors on the thyroid gland by autoantibodies; TSH-secreting tumors; thyroiditis, which releases large amounts of T_3 and T_4 into the circulation; and various tumors of the thyroid gland. Hyperthyroid patients have elevated metabolic activities with excess protein and fat catabolism and caloric malnutrition despite a good appetite. Treatment for hyperthyroidism involves surgical intervention, destruction of thyroid tissue by radioactive I^-, and antithyroid drugs. Among the latter are inhibitors of I^- oxidation and uptake by the thyroid gland, such as perchlorates and thiocyanate, and inhibitors of iodine incorporation into tyrosine, such as propylthiouracil and methimazole. The former also blocks the conversion of T_4 to T_3 in peripheral tissue.

There are numerous thyroid gland function tests, each designed to determine the etiology of thyroid dysfunction. In general, though, when hypothyroidism is present, circulating T_3 and T_4 levels are down and TSH is up. The opposite is true of hyperthyroidism. In addition, free (non–protein-bound) T_4 and TBG may be determined to clarify inconclusive results. In hyperthyroidism, free T_4 is increased but total T_4 may be normal. It is the free serum T_4 that has been correlated with clinical symptoms rather than total T_4.

16.4.2 Epinephrine and Other Catecholamines

Epinephrine (adrenaline) is a "stress" hormone, even though it is not under any direct pituitary or hypothalamic control. By *stress* is meant an environmental insult that also causes the release of ACTH and the glucocorticoids. A stressful situation may be a sense of danger, confinement in small or crowded quarters, oxygen deprivation, lowering of blood glucose levels, and so on. Epinephrine is synthesized in the chromaffin cells of the adrenal medulla from tyrosine, as shown in Figure 16.10. It has a major effect on the various metabolic pathways, on cardiac function (increases force and rate of heartbeat), on smooth muscle function (relaxation), on blood pressure (increase), and on blood coagulation (decreases the time of clotting by aggregating platelets). The pathway shown in Figure 16.10 is active in nerve tissue in addition to adrenal medulla.

Chemically, epinephrine is categorized as a *catecholamine*, because its aromatic residue is catechol. Several other catecholamines are shown in Figure 16.10, and these are either intermediates in epinephrine biosynthesis or its degradation products. The most important catecholamines besides epinephrine are dopamine and norepinephrine. Both are neurotransmitters, and both work locally. *Parkinson's disease* is apparently caused by an inadequate supply of dopamine in the brain. An effective treatment is the oral administration of L-*dopa*, its metabolic precursor. Although one of the normal pathways of tyrosine metabolism in the brain is to generate dopamine and norepinephrine, it is also possible to obtain a false neurotransmitter called octopamine, as shown in Figure 16.10. This occurs when the quantity of aromatic amino acids entering the brain is larger than normal (as in hepatic encephalopathy), so that octopamine becomes a major tyrosine metabolite. The accumulation of octopamine induces coma.

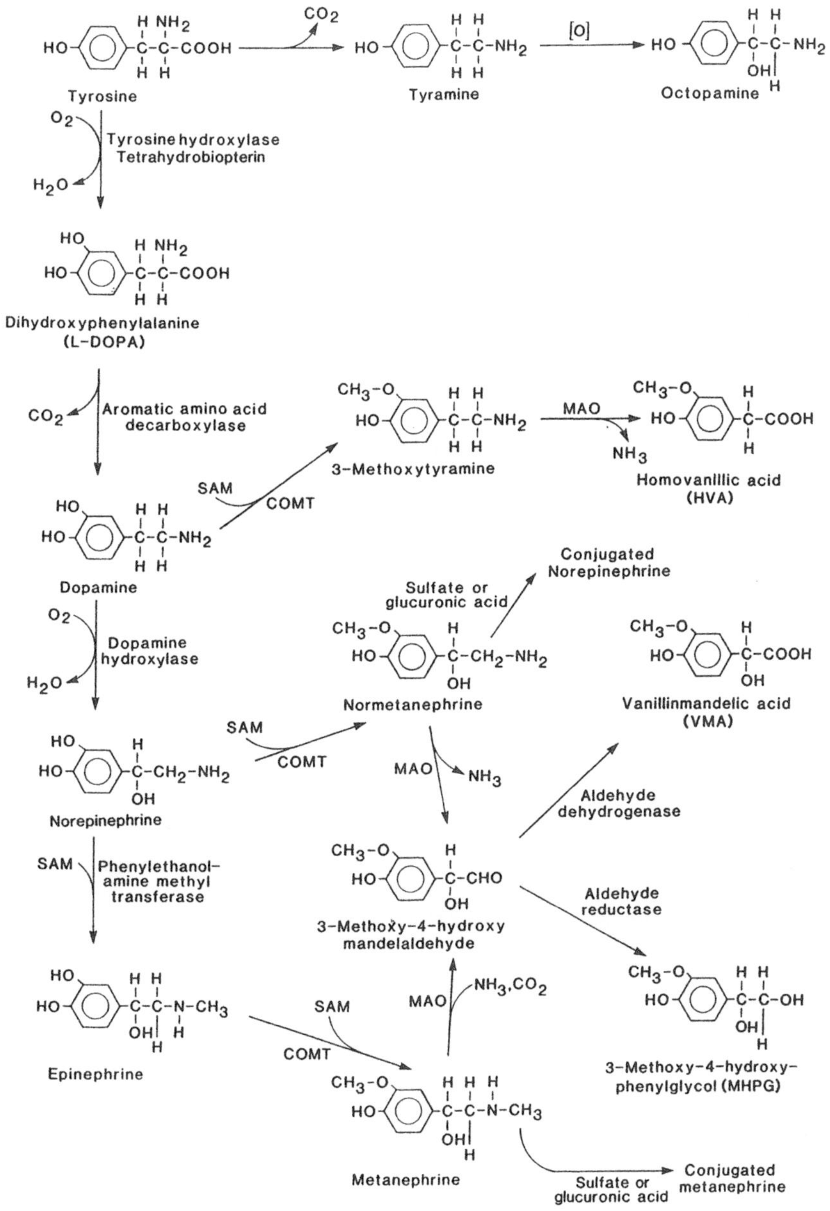

Figure 16.10 Catecholamine biosynthesis and metabolism. MAO, monoamine oxidase; COMT, catecholamine-*O*-methyltransferase; SAM, 5-adenosylmethionine.

The secretion of epinephrine by the adrenal medulla is controlled directly by nerve impulses and also by the other stress hormones, namely, corticosteroids. This is illustrated in Figure 16.11. Nerve impulses have a major stimulatory effect on tyrosine and dopamine hydroxylases, whereas glucocorticoids have a major effect on phenylethanolamine methyltransferase. Tyrosine hydroxylase is considered the rate-controlling enzyme in the biosynthesis

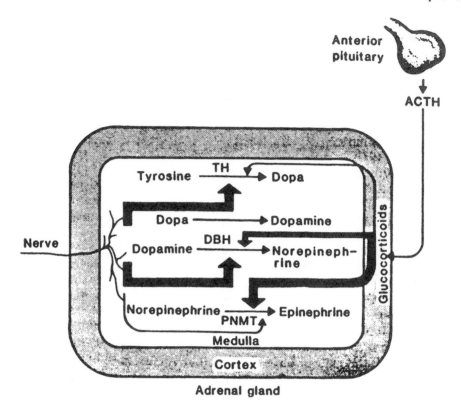

Figure 16.11 Control of catecholamine biosynthesis in the adrenal medulla. TH, tyrosine hydroxylase; DBH, dopamine hydroxylase; PNMT, phenylethanolamine methyltransferase; ACTH, adrenocorticotropic hormone. The heavy arrows indicate major sites of regulation. (Reproduced by permission from Axelrod, J. Reisine TD. Stress hormones: their interaction and regulation. Science 224:452–459, 1984.)

of catecholamines. It is an iron-containing enzyme, and an unusual redox cofactor, tetrahydrobiopterin, is required in this reaction. Its structure and properties are discussed in Chapter 20.

The degradation of catecholamines is also shown in Figure 16.10. Several enzymes are involved in the process: monoamine oxidase (MAO), a copper-containing flavoprotein; catecholamine-O-methyltransferase (COMT); and aldehyde oxidase and reductase. The action of COMT depends on the presence of S-adenosylmethionine (SAM), a carrier of methyl residues discussed in detail in Chapter 20. The order in which MAO and COMT work is immaterial: Figure 16.10 shows that the action of COMT precedes that of MAO, but this order may also be reversed. The end products of catecholamine metabolism are vanillylmandelic acid (VMA), homovanillic acid (HVA), 3-methoxy-4-hydroxyphenylglycol (MHPG), and free and conjugated metanephrines. These are all excreted in the urine and are indicators of certain pathologic states. Thus, in *pheochromocytoma*, a chromaffin cell tumor producing severe hypertension, VMA and the metanephrines are elevated in the urine. In *neuroblastoma*, a pediatric tumor, free dopamine and HVA are highly elevated in the urine. The latter is also increased in the urine of patients with *ganglioblastoma*. All catecholamine degradation products may appear in urine as glucuronic acid or sulfate conjugates. MAO inhibitors have been used as antihypertensive drugs. Best known among these is pargyline, which most likely works through Na^+ depletion.

16.4.3 Calcium and Phosphate Metabolism: Control by Parathormone and Calcitonin

The human organism contains 1–1.4 kg calcium, and about 1% of this is in the extracellular fluid. The rest is largely in bone. The serum calcium concentration is 9–11.5 mg/dL, of which 4.5–5.0 mg/dL is in the free, ionized, biologically active form. The rest is protein bound or complexed with a variety of chelators, such as citrate. The daily dietary calcium requirement is 400–500 mg, and each day, 300–400 mg calcium is lost in the urine and an additional 150 mg in the feces. Inorganic phosphorus (largely as HPO_4^{2-}) amounts to 2.7–4.5 mg/dL in adult serum.

Calcium and phosphate levels in the extracellular fluid are regulated by three factors: vitamin D (see Chapter 6), parathyroid hormone (PTH), and calcitonin (CT). Some properties of PTH and CT were discussed in Chapter 6. PTH secretion is controlled by serum $[Ca^{2+}]$; a low $[Ca^{2+}]$ increases [PTH]. The latter is initially synthesized as prepro-PTH, a 115 amino acid polypeptide. This is reduced proteolytically to pro-PTH, a 90 amino acid peptide, and finally to the 84 amino acid PTH. The active part of PTH is its N-terminal domain, consisting of amino acids 1–34. The action of PTH is to maintain serum $[Ca^{2+}]$ balance. At low concentrations, PTH maintains a steady state in bone mineral turnover. Hydroxyapatite $[Ca_{10}(PO_4)_6(OH)_2]$ is the principal mineral component of bone. Thus, both Ca and phosphate are necessary to build bone. PTH affects equally the activity of *osteoblasts*, which build bone, and *osteoclasts*, which destroy (resorb) bone. At high serum PTH levels, osteoblast activity is diminished and osteoclast activity is increased. In addition, PTH increases Ca reabsorption by the kidney tubules but, at the same time, increases phosphate excretion in the urine. It has been traditionally observed that those factors that increase serum $[Ca^{2+}]$ decrease serum P_i. This presumably maintains the solubility of $CaHPO_4$ (1 $\times 10^{-7}$) at a level that avoids its precipitation, thus maintaining Ca^{2+} in solution. There are numerous exceptions to this rule, however. PTH effects are achieved to a great extent through its action on vitamin D metabolism.

The hormone that opposes the action of PTH is CT. It is produced in the parafollicular cells of the thyroid gland, whereas thyroxine is produced by the follicular cells. Human CT is a 32 amino acid peptide with one disulfide bond. CT is secreted in response to increased serum $[Ca^{2+}]$, especially following a meal. Its role is to prevent hypercalcemia by decreasing the serum $[Ca^{2+}]$. This is achieved by counteracting the action of PTH on osteoclasts while having no effect on osteoblasts. In addition, CT affects the movement of serum Ca^{2+} into a labile Ca pool on the bone surface, which then releases Ca back into the circulation when $[Ca^{2+}]$ in serum declines.

Phosphate levels in the bloodstream are also controlled by the three factors just listed: vitamin D, CT, and PTH. These effects are summarized in Table 16.5.

Calcium determinations in serum are valuable in the diagnosis of a number of pathologic conditions. *Hypocalcemia* (low serum calcium) is seen in hypopara-

Table 16.5 Control of Ca and Phosphate Metabolism

Agent[a]	Uptake by bone	Intestinal absorption	Kidney tubule reabsorption	Fecal excretion
Vitamin D	$P_i \downarrow$ Ca $\downarrow$	$P_i \uparrow$ Ca $\uparrow$	$P_i \uparrow$ Ca $\uparrow$	
PTH	$P_i \downarrow$ Ca $\downarrow$	$P_i \uparrow$ Ca $\uparrow$	$P_i \downarrow$ Ca $\uparrow$	
CT	$P_i \uparrow$ Ca $\uparrow$	No effect	$P_i \downarrow$ Ca $\downarrow$	$P_i \uparrow$

[a]PTH, parathormone; CT, calcitonin.

thyroidism, dietary vitamin D deficiency (e.g., rickets), and fat malabsorption syndromes. In the last condition, not enough vitamin D is absorbed, and this may be because of chronic pancreatitis, among other diseases. Acute pancreatitis also results in hypocalcemia, although by a different mechanism. Hypocalcemia is usually accompanied by hyperphosphatemia. Free $[Ca^{2+}]$ is decreased in alkalosis, presumably because it is bound more avidly by serum proteins. Hypocalcemia may cause tetany and convulsions. *Hyperphosphatemia*, for example in renal failure, causes hypocalcemia. *Hypercalcemia* is caused by hyperparathyroidism or tumors, especially those that have metastasized to the bone. Milk alkali syndrome, induced by the ingestion of large amounts of $CaCO_3$ antacids and milk, causes both hypercalcemia and hyperphosphatemia.

16.5 INSULIN AND GLUCAGON

Insulin and *glucagon* are perhaps the most influential intermediary metabolism-regulating hormones. Both are produced by the *islets of Langerhans* of the pancreas: insulin in the β cells in response to high blood glucose levels (e.g., after a meal) and glucagon by the α cells in response to low blood glucose levels. A third group of cells, the D cells, produce *somatostatin*. All are peptides, and they are not under any major pituitary, hypothalamic, or neural control. The structures of insulin and glucagon are presented in Figures 16.12 and 16.13.

The biosynthesis of insulin, illustrated in Figure 16.14, involves the production of a single-chain polypeptide, *preproinsulin* (MW 11,500). The signal sequence, consisting of 23 amino acids, is removed proteolytically from the N terminus of the molecule, leaving the *proinsulin* structure shown in Figure 16.11. The proinsulin then loses a section called the C *peptide*, consisting of 33 amino acid residues, to give the circulating insulin. This molecule consists of two polypeptide chains joined by two disulfide bonds and containing a total of 51 amino acid residues. The overall MW is near 5700. The short chain (21 amino acids) is the A chain; the long chain (30 amino acids) is the B chain. The catabolism of insulin is initiated by the separation of the A and B chains via reduction with glutathione. The half-life of insulin is only about 5 minutes.

One of the functions of insulin is to stimulate the movement of glucose into cells. Only a limited number of tissues are sensitive to insulin, however, including the heart, skeletal muscle, and adipose tissue. Liver, kidneys, and brain are not sensitive to insulin, although they contain glucose transporters. Glucose transporters of insulin-sensitive tissues are normally stored in the microsomes

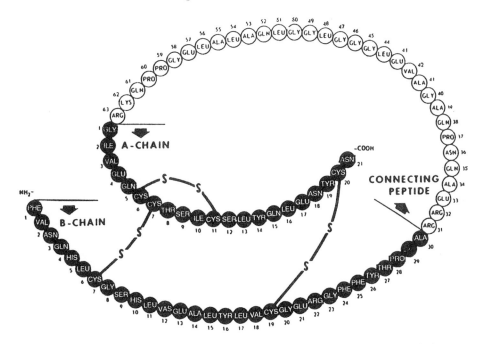

Figure 16.12 Structure of proinsulin, dark blocks representing the amino acids found in mature insulin. C peptide is the same as connecting peptide. (Reproduced by permission from Skillman T. Diabetes mellitus. In Kaplan A, Pesce AJ, eds. Clinical Chemistry. St. Louis: CV Mosby, 1984, p. 526.)

and appear on the membranes under the influence of insulin. As blood insulin levels recede, such transporters are rapidly returned to the microsomes.

In insulin-insensitive tissues, glucose transporters remain on the membrane surface throughout their life spans. They may be divided into four types: red blood cell and brain (GLUT 1), liver (GLUT 2), fetal muscle (GLUT 3), and small intestine (GLUT 5). These transporters, along with the insulin-sensitive transporters (GLUT 4), have molecular weights of about 55,000 and share extensive primary structure homologies. Their membrane topologies are also similar: multiple α-helical regions spanning the membrane in as many as 12 places.

Glucose transporters of both the insulin-sensitive and insensitive tissues do not require energy input. They are Na^+ independent and work in a facilitative capacity. These transporters should thus be distinguished from the Na^+-sensitive (insulin-insensitive) transporter that is dependent on the operation of the Na^+/K^+-ATPase and is utilized for glucose absorption from the intestinal tract and the glomerular filtrate. In addition to glucose, insulin stimulates the movement of amino acids and lipids into cells and enhances the biosynthesis of protein, storage lipid, and glycogen. For this reason, insulin is termed an anabolic hormone. Diabetes mellitus type I is a disorder involving a lack of insulin and high blood glucose levels. It is described in greater detail in Chapter 21.

Glucagon has the function of maintaining blood glucose levels, because certain tissues, such as brain and red blood cells, depend heavily on glucose for

| | Gastrin-Cholecystokinin Family | | | Secretin-Glucagon Family | | |
Gastrin-17	Synthetic Pentagastrin	Cholecystokinin	Glucagon	Secretin	GIP	VIP
		Lys	His	His	Tyr	His
		Ala	Ser	Ser	Ala	Ser
		Pro	Gln	Asp	Glu	Asp
		Ser	Gly	Gly	Gly	Ala
		Gly	Thr	Thr	Thr	Val
		Arg	Phe	Phe	Phe	Phe
		Val	Thr	Thr	Ile	Thr
		Ser	Ser	Ser	Ser	Asp
		Met	Asp	Glu	Asp	Asn
		Ile	Tyr	Leu	Tyr	Tyr
		Lys	Ser	Ser	Ser	Thr
		Ala	Lys	Arg	Ile	Arg
		Leu	Tyr	Leu	Ala	Leu
		Glu	Leu	Arg	Met	Arg
		Ser	Asp	Asp	Asp	Lys
		Leu	Ser	Ser	Lys	Gln
Glu		Asp	Arg	Ala	Ile	Met
Gly		Pro	Arg	Arg	Arg	Ala
Pro		Ser	Ala	Leu	Gln	Val
Tyr		His	Gln	Gln	Gln	Lys
Met		Arg	Asp	Arg	Asp	Lys
Glu		Ile	Phe	Leu	Phe	Tyr
Glu		Ser	Val	Leu	Val	Leu
Glu		Asp	Gln	Gln	Asn	Asn
Glu		Arg	Trp	Gly	Trp	Ser
Ala		Asp	Leu	Leu	Leu	Ile
Tyr-SO$_3$H	N-t-butyloxy-	Tyr-SO$_3$H	Met	Val	Ala	Asn
Gly	carbonyl	Met	Asn	NH$_2$*	Ala	NH$_2$*
Trp	β-Ala	Gly	Thr		Gln	
Met	Trp	Trp			Gln	
Asp	Met	Met			Lys	
Phe	Asp	Asp			Gly	
NH$_2$*	Phe	Phe			Lys	
	NH$_2$*	NH$_2$*			Lys	
					Ser	
					Asp	
					Trp	
					Lys	
					His	
					Asn	
					Ile	
					Thr	
					Gln	

Figure 16.13 Structures of glucagon and the digestive hormones, indicating their homologies. (Asterisk indicates amidation of C-terminal amino acid residue, which occurs with some gut hormones.) (Reproduced by permission from Tietz NW, Rinker AD, Henderson AT. Gastric, pancreatic, and intestinal function. In Tietz NW, ed. Textbook of Clinical Chemistry. Philadelphia: WB Saunders, 1986, p. 1439.)

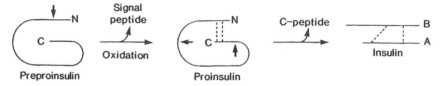

Figure 16.14 Biosynthesis of insulin. Dotted lines indicate disulfide linkages; arrows indicate sites of proteolytic cleavage. The drawing is not necessarily to scale.

survival. Its effects are therefore to move glucose from the cells into the bloodstream and to stimulate those metabolic processes that give rise to free glucose: glycogen degradation and the biosynthesis of glucose from small molecules, such as pyruvate, lactate, glycerol, and amino acids. Glucagon is also associated with protein degradation. In addition, it stimulates the breakdown of storage fat, whose function is to provide cellular fuel and thus spare glucose. Glucagon is considered a catabolic hormone.

The function of somatostatin in digestive processes is unclear. It inhibits the production of both insulin and glucagon, and these effects are believed to be local.

16.6 DIGESTIVE TRACT HORMONES

Both the stomach and the small intestine elaborate peptide hormones into the bloodstream, which is crucial in initiating food digestion. The most important hormones of this class are gastrin, secretin, and cholecystokinin. Their structures are displayed in Figure 16.13.

Gastrin is secreted by the G cells of stomach antrum in response to the ingestion of food. Gastrin migrates via the bloodstream to the fundic region of the stomach, which contains parietal cells and chief cells. The former proceed to secrete HCl, which acts on the chief cells to secrete a zymogen called *pepsinogen*. The same HCl then activates pepsinogen to *pepsin* by catalyzing the removal of a 42 amino acid peptide from it. Pepsin initiates protein digestion in the stomach. Its optimum pH is less than 2, generated by the HCl. The effects of gastrin are inhibited by several agents, such as the gastric inhibitory peptide (GIP) and vasoactive intestinal peptide (VIP), produced by the small intestine (see Figure 16.13 for structures).

Secretin is produced by the S cells of the duodenum in response to the acidic gastric contents entering the small intestine. The hormone migrates to the pancreas, where the release of a bicarbonate solution into the small intestine via the pancreatic duct is affected. The function of the bicarbonate is to neutralize the acidic gastric contents and to maintain the pH of the small intestine at 7.0–7.5, the optimum pH for small intestinal enzymes. Another hormone, *cholecystokinin* (CCK), is also released from small intestinal cells (the I cells) in response to the presence of food in the intestinal lumen. CCK causes contraction of the gallbladder to release bile into the small intestine via the bile duct and causes the release of zymogens by the pancreas. Secretin apparently potentiates the action of CCK on the pancreas. CCK may also inhibit the hunger sensation in mammals. The zymogens secreted by the pancreas into the duodenum via the pancreatic duct are activated in the small intestine to active enzymes, and these are described in Chapter 18 through 20.

Figure 16.13 illustrates that the peptide hormones described in this section may be divided into two homology groups: the gastrin and the secretin. Several gastrins are known, and of these, the so-called *little gastrin* (G_{17}) is shown in Figure 16.13. Although their structures are different, all share the N- terminal 14 amino acid peptide, as shown in Figure 16.13. The biologically active portion of all gastrins appears to be the N-terminal Phe-Asp-Met-Trp portion, however. A synthetic biologically active "pentagastrin" is also shown in Figure 16.13. CCK belongs to the gastrin homology group and has most if not all of the activities characteristic of the gastrins. The secretin group includes glucagon, secretin, GIP, and VIP.

16.7 MECHANISMS OF HORMONE ACTION

Hormones may be divided into two classes with respect to their mode of action on cells: one group, which is water soluble in nature and includes the peptide hormones and epinephrine, does not penetrate target cell membranes. Instead, these hormones interact with cell surface *receptors*, which are intrinsic membrane proteins. This generates a signal that is translated, in the cell interior, into the production of *second messengers*. Such second messengers then affect specific enzyme systems either in a positive (*activation*) or in a negative (*inhibitory*) way. In many cases, this involves protein phosphorylation, that is, covalent post-translational modification. This may either activate a zymogen or inactivate an enzyme.

The second group of hormones, the hydrophobic hormones, including the steroids and thyroxine, can easily penetrate the cell membrane. In the cytosol, the steroid hormones interact with specific receptor (*binding*) protein molecules. The hormone has no effect on the target cell, if such a specific cytoplasmic receptor does not exist there. Such receptors are proteins with molecular weights of about 200,000. When bound up with the hormone, the receptor molecule changes its conformation, which makes it possible to be translocated into the nucleus. The receptor-steroid complex interacts with a DNA-associated nonhistone protein, inducing the transcription of a specific mRNA. The latter is then translated into a specific protein or enzyme by the usual ribosomal mechanism. The situation with testosterone has a special feature: in target cells, testosterone is reduced to a more powerful androgen, *dihydrotestosterone*, by 5α-steroid reductase. This enzyme was mentioned in connection with the etiology of porphyrias in Chapter 7. The dihydrotestosterone then combines with its specific receptor protein in the cytosol.

Trioidothyronine from plasma, or that generated from T_4 in the cells, may interact with specific cell receptors. However, there seems to be an equilibrium between the free and bound T_3, and T_3 penetrates the nuclear membrane without being bound to the cytoplasmic receptor protein. In the nucleus, however, T_3 interacts with a chromatin-bound receptor and affects mRNA transcription. The responsiveness of various cells to T_3 is correlated with the presence of nuclear T_3 receptors. T_3 receptors are also present in mitochondria; O_2 consumption by mitochondria is increased under the influence of T_3. The function of cytosolic T_3 receptors may be simply to concentrate T_3 inside the cell rather than to serve as transporters. These processes are illustrated in Figure 16.15.

There are many ways in which hormone-receptor interactions may be studied, the classic method being the *Scatchard technique*, named in honor of George Scatchard. This technique is applicable to any protein–small molecule interaction, and it provides a means of determining the heterogeneity of binding sites, dissociation constants, and the number of binding sites per receptor unit. The last may be a protein molecule, a cell, a cell membrane fragment, or a unit volume of cytosol with a known protein content.

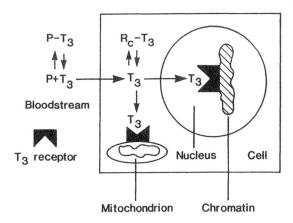

Figure 16.15 Effect of triiodothyronine on cells. In the bloodstream, protein-bound triiodothyronine (P-T_3) is in equilibrium with free T_3. The latter penetrates cell membranes with ease and may be concentrated in the cytosol by a T_3 binding protein (R_c). Free cytosolic T_3, in equilibrium with R_c-T_3, may interact with mitochondrial T_3 receptors or may penetrate the nuclear membrane to interact with a T_3 receptor on chromatin.

The following is a derivation of the Scatchard expression, where a hormone A reacts with its receptor P, assuming a 1:1 interaction:

$$P + A \rightleftharpoons PA \tag{16.3}$$

$$K_a = \frac{[PA]}{[P][A]} = \frac{1}{K_d} \tag{16.4}$$

where K_a is the association constant and K_d is the dissociation constant. Let us now define $\bar{V}$ as the fraction of P bound up with A; then,

$$\bar{V} = \frac{[PA]}{[PA] + [P]} \tag{16.5}$$

Substituting Equation (16.4) into (16.5), we have

$$\bar{V} = \frac{K_a[A]}{K_a[A] + 1} \tag{16.6}$$

If there is more than one binding site for A on P, then Equation (16.6) becomes

$$\frac{\bar{V}}{n} = \frac{K_a[A]}{K_a[A] + 1} \tag{16.7}$$

Rearranging Equation (16.7), we obtain the working Scatchard equation,

$$\frac{\bar{V}}{[A]} = nK_a - \bar{V}K_a \tag{16.8}$$

This equation has a straight-line character: a plot of $\bar{V}/[A]$ versus $\bar{V}$ yields a straight line if the binding sites for A are all equivalent and independent. $\bar{V}$ is the amount of A bound per unit receptor protein, and $[A]$ is the concentration of unbound (free) hormone. Both are experimentally determinable. The slope of

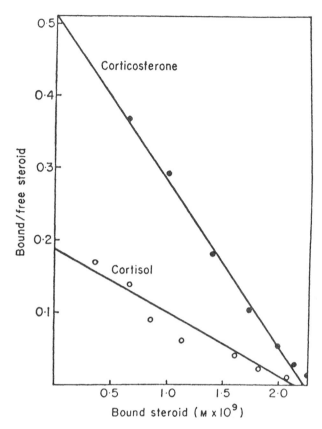

Figure 16.16 Scatchard plot representing the interaction between cortisol and corticosterone with their receptor in hepatoma cell cytosol. (Reproduced by permission from Rousseau GG, Baxter JD, Tomkins GM. Glucocorticoid receptors: relations between steroid binding and biological effects. J Mol Biol 67:99–115, 1972.)

such a curve indicates K_a, and both n and K_a can be determined from the y intercept.

Figure 16.16 is a Scatchard plot of cortisol and corticosterone (glucocorticoid) binding by hepatoma cell cytosol glucocorticoid receptors. The x axis is $\bar{V}$, whereas the y axis is $\bar{V}/[A]$. For both steroids straight lines are obtained, indicating a single class of noninteracting receptors. Both lines cross the x axis at the same point, indicating that at 0 free hormone concentration (all binding sites of P occupied), there are the same numbers of receptors for both cortisol and corticosterone. The conclusion was that the same receptor molecule was responsible for binding the two hormones and that its concentration in the cytosol was about 0.65 pmol/mg protein. Calculation of the association constant K_a from either the slope or the y intercept yielded 0.91×10^8 for cortisol and 2.3×10^8 for corticosterone. The corresponding $\Delta G'_0$ would be –11.2 Kcal/mol and –11.8 kcal/mol respectively. Thus, the receptor has a higher affinity for corticosterone than it has for cortisol. Rousseau and coworkers, who did this work, were able to correlate these data with the ability of these two steroids to induce the appearance of tyrosine aminotransferase (transaminase) in the cell: corticosterone showed half-maximal activity at $1.3 \times 10^{-7}M$, whereas cortisol was half-maximally active at a concentration of $1.9 \times 10^{-7}M$.

16.7.1　Cell Surface Hormone Receptors

All hormones, other than the steroids and thyroid hormones, as well as many neurotransmitters, act on cellular metabolism by interacting with membrane receptors. The extent of hormone action in a cell line or tissue depends on both the number of receptors per cell as well as the affinity of the receptor for the hormone. Very often, the circulating hormone concentration (e.g., for insulin) regulates the number of its tissue receptors in an inversely proportional manner.

The insulin receptor has been studied most extensively. A sketch is shown in Figure 16.17. The receptor molecule consists of two pairs of subunits: the α subunits, with a MW of 135,000 each, and the β subunits, MW 95,000 each. The α subunits are located on membrane surface and interact with insulin, whereas the β subunits are embedded in the membrane. Disulfide bonds hold the structure together, as shown in Figure 16.17. Both subunits are glycosylated. When insulin interacts with the α subunits, a signal is transmitted to the β subunits to phosphorylate (using ATP) some of its own tyrosyl residues. Such activity is termed *tyrosine kinase*. What happens beyond this is not entirely clear. However, a great deal of evidence suggests that β subunit tyrosine phosphorylation is a *sine qua non* for the effect of insulin on cell metabolism: glycogen biosynthesis, protein biosynthesis, activation of the pyruvate dehydrogenase enzyme, and so on. The glucose transporter and insulin receptor are not one and the same molecule.

There are two kinds of catecholamine receptors, the α and β receptors. The former respond best to norepinephrine, whereas the latter prefer epinephrine. Norepinephrine is normally associated with neurotransmission, and α-adrenergic receptors are indeed found in tissues serviced by the sympathetic nervous system. An example is the smooth muscle, which contracts in response to stimulation by

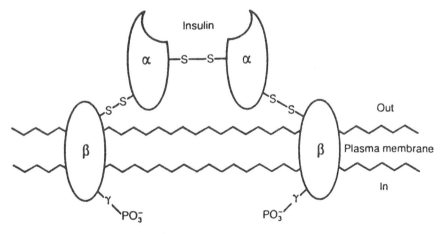

Figure 16.17　The insulin receptor. γ signifies the tyrosyl residues that become phosphorylated as a result of insulin action. (Reproduced by permission from Espinal J. What is the role of the insulin receptor tyrosine kinase? TIBS October:367–368, 1988.)

norepinephrine. The interaction of catecholamines with the β receptor relaxes smooth muscle. The reverse, however, is true of the heart muscle, in which epinephrine reacting with the β receptor increases cardiac output. β Receptor antagonists, such as *propranolol*, are therefore used to control hypertension. β Receptors are present in all tissues that play a major role in the energy metabolism of the organism, and epinephrine therefore has a profound effect on these processes. Examples are liver, adipose tissue, and skeletal muscle. Liver and adipose tissue, but not skeletal muscle, also have glucagon receptors on the cell surface. Although glucagon and epinephrine receptors are not the same, they nevertheless have the same effects on the metabolism of adipose tissue and liver.

16.7.2 Second Messengers

Most hormones influence cell metabolism through second messengers, as already stated. There are two major forms: the cyclic AMP (see Chapter 10) and the Ca^{2+} systems. The various hormones, neurotransmitters, and other metabolic mediators elicit the activation of either one or the other system by binding to their specific receptors. Table 16.6 summarizes the second messenger systems used by the various hormones. The details of the mode of action of each second messenger system are discussed here.

Cyclic AMP (cAMP) System

The interaction of such hormones as glucagon and epinephrine with their specific receptors increases cellular cAMP levels by activating *adenylate cyclase*,

Table 16.6 Second Messengers Involved in Hormone Action

Second messenger[a]	Hormone
cAMP[b]	β-Adrenergic catecholamines
	Glucagon
	ACTH
	LH
	FSH
	MSH
	TSH
	Vasopressin
	Calcitonin
	Parathyroid hormone
	Secretin
	Prostaglandin E_1
Ca^{2+}	Oxytocin
	α_1-Adrenergic catecholamines
	Cholecystokinin
	Angiotensin

[a]Second messenger unknown for insulin, prolactin, and GH.
[b]Target tissue cAMP or Ca^{2+} concentrations increase as a result of hormone action.

which converts ATP to cAMP. cAMP in turn activates certain protein kinases to affect the phosphorylation of various proteins. The process by which cellular cAMP levels are increased is quite complex and involves the so-called G_s protein. The other side of the coin is the existence of a number of substances that *inhibit* cAMP formation; that is, they *lower* cellular cAMP levels. These substances also interact with specific cell surface receptors and act, in an inhibitory fashion, on adenylate cyclase. This, too, occurs through the G-type proteins. Such inhibitory substances include the opiates, somatostatin, insulin, and some prostaglandins (see later). The function of G proteins in transmitting the signal generated by a hormone interacting with its specific receptor may be described as follows (Figure 16.18). As the hormone (H_s) interacts with its receptor (R), the membrane G_s protein containing bound GDP is induced to exchange the GDP for GTP. The binding of GTP causes dissociation of the G_s protein into the $G_{s\alpha}$ portion, which

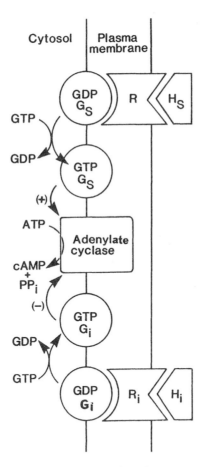

Figure 16.18 Overview of signal transmission from hormone-receptor interaction on the outside cell surface to cAMP production on the cytosol side of the membrane through stimulation of adenylate cyclase. H_s is the stimulatory hormone, and R is its receptor. G_s is the stimulatory G protein. H_i is an inhibitory hormone, and R_i is its cell surface receptor. G_i is the inhibitory G protein. The last inhibits adenylate cyclase when combined with GTP.

retains the bound GTP, and the $G_{s\beta\gamma}$ complex. The $G_{s\alpha}$-GTP complex activates adenylate cyclase. The GTP, however, is subject to hydrolysis to GDP via a GTPase activity intrinsic to the $G_{s\alpha}$ subunit. When this happens, the $G_{s\alpha}$-GDP and $G_{s\beta\gamma}$ complexes reassociate and the activity toward adenylate cyclase disappears. In the same fashion, when an inhibitor of adenylate cyclase combines with its specific receptor on the membrane surface, a G_i protein exchanges its GDP for GTP and dissociates into the $G_{i\alpha}$-GTP and $G_{i\beta\gamma}$ complexes. The $G_{i\alpha}$-GTP complex then inhibits adenylate cyclase. In addition, the activity of the $G_{s\alpha}$-GTP complex may be diminished by combination with the $G_{i\beta\gamma}$ complexes. The $G_{i\alpha}$-GTP complex may be diminished by combination with the $G_{s\beta\gamma}$ complex, because the β and γ subunits of G_s and G_i proteins are identical (Figure 16.19).

It is noteworthy that the properties of the $G_{s\alpha}$-GTP complexes depend in large part on their conformation. Thus, when GTP displaces GDP from the G_s protein, the α subunit loses its ability to interact with the hormone receptor and with the β subunit. When the $G_{s\alpha}$-GTP is hydrolyzed to the $G_{s\alpha}$-GDP complex, the ability to combine with the hormone receptor and the β subunit is restored.

cAMP levels in the cell can be downregulated by a number of processes. Some of them take place at the G protein level: the action of the G_i protein, the GTPase activity of the $G_{s\alpha}$ subunit, conformation of the $G_{s\alpha}$ subunit, and phosphorylation with protein kinase C, as described later. In addition, a group of enzymes called *phosphodiesterases* hydrolyze cAMP to 5'-AMP. Certain compounds, such as caffeine and theophylline, inhibit the activity of phosphodiesterases, causing increased blood sugar levels, muscle twitching, increased blood pressure, and numerous other pharmacologic effects. Cholera toxin is another agent that maintains cAMP at high levels in the intestinal tract cells. The high cAMP causes the intestinal tract to lose large volumes of isotonic salt solu-

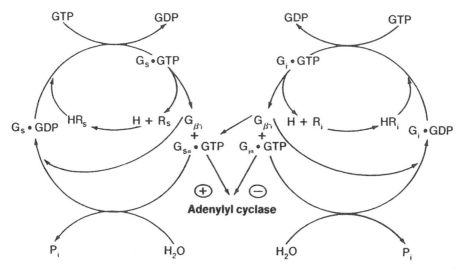

Figure 16.19 Function of G proteins in activating and inhibiting adenylate cyclase. See text for a detailed description of the process. (Reproduced by permission from Rawles RL. G-proteins; research unravels their role in cell communication. Chem Eng News December:30, 1987.)

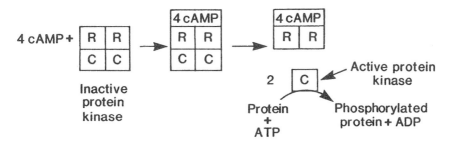

Figure 16.20 Activation of a typical protein kinase with cAMP. R, regulatory subunit; C, catalytic subunit.

tion. The mechanism of cholera toxin action is to inhibit the hydrolysis of $G_{s\alpha}$-bound GTP.

cAMP thus acts to activate cAMP-sensitive protein kinases, as shown in Figure 16.20. This group of enzymes usually consists of two regulatory and two catalytic subunits. As the regulatory subunits bind cAMP, dissociation of the catalytic subunits takes place. The free catalytic subunits catalyze the phosphorylation of various proteins using ATP as the phosphate donor. The phosphate residues normally esterify serine –OH groups and, less frequently, threonine –OH groups. Such phosphorylation is certainly not permanent, because a number of protein phosphatases exist that, under the influence of metabolic mediators, cause the loss of phosphate residues from phosphorylated proteins. As pointed earlier, phosphorylation may activate a zymogen to an enzyme, or it may inactivate an enzyme.

Ca^{2+} System

Many biologic processes, including muscle contraction and the process of vision, depend on Ca^{2+} fluxes. There are also several enzymes that are affeced by cellular $[Ca^{2+}]$, and such cell Ca^{2+} levels may be regulated by hormones. In the metabolic processes, the α_1-adrenergic receptors are perhaps the most prominent Ca^{2+} flow inducers. The mechanism of Ca^{2+} release is summarized in Figure 16.21 and may be described as follows: an interaction of the appropriate hormone or another agonist with its receptor (R_1) results in the activation of a phospholipase C. A G-type protein and hydrolysis of GTP may very well be involved as intermediates in this activation process. Phospholipase C, a phosphodiesterase, causes the removal of myoinositol-1,4,5-triphosphate (IP_3) from membrane-bound phosphatidylinositol-4′,5′-diphosphate [$PI(4,5)P_2$]. A diacylglycerol (DG) molecule is also produced. DG is also considered a second messenger, because it activates a kinase called protein kinase C. The last is capable of phosphorylating a number of metabolically important proteins. The IP_3 molecule then causes a release of Ca^{2+} from the endoplasmic reticulum, and it is also believed that exogenous Ca^{2+} enters the cell in response to IP_3 release. IP_3 is eventually dephosphorylated, as shown in Figure 16.21, and reacts with CDP-diglyceride to regenerate phosphatidylinositol. The latter is phosphorylated in the 4′ and 5′ positions to yield $PI(4,5)P_2$. It is noteworthy that Li^+, which is used to treat patients with manic depression, inhibits the reutilization of IP_3 for

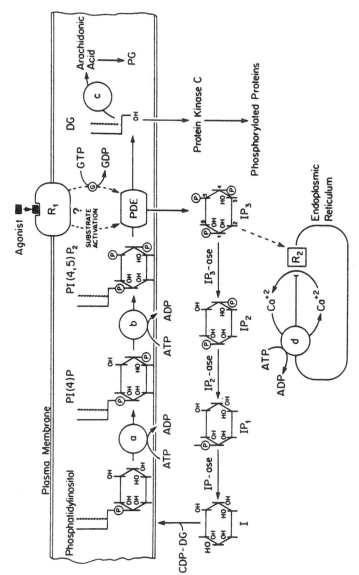

Figure 16.21 Operation of the Ca^{2+} second messenger system. For a detailed description and abbreviations, see the text. (Reproduced by permission from Berridge MJ, Irvine RF. Inositol triphosphate, a novel second messenger in cellular signal transduction. Nature 312:315–321, 1984; Holub BJ. The cellular forms and functions of the inositol phospholipids and their metabolic derivatives. Nutr Rev 45:65–71, 1987.)

PI(4,5)P$_2$ synthesis. This disease may thus be caused by a failure to control this second messenger pathway adequately.

The Ca^{2+} released from the endoplasmic reticulum by IP$_3$ may perform a number of functions. The metabolically most important action of Ca^{2+}, however, is to combine with a very ubiquitous protein called *calmodulin*. This protein has a molecular weight of about 17,500 and is in many ways similar to troponin. It has four Ca^{2+} binding sites and constitutes one of several subunits of several enzyme systems. Thus, as cellular [Ca^{2+}] rises, the calmodulin subunit binds Ca^{2+}. The result is that it changes its conformation to that of an α helix and thereby affects the catalytic activity of other constituent subunits. For instance, calmodulin is a component of *myosin kinase*, which phosphorylates one of the subunits of myosin. The structure of calmodulin is shown in Figure 16.22.

Diacylglycerol was mentioned as an activator of protein kinase C. In addition to diacylglycerol, protein kinase C is also activated by increased cellular calcium levels. Protein kinase C catalyzes, for example, the phosphorylation of G protein components: the β subunit of the $\beta\gamma$ complex and the α-GDP complex. Such phosphorylation apparently prevents the reassociation of the α-GDP with the $\beta\gamma$ complex to give the G$_{\alpha\beta\gamma}$-GDP protein. It is thus clear that phosphorylation via protein kinase C participates in the regulation of G protein function.

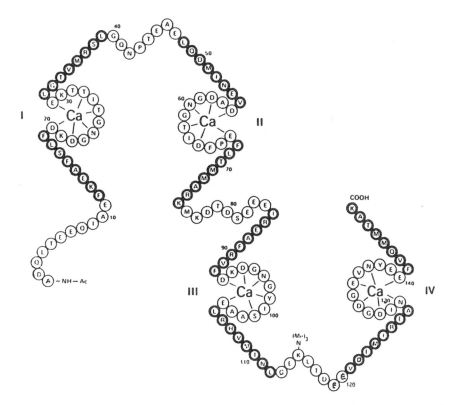

Figure 16.22 Structure of bovine brain calmodulin. See Chapter 4 for amino acid abbreviations. (Reproduced by permission from Klee CB, Crouch TH, Richman PG. Calmodulin. Annu Rev Biochem 49:489–515, 1980.)

16.8 PROSTAGLANDINS AND RELATED SUBSTANCES

Enzymatic oxidation of arachidonic acid (AA) and other C_{20} polyunsaturated acids leads to a multitude of important biochemical compounds with an extensive variety of actions. These compounds are known collectively as *eicosanoids*, that is, any 20-carbon fatty acid, including both cyclooxygenase (prostanoids) and lipooxygenase products (leukotrienes). Prostanoids include *prostaglandins* (PG), *prostacyclins* (PGI), and *thromboxanes* (TX). The *leukotrienes*, which are discussed later, constitute a group of fatty acid derivatives produced predominantly by various inflammatory cells. PGs were originally discovered in human semen and vesicular glands of sheep and were thought to be formed by the prostate gland. It is now known that they are produced by virtually all mammalian cells.

16.8.2 Structure of Prostaglandins

PGs are named from a hypothetical compound, *prostanoic acid*, a monocarboxylic acid with 20 carbon atoms, arranged with two side chains with 7 and 8 carbon atoms linked to a cyclopentane ring. PGs have functional groups with oxygen at carbons 9, 11, and 15 of prostanoic acid (see Figure 16.23) and one, two, or three double bonds in the side chain.

PGs of the 1 series have a trans double bond in the Δ^{13} position, whereas PGs of the 2 and 3 series have an additional cis double bond at Δ^{5}, and additional cis double bonds at both Δ^{5} and Δ^{17}, respectively. PGs are also classified by the functional groups attached to the cyclopentane ring, denoted A through I (Figure 16.23). TXs and PGIs are closely related to the PGs and can be of the 1, 2, or 3 series, depending on the fatty acid from which they are derived.

Important essential fatty acids in the diet are *linoleic acid* (*cis,cis*-9,12-octadecadienoic acid, $18:2\Delta^{9,12}$) and *α-linolenic acid* (all-*cis*-9,12,15-octadecatrienoic acid; $18:3\Delta^{9,12,15}$). The numbering in this conventional system begins with the *carboxyl group*. The "short hand," for example $18:2\Delta^{9,12}$, indicates 18 carbon atoms, with two double bonds located between carbon atoms 9 and 10 and 12 and 13. There is an alternative system of numbering in which fatty acids are numbered from the methyl (or ω) terminal. In this case, linoleic acid is designated ω-6,9-octadecadienoic acid ($18:2\omega^{6}$), and α-linolenic acid is ω-3,6,9-octadecatrienoic acid ($18:3\omega^{3}$). This serves to designate two unsaturated fatty acid families, the ω^{6} and the ω^{3} families.

The mammalian organism is unable to introduce double bonds at ω^{3} and ω^{6} of fatty acids, and this is probably why these families must be present in the diet. These fatty acids can be desaturated and elongated (see Chapter 19) to form *derived essential fatty acids*, dihomo-τ-linoleic acid ($20:3\omega^{6}$), arachidonic acid ($20:4\omega^{6}$), and eicosapentaenoic acid ($20:5\omega^{3}$), the three direct precursor acids of PGs. Dihomo-τ-linoleic acid, an intermediate in the biosynthesis of arachidonic acid from linoleic acid, is the precursor of PGs of the 1 series. Arachidonic acid and eicosapentaenoic acid are precursors of PGs of the 2 series and 3 series, respectively.

Interest in eicosapentaenoic acid (EPA, $20:5\omega^{3}$) arose from the observation that the Eskimos of Greenland have low incidences of acute myocardial infarction and atherosclerosis, and an increased tendency to bruise and bleed, includ-

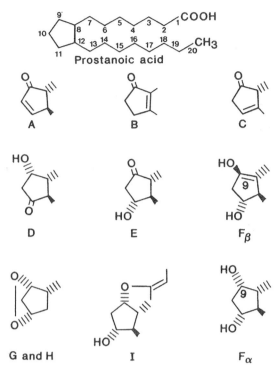

Figure 16.23   Structure of prostanoic acid and the cyclopentane ring of prostaglandins A through I; α and β indicate the orientation of the 9-hydroxy group.

ing cerebral hemorrhages. They consume a diet (fish oils) rich in ω^3 polyunsaturated acids, which leads to prostaglandins of the 3 series. Thus, PGI_3 and TXA_3 are formed instead of the arachidonic acid products PGI_2 and TXA_2 (Figure 16.24). PGI_3 is as potent an antiaggregating agent as PGI_2, whereas TXA_3 has a much weaker proaggregating activity than TXA_2. It was suggested that enrichment of the diet with EPA could reduce the incidence of thrombotic disorders. There is some additional experimental support for this contention. However, some caution should be exercised before one dashes to the local health food store for a supply of ω^3 polyunsaturated fatty acids, which can produce serious bleeding problems at improper doses.

Because arachidonic acid and compounds of the 2 series are predominant in humans, we direct our consideration primarily to these compounds, keeping in mind that biologically active 1 and 3 series compounds are also produced. Likewise, it is far beyond the scope of our discussion here to consider all the possible products of the C_{20} polyunsaturated fatty acids and their metabolites.

16.8.3   Biosynthesis of Prostaglandins

Very little free AA is found in unstimulated cells. AA, like other polyunsaturated fatty acids, is esterified almost exclusively to membrane phospholipids in the 2-acyl position. Different cells release AA in response to a number of stimuli, such

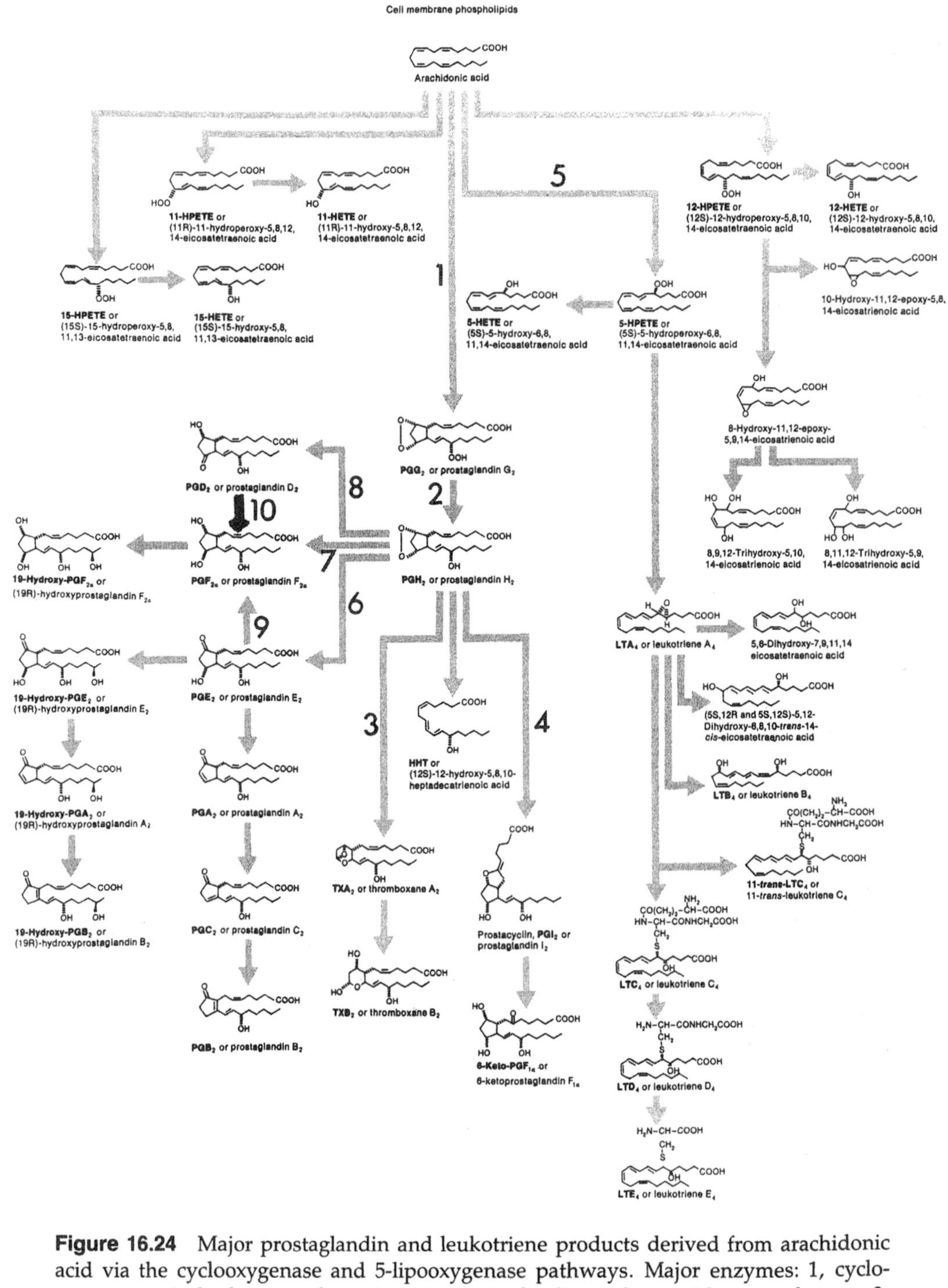

Figure 16.24 Major prostaglandin and leukotriene products derived from arachidonic acid via the cyclooxygenase and 5-lipooxygenase pathways. Major enzymes: 1, cyclooxygenase; 2, hydroperoxidase; 1 + 2, prostaglandin endoperoxidase synthetase; 3, thromboxane synthetase; 4, prostacyclin synthetase; 5, 5-lipooxygenase; 6, 9-ketoisomerase; 7, PGH-PGF$_{2\alpha}$ reductase; 8, 11-ketoisomerase; 9, PGE reductase; 10, PGD reductase. (Reproduced by permission from Nelson NA, Kelly RC, Johnson, RA. Prostaglandins and the arachidonic acid cascade. Chem Eng News August:30–44, 1982.)

as thrombin, bradykinin, angiotensin II, vasopressin, epinephrine, collagen, ADP, Ca^{2+}, calcium ionophores, and ischemia. The immediate source, at least in endothelial cells, appears to be phosphatidylethanolamine (Chapter 9). Although the mechanism is not clearly understood, it may involve a specific phospholipase A_2. Glucocorticoids (see earlier) inhibit the release of AA from membrane phospholipids, probably by the induction of the synthesis of a phospholipase inhibitory protein, *lipomodulin*, which combines in an approximate stoichiometry of 1:1 with the enzyme. Lipomodulin appears to be reversibly phosphorylated (inactive) and dephosphorylated (active) to provide a short-term regulation of phospholipase activity. Degradation and resynthesis of lipomodulin probably represents a longer term regulation mechanism.

Any reduction in the availability of free AA, by glucocorticoids or other agents, would virtually block all production of products via both the cyclooxygenase and lipooxygenase pathways.

Following release from membrane phospholipids, AA is converted by oxygenation and cyclization of C-8 to C-12 of arachidonate to form PGG_2, which contains both the endoperoxide (C-9 to C-11) and hydroperoxide moiety (at C-15). This activity is *fatty acid cyclooxygenase* (enzyme 1 in Figure 16.24). The next step is the reduction of the hydroperoxy group to a hydroxyl group by a *peroxidase* (enzyme 2) in a reduced glutathione (G-SH)-dependent reaction to yield PGH_2. Because it has not been possible to separate the two enzyme activities, it is believed that both reactions are catalyzed by the same enzyme, *prostaglandin endoperoxide synthetase*. Further transformations of PGH_2 into prostaglandins involves isomerization to PGD_2 (enzyme 8) and PGE_2 (enzyme 6) and reduction to $PGF_{2\alpha}$ (enzyme 7). PGE_2 may be converted to $PGF_{2\alpha}$ by reduction of the 9-keto group (enzyme 9), as can PGD_2 by reduction of the 11-keto group (enzyme 10).

PGH_2 is converted to thromboxane A_2 by the enzyme *thromboxane synthetase* (enzyme 3), which is located in the microsomal fraction of platelets, lung, spleen, and a number of other tissues. TXA_2 is the major prostaglandin of platelets and is a very powerful inducer of platelet aggregation and vasoconstriction. TXA_2 is very unstable and is readily and nonenzymatically hydrolyzed to the stable and virtually inactive TXB_2. TXB_2 is generally assayed as a measure of TXA_2 biosynthesis.

PGI_2 is formed by the action of PGI synthetase (enzyme 4), and it is the major prostaglandin produced by the vascular system. Its effects are opposite to those of TXA_2; it is a potent platelet antiaggregating agent and a vasodilator. PGI_2 is hydrolyzed spontaneously at physiologic pH to 6-keto-$PGF_{1\alpha}$, which is used for assay of PGI_2 levels.

Aspirin (acetylsalicyclic acid) causes irreversible acetylation of cyclooxygenase and inhibits the formation of PGs. Because mammalian platelets do not have a nucleus and the ability to carry out transcription and translation, they do not have the ability to resynthesize cyclooxygenase. New platelets must be formed, which takes several days. Other nonsteroidal antiinflammatory drugs (NSAIDs), such as indomethacin, ibuprofen, and phenylbutazone, also inhibit cylooxygenase by competing with the substrate AA at the active site.

We have already noted the effects of glucocorticoids that block AA release by inhibition of phospholipases. These include cortisol and certain synthetic steroids (prednisone and dexamethasone), which have antiinflammatory actions.

Since the discovery of TXA_2 and PGI_2, considerable effort has been expended to find selective inhibitors of thromboxane synthetase and prostacyclin synthetase. Simple derivatives of imidazole and pyridine inhibit the former, and hydroperoxides of various unsaturated fatty acids inhibit the latter. Because TXA_2 and PGH_2 are potent promoters of platelet aggregation and vasodilators, it was suggested that the balance between TXA_2/PGH_2 and PGI/PGD_2 might be an important physiologic regulator of hemostasis and thrombosis. Although TXA_2 and PGI_2 play a significant role in modulating platelet thrombus formation, it is clear that the functions of several other biologically active metabolites and their interactions must be known before we understand the regulation of hemostasis and thrombosis.

16.8.4 Prostaglandin Functions

Prostaglandins may be considered local hormones because they exert their actions primarily at the site of their production and at nearby cells. They probably constitute a modulating system for maintaining homeostasis. PGs are short-lived, from a few seconds to 1–2 minutes, are formed in most cells, and influence most biologic activities. They are produced on demand in extremely small amounts and are not organ localized or concentrated in specific cells. Circulating levels in blood plasma are in the range of 10^{-12}–10^{-9} g/mL. Different PGs may have opposite effects on the same organ, depending on the physiologic or pathologic conditions, and opposite effects with different concentrations of the same compound. Two PGs belonging to the same type but differing in degree of unsaturation may exert opposite effects.

Thus, the vast array of products formed by this arachidonic acid *cascade* produces an astonishing number of biologic responses, far beyond the scope of our discussion here.

Although the mechanism(s) whereby PGs exert their effects are not fully known, several appear to bind to specific receptor sites on cells and correlate with an activation or inhibition of adenylate cyclase. It has been shown in a large number of tissues that hormonal signal transmission involves both positive and negative modulation of the intracellular cAMP level. PGs play a role in this bidirectional regulation of cAMP levels. PGE_1 and PGI_2 *increase* the cAMP levels in platelets. The E-type PGs antagonize the lipolytic effects of such hormones as glucagon, catecholamines, corticotropin, and thyroid-stimulating hormone in human adipocyte cells by inhibiting adenylate cyclase. There is a dual action, however. Inhibition occurs in the nanomolar concentration range, and stimulation results with concentrations above 1 μM. Whether this is a result of the existence of two specific and independent receptor sites is not clear. Inhibition is dependent on GTP and is amplified by Na^+.

Here we discuss some of the numerous biologic actions of AA metabolites on various organs and systems, keeping in mind that there are numerous species variations.

Peripheral vasculature. PGI_2, PGE, and PGE_2 induce vasodilation in heart, kidney, skeletal muscle, and mesentery, lowering vascular resistance and blood pressure.

Heart. PGE_2 and PGF_{2r} contract human coronary arteries, whereas PGE_1 and PGI_2 induce relaxation. Ischemia increases the production of PGI_2 by the heart.

Platelets. PGI_2 (most important), PGE_1, and PGD_2 are inhibitors of platelet aggregation, presumably by increasing the concentration of cAMP. PGG_2 and PGH_2 are powerful inducers of platelet aggregation. Whether this is a result of conversion to TXA_2 is not known with certainty.

Gastrointestinal effects. PGE_1 and PGE_2 suppress gastric secretion in the human. PGI_2 is now known to be formed by gastric mucosa, where it is an inhibitor of gastric secretion. PGEs have a cytoprotective effect at doses that do not inhibit gastric acid secretion. They prevent the formation of and increase the rate of healing of duodenal ulcer in the human. The mucosa is protected by inhibition of acid secretion and by stimulation of bicarbonate secretion. PGI_2 has the former but not the latter activity. Prostaglandins of the E type stimulate the longitudinal muscles and relax the circular muscles of the intestine in humans and other animals. The F and D prostaglandins contract both muscle types. PGE_1, PGE_2, and $PGF_{2\alpha}$ inhibit the reabsorption of electrolytes and water in the small intestine, where PGD_2 and PGI_2 have the opposite effects.

Reproductive system. PGs of the E and F types given intravenously, intravaginally, or orally can induce labor or abortion and have been used for such purposes.

Pulmonary system. PGE_2, $PGF_{2\alpha}$, PGD_2, TXA_2, and PGI_2 are formed from the endoperoxides in lung. $PGF_{2\alpha}$ contracts and PGE_2 relaxes bronchial smooth muscle in the human and other species. TXA_2 and PGD_2 are also bronchoconstrictors, as are leukotrienes C and D, which are now believed to be primarily responsible for the symptoms of human asthma.

16.8.5 Structure and Function of Leukotrienes

Another important metabolic pathway for the metabolism of arachidonic acid the *5-lipooxygenase* pathway, which leads to a series of compounds calleɑ *leukotrienes* (LTs). These compounds appear to be essentially, but not exclusively, of a pathophysiologic nature and are formed in various inflammatory cells.

The name "leukotriene" was introduced originally for compounds that were non-cyclized C_{20} carboxylic acids, with *three* conjugated double bonds and one or two oxygen substituents. A, B, C, D, and E are used to distinguish structurally different leukotrienes, with a subscript to denote the number of double bonds. The structures and biosynthesis of LTA_1, and LTB_4 and of the sulfur-containing leukotrienes LTC_4, LTD_4, and LTE_4 are shown in Figure 16.24. The first step in the biosynthesis of leukotrienes is the oxidation of arachidonate (enzyme 5) to a hydroperoxide (5-HPETE), a reactive and unstable intermediate, which can be converted to LTA_4 or the more stable 5-HETE. LTA_4 can be converted to LTB_4 by enzymatic hydrolysis and to LTC_4 by addition of glutathione via a glutathione-5-transferase. LTC_4 is transformed by the enzymatic removal of the glycine residue.

Briefly summarized, the functions are as follows: HETE and LTB_4 mediate *chemotaxis* (directed cell movement), the degranulation of polymorphonuclear neutrophil leukocytes (PMN) and release of lysosomal hydrolytic enzymes, and the adhesion of cells to the endothelium of postcapillary venules; LTC_4, LTD_4, and LTE_4 are potent bronchoconstricters and vasoconstricters and increase vascular permeability. They are, in general, mediators of processes involved in inflammation and allergy and together comprise the slow-reacting substances of anaphylaxis (SRS-A).

QUESTIONS

16.1. The release of which pituitary gland hormone does not seem to be controlled by a long-loop system?
     a. α-MSH   c. ACTH   e. FSH
     b. TSH   d. LH

16.2. Which disorder is most likely to produce an alkaline urine (pH > 7)?
     a. Primary aldosteronism   d. Renal tubular acidosis
     b. Cushing's disease   e. Diabetes insipidus
     c. Addison's disease

16.3. Which condition is accompanied by hypernatremia?
     a. Addison's disease   d. SIADH
     b. Diabetes insipidus without thirst reflex   e. Uremia
     c. Diabetes mellitus

16.4. A protein, MW 35,000, at a concentration of 0.5 mg/mL, is *dialyzed* against a ligand at an initial concentration of $4 \times 10^{-5}M$. At equilibrium, the ligand concentration in the protein compartment is $2.3 \times 10^{-5}M$, and it is $1.7 \times 10^{-5}M$ in the initial compartment, which contains no protein. Calculate the association constant for the interaction. Assume a single protein–ligand binding site.
     a. 1.7×10^{-5} c. 3.7×10^7 e. 0.42×10^{-5}
     b. 4.3×10^4 d. 2.3×10^{-5}

16.5. What is serum sodium concentration in meq/L if $[Cl^-]$ = 85 meq/L, bicarbonate is 20 meq/L, and everything else is normal? Use values in Table 16.2 as "normal."
     a. 110   b. 115   c. 120   d. 125
     e. 130

16.6. In a uremic patient, what is serum $[Na^+]$ in meq/L if $[Cl^-]$ = 115 meq/L, bicarbonate is 5 meq/L, and phosphate is 6 meq/L? Everything else is normal. Use Table 16.2. (*Hint*: sulfate changes as phosphate does).
     a. 150   b. 128   c. 130   d. 138   e. 135

16.7. Which hormone does not interact with cell surface receptors?
     a. Insulin   c. Thyroxine   e. Epinephrine
     b. Glucagon   d. ACTH

A hormone receptor was isolated from plasma membranes of liver cells, and its molecular weight was found to be 120,000. It was incubated at a concentration of 2 mg/mL with various concentrations of the hormone, and this was followed by measurements at equilibrium of free and bound A (in mol/L) at 37 and 4°C. The data are presented here. Answer Questions 16.8 and 16.9 on the basis of this information.

Temperature (°C)	Free A (M)	Bound A (M)
37	1.25×10^{-5}	3.32×10^{-5}
	2.50×10^{-5}	4.98×10^{-5}
	5.00×10^{-5}	6.64×10^{-5}
	12.5×10^{-5}	8.30×10^{-5}
4	1.0×10^{-5}	1.66×10^{-5}
	2.5×10^{-5}	3.32×10^{-5}
	5.0×10^{-5}	4.98×10^{-5}
	10×10^{-5}	6.6×10^{-5}

16.8. Which set of constants determined from the preceding data is correct?

	Temperature (°C)	No. binding sites for A per mole protein	$\Delta G_o'$ of binding (kcal/mol)
a.	37	6	−7.3
	4	4	−3.6
b.	37	1	−2.0
	4	1	1.0
c.	37	2	5.3
	4	1	2.3
d.	37	6	−6.5
	4	6	−5.4
e.	37	5	−5.7
	4	3	−4.6

16.9. What are the ΔH (kcal/M) and ΔS (entropy units) values for the binding process, and what are the most likely binding forces involved (see Chapters 2 and 4 for calculations)?

	ΔH	ΔS	Bonding forces
a.	3.4	32	Hydrophobic and hydrogen bonds
b.	6.5	0	Hydrogen bonds only
c.	0	6.5	Hydrophobic bonds only
d.	5.4	3.4	Hydrophobic and hydrogen bonds
e.	7.4	2.9	Hydrophobic and hydrogen bonds

16.10. When cholecystokinin interacts with its receptors on pancreatic cell surface, the following set of events occurs in the order given:
a. Activation of phospholipase A_2, which then releases inositol phosphate from phosphatidylinositol. The latter then activates adenyl cyclase, which produces cyclic AMP from ATP.
b. Activation of phospholipase A_1, which releases inositol. The latter causes the release of Ca^{2+} from endoplasmic reticulum (ER), which then affects enzyme activities.
c. GTP substitutes for GDP in G_s protein, which dissociates into the α, β, and τ subunits. The G_α-GTP stimulates adenyl cyclase to produce cAMP from ATP.

    d. Activation of phospholipase C, which then releases inositol-1,4,5-triphos-phate from phosphatidylinositol diphosphate. The inositol-1,4,5-triphosphate releases Ca^{2+} from ER, which affects enzyme activities.

    e. Phospholipase A_2 is activated, which releases arachidonic acid from membrane lecithin. Arachidonic acid gives rise to prostaglandins, which affect enzyme activities.

16.11. Which process is *not* associated with the second messenger phenomenon?
    a. Phosphorylation of O-tyrosyl residues
    b. Action of phospholipase C
    c. Phosphorylation of phosphatidylinositol at positions 4 and 5
    d. Receptor-mediated endocytosis of a hormone
    e. Binding of Ca^{2+} by calmodulin

16.12. Phosphodiesterase activity is *not* associated with which of the following?
    a. Removal of phosphate residues from proteins
    b. Hydrolysis of cAMP
    c. Phospholipase C
    d. Inhibition by caffeine
    e. Controlling the level of cellular protein phosphorylation

16.13. High cellular cAMP levels are associated with which phenomenon?
    a. Action of insulin
    b. Interaction of an α_1-adrenergic mediator with its receptor
    c. Dissociation of G_s proteins into subunits and the binding of GTP
    d. Binding of Ca^{2+} by calmodulin
    e. Release of inositol-1,4,5-triphosphate by phospholipase C

16.14. Which is not a second messenger?
    a. Intracellular aldosterone binding protein
    b. Calmodulin
    c. Ca^{2+}
    d. Diacylglycerol
    e. Two of the above

16.15. Which of the following is not involved in the metabolism of catecholamines?
    a. Monoamine oxidase
    b. Vanillin mandelic acid
    c. Catecholamine-O-methyltransferase
    d. Homovanillic acid
    e. Indoleacetic acid

16.16. Let us assume that normal plasma $[HCO_3^-]$ = 27 meq/L and that the normal anion gap is 17 meq/L. Suppose an untreated diabetic has an anion gap of 30 meq/L, $[Na^+]$ = 144 meq/L, K^+ = 4 meq/L, $[Cl^-]$ = 100 meq/L, and pCO_2 = 40 mm. What is the blood pH?
    a. 7.20   b. 7.28   c. 7.35   d. 7.42
    e. 7.51

In Questions 16.17–16.23, mark as follows:
    a. Prostaglandins   b. Leukotrienes c. All
    d. None

16.17. Arachidonic acid is a precursor.
16.18. Products of lipooxygenase action.
16.19. Derived from eicosapentaenoic acid.
16.20. Biosynthesis inhibited by cortisol.
16.21. Biosynthesis inhibited by aspirin.

16.22. Products of cyclooxygenase enzyme action.
16.23. Products of phospholipase C action.

Answer Questions 16.24–16.29 by choosing from a through e:
- a. Growth hormone
- d. Calcitonin
- b. Cortisol
- e. Antidiuretic hormone
- c. Dopamine

16.24. Biosynthesis inadequate in congenital adrenal hyperplasia.
16.25. Acts via somatomedins.
16.26. Opposes the effects of parathyroid hormone.
16.27. Biosynthesis diminished in Parkinson's disease.
16.28. Produced in the hypothalamus.
16.29. Iron-containing enzyme controls rate of biosynthesis.

Answers

16.1. (a) The control of α-MSH secretion appears to involve dopamine, which in turn is controlled by nerve impulses from higher brain centers.

16.2. (d) In renal tubular acidosis, the mechanism for secreting protons into the urine is damaged.

16.3. (b) Large amounts of urine carry away inordinate quantities of sodium. If the water is not replaced through the thirst reflex, body sodium declines.

16.4. (b) First, the protein concentration is $0.5/35,000 = 1.42 \times 10^{-5}$ M. Next, remember that the ligand goes through the dialysis membrane, but the protein does not. Because ligand concentration in its initial chamber is 1.7×10^{-5} M, it follows that *free* ligand concentration in the protein chamber is also 1.7×10^{-5} M and *bound* ligand is $2.3 \times 10^{-5} - 1.7 \times 10^{-5} = 0.6 \times 10^{-5}$ M. $\bar{V}$ is therefore $0.6 \times 10^{-5}/1.42 \times 10^{-5} = 0.42$. Using the Scatchard equation, $K_a = \bar{V}/A(1 - \bar{V})$ $= 0.42/1.7 \times 10^{-5}(1 - 0.42) = 0.43 \times 10^{-5}$.

16.5. (b) Normal: $[Cl^-] = 107$ meq/L; $[HCO_3^-] = 27$ meq/L; $[Na^+] = 144$ meq/L; total normal anions are 134 meq/L; patient's anions are $85 + 20 = 105$ meq/L. There is a deficit of $134 - 105 = 29$ meq/L. $[Na^+]$ must be $144 - 29 = 115$ meq/L.

16.6. (e) Bicarbonate deficit is $27 - 5 = 22$ meq/L. Excess anions: $[Cl^-] = 115 - 107 = 8$ meq/L; $[PO_4^{3-}] = 6 - 2 = 4$ meq/L; $[SO_4^{2-}] = 1.5 - 0.5 = 1$ meq/L, for a total of $8 + 4 + 1 = 13$. There is a net anion deficit of $22 - 13 = 9$ meq/L, and therefore $[Na^+]$ must be $144 - 9 = 135$ meq/L.

16.7. (c) Thyroxine penetrates the cell membrane to produce T_3 inside the cell. T_3 then affects DNA transcription. All the other hormones listed act via second messengers.

16.8. (d) First, calculate the molarity of the protein: 2 mg/ml/120,000 mg/mmol = 1.66 $\times 10^{-5}$ M. Now, from bound A, calculate the corresponding $\bar{V}$. For the first set of data at 37°C, $\bar{V} = 3.32 \times 10^{-5}/1.66 \times 10^5 = 2$; for the second set, $\bar{V} = 4.98 \times 10^{-5}/1.66 \times 10^{-5} = 3$, and so on. Now, tabulate the corresponding $\bar{V}/A$ values. For the first point, we have $2/1.25 \times 10^{-5} = 1.6 \times 10^5$, and so on. Now plot the $\bar{V}/A$ values (y axis) against $\bar{V}$ (x axis). This is the Scatchard plot, and you should obtain a straight line intersecting the x axis at $\bar{V} = 6$. This is the n value in the Scatchard equation and the maximum number of binding sites for A on the receptor. To calculate K_a, take the y intercept, which is 2.4×10^5, equal to nK_a. K_a is then $2.4 \times 10^5/6 = 4 \times 10^4$. Calculate $\Delta G_0'$ from $-RT \ln K_a$. This is -6.5 kcal/mol. Repeat with data at 4°C, obtaining $n = 4$ and a $\Delta G_0''$ of -5.4 kcal/M.

16.9. (a) Use the data calculated for the two temperatures in the Gibbs-Helmholtz equation (Chapter 2), which can be written as $\ln K^2/k_1 = \Delta H/R\,(1/T_2 - 1/T_1)$ to calculate ΔH, which is independent of temperature. Remember to use degrees K. ΔH calculates to 3425 cal. Now use the expression $\Delta G = \Delta H - T\Delta S$ at either temperature. At 37°C, you obtain $-6500 = 3425 - 310\,\Delta S$; and $\Delta S = 32$ entropy units. The same result is obtained using 4°C (277 K) and a $\Delta G_0'$ of -5400 kcal/mol.

16.10. (d) Cholecystokinin works via the inositol triphosphate pathway, and this involves phospholipase C action.

16.11. (d) There is no hormone known that acts on target tissues through receptor-mediated endocytosis.

16.12. (a) Phosphatases remove P_i from proteins. Phosphodiesterases act on phosphate diesters

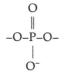

and control cellular cAMP levels.

16.13. (c) When a hormone interacts with its receptor, the G_s protein is induced to bind GTP and to dissociate into the $G_{s\alpha}$-GTP and $G_{s\beta\gamma}$ subunits. The former stimulates adenylate cyclase activity.

16.14. (e) Steroid binding receptors and calmodulin are not second messengers. Calmodulin is affected by a second messenger—Ca^{2+}.

16.15. (e) Indoleacetic acid is a metabolite of serotonin. Homovanillic acid is a metabolite of dopamine and vanillin mandelic acid of epinephrine and norepinephrine.

16.16. (b) Anion gap is $Na^+ + K^+ - Cl^- - HCO_3^-$; to determine HCO_3^-, we have $144 + 4 - 100 - 30 = 18$ meq/L. Using the Henderson-Hasselbach equation, $pH = 6.1 + \log 18/1.2 = 7.28$. The patient is acidotic.

16.17. (c) Both leukotrienes and prostaglandins can originate from arachidonic acid.

16.18. (b) Lipooxygenase initiates the formation of leukotrienes from arachidonic acid.

16.19. (a) Eicosapentaenoic acid is a precursor of series 3 prostaglandins, that is, prostaglandins with three double bonds in the side chains. Eicosapentaenoic acid is generated by linolenic acid, an essential fatty acid.

16.20. (c) Antiinflammatory steroids inhibit the release of arachidonic acid from membrane phospholipids by inhibiting a phospholipase A_2. If arachidonate is not released, it is not converted to either leukotrienes or prostaglandins.

16.21. (a) Aspirin, a synthetic antiinflammatory agent, inhibits cyclooxygenase but not lipooxygenase.

16.22. (a) Cyclooxygenase is involved in prostaglandin and thromboxane, not leukotriene, biosynthesis.

16.23. (d) Phospholipase A_2, not C, is involved in the release of arachidonic acid from membrane phospholipids.

16.24. (b) In congenital adrenal hyperplasia, progesterone is not hydroxylated in position 17, thus reducing cortisol biosynthesis.

16.25. (a) Growth hormone does not act directly on target tissues. It causes the production of somatomedins, which then proceed to affect tissues.

16.26. (d) Calcitonin acts to *decrease* plasma $[Ca^{2+}]$, an effect opposite to that of parathyroid hormone.

16.27. (c) Dopamine biosynthesis is diminished in Parkinson's disease. L-Dopa, a precursor of dopamine, is given in large doses as a therapeutic agent.

16.28. (e) ADH is produced in the hypothalamus and travels down the axons to the posterior pituitary gland.

16.29. (c) Tyrosine hydroxylase, an iron enzyme, is the rate-controlling and committing enzyme for the biosynthesis of all catecholamines.

PROBLEMS

16.1. You have two patients, both with blood pH 7.2. The following additional laboratory results are available:

	Patient 1	Patient 2	Normal
Na^+, meq/L	122	130	140
K^+, meq/L	6.0	3.0	4.5
Bicarbonate, meq/L	10.0	10.0	24.0
H_2CO_3, meq/L	0.79	0.79	1.2
Urine pH	4.5	8.0	6.0

Discuss the etiology of each disease (patients 1 and 2).

16.2. A 43-year-old woman developed high blood pressure and her doctor thought the diagnosis was diabetes. Her blood pressure kept increasing steadily until she developed cardiac arrhythmias and partial blindness. She was then sent to a university hospital, where a tumor on the adrenal gland was discovered. The tumor was removed, and she recovered completely. Answer the following:
   a. How was the tumor responsible for this patient's problems?
   b. Why was her blood sugar high? Did she really have diabetes?
   c. What test would have clinched the diagnosis before going to the university hospital?
   d. When one sees high blood pressure in a patient, does it usually come from a tumor?

16.3. A 33-year-old woman became progressively weak, her weight dropped, and her blood blood pressure went down significantly. Upon admission to the hospital, her blood chemistries showed the following: Na, 128 meq/L (normal 136–146); K, 6 meq/L (normal 3–5); BUN (blood urea nitrogen), 43 mg/dL (normal 7–18); Cl, 96 meq/L (normal 98–106); and bicarbonate, 20 meq/L. ACTH was 650 ng/L (normal less than 75). Identify the problem in this patient, and explain the laboratory values in terms of the underlying cause.

16.4. A 42-year-old male patient had been hypertensive for a number of years, and despite medication, including diuretics and potassium supplements, his blood pressure could not be brought under control, nor could his K level be maintained. He eventually developed obesity in the upper torso and developed muscle weakness and mental confusion. Based on these physical findings, the patient was given a cortisol suppression test, which involves the following: dexamethasone, an adrenocorticosteroid analog, was administered in the evening, and serum cortisol and its urinary excretion were measured the next morning. Normal individuals show a marked drop in both. The patient, however, had a serum cortisol level of 42 $\mu g/dL$ (normal 6–25 $\mu g/dL$). Address the following issues:
   a. What may be wrong with this patient? How does this case differ from that in Problem 16.3?

b. Why was there hypertension? What blood chemistries would you expect to in this patient relative to normal values (Na, K, BUN, Cl, and glucose)?

c. How would you treat this patient?

BIBLIOGRAPHY

Hadley ME. Endocrinology, 2nd ed. Englewood Cliffs: Prentice Hall, 1988.
Hoffman WS. The Biochemistry of Clinical Medicine, 4th ed. Chicago: Yearbook, 1970.
Keyes JL. Fluid, Electrolyte, and Acid–Base Regulation. Monterey: Wadsworth, 1985.
Shires TG. Fluids, Electrolytes, and Acid Bases. New York: Churchill Livingstone, 1988.

17

Overview of Metabolism and Oxidative Phosphorylation

After completing this chapter, the student should:

1. Be able to define glycogenesis, glycogenolysis, glycolysis, gluconeogenesis, the Krebs cycle, urea cycle, lipogenesis, lipolysis, and β oxidation and describe how these pathways interact with each other.
2. Be able to reproduce the oxidative phosphorylation process, and relate its physiology to the structure of mitochondria, including the pathway of electrons from NADH or $FADH_2$ to O_2, cofactors utilized, inhibitors, and where protons are extruded; explain the chemiosmotic hypothesis and how it explains the generation of ATP via proton flows, the F_0F_1 ATPase, and the various porters associated with this process; know the sites of action of the various inhibitors and proton ionophores; carry out calculations relating $\Delta G_0'$, protons extruded, and high-energy bonds synthesized.
3. Know how microsomal and mitochondrial monooxygenases operate and the components involved: FAD/FMN-containing reductases, ferredoxins, and cytochromes P_{450}.

17.1 INTRODUCTION

A living organism consumes food substances and oxygen and produces CO_2, water, nitrogen excretion products, and energy. Food is thus consumed for the purpose of energy production, which is in turn utilized for reproduction, locomotion, and other processes associated with life. The term "intermediary metabolism" has been applied to processes that produce energy or produce storage substances from which energy can be derived.

Substances arising from foodstuffs—glucose, fatty acids, amino acids, and others—yield energy by being oxidized; that is, they lose electrons. Such electrons are lost to the reduction-oxidation (redox) cofactors NAD^+ and FAD and, less commonly, to others. Because oxidation must take place at body temperature, that is, about 37°C in the human being, the organism uses a very complex series of enzymatic reactions, *metabolic pathways*. The products of these pathways are the reduced redox cofactors.

Reduced redox cofactors channel their electrons to O_2 via the process of *oxidative phosphorylation*. The products of this very complex pathway are H_2O and ATP. ATP is generated from ADP and P_i. The nature of high-energy phosphate bonds was discussed in some detail in Chapter 2, where the role of ATP in human biochemistry was introduced. ATP and related triphosphonucleosides may be used to drive various processes, such as muscle contraction, mainte- nance of ion gradients across membranes, or biosynthesis of macromolecules.

In addition to the degradative pathways that result in the production of reduced redox cofactors and, ultimately, ATP, the organism has biosynthetic processes that may require reduced cofactors and ATP. Degradative pathways are generally referred to as *catabolic*, whereas biosynthetic processes are *anabolic*. For instance, the degradation of glucose to CO_2 and water is a catabolic process, whereas the biosynthesis of proteins from amino acids is anabolism. In a normal organism, catabolism and anabolism are finely balanced, yet one may take prece- dence over the other in such conditions as starvation or the postfeeding state. A major regulatory mechanism of metabolic pathways and their interactions are the hormones, whose properties were discussed in Chapter 16.

The purpose of this chapter is to acquaint the student with the major metabolic events taking place in the various organs of the human organism and how they relate to oxidative phosphorylation. It is emphasized that the meta- bolic picture is like a symphony orchestra consisting of a number of interacting players. This should give the student the necessary introduction to the details of metabolism covered in Chapters 18 through 21.

17.2 MAJOR INTERMEDIARY METABOLIC PROCESSES

Glucose occupies the most prominent position in the world of metabolism, as shown in Figure 17.1. It is perhaps the most important fuel in the human organ- ism. Blood glucose levels are maintained at 80–120 mg/dL, which is necessary for supplying fuel to various tissues, especially the brain, retina, and red and white blood cells. When body glucose levels are high, as after a meal, the excess glucose is then converted to glycogen. This anabolic process is *glycogenesis*. Glyco- gen is present in all tissues, the most important being the liver and muscle. The reverse of glycogenesis is a catabolic process, *glycogenolysis*. Liver glycogen, via the glycogenolysis pathway, supplies glucose for the maintenance of normal blood glucose levels, whereas muscle glycogen serves largely as an energy source for rapid muscle contraction.

Practically all tissues can degrade glucose by the process of *glycolysis*. In this pathway, glucose is converted to two molecules of pyruvate, with the pro- duction of two ATP molecules. Two molecules of NAD^+ are also reduced to NADH. Pyruvate may proceed in at least two directions: toward the formation of lactate, in which case the glycolysis is *anaerobic*, or toward the formation of acetyl coenzyme A (acetyl-CoA) and oxidation via the *Krebs cycle* (also called the tricarboxylic acid cycle). In the former case, pyruvate is reduced by NADH and

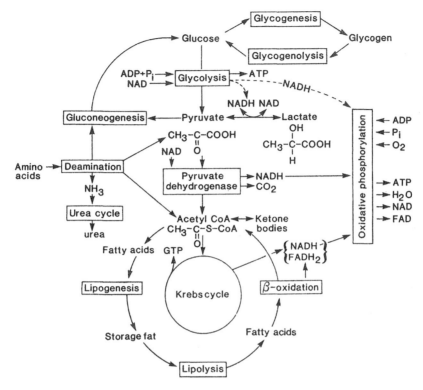

Figure 17.1 Major metabolic pathways in the human organism. For abbreviations, see list of Common Biochemical Abbreviations at the back of book.

lactate accumulates. Anaerobic glycolysis is thus self-contained, because NAD^+ is regenerated by the conversion of pyruvate to lactate. Many microorganisms ferment glucose in this manner, excreting lactic acid into the growth medium. Human beings, under hypoxic conditions, also generate excess quantities of lactate, which may accumulate in the bloodstream and cause lactic acidosis. Several tissues, such as the red blood cells, metabolize glucose via anaerobic glycolysis and are thus lactic acid producers even under normal circumstances.

The oxidative (*aerobic*) glycolytic pathway involves the conversion of pyruvate to acetyl-CoA via the multienzyme complex *pyruvate dehydrogenase* (Figure 17.1). A molecule of NADH is generated per molecule of pyruvate converted to acetyl-CoA. Acetyl-CoA, too, can go in several directions: it may be channeled into fatty acid (storage fat) biosynthesis—*lipogenesis*—or it may enter the Krebs cycle and become oxidized to CO_2, thus generating NADH and $FADH_2$. Lactic acidosis is also present in rare hereditary pyruvate dehydrogenase deficiency, when pyruvate cannot be converted to acetyl-CoA and must go to lactic acid.

In such physiologic conditions as fasting, glucose in the liver may be synthesized from pyruvate, glycerol, lactate, or amino acids. This glucose biosynthesis is *gluconeogenesis*, and it is, in part, a reversal of glycolysis. Gluconeogenesis does not operate in the muscle, because muscle lacks one of the gluconeogenesis enzymes. Brain, too, is a poor gluconeogenesis organ. The purpose of liver gluconeogenesis is to supply glucose for blood in the fasting state, especially after liver glycogen stores have been exhausted. Fatty acids are not glucose precursors, although fatty acids with an odd number of carbons are an exception.

Adipose and other tissues can degrade storage fat and release fatty acids into the bloodstream. This process is *lipolysis*. Fatty acids, in such target tissues as the heart and skeletal muscle, are oxidized to acetyl-CoA by the *β-oxidation* pathway. More than 50% of the energy requirement of muscle is derived from fatty acids. β-Oxidation yields both NADH and $FADH_2$. The acetyl-CoA produced is subject to oxidation by the Krebs cycle or, in the liver, to conversion into the ketone bodies. These are acetoacetate and β-OH-butyrate, and they are exported to other tissues to be used as fuels. By switching to fatty acids and ketone bodies as major energy-producing fuels under such stressful conditions as fasting or prolonged exercise, the organism spares glucose, which is absolutely required by the brain and other tissues. The brain cannot utilize fatty acids, although after prolonged starvation it can utilize ketone bodies. Normally the brain oxidizes glucose to CO_2 and water via aerobic glycolysis and the Krebs cycle and produces little if any lactate. It is thus extremely sensitive to O_2 deprivation.

In summary, the metabolism of carbohydrates, fats, and amino acids is closely interrelated by sharing many common intermediaries. There are significant organ differences with regard to fuel utilization. The catabolic processes include glycogenolysis, glycolysis, the Krebs cycle, lipolysis, and protein degradation. Some such pathways produce NADH and $FADH_2$, which are reoxidized by the oxidative phosphorylation system with ATP production. Among the anabolic pathways, one finds glycogenesis, gluconeogenesis, lipogenesis, and protein synthesis.

17.3 ELECTRON TRANSPORT AND ATP BIOSYNTHESIS

Figure 17.1 indicates that a number of metabolic pathways generate NADH and $FADH_2$. These reduced cofactors can give rise to ATP by being reoxidized by an *electron transport chain* (also known as respiratory chain) located in the inner membrane of the mitochondrion. The ultimate electron acceptor in this chain is O_2. Electron transport is very closely coupled to a system that phosphorylates ADP to form ATP. The latter is F_0F_1 *ATPase* or *ATP synthetase*. Oxidation of NADH and/or $FADH_2$ coupled with ATP production is *oxidative phosphorylation*. Some authorities have reserved the term "oxidative phosphorylation" for the process by which ADP is phosphorylated to ATP. Oxidative phosphorylation is also indicated in Figure 17.1.

Oxidative phosphorylation results in the creation of high-energy bonds. The energy required to form such bonds is provided by free energy generated by the passage of electrons from NADH and $FADH_2$, which possess relatively low redox potentials (see Chapter 2), to O_2, with its very high redox potential of 0.82 V. It is also possible to channel electrons from NADH or $FADH_2$ to O_2 without phosphorylating ADP. In this case, the energy that would normally be captured in the form of ATP is dissipated as heat.

As electrons are transferred to O_2 via the electron transport chain, protons are pumped from the mitochondrial interior into its surroundings, creating a

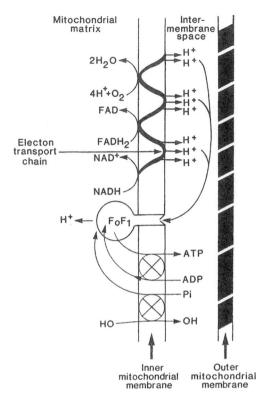

Figure 17.2 The chemiosmotic hypothesis. Electrons from NADH and/or $FADH_2$ are passed to O_2 via the electron transport chain. In the process, protons are extruded into the mitochondrial intermembrane space. The proton gradient thus created causes the movement of protons back into mitochondria through a channel in the F_0F_1 ATPase. In the process, one molecule of ATP is formed frm ADP and phosphate for every two to three protons channeled back into the mitochondria. ATP moves into the intermembrane space and cytosol in exchange for ADP moving in the opposite direction. Phosphate is taken up in exchange for OH^-.

proton gradient across the membrane. Proton flow back into the mitochondria is allowed only through specific particles, which harness the energy of the proton gradient to phosphorylate ADP. Such coupling of proton flow with ATP biosynthesis is the *chemiosmotic effect*. It was first proposed by Peter Mitchell, who won the Nobel Prize in 1978 for this discovery. Mitchell's hypothesis is summarized in Figure 17.2. This section discusses the details of the electron transport and phosphorylation pathways.

17.3.1 The Mitochondrion

Mitochondria are subcellular particles of varying sizes that are present in eukaryotic cells. A mitochondrial cross section is illustrated in Figure 17.3. There is an outer and an inner membrane, with an intermembrane space between them. The outer membrane is quite porous, permitting the passage of molecules with a molecular weight of 5000–10,000. The inner membrane is impermeable

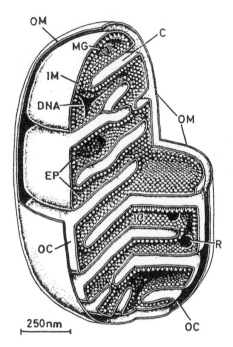

Figure 17.3 The mitochondrial structure: OM and IM, outer and inner membranes, respectively; IC, mitochondrial matrix; EP, "elementary particles" carrying the F_0F_1 ATPase; MG, mitochondrial granules; C, is crystae; OC, intermembrane space; and R, ribosomes. (Reproduced by permission from Kristic RV. Illustrated Encyclopedia of Human Histology. New York: Springer-Verlag, 1984, p. 265.)

and contains numerous folds called cristae that extend deep into the mitochondrial matrix. The oxidative phosphorylation system components are largely located on this inner mitochondrial membrane. This membrane is also the site of many other redox system enzymes. It is generally the inner mitochondrial membrane that we have in mind when we are concerned with the passage of various substances in and out of mitochondria.

Many authorities believe that mitochondria have prokaryotic origins because the inner mitochondrial membrane lacks cholesterol and contains cardiolipin. Moreover, mitochondrial DNA is circular and the ribosomes approximate the size of those from prokaryotic organisms.

17.3.2 Electron Transport

Electrons enter the electron transport chain from either NADH or $FADH_2$. As shown in Figure 17.4, the electron transport pathway may be divided into four groups of protein particles, complexes I–IV, even though the total number of individual steps involved to reach O_2 may be much higher. Several types of prosthetic groups are involved: iron-sulfur centers (ferredoxin-like proteins), iron-porphyrin groups, copper, riboflavin-containing groups, and quinones. Many of these factors are *cytochromes*, small proteins containing metalloporphyrin residues, which are present in three complexes. Cytochromes are classi-

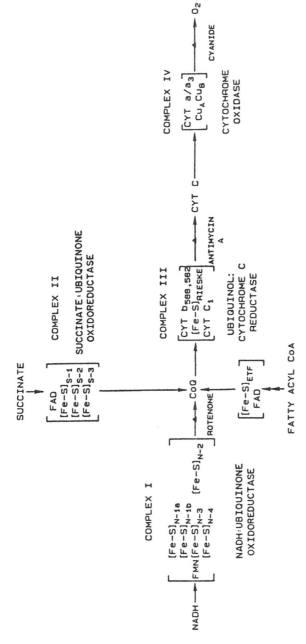

Figure 17.4 The electron transport chain of mitochondria. Triangles indicate sites of inhibition by various compounds. Cyt, cytochrome; ETF, electron transfer flavoprotein. (Reproduced with permission from Moreadith RW, Batshaw ML, Ohnishi T, Kerr D, Knox B, Jackson D, Hruben R, Olson J, Reynafarje B, Lehninger AL. Deficiency of the iron-sulfur clusters of mitochondrial reduced nicotinamide-adenine dinucleotide-ubiquinone oxidoreductase (complex I) in an infant with congenital lactic acidosis J Clin Invest 74:685–697, 1984.)

fied into the *a*, *b*, and *c* groups on the basis of their porphyrin structures. Those of the *b* type contain heme, whereas the others have porphyrins with different side chains. Cytochrome *c* was, in fact, the protein that served as a model for the formulation of evolutionary trees from protein amino acid sequences. Note that iron and copper associated with the various components of the electron transfer chain undergo continuous redox cycles: ferric to ferrous, cupric to cuprous, and vice versa. Electron transport stops if the metal becomes frozen in one of its oxidation states.

Oxidation of NADH begins with complex I, also termed NADH dehydrogenase or NADH:ubiquinone oxidoreductase. It contains 25 polypeptide chains, flavine mononucleotide (FMN), and several iron-sulfur centers. The function of this complex is to reduce a substance called ubiquinone (UQ or CoQ), whose structure is shown in Figure 17.5. UQ is not protein bound and can move about freely. In the process of reducing UQ, the NADH is oxidized to NAD^+. It is now accepted that in complex I, NADH first reduces FMN, and the resulting $FMNH_2$ then transfers its electrons through at least three iron-sulfur centers to UQ. As the electrons pass from NADH to UQ, two to four protons are extruded from the mitochondrial matrix across the inner membrane.

According to Figure 17.4, reduced UQ proceeds to reduce complex III, which contains *b* and *c* type cytochromes and an iron-sulfur protein called Rieske's protein. It is now well known that the *b* cytochromes of complex III are not in the direct electron transfer pathway, and the so-called Q cycle was proposed to explain their function. According to this scheme, UQ on the matrix side of the inner mitochondrial membrane is reduced to a semiquinone Q free radical, often represented by $U\dot{Q}_i^-$, by reduced cytochrome b_{562}. Another electron is picked up from complex I to give ubiquinol, UQH_2. UQH_2 diffuses to the cytosol side of the inner mitochondrial membrane and is reoxidized there first by Rieske's protein (one electron), and then by cytochrome b_{566} (one electron). The two protons are left behind on the cytosol side of the membrane, and UQ is regenerated. Cytochrome b_{566} then reduces cytochrome b_{562}, thus completing the cycle. Because this accounts for only one electron from the initial NADH mole-

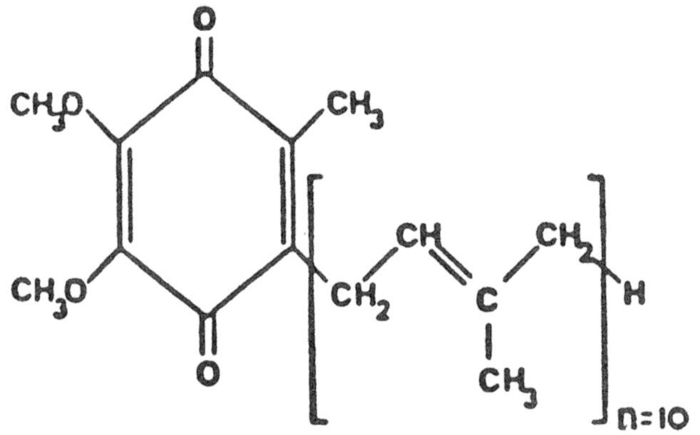

Figure 17.5 Structure of ubiquinone (oxidized). (Reproduced by permission from Greenberg SM, Frishman W. Coenzyme Q_{10}: a new drug for myocardial ischemia? Med Clin North Am 72:243–253, 1988.)

cule, the passage of the two electrons must therefore involve two UQ molecules, each extruding two protons from the mitochondrial matrix. Teleologically, the purpose of the Q cycle may be to maximize the extrusion of protons from mitochondria.

UQ may also be reduced by complex II (succinate:ubiquinone oxido-reductase, succinate dehydrogenase), which contains four polypeptide chains, molecular weights 70,000, 27,000, 15,500, and 13,500. The first two constitute bona fide succinate dehydrogenase, a Krebs cycle enzyme catalyzing reaction (17.1):

$$\text{Succinate} + \text{FAD} \rightleftharpoons \text{fumarate} + \text{FADH}_2 \tag{17.1}$$

Succinate dehydrogenase contains iron-sulfur centers and covalently bound FAD (both on the 70,000-dalton subunit). Iron-sulfur centers are also present on the 27,000-dalton subunit. The 15,500-dalton subunit of complex II is cytochrome b_{560}. Electrons from FADH_2 are channeled to UQ via cytochrome b_{560}.

UQ may also be reduced by FADH_2 generated from glycerol-3-phosphate by mitochondrial glycerol-3-phosphate dehydrogenase and from fatty acids by fatty acyl-CoA dehydrogenase. Glycerol-3-phosphate shuttles electrons from the cytosol to mitochondria (see Chapter 18), whereas fatty acyl-CoA dehydro-genase is an enzyme of the β-oxidation process. In both cases, FAD is covalently bound to the enzymes and an intermediary is necessary to carry electrons from FADH_2 to UQ. Such an intermediary is the elctron transfer flavoprotein (ETF), which is reduced by FADH_2 and oxidized by UQ in the presence of a specific enzyme, ETF:UQ oxidoreductase, an iron-sulfur center-containing protein. It is generally accepted that FADH_2 of whatever source donates its electrons to the electron transport chain at the UQ level (see Figure 17.4).

Complex III (UQH$_2$:cytochrome c reductase) transmits electrons gained from UQH$_2$ via Rieske's protein to cytochrome c_1 and then to cytochrome c. The latter is only loosely bound to the inner mitochondrial membrane. Cytochrome c then reduces complex IV (cytochrome c oxidase). This complex contains at least eight polypeptide chains designated I–VII-Ser and VII-Ile. These contain two heme molecules designated a and a_3 and two centers designated Cu_a and Cu_{a3}, as prosthetic groups. Polypeptide chains carrying the heme residues are often re-ferred to as cytochromes a and a_3. Cu_a is closely associated with heme a, and Cu_{a3} is associated with heme a_3. Both types of prosthetic groups are attached to only two polypeptide chains: I (molecular weight 56,000) and II (molecular weight 26,000). It is unclear, however, which subunit carries which prosthetic group.

Complex IV reduces molecular O_2, and it is apparently the a_3Cu_{a3} center that is the immediate donor of electrons to O_2. The aCu_a grouping oxidizes cyto-chrome c. The passage of electrons from Rieske's protein through complex IV to O_2 is summarized by Equation (17.2):

$$\tag{17.2}$$

The last reaction of (17.2) may proceed by the formation of an intermediate peroxide:

$$a_3^{2+}Cu_{a3}^{1+} + O_2 \rightarrow a_3^{3+} - \bar{O} - \bar{O} - Cu_{a3}^{2+} \xrightarrow[4H^{1+}]{2e^-} a_3^{3+}Cu_{a3}^{2+} + 2H_2O \qquad (17.3)$$

The intermediate peroxide is reduced further to $2O^{2-}$ as another pair of electrons is absorbed by the complex. Note that NADH, $FADH_2$, and UQH_2 are carriers of two electrons each. The heme molecules and copper are carriers of only one.

To form the relatively undissociated water, 2 protons per electron pair, transported through complex IV, are removed from the mitochondrial matrix. An additional 2 protons per electron pair transported are extruded from the matrix by complex IV. The total number of protons lost by the mitochondrial matrix through the action of complexes I, III, and IV is thus 8–10 per electron pair, depending on the authority cited. The reason protons are extruded across the inner mitochondrial membrane is 2-fold: complex IV apparently acts as a true proton pump with specific protein(s) of that complex acting as the transport particle(s). Complexes I and III, on the other hand, are associated with the so-called vectoral proton translocation process: those enzymatic reactions that release protons (e.g., reoxidation of UQH_2) take place at or near the intermembrane space surface on the inner mitochondrial membrane. This allows protons to be discharged into the intermembrane space rather than into the mitochondrial matrix. Overall, the pH differential between the cytosol and the mitochondrial matrix is about 1, or a 10-fold difference in [H$^+$] (alkaline inside).

Several inherited disorders are associated with faulty operation of the electron transport pathway. ATP production is diminished in such cases. These disorders are known as *mitochondrial myopathies,* and they are associated with the absence of specific polypeptide chains found in complexes I, III, or IV. In many cases, the problem may be traced to specific lesions in mitochondrial DNA, which codes for at least 13 polypeptide chains found in these complexes. Myopathies are tissue specific; some affect the heart, others the skeletal muscle. Many are accompanied by lactic acidosis, because the inability to reduce NADH normally results in its accumulation and the channeling of pyruvate toward lactic acid production. In complex I disorders, the oxidation of $FADH_2$ is not impeded. In complex III lesions, neither NADH nor $FADH_2$ can be oxidized. However, use has been made by B. Chance and colleagues of *menadione* (Chapter 6) and *ascorbic acid* in such cases. The former can oxidize UQH_2, whereas ascorbate can oxidize menadione and reduce cytochrome *c.* Marked clinical improvement in affected patients follows such treatment.

17.3.3 ATP Production

It is well established experimentally that a pair of electrons originating in NADH generates three ATP molecules via the oxidative phosphorylation pathway and that those from $FADH_2$ generate two. It is said that the P/O ratio is three for electrons from NADH and two for those from $FADH_2$, O referring to an atom of oxygen being reduced and P to a high-energy phosphate bond being synthesized. In the older literature, it was indicated that each of the complexes I, III, and IV was responsible for generating one ATP molecule from ADP and P_i. The more modern view is that complexes I, III, and IV are sites of proton extrusion and the reason $FADH_2$ produces only two ATP molecules rather than three is that its oxidation results in the extrusion of two to four fewer protons than that of NADH. It is generally accepted that some three protons must be extruded for each ATP molecule synthesized.

Why do electrons flow from NADH (or $FADH_2$) to O_2, and what is the thermodynamic origin of the high-energy bonds being created? The answer may be obtained by looking at the redox potentials of these coenzymes, on the one hand, and that of O_2, on the other. If one starts with NADH, with its redox potential of −0.32 V, and ends with O_2, redox potential 0.82, then one spans a total of 1.14 V (see Figure 17.6). Using Equation (2.6), this comes to a theoretical availability of about 52,000 cal/mol, and because three ATP molecules are synthesized for each pair of electrons channeled to O_2, oxidative phosphorylation recovers $8400 \times 3 = 25,200$ cal of the 52,000 available as ATP, for an approximate efficiency of 48%. Note also that the redox potential for the UQ system is 0.10.

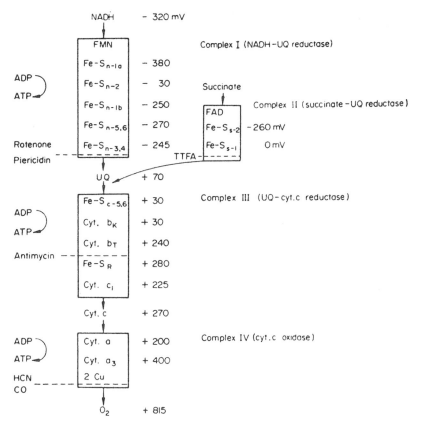

Figure 17.6 Electron transport chain showing redox potentials at each step. Note that electrons travel from components with a very negative redox potential (e.g., −0.32 V for NAD^+/NADH) to one with a very high one (0.82 V for O_2). With each step, the $\Delta E_0'$ increases. The overall $\Delta E_0'$ is 1.14 V. (Reproduced by permission from Hall DO, Rao KK, Cammack R. Science Prog Oxford 62:285–317, 1975.)

This translates to a $\Delta E_0'$ of 0.81–0.10 = 0.72 V and a $\Delta G_0'$ of –33,000 cal. This is theoretically available for electrons entering at the UQ level, as from FADH$_2$. With 48% efficiency, this leaves about 16,000 cal for ATP biosynthesis, corresponding to about two ATP molecules per electron pair.

It is also possible to approximate the number of protons necessary to export to generate 3 ATP molecules per electron pair. Assuming that the pH gradient across the inner mitochondrial membrane is about 1, that is, $[H^+]_{out}/[H^+]_{in} = 10$, and assuming that the transmembrane potential is 0.18 V (negative inside), we can use Equation (9.7) to calculate the $\Delta G_0'$ that becomes available per mol H$^+$ extruded by mitochondria:

$$\Delta G' = RT \ln 10 + nF \times 0.18 = 5500 \text{ cal} \tag{17.4}$$

If a total of about 52,000 cal becomes available by the passage of 2 electrons to O$_2$ and for each mol protons, 5500 cal is made available, then the total number of protons that must be extruded is 52,000/5500 = 9.5. This figure corresponds rather well with the experimentally determined figure of 8–10 protons cited earlier.

The mechanics of converting proton flow back into mitochondria into high-energy phosphate bonds is performed by the F$_0$F$_1$ ATPase. This complex enzyme system spans the inner mitochondrial membrane and appears as particles labeled EP in Figure 17.3. Structural details are given in Figure 17.7. The enzyme consists of two sections: the F$_0$ section is embedded in the membrane and forms a channel through which protons are permitted to enter the F$_1$ section. The latter is located on the matrix side of the membrane and is attached to the F$_0$ section. The ATPase catalyzes the formation of ATP from ADP and P$_i$. The reverse reaction, ATP → ADP + P$_i$, is carried out when F$_1$ is separated from F$_0$: hence the term ATPase.

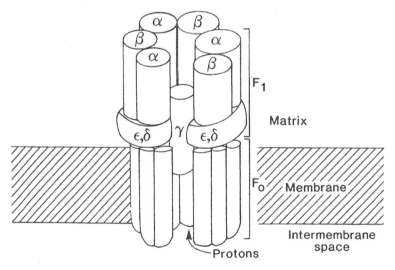

Figure 17.7 F$_0$F$_1$ ATPase. The F$_0$ section is embedded in the inner mitochondrial membrane, whereas F$_1$ section is located on the matrix side. The various subunits of F$_1$ are designated as α, β, γ, δ, and ϵ.

The F_1 section consists of five types of subunits with the following stoichiometry: α_3, β_3, γ, δ, ϵ (see Figure 17.7). The α and β subunits bind both ADP and ATP, and both are required for ATPase activity. The γ subunit serves as a stalk around which the other subunits are assembled and also as a point of attachment to the F_0 piece. It may act as a valve that controls the entry of protons from the F_0 section to the catalytic sites in the F_1 section. The function of the δ and ϵ subunits is not completely understood. The function of the F_0 section has been compared to the action of gramicidin, an antibiotic with ionophore properties. F_0, too, consists of a number of subunits, but their exact function is not known. It is known, however, that certain carboxyl groups are necessary for the transmittal of protons, because carboxyl group modifiers, such as dicyclohexylcarbodiimide (DCCD), inhibit the passage of protons through F_0. Two antiporters located in the inner mitochondrial membrane are associated with the action of F_0F_1 ATPases: The ADP/ATP and the P_i/OH^- porters. The former brings in ADP and exports ATP, whereas the latter brings in phosphate ions for ATP biosynthesis. These porters, together with the F_0F_1 ATPase, are often referred to as complex V.

ADP phosphorylation is tightly coupled to electron transport. Shutting down one shuts down the other. It is well known that if ADP phosphorylation is inhibited by such compounds as oligomycin, electron transport also ceases. If the proton gradient is broken by a proton ionophore, however, such as 2,4-dinitrophenol, electron transport resumes at a rapid pace and no phosphorylation takes place. Such proton ionophores are also termed "uncouplers" of electron transport and ADP phosphorylation. Under normal conditions, the factors limiting ATP production are the pH gradient across the inner mitochondrial membrane and the cellular ADP/ATP ratio. An increase in the proton gradient shuts down phosphorylation and electron transport, whereas an increase in the ADP/ATP ratio stimulates both. Stimulation of oxidative phosphorylation by increases in cellular ADP concentration is termed *respiratory control*.

17.3.4 Mitochondrial Membrane Transporters

Mitochondria perform a crucial series of reactions in the human organism. The inner mitochondrial membrane is relatively impermeable to charged substances, although uncharged substances, such as O_2 and CO, move across with ease. To perform their functions, however, mitochondria must transport various charged substances in and out of its matrix. This is done via transport particles called porters or translocases (see Chapter 9 for definitions). They are not directly associated with the hydrolysis of ATP; some depend for their operation on concentration gradients of one sort or another, and others depend on the mitochondrial membrane potential.

In the previous section we mentioned the ADP/ATP transporter, and it is also shown in Figure 17.2. This system allows the export of ATP and import of ADP. Because ATP and ADP have net charges of –4 and –3, respectively, at pH 7, the transport is not electroneutral and must occur at the expense of the membrane potential. Atractyloside and bongkrekic acid are inhibitors of this system, the former binding to the ADP binding site of the porter and the latter to the ATP site. Associated with ADP/ATP transport is the transport of P_i, which must enter the mitochondrion to participate in ATP formation. Several systems for transporting P_i in an electroneutral fashion are known: a $H_2PO_4^-/OH^-$ antiport mentioned earlier, a $HPO_4^{2-}/2H^+$ symport, a $H_2PO_4^-/H^+$ symport, and a $HPO_4^{2-}/malate$ antiport. The latter is also termed a dicarboxylate transporter. Malate is also associated with a citrate transporter. In this system, citrate with a H^+ is exchanged for malate in an electroneutral operation. This is *tricarboxylate transport*, in which citrate moves out of mitochondria as a means of exporting acetyl residues to the cytosol (see Chapter 19). The monocarboxylate transporter moves pyruvate into the mitochondrion and an OH^- ion out. A transporter moving glutamate in and aspartate out also exists, as does an antiporter moving malate in and α-ketoglutarate out.

An important mitochondrial membrane porter is used to move Ca^{2+} into the mitochondria while moving out two protons. Membrane potential is apparently the driving force.

It is often necessary to move electrons into mitochondria for disposal via oxidative phosphorylation. However, NADH and $FADH_2$ do not penetrate the inner mitochondrial membrane. Instead, such electrons may first be passed to dihydroxyacetone phosphate or to oxaloacetate to make glycerol-3-phosphate and malate, respectively. These compounds can penetrate the inner mitochondrial membrane via the porters described earlier and oxidized there by mitochondrial NAD^+ or FAD. These systems are termed the glycerol-3-phosphate and malate shuttles, respectively, and they are described in greater detail in Chapter 18.

17.3.5 Inhibitors and Uncouplers of Oxidative Phosphorylation

A number of substances inhibit oxidative phosphorylation at specific locations. These may be divided into agents that affect electron transport, those that affect complex V, and those that collapse proton gradients (proton ionophores). Such substances have been used as research tools to unravel the complexities of these pathways, as poisons, and as antibiotics. Inhibition of electron transport inhibits phosphorylation, the extent of which depends on the location of the inhibition site. Thus, if complex I is inactivated, electron transport can still take place using $FADH_2$ as an electron donor. The donor P/O ratio is then 2.

The action of some inhibitors is indicated in Figure 17.4. It is sometimes difficult to pinpoint exactly where an inhibitor may act, however, because our knowledge of the composition and function of the four complexes is far from complete. Complex I inhibitors, such as rotenone, piericidin A, and the barbiturates, are believed to inhibit the transfer of elctrons from the Fe-S centers to UQ. In complex III, antimycin appears to inhibit the reduction of UQ by cytochrome b_{562}. Myxothiazol and 2,3-dimercaptopropanol (BAL) inhibit the transfer of electrons from UQH_2 to Rieske's protein, because they destroy the Fe-S centers. The action of cyanide and azide on complex IV is also unclear, but it is believed that these substances combine with the Fe^{3+} moiety of the a_3 heme prosthetic group.

A proton ionophore "short-circuits" the proton current, so that both the proton gradient and membrane potential across the inner mitochondrial membrane are collapsed. No phosphorylation of ADP can take place, but electron

Table 17.1 Compounds Inhibiting Electron Transport and ADP Phosphorylation by Mitochondria

Compound	Site of inhibition	Notes
Inhibitors of electron transport		
Rotenone	Complex I	Fish poison, insecticide
Barbiturates (e.g., amytal)	Complex I	Sedatives
Piericidin A	Complex I	Antibiotic; accepts electrons instead of UQ
Myxothiazol	Complex III	—
Antimycin A	Complex III	Antibiotic
2,3-Dimercaptopropanol	Complex III	Reducing agent; metal chelator
N_3^- (azide)	Complex IV	Combines with Fe^{3+} in heme
CN^- (cyanide)	Complex IV	Combines with Fe^{3+} in heme
CO (carbon monoxide)	Complex IV	Combines with O_2 binding sites
Inhibitors of phosphorylation		
Dicyclohexylcarbodiimide	F_0 portion of F_0F_1 ATPase	Modifies essential –COOH groups
Oligomycin	F_0 portion of F_0F_1 ATPase	Antibiotic
Atractyloside	ADP/ATP porter	Alkaloid
Bongkrekic acid	ADP/ATP porter	Bacterial product
N-Ethylmaleimide	P_i/OH^- porter	Sulfhydryl group modifier
Aurovertin	F_1 portion of F_0F_1 ATPase	—
Proton ionophores		
2,4-Dinitrophenol	Collapses proton gradients	Used to control obesity in 1920s
Carbonyl cyanide-*m*-chlorophenylhydrazone (CCCP)	Collapses proton gradients	—
Carbonyl cyanide-*p*-trifluoromethoxyphenyl-hydrazone (FCCP)	Collapses proton gradients	—

transport proceeds at supernormal rate. Table 17.1 lists a number of oxidative phosphorylation inhibitors and their modes of action.

17.4 THE CYTOCHROME P_{450} ELECTRON TRANSPORT SYSTEMS

Cytochrome proteins participate in certain mitochondrial and nonmitochondrial reactions that involve the introduction of O_2 into organic substances. These are *hydroxylation reactions*; among the substrates, one finds steroids, various drugs, vitamin D intermediates, and other substances. The hydroxylation system uses molecular O_2 and is often referred to as monooxygenase, mixed-function oxygenase, or hydroxylase. One atom of oxygen is introduced into an organic compound from O_2 as an –OH group, and the other oxygen atom appears in H_2O [Equation (17.5)]. Monooxygenase components are membrane bound in eukaryotic systems: they may be associated with mitochondria or endoplasmic reticulum (microsomes) and, less often, with other subcellular particles. Microsomal oxygenase systems, especially those of the liver, are extremely nonspecific and may hydroxylate many hundreds of exogenous and endogenous hydrophobic compounds, the purpose being to render them more water soluble. Such solubility in water is further enhanced if the –OH group can be conjugated with gluc-uronic acid. Mitochondrial monooxygenases are much more substrate specific. Prokaryotic monooxygenases do not appear to be membrane bound.

Monooxygenase systems consist of several components, the most prominent of which is *cytochrome P$_{450}$*. Cytochromes P$_{450}$ are a group of proteins containing a *b*-type heme residue, which gives a maximum absorption at 450 nm when com-plexed with CO. Unlike hemoglobins, the proximal ligand of iron in these heme residues is an –SH group. The distal ligand may be O$_2$ or H$_2$O. In addition to cyto-chrome P$_{450}$, microsomal monooxygenases also contain NADPH-cytochrome P$_{450}$ reductases, which are proteins with FMN and FAD prosthetic groups. Mitochon-drial monooxygenases are associated with ferredoxins and ferredoxin reductases, which are also flavoproteins. The general monooxygenase-catalyzed reaction may be represented by Equation (17.5), where R is the substrate being hydroxylated.

$$RH + O_2 + NADPH + H^+ \rightarrow ROH + H_2O + NADP^+ \tag{17.5}$$

For example, we may examine the hydroxylation of steroids in the adrenal cortex. This is a very important hydroxylation site, because the adrenal cortex converts cholesterol to various hormones: mineralocorticoids, glucocorticoids, and male sex hormones. Certain hydroxylations take place in the mitochondria, others in the microsomes. The best known mitochondrial cytochromes P$_{450}$ are the P$_{450_{scc}}$ (molecular weight 51,000) and P$_{450_{11\beta}}$ (molecular weight 46,000). They are located on the matrix side of the inner mitochondrial membrane. P$_{450_{scc}}$ catalyzes the conversion of cholesterol to pregnenolone, and P$_{450_{11\beta}}$ catalyzes the conversion of 11-deoxycortisol to cortisol (Chapter 16). The ferredoxin involved in these hydroxylations is called adrenodoxin, a 12,000 dalton protein with two iron-sulfur centers of the 2Fe-2S type. Adrenodoxin reductase, an FAD-containing protein, has a molecular weight of 54,000. A typical adrenal mitochondrial hydroxylation is shown in Figure 17.8, which illustrates that the first reaction is the binding of the substrate by cytochrome P$_{450}$. This is then followed by two reduction steps with

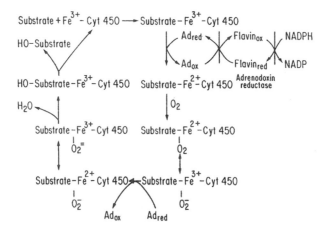

Figure 17.8 Typical hydroxylation reaction involving cytochrome P$_{450}$. Ad, adrenodoxin. The substrate is a steroid hormone biosynthesis intermediate. The location of the reaction is in the mitochondria of adrenal cortex. (Reproduced by permission from Bezkorovainy A. Biochemistry of Nonheme Iron. New York: Plenum Press, 1980, p. 380.)

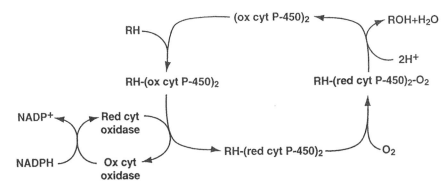

Figure 17.9 Microsomal (nonmitochondrial) hydroxylation sequence involving cytochrome P_{450}. RH is the substrate to be hydroxylated (ox, oxidized; red, reduced; cyt, cytochrome). Reduced cytochrome P_{450} has Fe^{2+}, oxidized cytochrome P_{450} has Fe^{3+}, reduced cytochrome oxidase has $FADH_2/FMNH_2$, and oxidized cytochrome oxidase has FAD/FMN.

adrenodoxin, which shuttles electrons from the adrenodoxin reductase to the substrate-P_{450} complex.

Microsomal hydroxylations do not involve adrenodoxin. The substrate-P_{450} complex is apparently reduced directly by the NADPH-cytochrome P_{450} reductase, a FMN-FAD (1:1) protein with a molecular weight of 78,000. The best known microsomal cytochromes P_{450} are the $P_{450_{C21}}$ and $P_{450_{7\alpha\,lyase}}$. The first catalyzes the hydroxylation of progesterone to 11-deoxycorticosterone and the 17α-hydroxyprogesterone to 11-deoxycortisol (Chapter 16). $P_{450_{7\alpha\,lyase}}$ catalyzes the hydroxylation of progesterone to 17α-hydroxyprogesterone. Figure 17.9 summarizes the microsomal hydroxylation sequence.

QUESTIONS

In Questions 17.1–17.7, use the following key:
- a. 1, 2, and 3 are correct.
- b. 1 and 3 are correct.
- c. 2 and 4 are correct.
- d. Only 4 is correct.
- e. All are correct.

17.1. The function of cytochromes b in complex III is to
1. Channel electrons from UQ to cytochrome c
2. Reduce UQ
3. Stabilize the inner mitochondrial membrane enzyme arrangement
4. Oxidize UQ

17.2. Mechanisms for proton removal from mitochondria include the following:
1. An ATPase to pump protons out while ATP is hydrolyzed.
2. There is no direct loss of protons; they are lost from mitochondria by being converted to H_2O.
3. Shuttle mechanisms remove protons via NADH.
4. The spatial arrangement of electron transport enzymes permits an easy exit of protons as they are released by various oxidative processes.

17.3. In a mitochondrial myopathy in which complex I is defective, the following symptoms are present in the patient:
1. Hypoglycemia (low blood sugar)
2. Lactic acidosis
3. High cellular NADH levels
4. Normal metabolism of succinate

17.4. Ferredoxin-like proteins are involved in
1. Mitochondrial hydroxylation reactions
2. Microbial redox reactions
3. Action of complex II
4. Action of complex IV

17.5. Cells or tissues that are normally the major lactic acid producers are
1. Red blood cells
2. Brain
3. Exercising muscle
4. Liver

17.6. The F_0F_1 ATPase
1. Is inhibited by oligomycin
2. Pumps protons from mitochondria, thus hydrolyzing ATP
3. Captures proton flow energy to synthesize ATP
4. Performs a redox function as part of the electron path from NADH to O_2

17.7. In an organism with a high level of gluconeogenesis
1. Glycogen synthesis is increased.
2. Glycolysis is increased.
3. Fatty acid biosynthesis is increased.
4. Ketone body production is increased.

17.8. The overall redox potential change as a pair of electrons passes from NADH to O_2 is about 1.14 V. This translates theoretically into about how many ATPs synthesized per proton extruded from the mitochondrial matrix? $R = 1.98$, $F = 23,000$, and $T = 37°C$.
    a. 0.3   c. 1   e. 3
    b. 0.6   d. 2

17.9. Which inhibitor would permit electron passage from $FADH_2$ to O_2 but not from NADH?
    a. Cyanide   c. 2,4-Dinitrophenol   e. Rotenone
    b. Oligomycin   d. Azide

17.10. A patient is severely acidotic and experiences serious muscle weakness. Her mitochondrial cytochrome b content is 0.1 nmol/mg protein (normal is 0.63), her creatine phosphate is low, and neither NADH nor succinate can reduce cytochrome c. The most likely problem is (see Nutr Rev 46:157–163, 1988)
    a. Complex I myopathy   d. Complex IV myopathy
    b. Complex II myopathy   e. Complex V myopathy
    c. Complex III myopathy

17.11. Which cannot be transported across the inner mitochondrial membrane?
    a. Malate   c. Pyruvate   e. H^+
    b. Aspartate   d. NADH

17.12. Which is *not* membrane bound in the human being?
    a. Adrenodoxin   d. Cytochrome P_{450} reductases
    b. Cytochrome P_{450} e. F_0F_1 ATPase
    c. Ferredoxin reductases

17.13. Which is *not* true about the monooxygenase group of enzymes?
    a. They generally use hydrophobic substances as substrates.

b. They introduce the entire O_2 molecule into organic substances.
c. They are generally associated with cytochromes P_{450}.
d. A flavoprotein participates in their reactions.
e. One of the products is H_2O.

Answers

17.1. (c) Cytochromes b are involved in the Q cycle and are not in the direct electron path from NADH to O_2. UQ is reduced by cytochrome b_{562}. Ubiquinol is reoxidized by cyt b_{566}, which then proceeds to reduce cytochrome b_{562} to complete the cycle.

17.2. (d) Protons are removed from mitochondria as electrons pass from NADH to O_2. This removal is facilitated by the location on the outer side of the inner mitochondrial membrane of those redox steps that result in proton release (e.g., from the reoxidation of ubiquinol).

17.3. (e) When complex I is defective, there is an excess of cellular NADH, which pushes the lactate dehydrogenase to form lactate from pyruvate (anaerobic glycolysis). This results in higher than normal utilization of glucose, causing hypoglycemia. Because succinate is oxidized at the complex II level, its oxidation is not affected.

17.4. (a) Ferredoxins are involved in many microbial redox reactions as well as in mitochondrial hydroxylation reactions in mammals. They are also components of complexes I, II, and III, but not complex IV.

17.5. (b) Muscle metabolizes glucose to lactic acid during exercise. Red blood cells depend upon anaerobic glycolysis for their energy source.

17.6. (b) The function of F_0F_1 ATPase is to convert proton flow from the outside into the mitochondrion into ATP. It has nothing directly to do with the electron flow.

17.7. (d) High gluconeogenesis activity means a high blood glucagon and/or epinephrine levels. Of the four choices, only ketone body production can coexist with gluconeogenesis.

17.8. (a) Dismiss information that is not required to solve the problem. We know that 8–10 protons are extruded by the mitochondria per 3 ATPs synthesized. Therefore, taking 9 protons as an average, we have 3/9 = 0.33 ATPs/proton.

17.9. (e) Rotenone inhibits complex I activity, but the others are unaffected.

17.10. (c) A low level of cytochromes b is consistent with complex III myopathy. If complex I myopathy existed, succinate would be able to reduce cytochrome c, and NADH would be able to reduce cytochrome c if a complex II myopathy were present.

17.11. (d) Redox cofactors cannot be transported across the inner mitochondrial membrane. To transport electrons across, shuttles are required.

17.12. (a) Adrenodoxin moves about freely, transporting electrons from the adrenodoxin reductase to cytochrome P_{450}. All others are membrane bound.

17.13. (b) Monooxygenases (hydroxylases) introduce only one oxygen atom of the O_2 molecule into organic substances. The other atom appears as water.

PROBLEM

A newborn male infant failed to thrive and develop normally immediately after birth. His most remarkable laboratory results were arterial pH 7.30, blood bicarbonate 16 meq/L, lactate 5 mM (normal less than 2.5), and an anion gap of 27 meq/L. By the age of 16 weeks, his lactate increased to 31 mM, blood pH dropped to less than 7.25, and plasma alanine level became highly elevated. Despite efforts to control his acidosis, the infant expired from cardiac arrest. Upon autopsy, tissue enzyme levels suspected of causing lactic acidosis were all normal; however, his tissues had abnormal accumulations of glycogen and fat. Electron paramagnetic resonance studies of his mitochondrial preparations showed absence of the Fe–S center signals normally observed in such preparations.

In a second case, a 15-year-old girl presented with a long-standing muscle weakness, exercise intolerance, hypoglycemia, lactic acidosis, and a high anion gap. For 2 subsequent years, she was treated by various methods in an effort to control her acidosis without success. At the age of 17, a muscle biopsy was collected, and her mitochondria were shown not to be able to oxidize reduced CoQ. She was then treated with vitamin K_3 and vitamin C with remarkable success.

Answer the following questions:

a. What was wrong with the two patients? How did one case differ from the other as to the causation of the disease?
b. Explain why blood lactate levels are high and glucose low in these diseases. Mention some other causes of lactic acidosis.
c. Why are blood alanine levels high in such cases?
d. Why did glycogen and fat accumulate in the infant's tissues?
e. What is the anion gap, and how can it be useful?
f. What was the action of vitamin K_3 and vitamin C? Would this treatment have helped the infant in the first case?

BIBLIOGRAPHY

Black SD, Coon MJ. P-450 cytochromes: structure and function. Adv Enzymol 60:35–75, 1987.

Capaldi RA. Mitochondrial myopathies and respiratory chain proteins. Trends Biochem Sci April:144–148, 1988.

Harold FM. The Vital Force: A Study of Bioenergetics. New York: Freeman, 1986.

Hatefi Y. The mitochondrial electron transport and oxidative phosphorylation system. Annu Rev Biochem 54:1015–1069, 1985.

Porter TD, Coon MJ. Cytochrome P-450: multiplicity of isoforms, substrates and catalytic and regulatory mechanisms. J Biol Chem 266:13469–13472, 1991.

Slater EC. The Q cycle: an ubiquitous mechanism or electron transfer. Trends Biochem Sci July:239–242, 1983.

18

Digestion and Metabolism of Carbohydrates

After completing this chapter, the student should

1. Know the names and modes of action of carbohydrate diges-
    tive enzymes found in the saliva and the small intestine, includ-
    ing the amylases and disaccharidases; review how glucose
    and other hexoses are absorbed.
2. Know the structures and names of all glycolytic and Krebs
    cycle intermediates, as well as enzymes catalyzing each reac-
    tion; follow the fate of each carbon atom of glucose through
    glycolysis and the Krebs cycle; explain hormone and energy
    charge effects on glycolysis and Krebs cycle and their mecha-
    nisms of action on the molecular level; understand organ differ-
    ences with respect to glycolysis regulation.
3. Understand the physiologic importance and mode of synthesis
    of glycerol-3-phosphate, 2,3-diphosphoglycerate, and acetyl-
    CoA; understand the mechanism of action and regulation of
    pyruvate dehydrogenase with all the cofactors involved.
4. Know the structures and names of gluconeogenic intermedi-
    ates, mechanisms for controlling gluconeogenesis, and organ
    differences with respect to gluconeogenesis.
5. Understand the physiologic importance of the hexose mono-
    phosphate shunt and understand reactions catalyzed by glu-
    cose-6-phosphate and 6-phosphogluconate dehydrogenases,
    transaldolase, and transketolase; discuss the importance of
    the hexose monophosphate shunt in red cell physiology.
6. Understand the chemistry and enzymes involved in glyco-
    gen biosynthesis and degradation and discuss the regulation
    of glycogen metabolism by hormones and other effectors;
    know the etiology of the common glycogen storage dis-
    eases; von Gierke's, Pompe's, McArdle's, Cori's, Ander-
    sen's, and Hers'.
7. Understand the mechanisms for N-acetylglucosamine biosyn-
    thesis and degradation of fructose and galactose, and inborn
    errors of metabolism associated with these pathways; Appreci-
    ate the physiologic role of the glucuronate pathway and the
    inborn errors of metabolism associated with its malfunction;

Understand how glycoproteins are synthesized and the role of dolichol in this process.

18.1 DIGESTION AND ABSORPTION OF CARBOHYDRATES

18.1.1 Digestion Enzymes

The most abundant carbohydrate ingested by humans is of the starch type— amylose and amylopectin (about 200 g/day). Smaller quantities of carbohydrate enter the digestive tract in the form of lactose (about 7 g) and sucrose (about 20 g; see Chapter 9 for structures). All dietary carbohydrates must be digested to monosaccharides to be absorbed.

Digestion of starches begins in the mouth, where salivary secretions contain the enzyme *amylase*. This enzyme is specific for α-1,4 nonterminal glycoside linkages. No digestion of carbohydrates takes place in the stomach. In the small intestine, however, digestion resumes via pancreatic amylase, which is manufactured in the pancreas and reaches the duodenum via the pancreatic duct. Both the salivary and pancreatic amylases have identical specificities and are often termed isoenzymes. They are expressions of separate genes, although there is about a 94% amino acid homology between them. Both enzymes are calcium metalloenzymes and have low molecular weights, 55,000–60,000. See Chapter 9 for additional information on amylases.

Amylases work most rapidly with large amylose sugar chains, releasing maltose, maltotriose, and, rarely, glucose molecules from them. Their action stops when the enzyme approaches the α-1,6 branch points (as in amylopectin and glycogen). Such branched products of amylase action are *limit dextrins*, which can be further digested by the action of an α-1,6-glucosidase termed isomaltase, dextrinase, or debranching enzyme. This enzyme catalyzes the hydrolysis of the α-1,6 branch points, allowing amylase then to complete the job. Isomaltase is a jejunal brush-border enzyme, as are various disaccharidases, maltase, sucrase, lactase (β-galactosidase), and trehalase. All but the last have been described in Chapter 9. Trehalose, α-D-glucopyranosyl-α-1,1-D-glucopyranoside, is a nonreducing disaccharide present in some mushrooms and is hydrolyzed to glucose via trehalase.

Absorption of glucose and galactose occurs via an active process described in Chapter 9. A similar process takes place when glucose is reabsorbed from the glomerular filtrate in the kidney tubules. It is interesting that, whereas glucose entry into the cell from gut lumen requires energy (in the form of Na^+/K^+ pump operation), its exit into the bloodstream on the transluminal (serosal) side of the intestinal cells is a facilitated process (see Chapter 9). The glucose transport particles in this system are inactivated by phloretin (phlorizin, less its glucose residue) and by cytochalasin B, a microfilament disrupting agent.

18.1.2   Organ Glucose Metabolism

Glucose and other monosaccharides absorbed by the small intestinal cells are transported into the liver via portal circulation. Liver cells are freely permeable to glucose arriving in this fashion. In the liver, glucose may enter the glycogenesis or the glycolysis pathways (see Chapter 17), or it may be exported into the circulation. Glucose leaves liver cells via a simple concentration gradient, because the liver cell glucose concentration is higher than that of the bloodstream, especially in the post-absorptive state, when glucagon levels are high and those of insulin are low. In the various organs, glucose is metabolized either aerobically (e.g., the heart or brain) or anaerobically. The latter results in lactate production, where the main lactate producers are the red blood cells, intestinal cells and white muscle cells. Lactate is extracted from the bloodstream largely by the liver and red muscle cells, which either convert it to glucose via gluconeogenesis (liver) or channel it into the Krebs cycle (red muscle). Glucose and lactate traffic is shown in Figure 18.1.

18.2   PATHWAYS OF GLUCOSE METABOLISM

18.2.1   Glycolysis

The glycolytic process takes place in the cytosol. It is summarized in Figure 18.2. The first reaction is catalyzed by hexokinase and/or glucokinase. The latter is a liver isoenzyme of hexokinase. Both utilize ATP to phosphorylate glucose in position 6 to yield glucose-6-phosphate. This reaction is irreversible, but glucose can be regenerated from glucose-6-phosphate by the hydrolytic enzyme glucose-6-phosphatase, an endoplasmic reticulum enzyme. This enzyme is present in the liver but is absent from muscle. The formation of glucose-6-phosphate serves to maintain glucose concentration outside the cells higher than those inside the cells, thus maintaining glucose flow into the cells. The two kinases, hexokinase and glucokinase, have K_m values of 0.1 and 10 mM, respectively, with regard to glucose. Glucokinase thus operates at those cellular glucose concentrations, where hexokinase runs at V_{max}. It is an enzyme whose biosynthesis in the liver is induced by insulin in response to high cellular glucose concentrations.

It is possible to ask a rhetorical question: why is glucose-6-phosphate formed by the action of hexokinase and glucokinase not immediately hydrolyzed back to glucose and phosphate by the action of glucose-6-phosphatase? This type of behavior is a *futile cycle*. The reason this particular futile cycle does not occur is twofold: first, intracellular glucose-6-phosphate concentrations are normally around 0.2 mM, whereas the K_m for this intermediate is 3 mM; second and more importantly, this enzyme is inhibited by the action of insulin and stimulated by the action of glucocorticoids and glucagon. Thus, in the fed state, when liver glycolysis is active and glucagon levels low, glucose-6-phosphatase activity is relatively low. The enzyme becomes active under conditions of gluconeogenesis, when blood insulin levels decrease and glucagon levels increase.

The next reaction in the glycolysis pathway is catalyzed by phosphoglucoisomerase and involves the isomerization of glucose-6-phosphate into fructose-6-

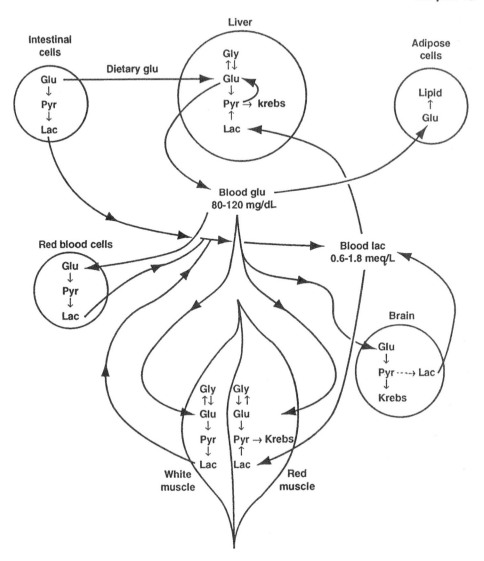

Figure 18.1 Glucose and lactate traffic in the human organism. Abbreviations: glu, glucose; gly, glycogen; lac, lactate; pyr, pyruvate; Krebs, Krebs cycle. Pyr is converted to lac, and vice versa, through lactate dehydrogenase (LDH). Although the action of LDH is reversible, the conversions shown indicate only the more prevalent direction. Pyr can be converted to glu via the gluconeogenesis pathway in the liver. Dotted arrow indicates a minor pathway.

phosphate. This step is reversible. The third step in the glycolysis pathway involves the phosphorylation of fructose-6-phosphate by ATP in position 1 to yield fructose-1,6-diphosphate. The enzyme catalyzing this reaction is phospho-fructokinase I (PFK I), which is the most important glycolytic enzyme from the regulatory point of view. It is an allosteric enzyme, which is inhibited in a feedback fashion (see Chapter 5) by ATP and citrate and is stimulated by ADP

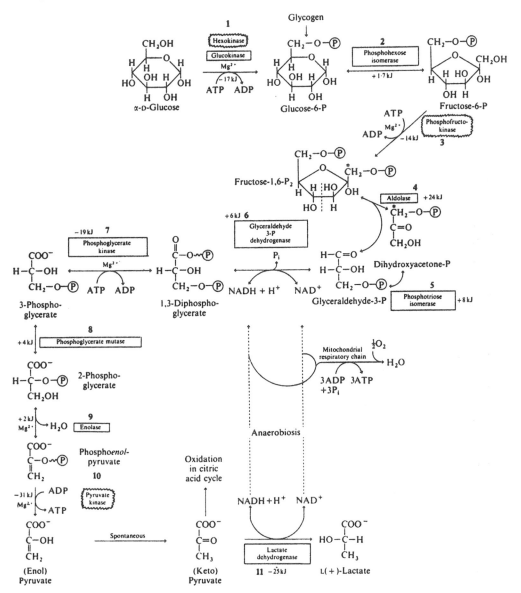

Figure 18.2 The glycolysis pathway. The $\Delta G_0'$ values for each reaction are given in kilojoules. Enzymes subject to various regulatory factors are indicated by jagged boxes. (Reproduced by permission from Wills ED. Biochemical Basis of Medicine Bristol: Wright, 1985, p. 584.)

and AMP. This enzyme thus responds positively to a low-energy status of the cell and negatively so to a high-energy status. The inhibition by ATP can be relieved by fructose-6-phosphate. This enzyme is also inhibited by high [H$^+$], which is important in muscle physiology. In a vigorously exercising muscle, as glucose is metabolized rapidly to lactate and protons, the organisms cannot remove the lactate and excess protons rapidly enough, and both accumulate. As the pH drops, it has the potential for damaging the cell machinery. Thus, to limit the further production of protons, the organism stops glycolysis by inhibiting PFK I. Chest pains experienced by angina pectoris patients are also caused by the inability of the bloodstream to carry away excess protons produced by the heart muscle and the subsequent drop in cellular pH. This is a result of blockage of coronary blood vessels, and relief is obtained by taking coronary blood vessel dilators, such as nitroglycerin or its derviatives.

By far the most important regulatory effect in liver glycolysis is achieved through cyclic AMP, whose cellular levels increase in response to high blood glucagon or epinephrine levels. PFK I absolutely requires an allosteric activator (positive effector), fructose-2,6-biphosphate. It increases the affinity of PFK I for fructose-6-phosphate but has no effect on its V_{max}. It is synthesized in small (catalytic) amounts from fructose-6-phosphate and ATP by the action of phosphofructokinase II (PFK II). Fructose-2,6-biphosphatase converts fructose-2,6-biphosphatase to fructose-6-phosphate and P_i. These latter two enzyme activities control cellular levels of fructose-2,6-biphosphate and, therefore, the activity of PFK I. Cyclic AMP activates a protein kinase (see Chapter 16), which then proceeds to catalyze the phosphorylation of both PFK II and fructose-2,6-biphosphatase. The latter becomes activated, whereas PFK II becomes inactivated by phosphorylation. The result is that new fructose-2,6-biphosphate is not synthesized and that present is converted to fructose-6-phosphate. Without fructose-2,6-biphosphate, PFK I does not work. Muscle PFK I responds weakly to fructose-2,6-biphosphate. In the muscle, the action of epinephrine results in the phosphorylation and activation of PFK II, thus increasing cellular fructose-2,6-biphosphate concentration. In the muscle, therefore, epinephrine has a slight stimulatory effect on glycolysis. Figure 18.3 summarizes the regulation of fructose-2,6-biphosphate levels in the liver cell.

PFK II and fructose-2,6-biphosphatase activities are carried by a single protein molecule, which is a homodimer with 470 amino acid residues in each subunit. The phosphatase activity resides in the C-terminal domain of each subunit, whereas the kinase activity is located in the N-terminal section.

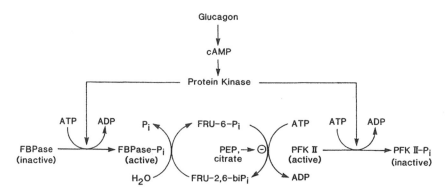

Figure 18.3 Regulation of cellular fructose-2,6-biphosphate levels by cAMP. Abbreviations: PEP, phosphoenolpyruvate; PFK, phosphofructokinase; FRU, fructose; FBPase, fructose-2,6-biphosphatase. (Reproduced by permission from Hers HG, Hue L, Van Schaftingen E. Fructose-2,6-biphosphate. Trends Biochem Sci September:330, 1982.)

The PFK I reaction is practically irreversible. As with glucose-6-phosphate, however, a fructose-1,6-diphosphatase exists in the liver that converts fructose-1,6-diphosphate to fructose-6-phosphate. The concerted actions of PFK I and fructose-1,6-diphosphatase are again capable of operating a futile cycle, the result of which would be the hydrolysis of ATP to ADP and P_i. This does not normally occur because of the hormone control systems involved: when blood insulin levels are high and glucagon levels low, liver PFK I is active but fructose-1,6-diphosphatase is inactive. This is so because fructose-2,6-biphosphate, whose cellular levels are high in this case, is a potent competitive inhibitor of the phosphatase. AMP is also a potent phosphatase inhibitor. On the other hand, when blood glucagon levels are high and cellular levels of fructose-2,6-biphosphate are diminished, fructose-1,6-diphosphatase becomes active just as the rate of glycolysis diminishes.

Fructose-1,6-diphosphate is cleaved into two trioses, dihydroxyacetone phosphate and glyceraldehyde-3-phosphate, by the action of aldolase, as indicated in Figure 18.2. The two trioses are interconvertible through the action of triose phosphate isomerase, and it is the glyceraldehyde-3-phosphate that is in the mainstream of the glycolytic pathway. It is oxidized, with the incorporation of an inorganic phosphate molecule, to 1,3-diphosphoglyceric acid, a high-energy phosphate compound. The enzyme involved is glyceraldehyde-3-phosphate dehydrogenase, which also uses NAD^+ as a substrate. This reaction is inhibited by arsenate, which substitutes for the P_i to give a very unstable arsenate analog of 1,3-diphosphoglyceric acid.

In the next reaction of the glycolytic pathway, 1,3-diphosphoglyceric acid transfers its high-energy phosphate residue to ADP to yield 3-phosphoglyceric acid and ATP under the influence of phosphoglycerate kinase. The biosynthesis of a high-energy nucleotide without the benefit of oxidative phosphorylation (Chapter 17) is substrate-level phosphorylation. Note that for each glucose molecule entering the glycolytic pathway, two ATP molecules are generated at the phosphoglycerate kinase level. 3-Phosphoglycerate next undergoes an isomerization reaction to 2-phosphoglycerate by the action of phosphoglycerate mutase, which then loses the elements of H_2O to give another high-energy phosphate compound, phosphoenolpyruvate (PEP). The enzyme catalyzing this reaction is enolase, which is apparently an Fe^{2+}-containing enzyme inhibited by F^-. PEP then transfers its high-energy phosphate group of ADP to give ATP and pyruvate, which is another example of substrate-level phosphorylation.

The enzyme that catalyzes the conversion of PEP to pyruvate is pyruvate kinase. Liver pyruvate kinase is stimulated allosterically by fructose-1,6-diphosphate, AMP, ADP, and glyceraldehyde-3-phosphate. It is inhibited by alanine, ATP, NADH, and, more importantly, by cAMP- and Ca^{2+}-calmodulin-controlled phosphorylation. High blood glucagon levels thus inhibit the activities of both PFK II and pyruvate kinase in the liver through phosphorylation. Transcription of pyruvate kinase is also decreased by glucagon and increased by insulin. Muscle pyruvate kinase is not subject to cAMP or Ca^{2+} regulation. The pyruvate kinase reaction is practically irreversible.

Note that Figure 18.2 provides information on $\Delta G_0'$ of each glycolytic step. The rate-limiting reactions, labeled "practically irreversible" here (hexokinase, glucokinase, PFK I, and pyruvate kinase), have negative $\Delta G_0'$ values, as does the phosphoglycerate kinase reaction. The others have positive $\Delta G_0'$ values, with the aldolase reaction especially favorable for the condensation of triose phosphates to fructose-1,6-diphosphate. The reason glycolysis moves forward toward pyruvate is because, under optimal physiologic conditions, reaction products are constantly removed by the subsequent reactions of the pathway. This is especially true of PEP, which is converted to pyruvate as soon as it is formed through the pyruvate kinase reaction. The overall $\Delta G_0'$ for glycolysis to pyruvate is about -8 kcal/mol of glucose, and the overall reaction to pyruvate may be represented by Equation (18.1):

$$\text{Glucose} + 2P_i + 2NAD^+ + 2ADP \rightarrow$$
$$2\text{pyruvate} + 2ATP + 2NADH + 2H_2O + 2H^+ \tag{18.1}$$

The fate of pyruvate is determined by various physiologic conditions. Under anaerobic glycolysis conditions, pyruvate is reduced reversibly to L-lactate through the action of lactate dehydrogenase (LDH), which also utilizes NADH as a substrate. In this final reaction, the anaerobic glycolysis pathway regenerates the NAD^+ that was utilized in the glyceraldehyde-3-phosphate dehydrogenase step. In tissues and microorganisms that utilize glucose via the anaerobic glycolysis pathway, lactate is either excreted into the medium (microorganisms), or exported into the bloodstream to be extracted by the liver. In yielding two lactate molecules, one glucose molecule thus generates a *net* gain of two ATP molecules through substrate-level phosphorylation: two each in the phosphoglycerate kinase and the pyruvate kinase steps, less the two ATP molecules used in the hexokinase or (glucokinase) and PFK I steps.

There are tissues, such as the red blood cells, that subsist on anaerobic glycolysis. They export lactate into the bloodstream, as does exercising muscle. It was stated earlier that lactate is extracted from the bloodstream by the liver, which can convert the lactate back to pyruvate and the latter to glucose by the process of *gluconeogenesis*. The glucose thus formed is free to migrate back to the muscle or to red blood cells. This behavior is the *Cori cycle*, illustrated in Figure 18.4 (see also Figure 18.1).

LDH [molecular weight (MW) about 150,000] occurs in most tissues and consists of isoenzymes whose electrophoretic pattern is tissue specific. There are

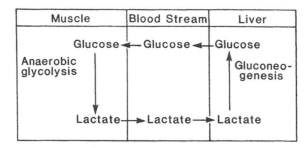

Figure 18.4 The Cori cycle. Glucose is metabolized anaerobically to lactate, as in white muscle fibers or red blood cells. Lactate is exported into the bloodstream, extracted from there by the liver, and reconverted to glucose via gluconeogenesis. Glucose is then returned to the muscle.

two types of polypeptide chains found in LDH molecules: the M and the H types, where M is muscle and H is heart. These are combined into tetramers in which the various combination possibilities include H_4, H_3M, H_2M_2, HM_3, and M_4. Most tissues contain all five LDH isoenzymes. In anaerobic tissues, however, such as skeletal muscle, there is a predominance of M subunits, whereas in the more aerobic tissues, the H subunit isoenzymes predominate. The physiologic reason is that pyruvate inhibits those isoenzymes in which the H subunits predominate; however, pyruvate does not inhibit those isoenzymes in which the M subunit predominates. In the latter case, pyruvate is readily converted into lactate, whereas the effect in the heart muscle is the opposite: lactate is largely converted to pyruvate. The use of LDH determinations is clinical diagnosis was mentioned in Chapter 5.

Many microorganisms recover the NAD^+ that is necessary for a continuous operation of the glycolysis pathway by ethanol production from pyruvate. The reaction may be written as

$$\text{Pyruvate} \xrightarrow{\quad CO_2 \quad} \text{Acetaldehyde} \xrightarrow{\quad NADH \quad NAD^+ \quad} \text{Ethanol} \qquad (18.2)$$

The NAD^+-requiring step is catalyzed by *alcohol dehydrogenase*, a Zn enzyme that is also present in humans, in whom its function is to convert ingested ethanol to acetaldehyde, which then is oxidized to acetate by NAD^+ in the presence of a ubiqitous enzyme, aldehyde dehydrogenase. Excess alcohol consumption thus generates enormous amounts of NADH, which in turn can cause a number of problems. For instance, excess NADH causes a shift of equilibrium in the LDH reaction, causing an accumulation of lactate, which in turn results in lactic acidosis, excretion of lactate with the concomitant loss of Na^+ from the organism, and hypoglycemia. One way to treat lactic acidosis is with dichloroacetate, which stimulates pyruvate dehydrogenase and thus shifts the LDH reaction equilibrium toward pyruvate production.

18.2.2 Synthesis of Some Physiologically Important Compounds from Glycolysis Intermediates

Glycerol-3-phosphate

Dihydroxyacetone phosphate may be reduced to glycerol-3-phosphate, and the latter can yield glycerol by a phosphatase reaction:

$$(18.3)$$

Glycerol-3-phosphate is a triglyceride biosynthesis intermediate (see Chapter 19), as well as a means of transporting electrons into the mitochondria. Remember that glycolysis takes place in the cytosol and that two NADH molecules per molecule glucose are produced in the glyceraldehyde-3-phosphate dehydroge-nase reaction. If conditions favor the aerobic oxidation of glucose, the NADH is not subject to reoxidation by LDH and must be oxidized in some other fashion. It cannot cross the inner mitochondrial membrane, but glycerol-3-phosphate can. The NADH is thus reoxidized to NAD$^+$, as shown in Equation (18.3). The glycerol-3-phosphate is transported into the mitochondria, where it is reoxidized to dihydroxyacetone phosphate by FAD in the presence of a mitochondrial membrane-bound glycerol-3-phosphate dehydrogenase. The dihydroxyacetone phosphate diffuses back into the cytosol, completing the cycle. This scheme is the *phosphoglycerate shuttle*, and it is illustrated in Figure 18.5. Note that the two electrons carried by cytosolic NADH are transferred to mitochondrial FAD in this scheme. The latter is firmly bound to the mitochondrial glycerol-3-phosphate dehydrogenase. As pointed out in Chapter 17, an electron transfer flavoprotein then carries the electrons from FADH$_2$ to ubiquinone (UQ). For this reason, cytosolic NADH is often said to yield only two rather than three ATP molecules/ molecule NADH when this shuttle is used. Another shuttle mechanism involves aspartate and malate (the malate-aspartate shuttle); this is discussed later in the chapter.

Another enzyme reaction, shown in Equation (18.3), is the phosphory-lation of glycerol by ATP through the action of glycerol kinase. This enzyme is absent from adipose tissue, and hence any glycerol-3-phosphate that may be necessary there for triglyceride biosynthesis must be made via the glycerol-3-phosphate dehydrogenase reaction. Glycerol kinase is abundant in the liver, however.

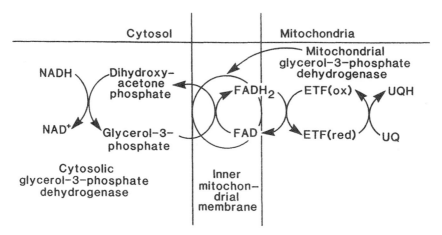

Figure 18.5 The glycerol-3-phosphate shuttle. This shuttle is used to bring electrons from cytosolic NADH into mitochondria. The mitochondrial glycerol-3-phosphate dehy-drogenase with its FAD prosthetic group is bound to the inner mitochondrial membrane. ETF is electron transfer flavoprotein, which extracts electrons from the FADH$_2$ of mitochondrial glycerol-3-phosphate dehydrogenase and with it reduces ubiquinone (UQ).

2,3-Diphosphoglycerate

2,3-Diphosphoglycerate (2,3-DPG) is an important mediator of hemoglobin physiology (see Chapter 7). It is synthesized from 1,3-diphosphoglycerate. The 2,3-DPG can be degraded to 3-phosphoglycerate by hydrolysis:

$$
\begin{array}{ccc}
\mathrm{O=C\text{-}O\text{-}Pi} & \mathrm{COOH} \quad \mathrm{H_2O} \;\; \mathrm{Pi} & \mathrm{COOH} \\
| & | \qquad \searrow\,\nearrow & | \\
\mathrm{HO\text{-}C\text{-}H} \xrightarrow{} & \mathrm{Pi\text{-}O\text{-}C\text{-}H} \xrightarrow[\text{Hydrolase}]{} & \mathrm{H\;O\text{-}C\text{-}H} \\
| \qquad \text{Diphospho-} & | & | \\
\mathrm{H_2C\text{-}O\text{-}Pi} \quad \text{glycero-} & \mathrm{H_2C\text{-}O\text{-}Pi} & \mathrm{H_2C\text{-}O\text{-}Pi} \\
\text{mutase} & &
\end{array}
\qquad (18.4)
$$

| 1,3-diphospho-glyceric acid | 2,3-diphospho-glyceric acid | 3-phospho-glyceric acid |

Cellular levels of 2,3-DPG can vary depending on the functioning of the glycolytic pathway. This is especially obvious in glycolytic enzyme deficiencies. For instance, in hexokinase deficiency, when cellular triose phosphate levels are low, a decrease in 2,3-DPG production is observed. This causes the stabilization of oxyhemoglobin in the R form, impeding O_2 release into the peripheral tissues. On the other hand, in pyruvate kinase deficiency, cellular triose phosphate levels are high and production of 2,3-DPG is excessive. Hemoglobin is stabilized in the T state, resulting in its inability to take up oxygen. Hypoxia, once again, is the result.

Conversion of Pyruvate to Acetyl Coenzyme A (Acetyl-CoA)

Pyruvate produced by the glycolytic pathway may be transported into the mitochondria (via an antiport with OH^-), where it is converted to acetyl-CoA by the action of the enzyme complex pyruvate dehydrogenase. The pertinent enzyme activities are pyruvate dehydrogenase (PD), lipoic acid acetyltransferase, and dihydrolipoic acid dehydrogenase. In addition, several cofactors are utilized: thiamine pyrophosphate (TPP), lipoic acid, NAD^+, CoA, and FAD. Only CoA and NAD^+ are used in stoichiometric amounts, whereas the others are required in catalytic amounts. Arsenite and Hg^{2+} are inhibitors of this system. The overall reaction sequence may be represented by Figure 18.5. The NADH generated may enter the oxidative phosphorylation pathway to generate three ATP molecules per NADH molecule reduced. The reaction is practically irreversible; its $\Delta G_0' = -9.4$ kcal/mol.

Pyruvate dehydrogenase is subject to regulation by phosphorylation as indicated in Figure 18.6, although the phosphorylation does not depend on cAMP effects. Pyruvate dehydrogenase kinase is activated by increased cellular levels of NADH and acetyl-CoA, products of the pyruvate dehydrogenase complex. On the other hand, pyruvate, NAD^+, and free CoA inhibit the kinase, that is, activate pyruvate dehydrogenase. The active pyruvate dehydrogenase complex per se is also inhibited by acetyl-CoA and NADH. Insulin and catecholamines are significant pyruvate dehydrogenase complex activators. A protein phosphatase reverses the effects of pyruvate dehydrogenase kinase. Insulin, especially in the adipose tissue, acts by stimulating the phosphatase. Both

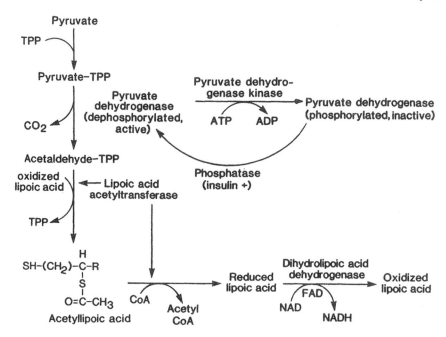

Figure 18.6 The pyruvate dehydrogenase pathway and its regulation. TPP is thiamine pyrophosphate.

pyruvate dehydrogenase kinase and the phosphatase are components of the pyruvate dehydrogenase complex, which has a molecular weight of 7–8 million and contains up to 100 polypeptide subunits.

18.2.3 The Krebs Cycle

Acetyl-CoA is oxidized to CO_2 by the *Krebs cycle*, also called the tricarboxylic acid cycle or citric acid cycle. The origin of the acetyl-CoA may be pyruvate, fatty acids, amino acids, or the ketone bodies. The Krebs cycle may be considered the terminal oxidative pathway for all foodstuffs. It operates in the mitochondria, its enzymes being located in their matrices. Succinate dehydrogenase is located on the inner mitochondrial membrane and is part of the oxidative phosphorylation enzyme system as well (Chapter 17). The chemical reactions involved are summarized in Figure 18.7. The overall reaction from pyruvate can be represented by Equation (18.5):

$$\text{Pyruvate} + 4NAD^+ + FAD + GDP + P_i + 2H_2O \rightarrow 3CO_2 +$$
$$4NADH + FADH_2 + GTP + 4H^+ \tag{18.5}$$

The overall $\Delta G_0'$ from pyruvate through the Krebs cycle calculates to about −22 kcal/mole. It is irreversible.

Four of the Krebs cycle reactions are considered irreversible: citrate synthase, isocitrate dehydrogenase, α-ketoglutarate dehydrogenase, and succinyl-CoA synthase. In two of these, CO_2 is evolved. In one reaction, succinyl-CoA synthase, a substrate-level phosphorylation takes place, in which a high-energy compound, GTP, is generated. Note that in three of the reactions NADH is

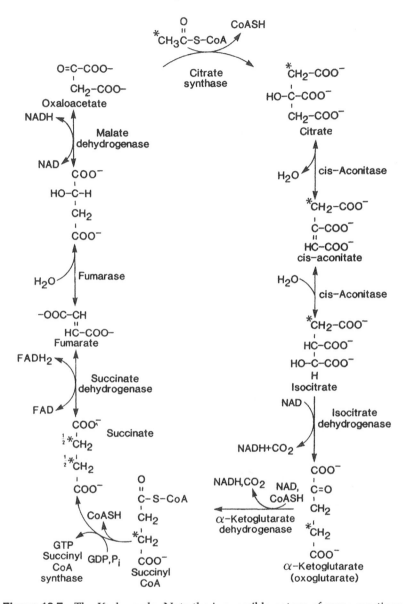

Figure 18.7 The Krebs cycle. Note the irreversible nature of some reactions.

produced, whereas in one FADH$_2$ is generated. α-Ketoglutarate dehydrogenase is very similar to pyruvate dehydrogenase: it requires the same cofactors (thiamine pyrophosphate, lipoic acid, FAD, NAD$^+$, and CoA–SH) and it catalyzes the same type of reaction-decarboxylation of an α-keto acid. However, it is apparently not subject to regulation by phosphorylation. The most important regulatory enzyme of the Krebs cycle is isocitrate dehydrogenase. It is subject to inhibition by NADH and ATP (sometimes referred to as a *high-energy charge*) and stimulation by ADP and NAD$^+$. When the cellular energy charge is high, cellular citrate levels become high and citrate exerts an inhibitory effect on PFK I (citrate

Table 18.1   ATP Yield per Molecule of Glucose Degraded

Pathway	Enzyme reaction	Cofactor	ATP yield
Glycolysis	Hexokinase	ATP	−1
	PFK I	ATP	−1
	Glyceraldehyde-3-phosphate dehydrogenase, glycerol-3-phosphate shunt	NAD	4
	Phosphoglycerate kinase	ADP	2
	Pyruvate kinase	ADP	2
Pyruvate dehydrogenase		NAD	6
Krebs cycle	Isocitrate dehydrogenase	NAD	6
	α-Ketoglutarate dehydrogenase	NAD	6
	Succinyl-CoA synthase	GDP	2
	Succinate dehydrogenase	FAD	4
	Malate dehydrogenase	NAD	6
Total			36[a]

[a]Using the malate–aspartate shuttle, total ATP yield is 38.

moves across the inner mitochondrial membrane with ease). There are no cAMP regulatory steps in the Krebs cycle.

There are two Krebs cycle inhibitors that are worth mentioning. Malonate inhibits succinate dehydrogenase because of its very similar structure. Fluoroacetate inhibits *cis*-aconitase, which is an Fe-S enzyme. The fluoroacetate replaces acetate as a substrate in the citrate synthase reaction; when this combines with *cis*-aconitase, however, no further reaction becomes possible.

We now calculate the number of ATP molecules that become available when one molecule of glucose is metabolized to CO_2 and H_2O via glycolysis, pyruvate dehydrogenase, the Krebs cycle, and the oxidative phosphorylation pathway. These data are summarized in Table 18.1. Glycolysis to pyruvate thus generates a net of 6 ATP molecules, whereas the Krebs cycle generates 12 molecules of ATP per molecule of acetyl-CoA oxidized. Compared with anaerobic glycolysis, the oxidative pathway thus yields 18 times more energy in the form of ATP. It has been observed, in fact, that a tissue or microorganism under anaerobic conditions utilizes much more glucose than a tissue or microorganism under aerobic conditions. This is the *Pasteur effect*.

18.2.4   Gluconeogenesis

Gluconeogenesis is the biosynthesis of glucose from small-molecular-weight compounds, such as pyruvate, glycerol, lactate, and amino acids. Liver is the principal gluconeogenesis organ of the organism. The purpose of gluconeogenesis is to maintain normal blood glucose levels, which in turn provide fuel for the brain and other organs. The brain uses about 120 g glucose per day, whereas other glucose-requiring tissues use 40 g/day. Gluconeogenesis is necessary, because glycogen can provide glucose for only a limited amount of time. The main hormone promoters of gluconeogenesis are glucagon, epinephrine, and the glucocorticoids. It may be said that liver glycolysis is shut down when gluconeogenesis is active, and vice versa.

Gluconeogenesis is essentially a reversal of glycolysis. To avoid the relatively irreversible glycolytic steps and to be able to affect hormonal control, however, there exist four enzymes (principally in the liver, adipose tissue, and kidney) that are unique to gluconeogenesis: pyruvate carboxylase (PC), phosphoenolpyruvate carboxykinase (PEPCK), fructose-1,6-diphosphatase, and glucose-6-phosphatase. The latter two were discussed earlier in the context of glycolysis. Of these two, fructose-1,6-diphosphatase is especially important because it is inhibited in a glycolysis climate by fructose-2,6-biphosphate and derepressed in a gluconeogenesis environment. The activity of all four enzymes is controlled at the transcription level by glucagon, epinephrine, T_3, and the glucocorticoids (positive effectors) and by insulin (negative effector). The gene of the most important regulatory enzyme, PEPCK, has a 520 base pair section at its 5' end, which is sensitive to cAMP and T_3 and under whose influence transcription of the gene increases dramatically. All four enzyme activities are increased in the fasting state and decreased in the fed state.

Glucocorticoids also increase the activity of transaminases (aminotransferases), especially in the skeletal muscle. Aminotransferases serve to transfer the amino groups from amino acids to be metabolized to α-keto acids, especially pyruvate. In the latter case, the alanine thus formed is transported from the muscle into the bloodstream and extracted from there by the liver. In the liver, alanine is converted to glucose, and glucose may then return to the muscle as it does in the Cori cycle (Figure 18.4). This is the *alanine cycle*, and more about this is discussed in Chapter 20. Branched-chain amino acids are the principal donors of nitrogen to pyruvate in the muscle and are thus important actors in the alanine cycle.

The gluconeogenesis pathway is summarized in Figure 18.8. Note that both the mitochondria and cytosol are involved. In the mitochondria, pyruvate is carboxylated by PC to oxaloacetate, as shown in Equation (18.6):

$$\text{Pyruvate} + \text{ATP} + \text{HCO}_3^- \xrightarrow{\text{PC}} \text{oxaloacetate} + \text{ADP} + \text{P}_i \qquad (18.6)$$

PC requires biotin for activity. Biotin is bound to the enzyme via a peptide-like linkage involving ϵ-NH_2 groups of certain lysine residues. This type of biotin complex is biocytin (see Chapter 6). Another compound necessary for PC activity is acetyl-CoA, a positive effector. PC is activated as cellular levels of acetyl-CoA increase, as when extensive lipolysis takes place. Acetyl-CoA is produced in large amounts from fatty acids via the β-oxidation reaction (see Chapter 19). PC can also be considered an *anaplerotic reaction*, those reactions that replenish crucial intermediates for metabolic pathways. In this case, oxaloacetate, an important intermediate in the Krebs cycle, is replenished by a reaction catalyzed by PC.

Figure 18.8 indicates that oxaloacetate may proceed in three directions toward glucose biosynthesis. It may be converted to phosphoenolpyruvate by a mitochondrial PEPCK, as shown in Equation (18.7):

$$\text{Oxaloacetate} + \text{GTP} \xrightarrow{\text{PEPCK}} \text{phosphoenolpyruvate} + \text{GDP} + \text{CO}_2 \qquad (18.7)$$

The phosphoenolpyruvate may then transport out of the mitochondria and yield glucose by the reversal of glycolysis, with the exception of the PFK I and

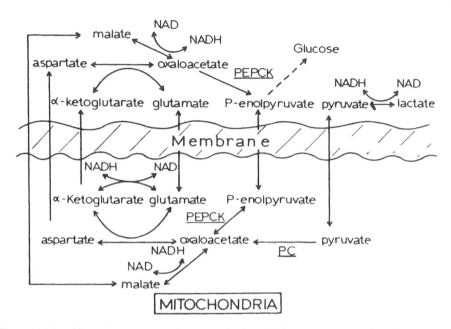

Figure 18.8 Gluconeogenesis pathway in the liver. PC is pyruvate carboxylase; PEPCK is phosphoenolpyruvate carboxykinase. (Reproduced by permission from Vidues J, Sovik O. Gluconeogenesis in infancy and childood. Acta Paediatr Scand 65:307–312, 1976.)

hexokinase reactions. To get around these glycolytic reactions, the gluconeogenesis pathway uses fructose-1,6-diphosphatase and glucose-6-phosphatase, respectively. A second pathway is for oxaloacetate to be converted to malate via the normal Krebs cycle enzyme, malate dehydrogenase. Malate then crosses the mitochondrial membrane to the cytosol via the malate/HPO_4^{2-} antiport (see Chapter 17), where it is reconverted to oxaloacetate by a cytosolic malate dehydrogenase. Alternatively, oxaloacetate may become transaminated, that is, acquire an amino group from glutamate, thus being converted to aspartate. Aspartate is then transported across the inner mitochondrial membrane to the cytosol, where it is reconverted to oxaloacetate by a cytosolic aminotransferase. This is a minor pathway compared with the other two. Cytosolic oxaloacetate is then converted to phosphoenolpyruvate by a cytosolic PEPCK according to Equation (18.7). Such roundabout ways of getting oxaloacetate to cytosol are necessary because it cannot cross the inner mitochondrial membrane.

　　Let us now focus on a specific aspect of gluconeogenesis, namely, the availability of NADH necessary to affect a reversal of the glyceraldehyde-3-phosphate dehydrogenase reaction. Figure 18.8 indicates that the source of mitochondrial pyruvate is cytosolic lactate. When the latter is oxidized to pyruvate in the cytosol, NADH is generated, which can then be used in the glyceraldehyde-3-phosphate dehydrogenase reaction. What if the source of mitochondrial pyruvate is something else, such as an amino acid? Cytosolic NADH would soon be exhausted and gluconeogenesis would stop. Under such circumstances, the mitochondrial oxaloacetate can be reduced with NADH to malate via malate dehydrogenase (Krebs cycle enzyme). There is plenty of NADH in the mitochondria in a gluconeogenesis environment because of the operation of the β-oxidation pathway for fatty acids. Malate can then cross the inner mitochondrial membrane into cytosol, where a cytosolic malate dehydrogenase can reoxidize the malate to oxaloacetate with the concomitant reduction of NAD^+ to NADH.

Malate may be transported in and out of the mitochondrial compartment using an antiporter with phosphate to get out and α-ketoglutarate, the α-keto analog of glutamic acid, to get in. Glutamic acid, in turn, can be transported into the mitochondria using an antiporter with aspartic acid (amino acid analog of oxaloacetate). These porters not only provide the means of getting aspartate and malate across mitochondrial membrane, but they also provide a means of transporting reducing equivalents into the mitochondria from cytosol, complementing the glycerol-3-phosphate shuttle. Thus cytosolic NADH can reduce oxaloacetate to malate; malate could then cross the inner mitochondrial membrane (antiport with α-ketoglutarate) into the mitochondrion, where it would be oxidized to oxaloacetate, generating NADH. Oxaloacetate could then transaminate to aspartate, which would exit the mitochondrion using the glutamate antiporter. In the cytosol, the aspartate would transaminate (lose the nitrogen) with α-ketoglutarate to regenerate oxaloacetate. This is the *malate-aspartate shuttle*, and its use generates the full three ATP molecules per pair of electrons acquired in the cytosol. It is summarized in Figure 18.9 and exhibits many similarities to events described in Figure 18.8.

Pyruvate is a crucial intermediate in gluconeogenesis. Glucose may be synthesized from pyruvate only if the latter fixes CO_2 to generate oxaloacetate. If pyruvate is converted to acetyl-CoA via the pyruvate dehydrogenase reaction, no net glucose synthesis can occur. This is true of all other substances whose degradation yields acetyl-CoA, such as leucine, lysine, and the ketone bodies. The reason is that acetyl-CoA must enter the Krebs cycle to generate oxaloacetate, the gluconeogenesis intermediate, but in doing so, two CO_2 molecules are lost, leaving no *net* carbon atom supply to generate glucose.

It may also be possible to set up a futile cycle, as in Equation (18.8):

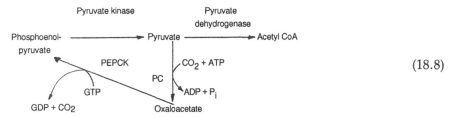

$$(18.8)$$

whose only effect would be to hydrolyze ATP and GTP to ADP and GDP, respectively. Again, this does not happen, first because of compartmentation of enzymes (PG is mitochondrial, pyruvate kinase is cytosolic) and, second because under physiologic conditions in which gluconeogenesis is active and PC and PEPCK are active, whereas pyruvate kinase is inactive. Conversely, when glycolysis is active, pyruvate kinase is active, but PC and PEPCK are inactive and pyruvate is channeled into acetyl-CoA production.

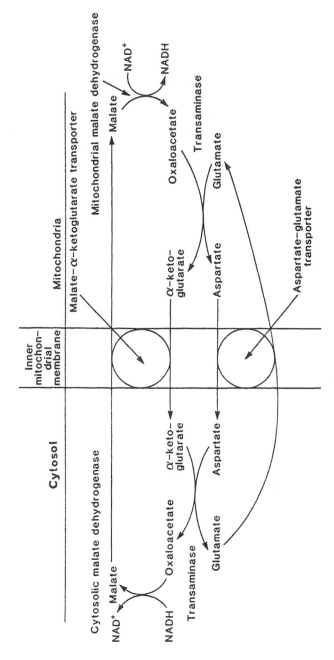

Figure 18.9 The malate-aspartate shuttle to bring cytosolic NADH electrons into mitochondria. This shuttle is more common in the human being than the glycerol-3-phosphate shuttle (Figure 18.5). It depends on two antiporters: malate/α-ketoglutarate and glutamate/aspartate. Electrons are brought into mitochondria via malate. Oxaloacetate cannot penetrate the inner mitochondrial membrane; hence it must be converted to aspartate.

The overall gluconeogenesis pathway has a $\Delta G_0'$ of about −9 kcal/mol and may be represented by Equation (18.9):

$$2\text{Pyruvate} + 4\text{ATP} + 2\text{GTP} + 2\text{NADH} + 2\text{H}^+ + 2\text{H}_2\text{O} \rightarrow \text{glucose} + 4\text{ADP} + 2\text{GDP} + 2\text{NAD}^+ + 6\text{P}_i \tag{18.9}$$

18.2.5 Hexose Monophosphate Shunt

The *hexose monophosphate shunt* (HMPS), also termed the pentose cycle, operates in the cytosol and represents an alternative way of catabolizing the glycolysis intermediate glucose-6-phosphate to fructose-6-phosphate and the trioses. HMPS is active in the skin, the red blood cells, the liver, and especially the adipose tissue. The purpose of HMPS is to generate NADPH, which is required for fat biosynthesis (see Chapter 19), and pentoses, which are necessary for nucleic acid biosynthesis. Because HMPS provides the NADPH for fatty biosynthesis and because the latter is stimulated by insulin, insulin also stimulates the activity of HMPS, albeit indirectly. The overall reaction of HMPS may be represented by Equation (18.10):

$$3\text{-Glucose-6-phosphate} + 6\text{NADP}^+ \rightarrow 2\text{fructose-6-phosphate} + \text{glyceraldehyde-3-phosphate} + 3\text{CO}_2 + 6\text{NADPH} + 6\text{H}^+ \tag{18.10}$$

The HMPS is summarized in Figure 18.10. All carbohydrate structures are written in the open form to make the mechanism more comprehensible. The pathway may be divided into two phases: the oxidative, which includes the first three reactions, and the nonoxidative. The purpose of the oxidative branch is to generate NADPH, that of the nonoxidative to generate ribose-5-phosphate. The rate-controlling enzyme of HMPS is glucose-6-phosphate dehydrogenase, which catalyzes the oxidation of glucose-6-phosphate to the corresponding aldonic acid, 6-phosphogluconic acid. A molecule of NADP^+ is reduced in the process. This enzyme is controlled by cellular $\text{NADPH}/\text{NADP}^+$ ratios (normal is about 80), where an increase in the ratio inhibits the enzyme. Another molecule of NADPH is formed in the 6-phosphogluconate dehydrogenase reaction, in which a molecule of CO_2 is also released. Enzymes that are unique to HMPS are transketolases and the transaldolase. The latter transfers a three-carbon section from sedoheptulose-7-phosphate to the aldose, glyceraldehyde-3-phosphate, to give erythrose-4-phosphate and fructose-6-phosphate. The transketolases, thiamine pyrophosphate-requiring enzymes, transfer two-carbon sections from a ketose to an aldose: from xylulose-5-phosphate to ribose-5-phosphate, on the one hand, and from xylulose-5-phosphate to erythrose-4-phosphate, on the other. In Wernicke-Korsakoff syndrome, a psychiatric disorder occurring in some individuals with alcoholism who are mildly thiamine deficient, the transketolase has a lower affinity for TPP: 16 versus 195 μM in normal subjects. The V_{max} values for both types of enzymes are virtually the same. This disease is an example of a genetic disorder that is exacerbated by excessive consumption of alcohol, an environmental factor.

The NADPH generated by HMPS in the red cell is important in the maintenance of normal reduced glutathione (GSH) levels, which in turn are required for the maintenance of red cell membrane integrity and the −SH groups of

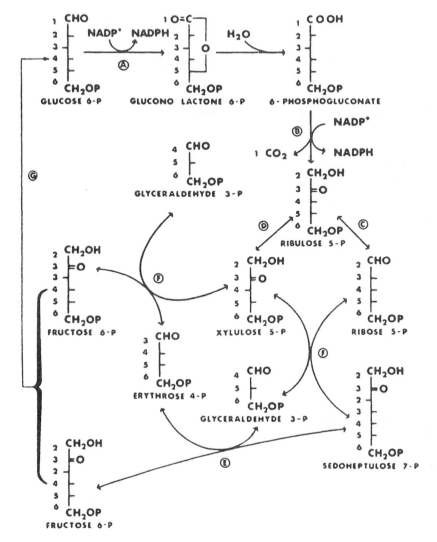

Figure 18.10 The hexose monophosphate shunt pathway. A, glucose-6-phosphate dehydrogenase; B, 6-phosphogluconate dehydrogenase; C, pentose-5-phosphate isomerase; D, pentose phosphate epimerase; E, transaldolase; F, transketolase; G, phosphohexoseisomerase. (Reproduced by permission from Williams JF. A critical examination of the evidence for the reactions of the pentose pathway in animal tissues. Trends Biochem Sci December:316, 1980.)

hemoglobin. Reduced glutathione mops up the extremely toxic H_2O_2. The pertinent reactions are shown in Equations (18.11) and (18.12):

$$GSSG + NADPH + H^+ \xrightarrow[\text{glutathione reductase}]{\text{FAD}} 2G\text{–}SH + NADP^+ \qquad (18.11)$$

$$2G\text{–}SH + H_2O_2 \xrightarrow[\text{glutathione peroxidase}]{} G\text{–}S\text{–}S\text{–}G + 2H_2O \qquad (18.12)$$

Glutathione peroxidase is a selenium enzyme and the reason that selenium is required in the diet. H_2O_2 most often comes from the superoxide anion (O_2^-) by the action of *superoxide dismutase*, which is generated when hemoglobin is oxidized to methemoglobin:

$$\text{Hemoglobin} + O_2 \rightarrow \text{methemoglobin} + O_2^- \tag{18.13}$$

and

$$2O_2^- + 2H^+ \xrightarrow[\text{dismutase}]{\text{superoxide}} H_2O_2 + O_2 \tag{18.14}$$

It has been estimated that as many as 10^7 superoxide anions are produced by the red cells each day. Superoxide dismutases of eukaryotic cytosol are Cu-Zn enzymes, whereas the mitochondrial enzymes contain Mn.

Glucose-6-phosphate dehydrogenase deficiency is relatively common among several population groups. This leads to lower cellular GSH levels and subsequent hemolysis of the red cells. Hemolysis episodes are precipitated by various forms of stress, such as infection, or ingestion of certain types of drugs, such as the antimalarial primaquine.

It is necessary to go through the oxidative part of HMPS to generate NADPH, but ribose-5-phosphate can be generated by a reversal of the HMPS starting with fructose-6-phosphate. The two fructose-6-phosphate and one glyceraldehyde-3-phosphate molecules can theoretically give rise to three ribose-5-phosphate molecules (Figure 18.10). The latter is a precursor of phosphoribosyl pyrophosphate, which is used in purine biosynthesis and nucleotide salvage pathways (Chapter 10).

18.2.6 Glycogen Metabolism

Glycogen is a polysaccharide and a storage form of glucose. It is very similar to amylopectin (Chapter 9), although it is more heavily branched. Each nonreducing end has 7–12 glucose residues (α-1,4 linked), and there are 3–4 glucose residues between branching points. Some 8–10% of all glycogen glucose residues are at the nonreducing ends of the molecule.

The liver contains some 150 g glycogen, some 10% liver weight. The purpose of liver glycogen is to maintain blood glucose levels, but the 150 g just mentioned is sufficient for up to 12–24 h of fasting. Muscle glycogen may account for as much as 1–2% of its total weight and may amount maximally to about 400 g. The purpose of muscle glycogen is to provide energy for muscle contraction. Glycogen is stored principally in the white muscle fibers, which are largely anaerobic metabolically because they contain few if any mitochondria. The white muscle fibers are concerned with short-term spurts of work.

Biosynthesis of Glycogen

Because glycogen is such an important regulator of homeostasis, it is synthesized and degraded very rapidly. Glycogen biosynthesis may be initiated *de novo* through the transfer of glucose residues from UDP-glucose to a glycogen initiator protein, followed by a growth of the amylose chain, or by the addition of glucose residues from UDP-glucose to the nonreducing ends of an incomplete glycogen molecule, *glycogen primer*. The stepwise growth of the amylose chain is catalyzed by glycogen synthase, which catalyzes the formation of α-1,4 glycosidic linkages. When the amylose chain is about 11 residues long, a 7-residue oligosaccharide section is transferred to an existing section of the growing glycogen molecule, forming an α-1,6 linkage and creating a branch point. The enzyme responsible for this step is glucosyl-4:6-transferase, or *branching enzyme*. These biosynthetic steps are illustrated in Figure 18.11.

Degradation of Glycogen

The degradation of glycogen occurs by phosphorolysis of the α-1,4 linkages and hydrolysis of the α-1,6 linkages. The enzyme that breaks the α-1,4 linkages phosphorolytically in a stepwise fashion is phosphorylase *a*. It removes glucose units from glycogen to within four residues of a branching point. Another enzyme, a 4:4-transferase, then transfers a three-residue section to a nonreducing end of the glycogen molecule, allowing an α-1,6-glucosidase to remove the α-1,6-linked glucose hydrolytically. The glucose-1-phosphate formed phosphorolytically is converted to glucose-6-phosphate and then to glucose via liver glucose-6-phosphatase, or it may enter the glycolytic pathway. The steps involved in glycogenolysis are summarized in Figure 18.12.

Regulation of Glycogen Biosynthesis and Degradation

The glycogenesis and glycogenolysis enzymes subject to hormonal control are glycogen synthase and phosphorylase, respectively. Briefly, glycogen synthase is inhibited by high cellular cAMP and Ca^{2+} levels, whereas phorphorylase is stimulated. The mechanisms for accomplishing this are quite complex.

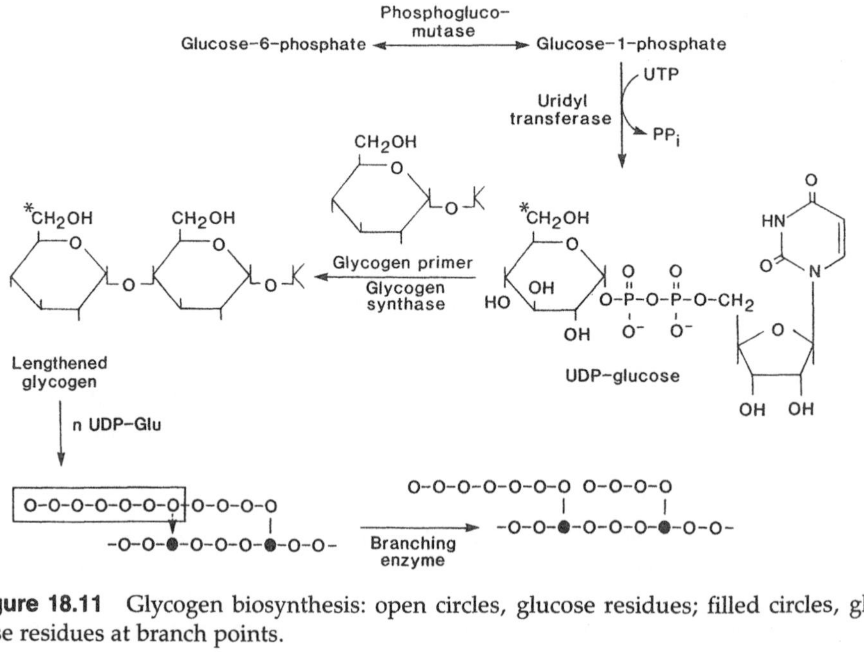

Figure 18.11 Glycogen biosynthesis: open circles, glucose residues; filled circles, glucose residues at branch points.

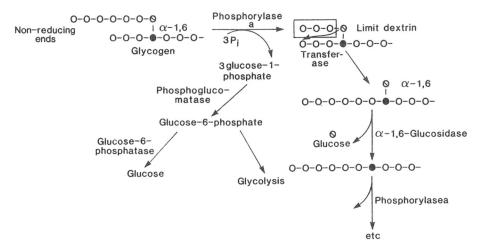

Figure 18.12 Glycogen degradation. P_i indicates inorganic phosphate. Designation of glucose molecules as in Figure 18.11.

Using the cardiac glycogen synthase as the prototype, we note that it is stimulated by insulin, which apparently does not alter either the cAMP or Ca^{2+} levels in the cell. Epinephrine acts as an agonist on both the α and β receptors of the heart muscle cells, activating both the Ca^{2+}- and cAMP-dependent protein kinases. These inactivate glycogen synthase. In addition, glycogen synthase is subject to inactivation of Ca^{2+} and cAMP-independent kinases (pyruvate dehydrogenase kinase) and by diacylglycerol-dependent kinase (kinase C). Phosphorylation occurs at up to eight different sites on the glycogen synthase molecule. The effects of epinephrine may be mimicked by α- and β-adrenergic receptor agonists, as indicated in Figure 18.13, and inhibited by the respective antagonists. Liver glycogen synthase is also inhibited by glucagon. Active glycogen synthase is often referred to as the I form, whereas the phosphorylated inactive form is the D form. The D form may be activated by glucose-6-phosphate.

The degradation of glycogen is also regulated via phosphorylation. The cAMP-dependent protein kinase, mentioned earlier in connection with glycogen synthase, catalyzes the phosphorylation of the inactive *phosphorylase kinase*, an enzyme consisting of four types of subunits that can be represented as $\alpha_4\beta_4\gamma_4\delta_4$. The α and β subunits are regulatory and are phosphorylated in the activation process. The τ subunit is catalytic, whereas the δ subunit is calmodulin, a calcium binding protein (see Chapter 16). Ca^{2+} bound to the δ subunit is necessary to affect phosphorylation of the α and β subunits. The phosphorylated phosphorylase kinase then catalyzes the phosphorylation of phosphorylase b to the active phosphorylase a. It is the only enzyme capable of phosphorylating phosphorylase b. The latter is a dimer with MW 185,000, and phosphorylase a is a tetramer with a MW of 370,000. Activation of b, albeit to a smaller extent, may be accomplished by increases in cellular AMP levels. This is understandable, because in a high-AMP/low-ATP environment, generation of glucose-6-phosphate for glycolysis and energy production would be desirable.

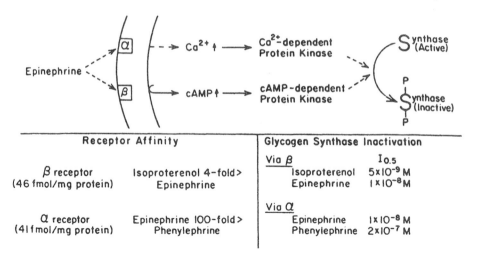

Receptor Affinity		Glycogen Synthase Inactivation	
		Via β	$I_{0.5}$
β receptor	Isoproterenol 4-fold>	Isoproterenol	5×10^{-9} M
(46 fmol/mg protein)	Epinephrine	Epinephrine	1×10^{-8} M
		Via α	
α receptor	Epinephrine 100-fold>	Epinephrine	1×10^{-8} M
(41 fmol/mg protein)	Phenylephrine	Phenylephrine	2×10^{-7} M

Figure 18.13 Regulation of glycogen synthase by epinephrine and the action of various adrenergic agonists and antagonists on the cardiac cells. (Reproduced by permission from Ramachandran C, Angelos KL, Sivaramakrishnan S, Walsh DA. Regulation of cardiac glycogen synthase. Fed Proc 42:9–13, 1983.)

The effects of protein kinases and phosphorylase kinase are opposed by a phosphoprotein phosphatase, which catalyzes the removal of phosphate residues from glycogen synthase, thus activating it, and from phosphorylase kinase and phosphorylase *a*, thus inactivating them. Glucose is bound by phosphorylase *a* when its levels in the bloodstream and liver increase. The bound glucose promotes the action of the phosphatase on phosphorylase *a*. ATP also has an inhibitory effect of phosphorylase *a*, and this is again consistent with the fact that no energy, that is, glucose-6-phosphate, is required if cellular ATP levels are high. The phosphatase is in turn regulated by an inhibitory protein. Phosphorylated inhibitory protein inhibits the phosphatase, whereas it is inactive in its dephosphorylated form. The inhibitory protein is phosphorylated as a result of high cellular cAMP levels, thus keeping the phosphatase inactive in gluconeogenesis/glycogenolysis environment. Glycogen metabolism regulation is illustrated in Figure 18.14.

The process of degrading glycogen has been often referred to as a cascade, because the signal given by only a limited number of hormone molecules is amplified manyfold by the various steps leading to the activation of phosphorylase *b*. This is illustrated in Figure 18.15, which shows the cascade effect of the action of epinephrine on a liver or muscle cell.

Glycogen Storage Diseases

Hereditary disorders exist in which one of the glycogen metabolism enzymes is defective, resulting in glycogen accumulation in the liver or muscle. These are the *glycogen storage diseases*. Most of them are autosomal recessive. Examples are von Gierke's disease (type I), Pompe's disease (type II), Cori's disease (type III), Andersen's disease (type IV), McArdle's disease (type V), and Hers' disease (type VI). In von Gierke's disease (type Ia), liver glucose-6-phosphatase is defi-

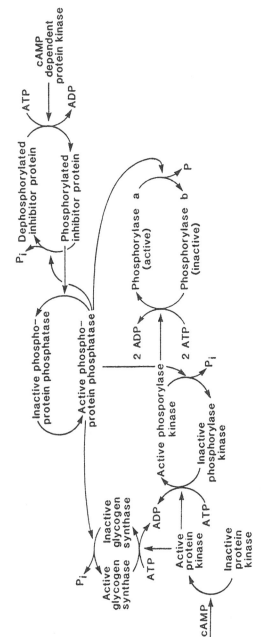

Figure 18.14 Glycogen biosynthesis and degradation regulation. cAMP activates cAMP-dependent protein kinases. They cause the phosphorylation of glycogen synthase (inactivation), phosphorylase kinase (activation), and the inhibitory protein. The last inhibits phosphoprotein phosphatase. Activated phosphorylase kinase causes the phosphorylation of phosphorylase *b*, thus activating it to phosphorylase *a*. Phosphoprotein phosphatase is inhibited by the phosphorylated inhibitor protein. Such inhibition is released when the inhibitor protein is dephosphorylated. The phosphatase then reactivates glycogen synthase and inactivates phosphorylase kinase and phosphorylase *a*.

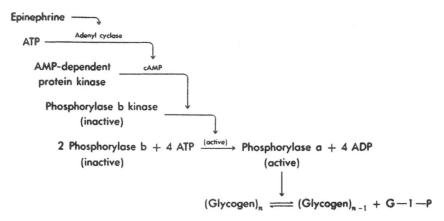

Figure 18.15   The glycogen degradation cascade.

cient, resulting in hypoglycemia. A variant of this disease (type Ib) is characterized by a defective glucose-6-phosphate translocase, which delivers glucose-6-phosphate to endoplasmic reticulum, where the phosphatase is located. In Pompe's disease, lysosomal α-1,4-glucosidase (maltase) is defective, so that glycogen accumulates in the lysosomes. Lysosomal α-1,4-glucosidase is apparently important in cellular turnover processes rather than carbohydrate metabolism pathways. In Cori's disease, the α-1,6-glucosidase is defective, resulting in limit dextrin-like substance accumulation. In Andersen's disease, the branching enzyme (glucose-4,6-transferase is defective). Glycogen with long reducing ends accumulates. In McArdle's and Hers' diseases, muscle and liver phosphorylases are defective. Individuals with McArdle's disease have a very low capacity for exercise.

18.3   METABOLISM OF MISCELLANEOUS BIOLOGICALLY IMPORTANT CARBOHYDRATES

18.3.1   Hexoses

Galactose, mannose, and fructose are absorbed and metabolized to glucose in the human being. The pathways involved are given in Figure 18.16. Of special importance is the conversion of galactose to glucose, because of the existence of galactosemia, a serious hereditary disorder, in which this conversion cannot take place. Galactose is first phosphorylated to galactose-1-phosphate and then converted to UDP-galactose by the action of phosphogalactose uridyltransferase:

$$\text{Galactose-1-P}_i + \text{UDP-glucose} \rightleftharpoons \text{UDP-galactose} + \text{glucose-1-P}_i \qquad (18.15)$$

It is this transferase that is missing in galactosemia. UDP-galactose is normally transformed to UDP-glucose by UDP-galactose epimerase, and UDP-glucose may then form glycogen.

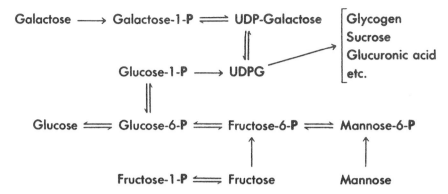

Figure 18.16   Interconversions of the various hexoses in mammals.

Fructose may be phosphorylated to either fructose-6-phosphate, the glycolysis intermediate, or to fructose-1-phosphate, which may be metabolized by a specific fructose-1-phosphate aldolase:

Fructose-1-$P_i \rightleftharpoons$ dihydroxyacetone phosphate (DHAP)
   + glyceraldehyde   (18.16)

DHAP is a glycolysis intermediate, whereas glyceraldehyde must be reduced by a mitochondrial enzyme, glyceraldehyde dehydrogenase, to glycerol, which is then subject to action by glycerol kinase in the liver. The aldolase seems to be the principal pathway of metabolizing fructose and depends on the initial phosphorylation step catalyzed by fructokinase, which produces fructose-1-phosphate. Fructokinase is defective in an inherited disorder, essential fructosuria. Fructose-1-phosphate aldolase is deficient in the hereditary disorder fructose intolerance.

18.3.2   *N*-Acetylglucosamine

N-acetylglucosamine (see Chapter 9) is a component of glycoproteins, connective tissue proteoglycans, and complex lipids. It may be synthesized in the human organism from fructose-6-phosphate, as indicated in Figure 18.17. *N*-acetylglucosamine is also a precursor of *N*-acetylmannosamine, which along with pyruvic acid participates in the biosynthesis of sialic acid.

18.3.3   The Glucuronate Pathway

Glucuronic acid may be synthesized from glucose and yield various pentoses by the glucuronate pathway. The pentoses form a common link with the HMPS pathway (Figure 18.18). Although the glucuronate pathway provides a way of circumventing glycolysis, it is apparently not in heavy use, because persons suffering from idiopathic pentosuria (failure to convert L-xylulose to xylitol) suffer no adverse effects other than excreting large amounts of L-xylose. The glucuronate pathway also provides a means of synthesizing ascorbic acid (vitamin C) in nonprimates. In primates, gulonolactone oxidase is missing, and vitamin C must be obtained from exogenous sources.

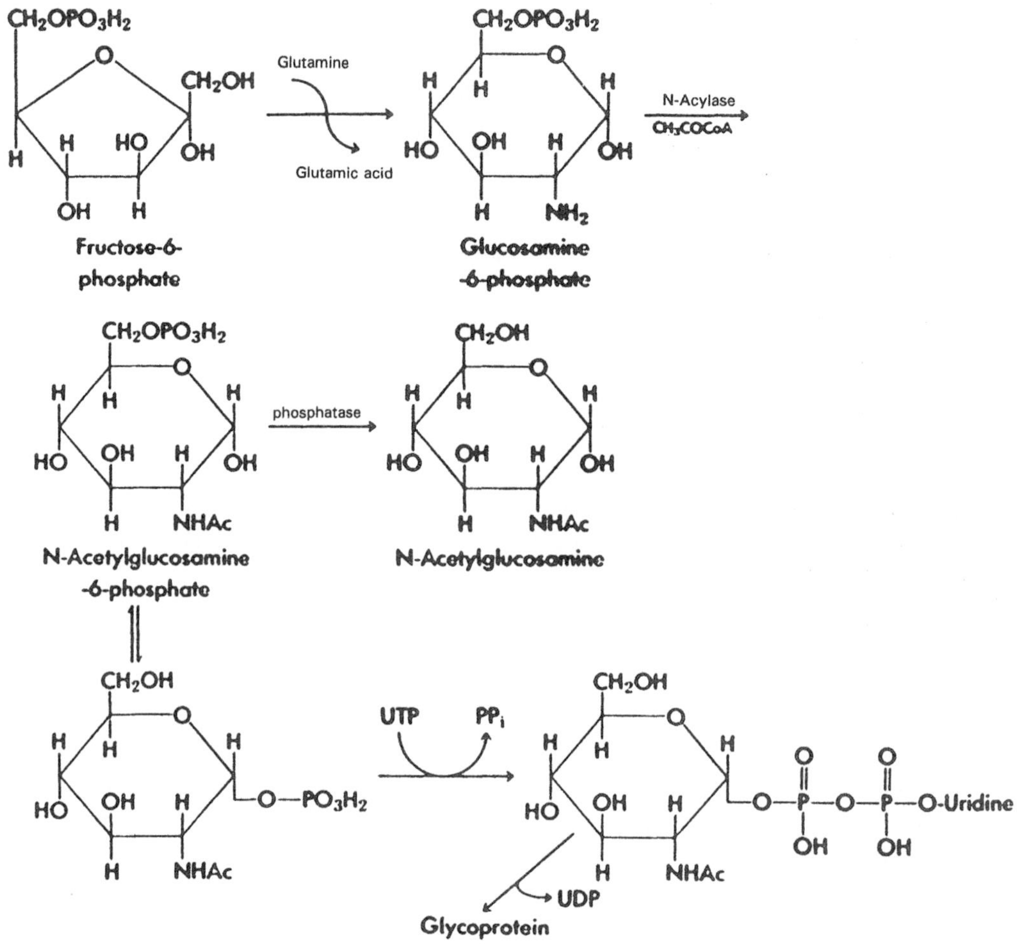

Figure 18.17 Conversion of fructose-6-phosphate to *N*-acetylglucosamine. Note that the amino group of glucosamine comes from the amide residue of glutamine.

18.3.4 Glycoprotein Biosynthesis

The basic structure of glycoproteins was described in Chapter 9. These are proteins to which are attached oligosaccharide units in either the *O*-glycoside (serine or threonine residues) or *N*-asparaginyl linkages. The former are synthesized by the stepwise addition of sugars in their diphosphonucleoside form, first to the –OH group of serine or threonine and then to the nonreducing end of the growing oligosaccharide chain. A number of glycosyltransferases, specific for each sugar, catalyze these reactions. GlcNAc and GalNAc, galactose, and glucose are used as their UDP derivatives. Mannose and L-fucose are used as GDP derivatives, whereas sialic acid is used as a CDP derivative.

The asparaginyl glycoproteins are synthesized through the use of dolichol phosphate, a member of the isoprenoid family, which is attached through its hydrophobic residue to endoplasmic reticulum. Other isoprenoid compounds or their derivatives are natural rubber, the steroids, including cholesterol, and vita-

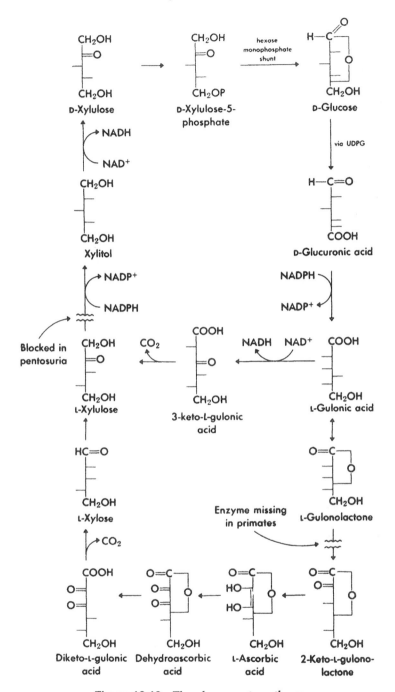

Figure 18.18 The glucuronate pathway.

min A. Dolichol, an alcohol, has 16–21 isoprene units (80–100 carbon atoms), whose –OH residue is esterified by phosphate (see Figure 18.19). It serves as an anchor for the growing oligosaccharide chain, which is also represented in Figure 18.19. Note that in the initial step, a molecule of GlcNAc is transferred to dolichol phosphate from UDP-GlcNAC. This reaction is blocked by the antibiotic tunicamycin. Next, another GlcNAc is transferred to the bound GlcNAc molecule, followed by a number of mannose residues from GDP-mannose and glucose from UDP-glucose. The addition of mannose and glucose requires the participation of monosaccharide derivatives of other dolichol phosphate molecules, as shown in Figure 18.19. Following the addition of mannose and glucose, the entire oligosaccharide chain is transferred to a protein molecule. Glucose and certain mannose residues are then trimmed off by the action of α-glucosidases and α-mannosidases, and the oligosaccharide chain is completed by the stepwise addition of monosaccharides via their UDP, GDP, or CDP derivatives. The initial presence of glucose is apparently necessary to affect a transfer of the oligosaccharide chain unto the polypeptide chain. Note that the dolichol-oligosaccharide complex flip-flops from the outer surface of the ER membrane structure into its lumen following the addition of the first five mannose residues. The addition of the last four mannose and all the glucose residues, as well as the

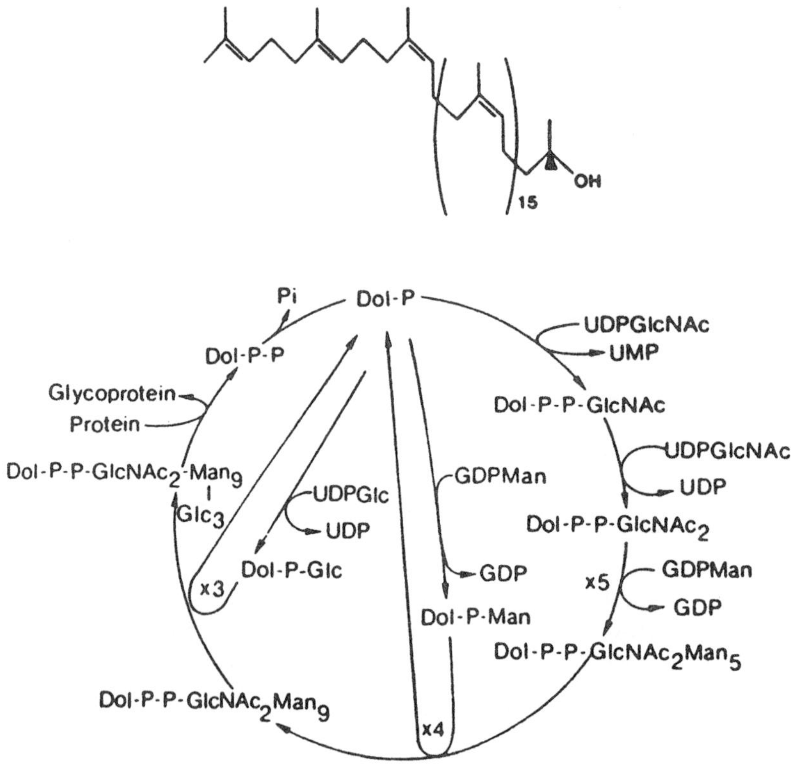

Figure 18.19 Dolichol structure (upper) and its function in glycoprotein biosynthesis (lower). Dolichol is shown in its dephosphorylated state. (Reproduced by permission from Keller RK. Dolichol metabolism in the rat. Trends Biochem Sci November:443, 1987.)

transfer of the carbohydrate to a polypeptide chain, takes place on the luminal side of the system.

18.4   SYNOPSIS OF HORMONE EFFECTS ON CARBOHYDRATE METABOLISM

Glucose metabolism is closely regulated by blood hormone levels, most significantly by insulin and glucagon/epinephrine. In the fed state, when the insulin/glucagon ratio is high, glucose enters the cells and is converted to glucose-6-phosphate via hexokinase and/or glucokinase. This can be channeled into glycogen biosynthesis or glycolysis. Glycogen biosyntheses is stimulated because glycogen synthase is activated by insulin. Glycolysis in the liver is stimulated because a high insulin/glucagon ratio derepresses PFK I (increases the concentration of fructose-2,6-biphosphate) and pyruvate kinase. At the same time, the activities of glucose-6-phosphatase and fructose-1,6-phosphatase are very low because of a low blood glucocorticoid level in the first case and the presence of high levels of fructose-2,6-biphosphate in the second.

Pyruvate dehydrogenase, especially in the adipose tissue, is stimulated by a high insulin/glucagon ratio. This leads to the production of acetyl-CoA, which may enter the Krebs cycle in the fed state. The more likely possibility is the biosynthesis of fatty acids from acetyl-CoA. The latter requires NADPH, and for this reason, the hexose monophosphate shunt is also activated.

When the insulin/glucagon ratio is low and/or the epinephrine level is high, liver glycolysis is shut down, largely because PFK II is inactivated by cAMP-dependent phosphorylation and the phosphatase specific for fructose-2,6-biphosphate is activated. PFK I ceases to function. Phosphorylation also inactivates pyruvate kinase, and pyruvate dehydrogenase is also inactivated. cAMP and Ca^{2+}-dependent protein kinases inactivate glycogen synthase and activate phosphorylase kinase. The latter activates phosphorylase, causing glycogen degradation. In the liver, this leads to glucose formation and export. In the muscle, which is sensitive to epinephrine but not glucagon, glycolysis is activated.

In the liver but not muscle, the action of glucagon and/or epinephrine induces gluconeogenesis from such starting compounds as lactate, glycerol, and alanine. Under the influence of the glucagon and glucocorticoids, PC, PEPCK, glucose-6-phosphatase, and fructose-1,6-diphosphatase activities show an increase. Substrates from gluconeogenesis are provided by the Cori and alanine cycles. Physiologic and pathologic conditions arising from high or low insulin/glucagon ratios are discussed more fully in Chapter 21.

QUESTIONS

For Questions 18.1–18.8, use the following answers:
- a.   1, 2, and 3 are correct.
- b.   1 and 3 are correct.
- c.   2 and 4 are correct.
- d.   Only 4 is correct.
- e.   All are correct.

18.1. Glucose-6-phosphate dehydrogenase
    1. Converts glucose-6-phosphate to glucose
    2. Has a role in the maintenance of red blood cell glutathione levels
    3. Rate-controlling enzyme in the gluconeogenesis pathway
    4. Deficiency results in decreased ability of the organism to detoxify peroxides
18.2. The degradation of glycogen in human cells requires the action of
    1. Phosphorylated phosphorylase
    2. Phosphorylated phosphoprotein phosphatase inhibitor protein
    3. Phosphorylated phosphorylase kinase
    4. 1,6-Glucosidase, a hydrolytic enzyme
18.3. Biosynthesis of glycogen involves
    1. Activation by Ca^{2+}-dependent kinases
    2. Low cellular cyclic AMP levels
    3. Phosphorylation of glycogen synthase
    4. Transfer of an oligosaccharide from the α-1,4 linkage to an α-1,6 linkage
18.4. In an organism with a high level of gluconeogenesis
    1. Glycogen synthesis is increased.
    2. Glycolysis is increased in the liver.
    3. Pyruvate dehydrogenase activity is increased.
    4. Glycogen degradation is increased.
18.5. Cellular levels of fructose-2,6-biphosphate are higher than normal when
    1. Blood insulin levels are high.
    2. Blood glucagon levels are high.
    3. Phosphofructokinase II is dephosphorylated.
    4. Phosphofructokinase I is inactive.
18.6. Dolichol phosphate
    1. Is a mitochondrial component
    2. Has numerous isoprenoid sections
    3. Is a carbohydrate molecule
    4. Acquires an N-acetylglucosamine from UDP-GlcNAc
18.7. The following enzymes are phosphorylated as a result of high cellular cAMP levels:
    1. Phosphorylase kinase
    2. Pyruvate kinase
    3. Glycogen synthase
    4. Pyruvate dehydrogenase
18.8. Dihydroxyacetone phosphate
    1. Participates in the transfer of electrons from cytosol to mitochondria
    2. Product of fructose-1-phosphate aldolase reaction
    3. Substrate of triose isomerase
    4. Substrate of aldolase

For Questions 18.9–18.12, choose answers from the following, which represent the numbers of ATPs generated. Use the aspartate–malate shuttle wherever necessary.
    a. 2
    b. 3
    c. 18
    d. 36
    e. 38

18.9.   Oxidation of one glucose molecule to CO_2 and H_2O.
18.10. Degradation of one glucose molecule via anaerobic glycolysis
18.11. Degradation of one lactate molecule to CO_2 and H_2O

18.12. Degradation of one glucose unit (α-1,4 linked) in glycogen to lactic acid

18.13. If glucose-1-^{14}C was metabolized by the hexose monophosphate shunt, the ^{14}C would be found in
   a. CO_2
   b. Fructose-6-phosphate carbon 1 (anomeric)
   c. Fructose-6-phosphate carbon 6 (phosphorylated)
   d. Glyceraldehyde-3-phosphate, carbon 1 (anomeric)
   e. A pentose

18.14. If glucose-1-^{14}C is converted to acetyl-CoA via glycolysis and the pyruvate dehydrogenase reaction and enters the Krebs cycle, then where is radioactivity found in succinate before the first run of the Krebs cycle is completed?

   1. COOH   a. Carbons 1 and 4
         |
   2. CH_2 b. Carbons 2 and 3
         |
   3. CH_2 c. Carbons 1 and 2
         |
   4. COOH   d. Carbons 3 and 4
     Succinate e. All carbons

18.15. Fructose-6-phosphate in the human being serves as a precursor of
   a. Galactose
   b. Glucuronic acid
   c. UDP-N-acetylglucosamine
   d. Sucrose
   e. Ascorbic acid

18.16. If glucose is labeled with ^{14}C in position 1 and metabolized by glycolysis, where is the label in pyruvate?

   1 COOH   a. Carbon 1
          |
   2 C = 0   b. Carbon 2
          |
   3 CH_3 c. Carbon 3
     Pyruvate d. Carbons 1 and 3
              e. Carbons 1 and 2

18.17. Lactate dehydrogenase of the heart muscle cells
   a. Consists largely of the M subunits
   b. Has a high affinity for lactate
   c. Has the same subunit structure as the skeletal muscle LDH
   d. Has a high affinity for pyruvate
   e. None of the above

18.18. Which description is not shared by pyruvate and α-ketoglutarate dehydrogenases?
   a. NADH a product
   b. Involvement of thiamine pyrophosphate in catalytic amounts
   c. Decarboxylation
   d. Use of lipoic acid in catalytic amounts
   e. Control via phosphorylation

18.19. Which enzyme is not present in the muscle?
   a. Glycogen synthase
   b. Hexokinase
   c. Phosphorylase b
   d. Glucose-6-phosphatase
   e. Isocitrate dehydrogenase

18.20. Which is a *positive* effector in gluconeogenesis?
    a. ADP
    b. Acetyl-CoA
    c. Insulin
    d. Fructose-2,6-phosphate
    e. 2,3-Diphosphoglycerate

18.21. Which compound is generated when NAD^+ is reduced in the glycolytic pathway?

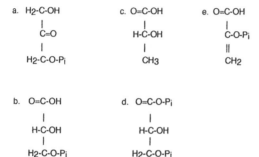

Answers

18.1. (c) Glucose-6-phosphate dehydrogenase is the first enzyme in the HMPS pathway; it generates NADPH. The latter is required in the glutathione reductase reaction, which produces GSH. GSH destroys H_2O_2, which is detrimental to the red blood cell membrane.

18.2. (e) Glycogen degradation requires phosphorylated (active) phosphorylase kinase to maintain the production of phosphorylated (active) phosphorylase a; the α-1,6-glucosidase is required to remove branch molecules from partially degraded glycogen, and phosphorylated (active) inhibitor protein is required to inactivate phosphoprotein phosphatase.

18.3. (c) Biosynthesis of glycogen requires dephosphorylated (active) glycogen synthase and an enzyme that creates branch points in the growing glycogen molecule, glucosyl-4,6-transferase.

18.4. (d) All processes except 4 go in the opposite direction. Glycogen is degraded because of the high cellular cAMP level.

18.5. (b) Cellular levels of fructose-2,6-biphosphate, the positive effector of PFK I, are increased when blood insulin levels are high because PFK II is active as a result of a suppression of fructose-2,6-biphosphate phosphatase (dephosphorylation) and activation (dephosphorylation) of PFK II.

18.6. (c) Dolichol phosphate is an amphipathic lipid of the endoplasmic reticulum consisting of isoprenoid units and initiating the biosynthesis of the oligosaccharide portion of glycoproteins.

18.7. (a) cAMP catalyzes the phosphorylation of all enzymes but pyruvate dehydrogenase. The latter is phosphorylated by a cAMP-independent kinase.

18.8. (e) DHAP, a glycolysis intermediate, is reduced by NADH to glycerol-3-phosphate. Triose isomerase converts it to glyceraldehyde-3-phosphate, and it is a product of the fructose-1-phosphate aldolase reaction.

18.9. (e) See Table 18.1 for an explanation. Use of the malate-aspartate shuttle permits the generation of three ATP molecules from each cytosolic NAD^+ molecule.

18.10. (a) See Figure 18.2 for an explanation.

18.11. (c) Lactate and pyruvate dehydrogenases generate 3 ATPs each, whereas acetyl-CoA generates 12 ATPs for a total of 18.

18.12. (b) A glucose unit in glycogen bypasses the hexokinase reaction, giving an additional ATP molecule in anaerobic glycolysis.

18.13. (a) The anomeric carbon of glucose is lost as CO_2 through the action of the 6-phosphogluconate dehydrogenase reaction.

18.14. (b) The anomeric carbon of glucose ends up in position 3 (methyl) of pyruvate and then in the methyl group of acetyl-CoA. From this point on, follow the starred carbon atom marked by an asterisk in Figure 18.7.

18.15. (c) See Figure 18.17.

18.16. (c) Follow the anomeric carbon in Figure 18.2.

18.17. (b) Heart muscle in aerobic. It is likely to be converting lactate to pyruvate, rather than the other way around. Skeletal muscle has M subunits, heart muscle H type.

18.18. (e) Both enzymes use the same cofactors and catalyze the decarboxylation of an α-keto acid. α-Ketoglutarate dehydrogenase is apparently not regulated by phosphorylation.

18.19. (d) Muscle is not capable of carrying out gluconeogenesis, in part because it lacks glucose-6-phosphatase.

18.20. (b) Acetyl-CoA is a positive effector of pyruvate carboxylase, a biotin enzyme.

18.21. (d) The correct answer is 1,3-diphosphoglyceric acid. It is produced by the oxidation of glyceraldehyde-3-phosphate in the presence of P_i.

PROBLEMS

18.1. A 58-year-old man was brought to the emergency room in a comatose state, with hypotension and severe acidosis: blood pH 6.63–7.03 and an anion gap of 35–40 meq/L. His hemoglobin was well saturated with O_2 and he showed no sign of infection. Despite supportive measures, he died within 10 h of being admitted. Follow-up investigation revealed that he had been on a drinking binge for about 1 month, and that his blood thiamine level had dropped to 5 μg/L (normal 12–26) upon admission. Address the following:

    a. Suggest reason that this patient developed a severe acidosis: the compound involved, the reason for the large anion gap, and biochemical basis for this.

    b. Suggest several possible diagnostic tools to detect this type of problem in patients presenting with these symptoms.

    c. What, if anything, did the drinking binge have to do with his condition?

    d. How would you treat this patient?

18.2. A newborn boy appeared to be healthy and was discharged from the hospital. He was breast-fed by his mother. A blood sample collected for galactosemia and phenylketonuria testing per state law indicated lowered levels of galactose-1-phosphate uridyltransferase in the child's red blood cells. Discuss the following:

    a. Does the baby have lactose intolerance? If not, what does a low galactose-1-phosphate uridyltransferase level in red blood cells indicate?

    b. Suggest clinical and/or laboratory tests to confirm a diagnosis of galactosemia.

    c. Should the baby's mother continue to breast-feed?

    d. Discuss galactose metabolism in detail, and show which metabolic lesions could lead to galactosemia.

    e. Why is untreated galactosemia dangerous?

18.3. If [^{14}C]acetate (or [^{14}C]acetyl-CoA) were injected into an animal, would radioactive carbons be found in glucose? Explain your answer in terms of acetyl-CoA metabolism.

18.4. List as many enzyme defects as you can that can result in lactic acidosis. Defend your selections on the basis of known pathways of carbohydrate metabolism.

BIBLIOGRAPHY

Behal RH, Buxton DB, Robertson JG, Olson MS. Regulation of the pyruvate dehydrogenase multienzyme complex. Annu Rev Nutr 13:497–520, 1993.

Cunningham, EB. Biochemistry Mechanisms of Metabolism. New York: McGraw-Hill, 1975.

McGany JD, Kuwajima M, Newgard CB, Foster DW, Katz J. From dietary glucose to liver glycogen. Annu Rev Nutr 7:51–53, 1987.

Parker PH, Ballew M, Greene HL. Nutritional management of glycogen storage disease. Annu Rev Nutr 13:83–109, 1993.

Pilkis SJ, Claus TH. Hepatic gluconeogenesis/glycolysis: regulation and structure/function relationships of substrate cycle enzymes. Annu Rev Nutr 11:465–515, 1991.

Van Schaftingen E. Fructose-2,6-biphosphate. Adv Enzymol 59:315–385, 1987.

19

Lipid Digestion and Metabolism

After completing this chapter, the student should

1. Understand the mechanisms involved in lipid digestion and absorption, including bile salt metabolism.
2. Know lipid transport systems throughout the organism: the different types of lipoproteins and their properties, their metabolism, their component apoproteins, and the functions of each individual lipoprotein and apoprotein.
3. Understand the utility of (apo)lipoprotein analysis in clinical medicine, and understand the various types of primary lipoproteinemias.
4. Understand hormonal regulation of lipid metabolism, and for each metabolic pathway, be able to identify the rate-controlling step and its mode of regulation.
5. Know pathways of triglyceride biosynthesis and catabolism, the β-oxidative pathway, and pathways for the degradation of propionyl-CoA, branched fatty acids, and unsaturated fatty acids; identify cofactors required; calculate ATP yields for fatty acid oxidation; know the identity of key enzymes in each pathway.
6. Know pathways and attendant cofactors and key enzymes for fatty acid biosynthesis; ketone body biosynthesis, utilization, and clinical implications; and fatty acid elongation and unsaturation mechanisms.
7. Understand pathways for the biosynthesis of phosphoglycerides and factors that control this process.
8. Understand the biosynthesis of cholesterol; compare this process with that of ketone body production; know what controls cholesterol biosynthetic reactions.

19.1 DIETARY LIPID DIGESTION

19.1.1 Emulsification of Fats

A human being normally ingests 90–150 g fat per day. About 90% of this is triglyceride. In addition, bile brings into the intestinal tract 1–2 g cholesterol and

4–5 g phosphoglyceride daily. Dietary fat is largely water insoluble, and it is therefore necessary to break it up into the smallest possible particles for digestive enzyme action. The smaller and the more numerous the particles, the greater is their total surface area and faster and more effective is their digestion. Surface area A can be represented by Equation (19.1), where R is the particle radius, n is the number of particles, and K_1 and K_2 are constants:

$$A = \frac{K_1}{R} = K_2\sqrt[3]{n} \tag{19.1}$$

The emulsifying agents (biologic detergents) that allow for lipid digestion are the phosphoglycerides (both endogenous and exogenous) and, more importantly, the *bile salts*. The latter are amphipathic derivatives of cholesterol (see later) synthesized in the liver. There is a total pool of about 3–5 g bile salts in the organism, which enter the small intestine via the bile duct. Bile, which includes bile salts, may be stored in the gallbladder and released upon the action of cholecystokinin. The bile salts and lipid digestion products form micelles that are 3–10 nm in diameter, and these micelles present lipid digestion products to the intestinal mucosal cells for absorption. This occurs largely in the duodenum and jejunum, leaving bile salts behind. Bile salts are then resorbed in the ileum and make their way back to the liver, although about 500 mg per day may appear in the feces. During a single day, a total of 40–50 g bile salts may circulate through the small intestine: *enterohepatic circulation*.

About 500 mg cholesterol is converted every day to bile salts. This may be increased if the patient is given bile salt binding resins, such as cholestyramine, which diminishes bile salt resorption, causing increased bile salt excretion in the feces. Cholestyramine and similar substances are given to individuals with high serum cholesterol levels. Most of the cholesterol that enters the small intestine via bile (see earlier) is also excreted. Fecal cholesterol amounts to about 1 g/day and is a major means of removing cholesterol from the organism.

19.1.2 Lipases in the Small Intestine

Dietary triglycerides are hydrolyzed in the small intestine by pancreatic lipase. This enzyme action is associated with a cofactor, *colipase*, also a pancreatic protein, molecular weight (MW) 12,000, which helps to anchor lipase to the fat droplets. Without colipase, lipase is rapidly denatured. Colipase is apparently secreted by the pancreas as a zymogen and is activated to its active form in the small intestine by trypsin. Pancreatic lipase appears in the circulation in large amounts during acute pancreatitis.

Pancreatic lipase is specific for ester linkages at positions 1 and 3 of triglycerides, whose fatty acids are at least 10 carbons in length. Its hydrolysis products are therefore 2 fatty acid molecules and one molecule of 2-monoglyceride per molecule triglyceride. Although the last may be slowly hydrolyzed to glycerol and a fatty acid, the fat digestion products absorbed are largely 2-monoglycerides and fatty acids. Pancreatic juice contains other lipases as well: a nonspecific lipid esterase that acts on cholesterol esters and 2-monoglycerides, among other compounds, and phospholipase A_2 (see Chapter 9), which is also activated in the intestinal tract by trypsin. There is also an esterase that acts on triglycerides with short fatty acids.

19.1.3 Absorption of Lipids and Fat Malabsorption Syndromes

Fatty acids and 2-monoglycerides are absorbed by the intestinal mucosal cells from micelles stabilized by bile salts. In the absence of such micellar structure, lipid digestion products are absorbed at only 1/1000 the normal rate. There are apparently no specific carriers involved. The intestinal mucosal cells channel the short-chain fatty acids into the portal circulation and then to the liver. Fatty acids with 12 or more carbons, as well as 2-monoglycerides and their hydrolysis products, are used once again to form triglycerides. These, along with other lipids and polypeptide chains termed *apolipoproteins*, are assembled into particles called *chylomicrons*. Chylomicrons then enter the lymphatic system, which via the thoracic duct connects with the general circulation. Chylomicrons thus enter the circulation without being processed by the liver.

Normally there is very little fat in the feces. However, fat content in stools may increase because of various fat malabsorption syndromes. Such increased fat excretion is *steatorrhea*. Decreased fat absorption may be the result of failure to emulsify food contents because of a deficiency in bile salts, as in liver disease or bile duct obstruction (stone or tumor). Pancreatic insufficiency may result in an inadequate pancreatic lipase supply. Finally, absorption itself may be faulty because of damage to intestinal mucosal cells through allergy or infection. An example of allergy-based malabsorption is celiac disease, which is usually associated with gluten intolerance. Gluten is a wheat protein. An example of intestinal infection is tropical sprue, which is often curable with tetracycline. Various vitamin deficiencies may accompany fat malabsorption syndromes.

19.1.4 Biosynthesis of Bile Salts

Bile salts are produced in the liver from cholesterol. These are primary bile salts, as distinguished from secondary bile salts generated in the intestinal tract from primary bile salts. Primary bile salts are synthesized in part in the endoplasmic reticulum and in part in mitochondria. The former is the location for hydroxylation reactions, whereas the latter is where the side chain is shortened. Figure 19.1 illustrates the biosynthesis of the two primary bile salts, taurocholic (or glycocholic) and chenodeoxyglycocholic (or chenodeoxytaurocholic) acids, from cholesterol. The rate-controlling enzyme is the 7α-hydroxylase, which is a cytochrome P_{450} enzyme that requires vitamin C and is inhibited by bile salts. The pathway can proceed in two directions after the formation of 7α-hydroxycholestenone: with an additional hydroxylation to the 12 position to yield cholic acid derivatives eventually or, without further hydroxylation, to yield chenodeoxycholate derivatives. The final step in both branches of the pathway is conjugation with either taurine or glycine. Glycine conjugates generally predominate by a margin of 3:1. The taurine derivatives are more acidic than glycine conjugates: pK values are about 1.5 versus 3.5, respectively.

In the intestinal tract, a substantial portion of the primary bile salts is deconjugated by bacterial enzymes and reduced (dehydroxylated), whereby

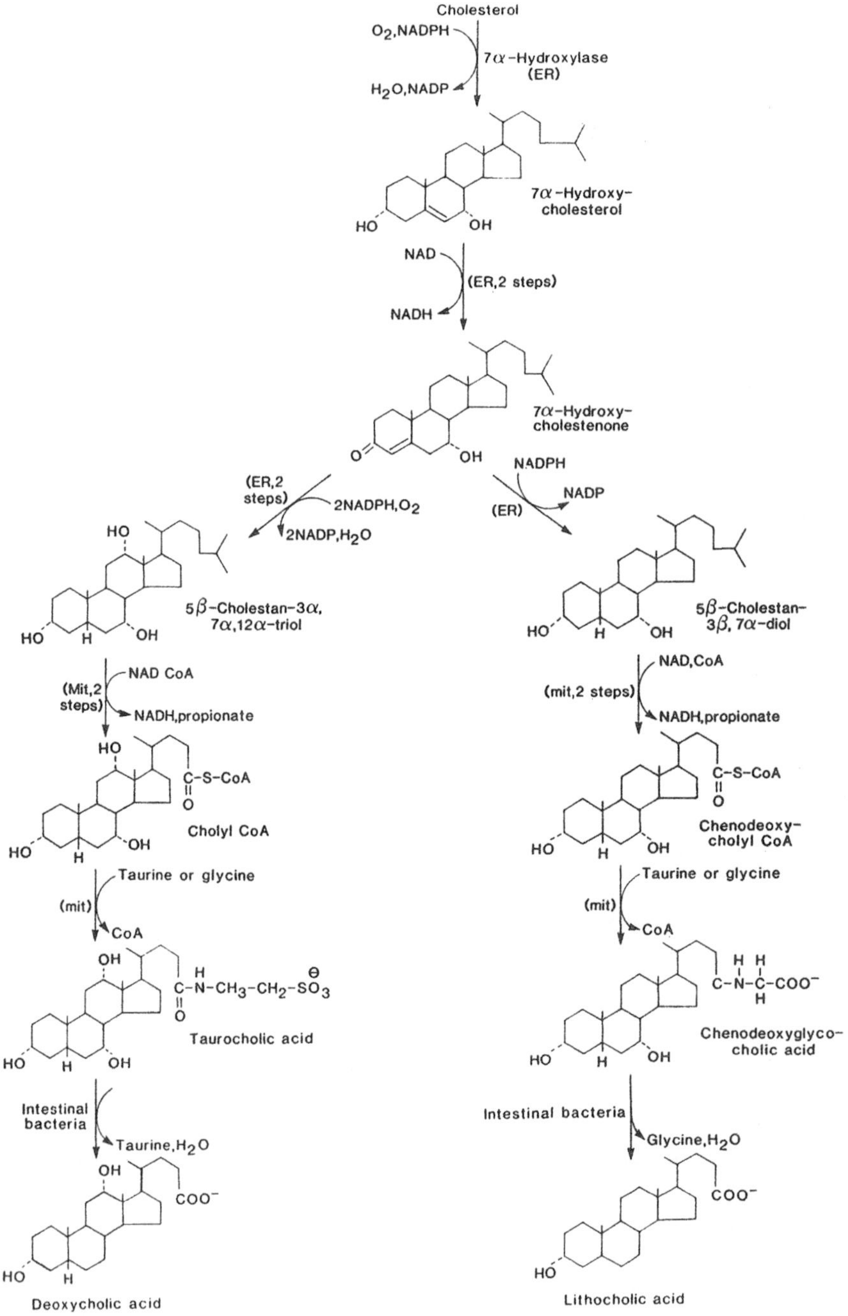

Figure 19.1 Biosynthesis of bile salts from cholesterol. Mit, mitochondria; ER, endoplasmic reticulum.

they lose their −OH group at position 7. The products are secondary bile acids: deoxycholate from conjugated cholate and lithocholate from conjugated chenodeoxycholate. Lithocholate is only sparsely soluble in water, and much of it is excreted in the feces. The conjugated primary bile salts and deconjugated secondary bile salts remaining in the gut are resorbed in the ileum and travel back to the liver via the enterohepatic system, where the secondary unconjugated bile salts may also be conjugated with glycine or taurine and then reappear in the intestinal lumen.

19.2 TRANSPORT OF LIPIDS AND LIPOPROTEIN DYNAMICS

19.2.1 Chemistry of Lipoproteins

When a nonfasting serum sample is subjected to electrophoresis and stained with a lipid-positive dye, four bands become visible. These are termed, of increasing mobility, the chylomicrons (immobile), the β, the pre-β, and the α-lipoproteins. The last has an electrophoretic mobility approximately that of the α_1-globulins, whereas pre-β is approximately in the α_2-globulin area. Likewise, when such a serum sample is subjected to ultracentrifugation, four components are noted. These are, in the direction of increasing density, the chylomicrons, very low density lipoproteins (VLDL), low-density lipoproteins (LDL), and high-density lipoproteins (HDL). The latter correspond to the electrophoretically distinguishable α-lipoproteins; the LDL corresponds to β-lipoproteins, and VLDL corresponds to pre-β-lipoproteins. Occasionally, an additional component may be seen in pathologic specimens, the intermediate-density lipoprotein (IDL), which moves electrophoretically between the β- and pre-β-lipoproteins. In normal fasting serum, chylomicrons are not observed either electrophoretically or ultracentrifugally.

The chemical-physical properties of lipoproteins are listed in Table 19.1. It is seen that the density of lipoproteins is lowest for chylomicrons, followed by VLDL, IDL, LDL, and HDL. As density increases, the amount of lipid de-

Table 19.1 Chemical-Physical Properties of Lipoproteins

Property	Chylomicron	VLDL	IDL	LDL	HDL
Density	0.94	0.97	1.003	1.034	1.1–1.2
Diameter, Å	$\sim 10^3$	250–750	~ 230	200–230	50–130
Molecular weight	10^9–10^{10}	10^6–10^7	4–5×10^6	$\sim 3 \times 10^6$	2–4×10^5
Total lipid, %	97–99	90–95	—	75–80	45–55
Cholesterol	5	11–14	22	49	38
Cholesterol, unesterified	2	5–8	8	13	10
Triglyceride	84	44–60	30	11	9
Phospholipid	7	20–23	25	27	22
Protein	2	4–11	15	23	45–55

Source: Largely from Stein E. Lipids, lipoproteins, and apolipoproteins. In Tietz NW, ed. Textbook of Clinical Chemistry. Philadelphia: Saunders, 1986, p. 849.

creases and that of protein increases. Chylomicrons and VLDL are considered triglyceride carriers, and LDL and HDL are considered cholesterol carriers. Lipoprotein components are arranged in the lipoprotein particle in such a way that the hydrophobic residues are in the particle interior and those of hydrophilic nature are on the surface in contact with the aqueous environment, as shown in Figure 19.2.

Several types of proteins are associated with lipoproteins. These are termed apolipoproteins, or simply apoproteins. Table 19.2 shows the various apolipoproteins (Apos), their chemical properties and occurrence, and their function, which is discussed later. Note that the A apoproteins are found largely in HDL, the B-100 is found largely in LDL, VLDL, and IDL, and C apoproteins are largely seen in chylomicrons. Nevertheless, there is a large degree of apoprotein overlap among the various lipoprotein classes.

19.2.2 Lipoprotein Metabolism

Lipoproteins are fat carriers in the circulation. Figure 19.3 summarizes human lipoprotein traffic. We focus first on the chylomicrons, which are produced in the intestinal cells and are exported into the general circulation via lymph. Chylomicron metabolism is often referred to as *exogenous lipoprotein metabolism*.

Chylomicrons are triglyceride rich and contain apolipoprotein B-48 and the A types. The latter are synthesized in the intestinal tract cells. Additional apoproteins are transferred to the chylomicrons from HDL in circulation: the apoE and apoC types. Their site of synthesis is the liver. The chylomicrons are subject to degradation by lipoprotein lipase in the peripheral tissue, especially adipose tissue. Lipoprotein lipase activity is increased by increased blood insulin levels. This enzyme is extracellular, attached to the capillary endothelial cells, and activated by ApoC-II, which is present in the chylomicrons. Lipoprotein lipase causes the hydrolysis of triglycerides, thus decreasing chylomicron size

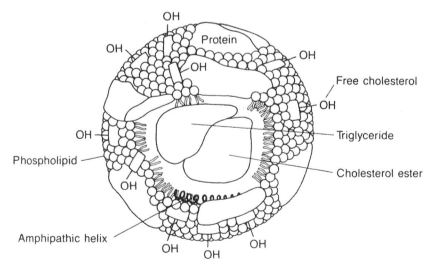

Figure 19.2 A lipoprotein particle. (Reproduced with permission from Warnick GR. Apolipoproteins. Clin Chem News September:8, 1985.)

Table 19.2 Human Apolipoproteins[a]

Apolipoprotein designation	Lipoprotein class	Molecular weight	Mean plasma concentration (mg/dL)	Function
A-I	C, HDL	28,300	120	Activates LCAT
A-II	C, HDL	17,000	35	Cofactor with hepatic lipase
B-100	LDL, VLDL, IDL	250,000	100	LDL, VDL receptor recognition
B-48	C	120,000	Trace	Required for secretion of Cs
C-I	C, VLDL, HDL	6,300	7	Cofactor with LCAT
C-II	C, VLDL, HDL	8,800	4	Activates LPL
C-III	C, VLDL, HDL	8,800	13	LPL inhibitor
D	HDL	33,000	6	Concerned with transfer of cholesterol esters
E	C, VLDL, HDL, IDL	38,000	4	C remnant, IDL and VLDL receptor recognition
Lp(a)	LDL, HDL	900,000	10	Similar to plasminogen; may have a role in the clotting mechanism
F	HDL	30,000	2	—
G	HDL	72,000	—	—
H	C	43,000	10	Cofactor with LPL

[a]Major protein component of that lipoprotein class. C, chylomicrons; LCAT, lecithin-cholesterol acyltransferase; LPL, lipoprotein lipase.
Source: Especially from Schaefer EJ and Levy RI. Pathogenesis and management of lipoprotein disorders. N Engl J Med 312:1300–11310, 1985.

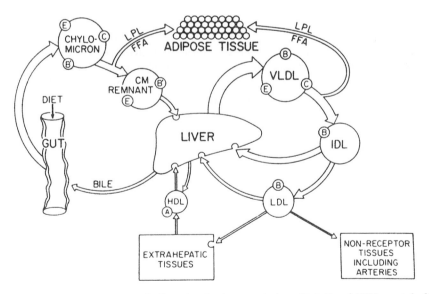

Figure 19.3 Lipoprotein metabolism in the human being. Details of HDL metabolism have been omitted. LPL, lipoprotein lipase; FFA, free fatty acids; CM, chylomicrons; A–E, apoproteins A–E; HDL, LDL, IDL, and VLDL are high-density, low-density, intermediate-density, and very low density lipoproteins. (Reproduced by permission from Staff writers. Heart-liver transplantation in a child with homozygous familial hypercholesterolemia. Nutr Rev 43:274–278, 1985.)

and providing fatty acids for tissue metabolism. Another extracellular enzyme that may act to hydrolyze triglycerides of chylomicrons is hepatic lipase, which is present in liver and kidney. In the process of losing triglyceride, chylomicrons also lose apoCs and apoAs to HDL. The particle that remains is the *chylomicron remnant*, which is removed from circulation by the liver. Liver cells have receptors that recognize ApoE, enabling them to internalize and degrade chylomicron remnants.

Another triglyceride-rich glycoprotein, the VLDL, is produced in the liver from lipid generated endogenously. For this reason, VLDL and LDL metabolisms are referred to as *endogenous lipoprotein metabolism*. VLDL is synthesized in the endoplasmic reticulum (ER) and the Golgi apparatus of hepatocytes. If a defect in VLDL formation exists, or in such conditions as poisoning by organic solvents or methionine deficiency (see Chapter 20), the liver may not form VLDL and may not be able to export lipid. Lipid then accumulates in the liver, resulting in a condition known as fatty liver. It is very damaging to normal liver function. VLDL carries ApoB-100 when it is released by the liver and picks up ApoE and ApoCs from HDL in the circulation. As with chylomicrons, VLDL is a substrate for lipoprotein and hepatic lipases. As triglyceride is removed from VLDL, IDL is produced and IDL is further degraded to LDL. As VLDL is degraded it loses its ApoCs and ApoE to HDL. IDL and LDL may receive cholesterol esters from HDL (see later), so that LDL eventually emerges as a triglyceride-poor and cholesterol-rich particle.

Both IDL and LDL can be removed from the circulation by the liver, which contains receptors for ApoE (IDL) and ApoB-100 (IDL and LDL). After IDL or LDL interacts with these receptors, they are internalized by the process of *receptor-mediated endocytosis*. Receptors for ApoB-100 are also present in peripheral tissues, so that clearance of LDL occurs one-half by the liver and one-half by other tissues. In the liver or other cells, LDL is degraded to cholesterol esters and its other component parts. Cholesterol esters are hydrolyzed by an *acid lipase* and may be used for cellular needs, such as the building of plasma membranes or bile salt synthesis, or they may be stored as such. Esterification of intracellular cholesterol by fatty acids is carried out by *acyl-CoA-cholesterol acyltransferase* (ACAT). Free cholesterol derived from LDL inhibits the biosynthesis of endogenous cholesterol. B-100 receptors are regulated by endogenous cholesterol levels. The higher the latter, the fewer ApoB-100 receptors are on the cell surface, and the less LDL uptake by cells takes place.

A few words about HDL: these lipoproteins are synthesized largely by the liver. They act as ApoE, ApoC, and ApoA traffickers, but in addition, they also serve as a factory for the synthesis of cholesterol esters. HDL may absorb free cholesterol from various peripheral tissues, including arteries. Cholesterol is then converted to a large extent to fatty acyl esters by the action of the enzyme *lecithin-cholesterol acyltransferase* [LCAT; see Equation 19.2)]. LCAT is activated by ApoA-I. Inactive LCAT is a plasma component.

$$\text{Cholesterol + lecithin} \xrightarrow{\text{LCAT}} \text{cholesterol ester + lysolecithin} \qquad (19.2)$$

Cholesterol esters may be transferred to IDL, chylomicron remnants, and to LDL via a transfer protein (ApoD) or nonspecifically. In addition, HDL carrying the cholesterol esters may be cleared by the liver, which recognizes HDL via its ApoA-I. HDL can also be metabolized by other tissues. It is an especially good substrate for the hepatic lipase.

19.2.3 Pathology Associated with Lipoprotein Metabolism

Increases in circulatory VLDL and LDL predispose affected individuals to cardiovascular disease. When there is an increase in serum LDL, increasing amounts are taken up by macrophages. LDL may be altered, possibly by free radicals, to an "oxidized" form, and it is the oxidized LDL that is especially well bound by macrophages. These cholesterol-laden macrophages then enter the blood vessel walls and contribute to the formation of plaque. It is thus desirable to lower circulating VLDL and LDL to lower the risk of cardiovascular disease.

Lipoproteinemias (increase in circulating lipoproteins) may be secondary to some other disease (e.g., diabetes and multiple myeloma), or they may be "primary." The latter are usually hereditary. Frederickson has cataloged primary lipoproteinemias into six categories, each characterized by an increase in specific lipoprotein(s). These are also reflected by increases in circulating cholesterol and triglyceride levels, as shown in Table 19.3. It is seen that, as the triglyceride carriers—chylomicrons and VLDL—are increased, circulating triglyceride is also increased. Cholesterol levels, on the other hand, reflect LDL levels.

Type I lipoproteinemia is generally caused by the inability of the organism to clear chylomicrons. The problem may be defective ApoC-II or a defective lipoprotein lipase. Very often, chylomicron clearance may be affected by injection of heparin, which apparently releases hepatic lipase from the liver into the circulation. ApoE disorders may be associated with type III lipoproteinemia, in which clearance of IDL is impeded. Increases in circulatory LDL are usually caused by a decrease in tissue receptors specific for ApoB-100. An extreme case of type IIa hyperlipoproteinemia is familial hypercholesterolemia, in which serum cholesterol levels may be as high as 1000 mg/dL and the subjects may die in adolescence from cardiovascular disease. There is total absence of ApoB-100 receptors. Mild type IIa and IIb lipoproteinemias are the most commonly occurring primary lipoproteinemias in the general population.

Increases in chylomicrons, VLDL, and LDL have been associated with increased risk of cardiovascular or other diseases, but increased circulating HDL levels are thought to provide protection against cardiovascular disease. Premeno-

Table 19.3 Primary Lipoproteinemias

Type	Lipoprotein type increased	Serum triglyceride	Serum cholesterol
I	Chylomicrons	Increased	Normal
IIa	LDL	Normal	Increased
IIb	LDL, VLDL	Increased	Increased
III	IDL	Increased	Normal
IV	VLDL	Increased	Normal
V	Chylomicrons and VLDL	Increased	Normal

pausal women, vegetarians, and physically active persons have high serum HDL levels; obesity, inactivity, and smoking have been associated with low HDL levels. Persons with familial HDL deficiency, as in *Tangier disease*, may develop premature cardiovascular disease. Tangier disease is caused by an ApoA-I defect.

There have been numerous attempts to discover diagnostic procedures that would accurately predict cardiovascular disease risks in the general population. "Phenotyping" (i.e., electrophoresis) of lipoproteins has been used, as have determinations of total cholesterol, HDL cholesterol, triglyceride, and LDL cholesterol. "Normal" although not optimal values for these parameters are 140–310, 30–70, 60–300, and 90–200 mg/dl, respectively. These values are both age and sex related. LDL cholesterol cannot be determined directly but can be calculated from Equation (19.3):

$$\text{LDL cholesterol} = \text{total cholesterol} - \text{HDL cholesterol} - \frac{\text{triglyceride}}{5} \qquad (19.3)$$

The latter term really represents VLDL cholesterol. It is now recognized that serum apoprotein determinations provide the best cardiovascular disease risk evaluation: high levels of ApoB-100, especially ApoLp(a), are associated with a high disease risk, but high levels of ApoA-I are associated with a low risk. The optimal LDL/HDL cholesterol ratio is 3 or less.

Therapy aimed at improving cardiovascular disease risk is aimed at lowering circulating lipid levels, especially that of cholesterol. Dietary intervention (low saturated triglyceride and cholesterol) is effective. Circulating cholesterol can in fact be determined from daily fat intake by the *Hegstedt formula*:

$$\text{Total cholesterol} = 2.1 \text{ saturated fat} - 1.6 \text{ polyunsaturated fat} \\ + 0.7 \text{ cholesterol} \qquad (19.4)$$

It is clear from Equation (19.4) that saturated fat, not cholesterol, is the single most important factor that raises serum cholesterol. Some cases of hyperlipoproteinemia type IV (high VLDL) respond to low-carbohydrate diets, because the excess of VLDL comes from intestinal cells, where it is produced from dietary carbohydrate. Resins, such as cholestyramine and cholestipol, bind and cause the excretion of bile salts, forcing the organism to use more cholesterol. Lovastatin decreases endogenous cholesterol biosynthesis (see later), and niacin (nicotinic acid) apparently decreases the production of VLDL and, consequently, LDL. It also results in an HDL increase. Antioxidants that inhibit the conversion of LDL to oxidized LDL have also been used with some success. These are high doses of vitamin E and the drug probucol.

19.3 TRIGLYCERIDE METABOLISM

Fatty acids released by lipoprotein lipase are taken up by the tissue where this enzyme is located, where they may be oxidized (see later) or stored in the form of triglycerides, such as adipose tissue. Triglyceride biosynthetic enzymes are located in the endoplasmic reticulum. Triglyceride biosynthesis is summarized in Figure 19.4. It is seen that dihydroxyacetone phosphate (see Chapter 18) is a key intermediate. It can combine with an acyl residue carried by acyl coenzyme A

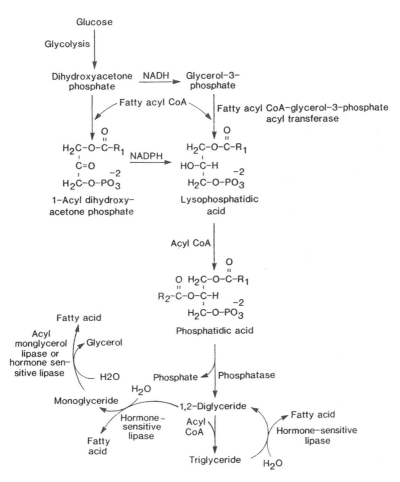

Figure 19.4 Biosynthesis and degradation of triglycerides.

(acyl-CoA), or it can give rise to glycerol-3-phosphate, which then proceeds to form a lysophosphatidic acid. Glycolysis is thus an essential process in the biosynthesis of fats. The fatty acid must be activated by CoA in the presence of fatty acyl-CoA synthetase before it reacts:

$$\text{Fatty acid + CoA} \xrightarrow[\text{ATP} \quad \text{AMP + PP}_i]{} \text{fatty acyl-CoA} \tag{19.5}$$

Activation of the fatty acid thus requires two ATP equivalents, because the high energy of inorganic pyrophosphate (PP_i) is not recoverable. It is hydrolyzed to phosphate by a ubiquitous enzyme called pyrophosphatase.

In human adipose tissue, palmitoyl-CoA is usually used in the first glycerol-3-phosphate acylation reaction. The next two acyl residues are normally unsaturated fatty acids: oleic acid and, less commonly, linoleic acid. Triglyceride biosynthesis is stimulated by insulin, most likely via its activation of lipoprotein lipase and its activity in moving glucose into the cells.

The degradation of tissue triglycerides (*lipolysis*) takes place hydrolytically and via different enzymes. This process is also shown in Figure 19.4. The main enzyme responsible for triglyceride degradation is the hormone-sensitive lipase, which is subject to activation by cAMP-sensitive protein kinases and deactivation by phosphoprotein phosphatases. High cellular cAMP levels also cause the inactivation of fatty acyl-CoA–glycerol-3-phosphate acyltransferase, thus favoring triglyceride degradation rather than biosynthesis. The removal of the first fatty acid is the slowest, and this step is thus rate controlling. The last step, hydrolysis of the monoglyceride, is also catalyzed by the hormone-insensitive monoacyl-glycerol lipase. Glycerol is a product of the latter reaction. It may be utilized in the liver, where it is phosphorylated by ATP to glycerol-3-phosphate in the presence of glycerol kinase. This enzyme is absent from adipose tissue. Glycerol-3-phosphate may be converted to dihydroxyacetone phosphate via the action of glycerol-3-phosphate dehydrogenase using NAD^+ as a cofactor. Glycerol-3-phosphate may thus participate in gluconeogenesis. Fatty acids leave adipose tissue and are distributed throughout the organism by being bound to serum albumin. Normally, 0.18–1.65 mmol fatty acids is bound to albumin per liter serum.

19.4   OXIDATION OF FATTY ACIDS

19.4.1   Activation of Fatty Acids

Fatty acids are utilized as fuels by most tissues, although the brain, red and white blood cells, the retina, and adrenal medulla are important exceptions. Catabolism of fatty acids requires extramitochondrial activation, transport into mitochondria, and then oxidation via the β-oxidative pathway. The initial step is catalyzed by fatty acyl-CoA synthetase (also called thiokinase and fatty acyl-CoA ligase), as shown in Equation (19.5). The product, fatty acyl-CoA, then exchanges the CoA for carnitine, as shown in Equation (19.6):

$$(CH_3)_3\overset{\oplus}{N}-CH_2CHCH_2-COOH + \text{acyl-CoA} \rightarrow (CH_3)_3\overset{\oplus}{N}CH_2CHCH_2COOH + CoA$$

$$\underset{\text{HO}}{|} \qquad\qquad\qquad\qquad\qquad\qquad\qquad \underset{\underset{R-C=O}{|}}{\overset{|}{O}} \qquad (19.6)$$

$$\text{Carnitine} \qquad\qquad\qquad\qquad\qquad \text{Acylcarnitine}$$

The reaction is catalyzed by palmitoyl-CoA-carnitine acyltransferase, which is inhibited by malonyl-CoA (see later), and is the limiting reaction of the fatty acid oxidation process.

Acylcarnitine then moves across the mitochondrial membrane via an antiport, which also transports carnitine in the opposite direction. In the mitochondria, carnitine is once more exchanged with CoA, which is a reversal of Equation (19.6), yielding acyl-CoA. Free carnitine is then returned to the extramitochondrial space by the antiport. The carnitine shuttle is shown in Figure 19.5. Carnitine is synthesized in the organism from lysine. The symptoms of carnitine deficiency are muscle weakness, cardiac myopathy, and hypertriglyceridemia. These are observed in certain genetic disorders, alcoholism, hemo-

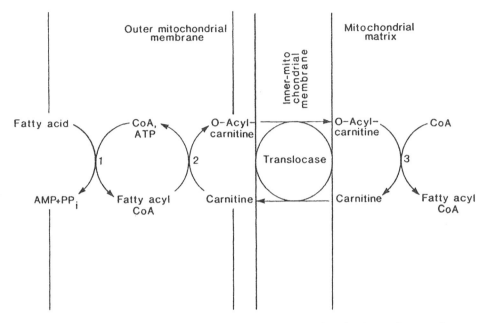

Figure 19.5 Movement of fatty acids across inner mitochondrial membrane. The enzymes involved are designated as follows: (1) fatty acyl-CoA synthetase; (2) palmitoyl-CoA–carnitine acyltransferase on the cytosol side of the inner mitochondrial membrane; and (3) the same enzyme on the mitochondrial matrix side of the membrane.

dialysis patients, and premature newborns. Fatty acids with 4–12 carbon atoms can diffuse across the inner mitochondrial membrane without being bound to carnitine, where they are converted to their CoA derivatives by butyryl-CoA synthetase.

19.4.2 The β-Oxidation Pathway

Enzymes involved in the β-oxidation pathway are located on the inner side of the inner mitochondrial membrane or in the peroxisomes. The design of this pathway involves the oxidative and stepwise removal of acetyl-CoA units from the shrinking fatty acid chain, the acetyl-CoA molecules being fed into the Krebs cycle (Chapter 18) or forming ketone bodies (see later). The overall reaction, involving palmitic acid, may be represented by Equation (19.7):

Palmitic acid + ATP + 8CoA + 7NAD$^+$ + 7FAD + 7H$_2$O →

8acetyl-CoA + AMP + PP$_i$ + 7NADH + 7FADH$_2$ + 7H$^+$ (19.7)

Figure 19.6 indicates the oxidation of palmitoyl-CoA to myristoyl-CoA with the production of an acetyl-CoA molecule. The myristoyl-CoA molecule can undergo another oxidative cycle, and so on. Note that the β-hydroxyacyl-CoA dehydrogenase is specific for the L isomer of β-hydroxyacyl-CoA. Also note that at least three acetyl-CoA dehydrogenases exist, one favoring short-chain fatty acids, another intermediate-length fatty acids, and the third long-chain fatty acids.

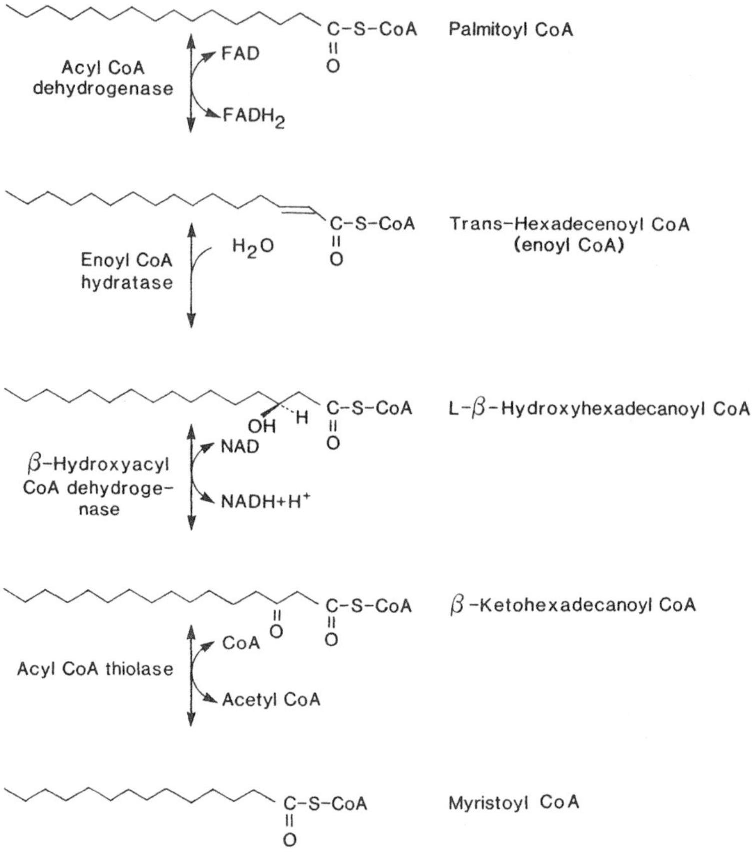

Figure 19.6 β-Oxidative degradation of palmitoyl-CoA.

The oxidation of palmitic acid to acetyl-CoA requires seven β-oxidation cycles, each producing 1 $FADH_2$ molecule (2 ATP) and 1 NADH molecule (3 ATP). This is 35 ATP for the seven cycles. Because each palmitic acid molecule requires an equivalent of 2 ATP molecules to become activated [Equation (19.5)], the net ATP yield is 33. Because each acetyl-CoA yields 12 ATP via the Krebs cycle (Chapter 18), the total ATP yield from the oxidation of one palmitic acid molecule is 12(8) + 33 = 129.

Because reduced redox cofactors, NADH and $FADH_2$, are produced in the mitochondria, there is no need for shuttle mechanisms to reoxidize them via oxidative phosphorylation. NADH is reduced directly by complex I. $FADH_2$ is reduced by the electron transfer flavoprotein, which then reduces ubiquinone. See Chapter 17 for details.

A significant amount of β oxidation takes place in the peroxisomes. These structures specialize in the oxidation of "very long chain" fatty acids (20 carbons or more). They enter the peroxisomes as CoA derivatives, and no carnitine is required for the transfer from cytosol. Peroxisomal β-oxidation enzymes differ from those of mitochondria, although they perform the same functions except for the first (unsaturation) step. Instead of using mitochondria-like FAD-dehydrogenases, peroxisomes utilize FAD-containing oxidases that use O_2 as an electron acceptor, thereby generating H_2O_2. The most important enzyme in this group is palmitoyl-CoA oxidase. Thus, each β-oxidation cycle in the peroxisomes yields, not 5, but only 3 ATPs. NADH can apparently move across peroxisomal membrane without requiring a shuttle mechanism to transfer its electrons to the cytosol. The end products of peroxisomal β oxidation are usually shorter fatty acyl-CoAs, so that β oxidation is then completed in the mitochondria. It has been said that the main purpose of peroxisomal β oxidation is to shorten very long chain fatty acids, rather than to extract the maximum number of ATP equivalents from them.

19.4.3   Oxidation of Odd-Carbon Chain Fatty Acids

The β-oxidation pathway converts even-carbon fatty acids (by far the most abundant fatty acids in the human organism) to acetyl-CoA. If a C_{17} fatty acid were catabolized, however, seven acetyl-CoA molecules and one propionyl-CoA molecule would result after seven cycles of the β-oxidation process. The latter is catabolyzed to succinyl-CoA, a Krebs cycle intermediate, as shown in Figure 19.7. In this series of reactions, bicarbonate (sometimes referred to as CO_2) is incorporated into propionate in the presence of the biotin-containing propionyl-CoA carboxylase enzyme to give D-methylmalonyl-CoA (also called S-methylmalonyl-CoA). The latter is isomerized to L-methylmalonyl-CoA (also termed R-methylmalonyl-CoA) and then converted to succinyl-CoA in the presence of a vitamin B_{12} coenzyme-containing mutase. Odd-carbon fatty acids can therefore give net biosynthesis of glucose through propionyl-CoA. Propionic acidemia results when, because of a genetic lesion, propionyl-CoA carboxylase is not present in the organism. L-Methylmalonic acid is excreted in the urine (methylmalonic aciduria) when the methylmalonyl-CoA mutase is defective as a result of a genetic lesion or in vitamin B_{12} deficiency. Methylmalonic aciduria may also result if the coenzyme of vitamin B_{12}, deoxyadenosylcobalamine, cannot be formed from the vitamin because of a genetic lesion.

19.4.4   Oxidation of Unsaturated Fatty Acids

Unsaturated fatty acids are also oxidized by the β-oxidation pathway in both the mitochondria and peroxisomes, although at least one and, in some cases, two additional enzymes are required. The oxidation of linoleyl-CoA is shown in Figure 19.8. This fatty acid has 18 carbon atoms with cis double bonds in positions 9 and 12. After three β-oxidation cycles, carbons 3 and 4 of the resulting cis,cis-3,6-dodecadienoyl-CoA (II) are joined by a cis double bond. For β oxidation to proceed, we need a trans double bond between carbons 2 and 3, as in enoyl-CoA in Figure 19.6. This problem may be taken care of by the action of a 3 cis → 2 transisomerase, as shown in Figure 19.8. Alternatively, the double bond originally in position 9 of the fatty acid may be reduced by an NADPH-dependent reductase as the 5-enoyl-CoA intermediate is generated. Following such reduction, β oxidation may proceed unimpeded.

If the unsaturated fatty acid were oleic acid, the double-bond obstacle would be encountered only once and overcome as described earlier. Linoleic

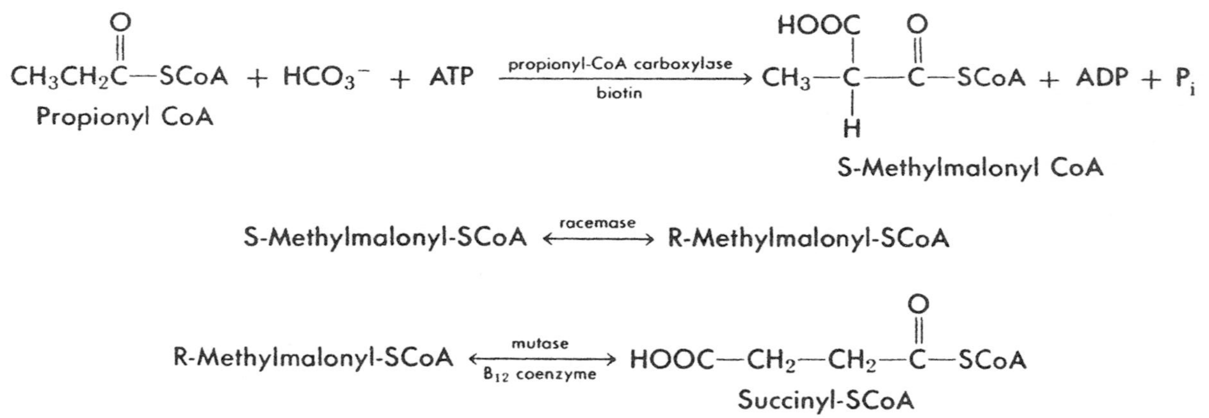

Figure 19.7 Metabolism of propionyl-CoA. S designates the L isomer, and R designates the D isomer of methylmalonyl-CoA.

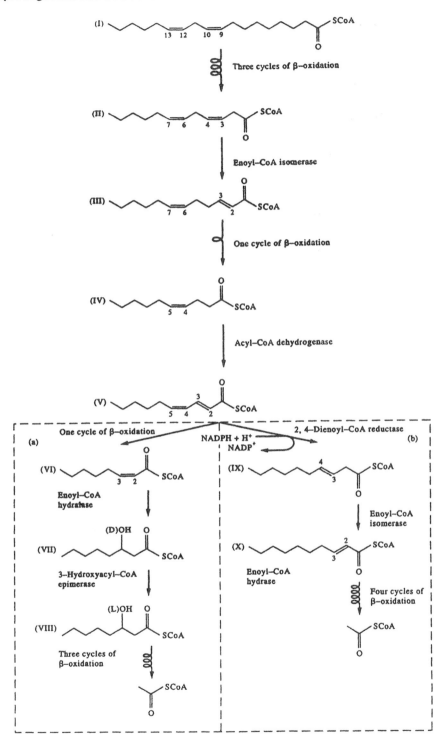

Figure 19.8 Oxidation of linoleoyl-CoA. Pathway labeled b predominates. (Reproduced by permission from d'Andrea G. β-Oxidation of polyunsaturated fatty acids. Biochem Educ 22:89–91, 1994.)

acid, on the other hand, has a second double bond, originally in position 12, and this, too, must be taken care of. This may be done in two ways, as shown in Figure 19.8. The more prevalent system uses NADPH-specific 2,4-dienoyl-reductase plus an enoyl-CoA isomerase to convert 2,4-decadienoyl-CoA (structure V, Figure 19.8) into 2-*trans*-decaenoyl-CoA (X), from which point β oxidation can proceed normally. In the second system, 2,4-decadienoyl-CoA (V) undergoes a β-oxidation cycle to give 2-*cis*-octaenoyl-CoA (VI), which is then hydrated to give the D-β-hydroxyoctanoyl-CoA (VII), an unnatural intermediate not subject to β-hydroxyacyl-CoA dehydrogenase action. An epimerase, however, can convert the D epimer to the L epimer, the natural substrate, and β oxidation can then be completed. It is clear that, regardless of which system is used to overcome the double-bond obstacles, the unsaturated fatty acids would yield fewer ATP equivalents than a saturated bond with the same number of carbons. Traditionally, two ATP equivalents have been subtracted for each double bond.

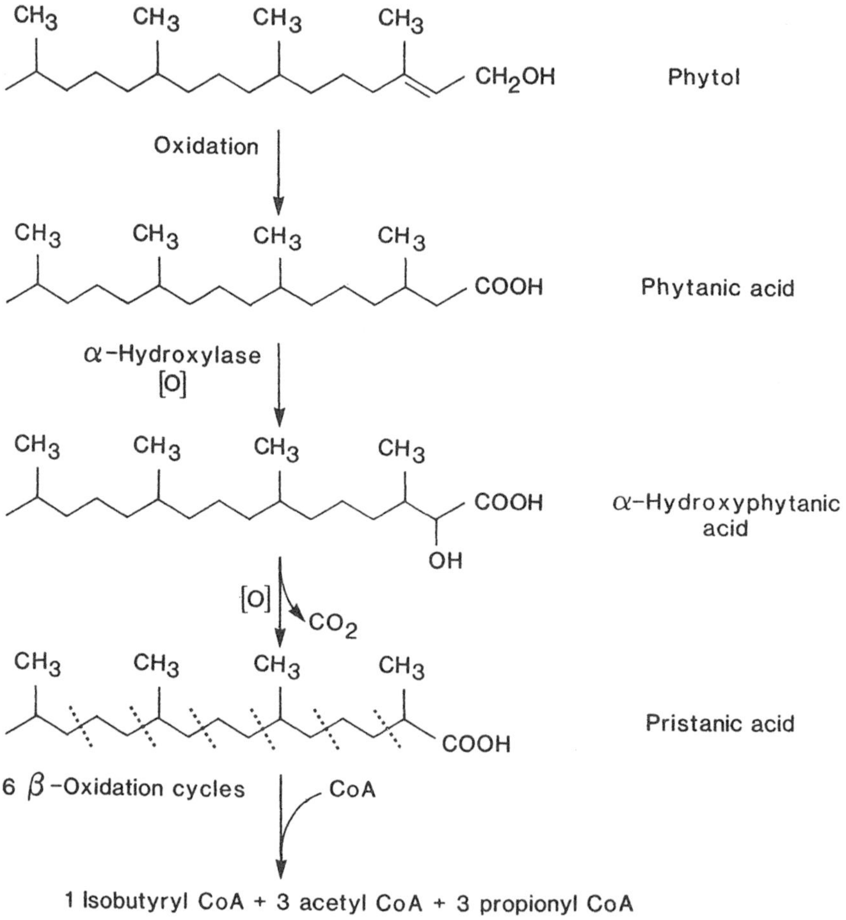

Figure 19.9   The α-oxidation pathway of phytol.

19.4.5 ω Oxidation

Fatty acids may be oxidized in the endoplasmic reticulum at the terminal methyl groups to dicarboxylic acids. This is done using cytochrome P-450 systems (Chapter 17), where the initial product is ω-hydroxy fatty acid. These dicarboxylic acids may undergo β oxidation at either end to yield shorter dicarboxylic acids. ω Oxidation occurs to a minor extent in humans.

19.4.6 α Oxidation

β Oxidation focuses on the β carbon of the fatty acid. In some instances, it is impossible to form a ketone on the β carbon, for example, if the β carbon is methylated. In such cases, the α carbon may be oxidized to initiate the oxidation process. α Oxidation is useful in the degradation of certain plant materials, such as phytol. The degradation of this compound is illustrated in Figure 19.9. In Refsum disease, caused by a genetic lesion, the enzyme hydroxylating phytanic acid is absent and phytanic acid accumulates in tissues.

19.5 KETONE BODY PRODUCTION AND METABOLISM

When the blood insulin/glucagon ratio is low, in fasting or in a patient with untreated diabetes, the flow of fatty acids is away from adipose tissues and into the liver. In the liver, the β-oxidation results in a depletion of oxaloacetate, because the excess of NADH produced converts it to malate. The dearth of oxaloacetate is exacerbated by a high level of gluconeogenesis activity. All this results in decreased activity of the Krebs cycle, and much of the acetyl-CoA produced by β oxidation must find another outlet. Fatty acid biosynthesis is largely shut down under such circumstances (see later), and acetyl-CoA is instead channeled into ketone body production, as shown in Figure 19.10. Ketone bodies are acetoacetate, β-D-hydroxybutyrate, and acetone. The first two only are organic acids. They are produced largely in the liver but utilized elsewhere. In addition to starvation and untreated diabetes, excessive quantities of ketone bodies are present in the circulation of patients with alcoholism, carbohydrate deficiency, toxemia of pregnancy, and other disorders.

Ketone bodies are normally present in the bloodstream in concentrations of about 0.3 mM, and a 3 day fast produces a *ketosis*, with ketone bodies amounting to 2–3 mM. In untreated diabetes, this may rise to 25 mM. β-D-Hydroxybutyrate always predominates. Under normal circumstances, the various organs can efficiently extract ketone bodies from the circulation, so that their levels remain relatively low. This does not happen in situations with severe lipolysis, even though in such conditions as starvation, ketone bodies may become the principal fuel for several tissues and are used quite extensively. For example, after prolonged starvation, more than half of the brain energy requirement may be met by ketone bodies. Ketone bodies may also provide a major source of energy for the cardiac and skeletal muscle, the kidney, and the gastrointestinal tract. The use of ketone bodies as an energy source is designed to spare glucose and therefore protein.

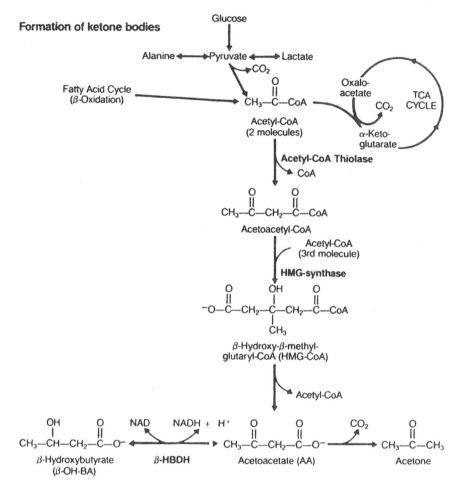

Figure 19.10 Ketone body biosynthesis in the mitochondria. HBDH is β-hydroxybutyrate dehydrogenase. (Reproduced by permission from Li PK. β-Hydroxybutyrate. Clin Chem News February:13, 1985.)

Tissues other than liver utilize ketone bodies by first reoxidizing β-D-hydroxybutyrate to acetoacetate (see Figure 19.10) and then converting acetoacetate to acetoacetyl-CoA. The latter occurs via a mitochondrial thiophorase reaction [Equation (19.8)] or a cytosolic acetoacetate CoA synthetase reaction [Equation (19.9)]:

$$\text{Acetoacetate} + \text{succinyl-CoA} \rightarrow \text{acetoacetyl-CoA} + \text{succinate} \qquad (19.8)$$

$$\text{Acetoacetate} + \text{ATP} + \text{CoA} \rightarrow \text{acetoacetyl-CoA} + \text{ADP} + \text{P}_i \qquad (19.9)$$

Enzymes catalyzing reactions (19.8) and (19.9) are present in very minor amounts in the liver, and hence liver is a ketone body exporter rather than user. Acetoacetyl-CoA is converted to two acetyl-CoA molecules by the action of a thiolase, and the acetyl-CoA is used in the Krebs cycle. 1 mol β-D-hydroxybutyrate can thus yield a total of 27 mol ATP using β-hydroxybutyrate dehydrogenase to generate acetoacetate, then thiophorase, and thiolase to yield 2 mol acetyl-CoA.

Ketosis is undesirable because it causes a loss of Na^+ and K^+ from the organism and may cause severe metabolic acidosis. Large amounts of ketone bodies are excreted in the urine during spells of ketosis, and being anions, they also carry away Na^+ and K^+ ions. Loss of circulatory Na^+ may cause acidosis, because the loss of Na^+ often results in a decrease in circulatory HCO_3^-. Alternatively, one may view this problem in terms of ketone bodies displacing HCO_3^-, even if the $[Na^+]$ remains constant. Assuming normal Na^+, K^+, HCO_3^-, and Cl^- distribution of 140, 4, 25, and 100 meq/L, the infusion of 10 meq/L of ketone bodies into the circulation displaces 10 meq/L of bicarbonate, leaving only 15 meq/L of bicarbonate. Assuming a lack of compensation and a normal pCO_2 of 40 mm Hg, the plasma pH of the subject would be down to 7.2.

19.6 BIOSYNTHESIS OF LIPIDS

19.6.1 Fatty Acid Biosynthesis

The biosynthesis of fatty acids occurs extramitochondrially and by a set of enzymes that are different from those of fatty acid degradation. Nevertheless, both processes may involve the same, although not exchangeable, intermediates. Acetyl-CoA forms the building blocks of the newly synthesized fatty acid. It may be derived from glucose, amino acids, or ethanol.

More likely than not, acetyl-CoA originates in the mitochondria. It cannot be transported across the mitochondrial membrane to cytosol, where fatty acid synthesis takes place. Instead, acetyl-CoA condenses with oxaloacetate to form citrate (see Chapter 18), and citrate is then transported into the cytosol. In the cytosol, citrate is cleaved to oxaloacetate and acetyl-CoA via citrate lyase, also termed citrate cleavage enzyme. It is an energy-requiring reaction. The oxaloacetate is reduced to malate by a cytosolic malate dehydrogenase, and the malate is converted to pyruvate, with the loss of CO_2 by malic enzyme, generating NADPH from NADP in the process. Citrate becomes available for fatty acid biosynthesis when the Krebs cycle is relatively inactive. This happens when isocitrate dehydrogenase is inhibited by high cellular ATP and low ADP levels. Participation of citrate in fatty acid biosynthesis is summarized in Figure 19.11.

The acetyl-CoA generated from citrate is then used for fatty acid biosynthesis. In the human being, only two multifunctional enzymes are involved: acetyl-CoA carboxylase (also termed malonyl-CoA synthetase) and fatty acid synthetase, with a molecular weight of 500,000, and coded by a single gene. The product of the two enzymes is palmitate. Other fatty acids may be made from palmitate by chain unsaturation, or elongation, or both (see later). The initial reaction involves the carboxylation of acetyl-CoA in two steps by acetyl-CoA carboxylase. Biotin is a cofactor, and one molecule of ATP is hydrolyzed to ADP and P_c:

$$\text{Biotin-enzyme} + HCO_3^- \xrightarrow[\quad]{\text{ATP} \quad \text{ADP} + P_c} \text{Enzyme-biotin-}CO_2 \qquad (19.10)$$

$$\text{Enzyme-biotin-}CO_2 + \text{acetyl-CoA} \rightarrow \text{malonyl-CoA} + \text{biotin-enzyme} \qquad (19.11)$$

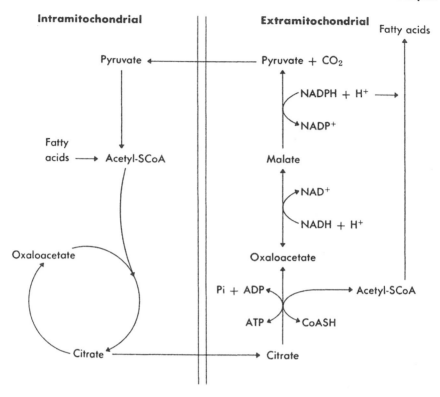

Figure 19.11   Relationship between extra- and intramitochondrial acetyl-CoA and the transport of acetyl-CoA in the form of citrate across the mitochondrial membrane.

Acetyl-CoA carboxylase is the major rate-controlling enzyme in fatty acid biosynthesis. It is stimulated by citrate and CoA and inhibited by phosphorylation and fatty acyl-CoA. The active enzyme consists of multimers of a polypeptide chain containing 2345 amino acids (MW 265,220). The formation and maintenance of the multimeric state of the enzyme apparently depends on the presence of citrate and CoA. The mode of phosphorylation of acetyl-CoA carboxylase is a matter of some disagreement: some authorities report that both cAMP-dependent and independent kinases are involved, along with Ca^{2+}-dependent kinases, whereas others insist that only an AMP-dependent kinase regulates the activity of acetyl-CoA carboxylase. The latter view is presented in Figure 19.12. According to this scheme, as cellular levels acyl-CoA rise, a kinase kinase enzyme is activated, which in turn catalyzes the phosphorylation of AMP-dependent protein kinase. The latter uses AMP as a positive allosteric effector. The activated (phosphorylated) AMP-dependent kinase then causes the phosphorylation and inactivation of acetyl-CoA carboxylase. Figure 19.12 also indicates the regulation of cholesterol biosynthesis, and this topic is discussed later in this chapter.

Even though AMP, not cAMP, may be the protein kinase activator, glucagon causes its activation and insulin, inactivation. Details on such hormone effects are lacking. Also recall that malonyl-CoA inhibits palmitoyl-CoA–carnitine acyltransferase, the rate-controlling enzyme in the β-oxidation process. Thus, lipid oxidation is inhibited in an environment that favors lipid synthesis, as in the fed state, whereas lipid biosynthesis is inhibited in an environment favoring lipid oxidation, as in fasting.

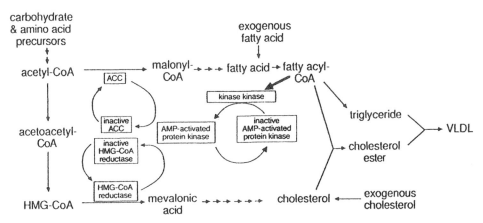

Figure 19.12 Regulation of liver acetyl-CoA carboxylase and cholesterol biosynthesis by phosphorylation. ACC indicates acetyl-CoA carboxylase. Bold arrow indicates activation of kinase kinase by fatty acyl-CoA. (Reproduced by permission from Hardie DG, Carling D, Sim ATR. The AMP-activated protein kinase: a multi-substrate regulator of lipid metabolism. Trends Biochem Sci 14:20–23, 1989.)

The next series of reactions is carried out by fatty acid synthetase, a two-subunit enzyme, in which both subunits are absolutely necessary for enzyme activity. Each enzyme molecule builds two fatty acyl residues at the same time. The enzyme has pantothenic acid as prosthetic groups and uses NADPH as a reducing agent. Sulfhydryl groups are an essential feature of this enzyme activity. Two are supplied by the pantothenic acid and two by component cysteine residues. The *de novo* biosynthetic reaction is initiated by acetyl-CoA, which combines with the –SH group of pantothenate. The acetyl group is then moved to the –SH residue of a cysteine group of the other subunit (see Figure 19.13). The freed pantothenate residue then combines with a molecule of malonyl-CoA. Acetyl-CoA then moves into the methylene carbon of the malonyl residue, displacing CO_2 and creating an acetoacetyl group. This is then reduced in several steps to a butyrate residue, which is transferred for temporary storage to the cysteinyl residue, so that the pantothenate can combine with the next malonyl-CoA group. The overall reaction represented in Figure 19.13 can be summarized by Equation (19.12):

$$\text{Acetyl-CoA} + 7\text{malonyl-CoA} + 14\text{NADPH} + 14\text{H}^+ \rightarrow \text{palmitate}$$
$$+ 7\text{CO}_2 + 8\text{CoA} + 14\text{NADP}^+ + 6\text{H}_2\text{O} \tag{19.12}$$

If we start with acetyl-CoA only, then reaction (19.12) becomes (19.13):

$$8\text{acetyl-CoA} + 7\text{ATP} + 14\text{NADPH} + 14\text{H}^+ \rightarrow \text{palmitate} + 8\text{CoA}$$
$$+ 7\text{ADP} + 7\text{P}_i + 6\text{H}_2\text{O} + 14\text{NADP}^+ \tag{19.13}$$

A total of 14 NADPH molecules are utilized to make each palmitate molecule. It comes from three sources: the malic enzyme (see earlier) provides one NADPH molecule for every acetyl-CoA molecule generated from citrate. For palmitate, this accounts for eight NADPH molecules. The rest must be derived largely from the hexose monophosphate shunt (see Chapter 18). A minor source of NADPH is cytosolic isocitrate dehydrogenase (see Chapter 18). The synthesis of one palmitate molecule thus requires an equivalent of 7 + (3)14 = 49 ATP molecules.

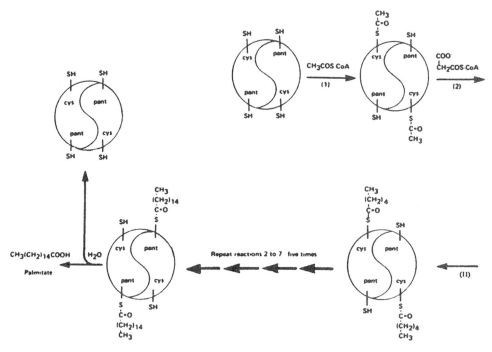

Figure 19.13   Biosynthesis of palmitate via fatty acid synthetase. The numbered enzyme activities (steps) are as follows: (1) acetyl-CoA transacylase; (2) malonyl-coA transacylase; (3) β-ketoacylsynthetase; (4) β-ketoacylreductase; (5) β-hydroxyacyldehydratase; (6) enoyl reductase; (7) fatty acyltransacylase. (Reproduced by permission from Wakil SJ, Stoops JK, Joshi VC. Fatty acid synthesis and its regulation. Annu Rev Biochem 52:537–579, 1983.)

Fatty acid synthetase is not controlled directly by phosphorylation; however, insulin, glucagon, and thyroxine have an effect on its activity by controlling its cellular concentration. Both insulin and thyroxine increase the biosynthesis of the enzyme, whereas glucagon is inhibitory. Thyroxine and glucagon appear to regulate the biosynthesis at the transcription level, whereas insulin affects the enzyme activity at the translation level. It has no effect on cellular fatty acid synthetase mRNA concentration. In summary, fatty acid synthetase levels are up in the fed state and down in the fasting state.

19.6.2   Fatty Acyl Chain Elongation and Unsaturation

Palmitate can serve as a precursor for both longer and unsaturated fatty acids. Chain elongation takes place in both the endoplasmic reticulum and mitochondria. In the latter, this is a simple reversal of the β-oxidation reaction sequence, except that the step that would normally require $FADH_2$ requires NADPH instead. This system is designed for the elongation of short-chain acids. There is no activity with palmitate.

The ER elongation system works similarly to the fatty acid synthetase sequence, except that individual enzymes (gene products) are involved: palmitoyl-CoA reacts with malonyl-CoA to give CO_2 and β-ketooctadecanoyl-CoA. The

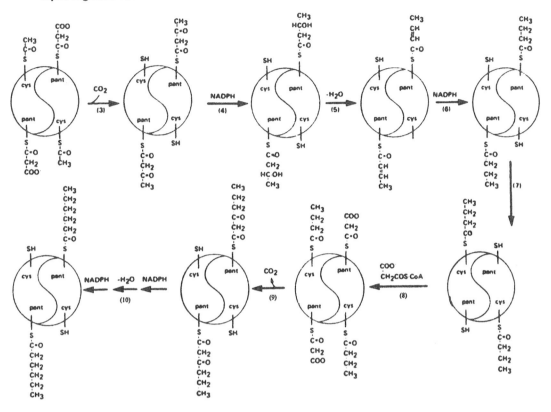

latter is then reduced by NADPH to stearoyl-CoA. The formation of oleyl-CoA takes place from stearoyl-CoA first through a lipoxygenase reaction, which hydroxylates position 9 of stearoyl-CoA, and then a dehydratase removes the elements of water to create the cis double bond and hence oleyl-CoA. Figure 19.14 indicates how the two processes are combined to form arachidonoyl-CoA, a precursor of prostaglandins, from linoleyl-CoA. In essential fatty acid deficiency, the unsaturation-elongation system uses oleyl-CoA instead of linoleyl-CoA. After the usual two unsaturation and one elongation steps, the system stops at 5,8,11-eicosatrienoyl-CoA. It is a useless product and accumulates in the fatty tissues of the animal.

The mechanism of fatty acid unsaturation (e.g., stearic acid → oleic acid) utilizes a system similar to that involving cytochrome P-450 (Chapter 17): it is microsome bound, and it includes a heme-containing protein (cytochrome b_5), an FAD-containing reductase, and an iron-sulfur center-containing "desaturase." The electron source is NADH or NADPH. Equation (19.14) summarizes this process:

NADH   FAD   2 cyt b_5 - Fe^{2+} 2 Fe^{3+} - S   2 H_2O + oleyl CoA

(19.14)

NAD^+ $FADH_2$ 2 cyt b_5 - Fe^{3+} 2 Fe^{2+} - S O_2 + 4 H^+ + stearoyl CoA

Reductase   Desaturase

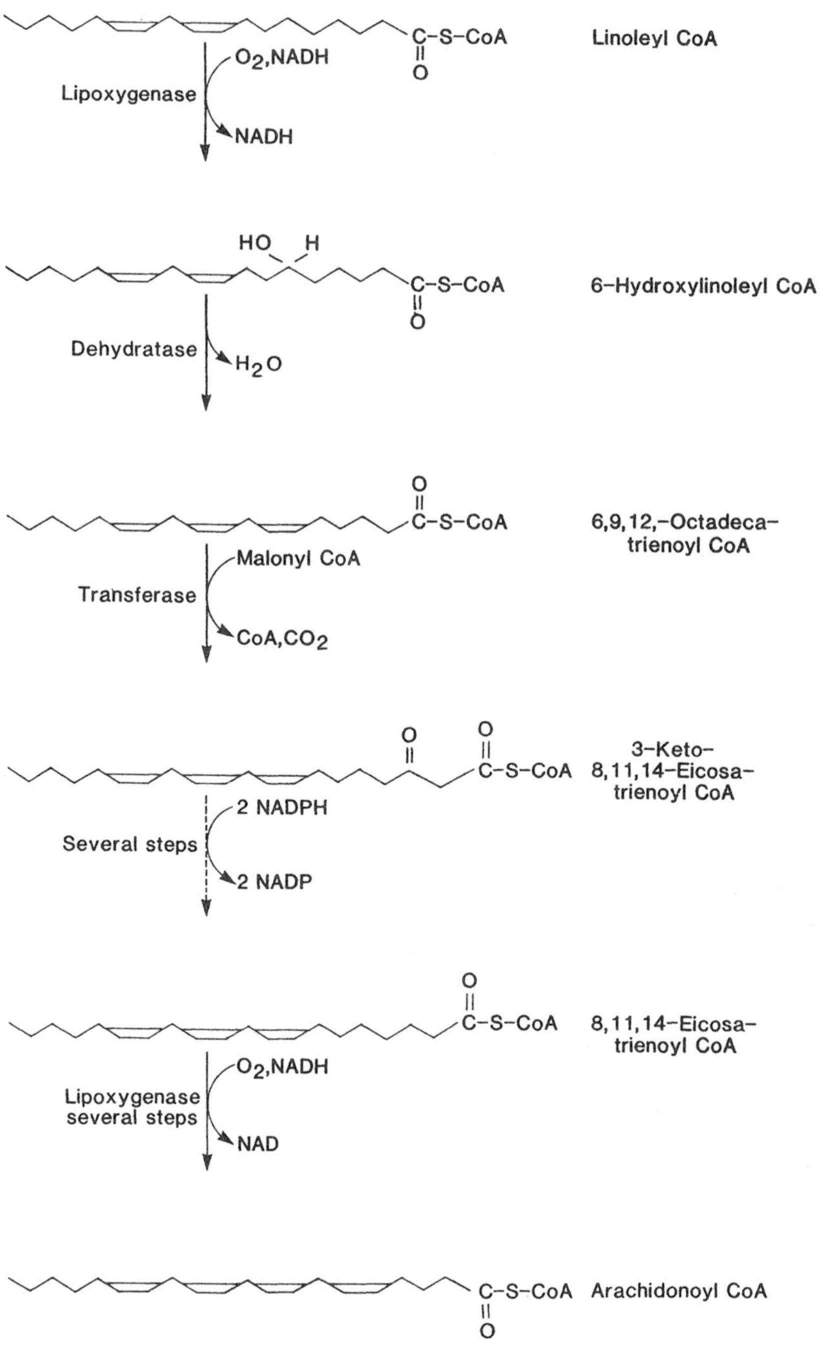

Figure 19.14 Biosynthesis of arachidonoyl-CoA from linoleoyl-CoA: fatty acid unsaturation and elongation.

19.6.3 Biosynthesis of Phosphoglycerides

Phosphoglycerides may be synthesized either from phosphatidic acid or by the so-called salvage pathway. Phosphatidic acid is also an intermediate in triglyceride biosynthesis (Figure 19.4). The phosphatidic acid pathway is relatively minor in eukaryotes: phosphatidic acid reacts with CTP to form CDP diglyceride (see Figure 19.15), and the latter may then react with choline or inositol to form phosphatidylinositol or phosphatidylcholine, as in Equations (19.14) and (19.15).

$$\text{Phosphatidic acid} + \text{CTP} \rightarrow \text{CDP-diglyceride} + \text{PP}_i \tag{19.15}$$

$$\text{CDP-diglyceride} + \text{inositol} \rightarrow \text{phosphatidylinositol} + \text{CMP} \tag{19.16}$$

The major (salvage) pathways for the formation of phosphatidylcholine and ethanolamine are illustrated in Figure 19.16. Free (dietary) choline and ethanolamine are converted to their CDP derivatives, which then react with diacylglycerol to form phosphatidylcholine and ethanolamine. In the lungs, another pathway forms dipalmitoyl phosphatidylcholine, a powerful surfactant. Phosphatidylethanolamine may be methylated by S-adenosylmethionine (SAM; see Chapter 20) to yield phosphatidylcholine. The reaction is catalyzed by two enzymes: the first methyl group is transferred via phosphatidylethanolamine N-methyltransferase I. The other two methyl groups are transferred by phosphatidylethanolamine N-methyltransferase II. Some authorities believe that the two enzymes are identical. It has also been proposed that methylation of phospha-

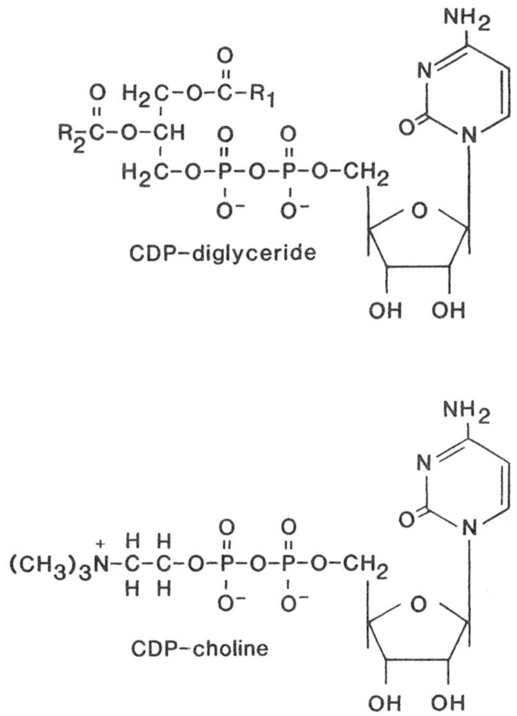

Figure 19.15 Structures of CDP-diglyceride and CDP-choline.

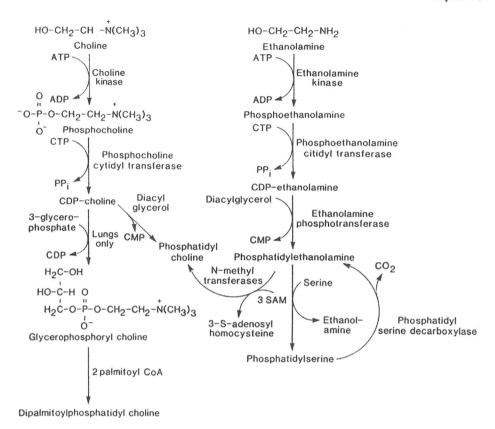

Figure 19.16 "Salvage" pathways for phosphatidylcholine and ethanolamine and related biosynthetic reactions. SAM is *S*-adenosylmethionine and PP_i is pyrophosphate.

tidylethanolamine to form lecithin increases membrane fluidity and thus enhances the lateral movement of plasma membrane proteins, especially during receptor–hormone processes.

Another reaction shown in Figure 19.16 is the formation of phosphatidylserine from phosphatidylethanolamine. This reaction also serves to make more phosphatidylethanolamine by decarboxylating the phosphatidylserine. The net reaction is thus

$$\text{Serine} \rightarrow CO_2 + \text{ethanolamine} \tag{19.17}$$

The rate-controlling enzymes in the salvage pathways are the phosphocholine and phosphoethanolamine citidyltransferases. Thus, rat liver cell choline, phosphocholine, and CDP-choline concentrations are 0.23, 1.3, and 0.03 mM, respectively. For the ethanolamine derivatives, these are 1.09, 3.83, and 0.24 mM, respectively. The bottlenecks are clearly in the formation of the CDP derivatives. Phosphocholine citidyltransferase of cytosol is phosphorylated and inactive. Phosphorylation prevents its interaction with the ER. It is activated when it is dephosphorylated and translocated to the ER. cAMP-dependent phosphorylation then promotes its removal from the ER and its inactivation. Ethanolamine levels are closely controlled by choline. Increases in cellular choline levels depress those of ethanolamine, whereas choline deficiency increases cellular ethanolamine levels.

19.6.4 Cholesterol Biosynthesis

The first two steps in cholesterol biosynthesis from acetyl-CoA are identical to those of ketone body formation (Figure 19.10). The difference is that ketone bodies are formed in the mitochondria, whereas cholesterol synthesis initially takes place in the ER. A thiolase catalyzes the condensation of two acetyl-CoA molecules to acetoacetyl-CoA, and the combination of a third acetyl-CoA with acetoacetyl-CoA to form β-hydroxymethylglutaryl-CoA (HMG-CoA) is catalyzed by HMG-CoA synthase. Although HMG-CoA is split into acetoacetate and acetyl-CoA in the mitochondria, in cholesterol biosynthesis, HMG-CoA is reduced by a microsomal enzyme, HMG-CoA reductase, to mevalonate (see Figure 19.17). The reducing agent is NADPH.

Mevalonate gives rise to various substances of the isoprenoid class, including cholesterol and dolichol. It is changed through a series of steps to isopentenyl pyrophosphate, a 5-carbon compound that condenses with itself to form the 10-carbon geranyl pyrophosphate. Another isopentenyl pyrophosphate molecule condenses with geranyl pyrophosphate to form the 15-carbon farnesyl pyrophosphate. Two of the latter form the 30-carbon squalene molecule. Squalene, a noncyclic hydrocarbon, may be represented by a "folded" structure resembling the steroid molecule, as shown in Figure 19.18. A microsomal oxygenase introduces an oxygen residue into squalene, and then cyclization takes place to form the steroid lanosterol. The latter is converted to cholesterol by various microsomal enzymes. Some 800 mg cholesterol is synthesized per day in an average adult by this pathway.

The control of cholesterol biosynthesis occurs at the transcription level (changes in functional RNA levels) and via phosphorylation. HMG-CoA reductase is inactivated by phosphorylation with AMP-dependent protein kinase in a process similar to that of acetyl-CoA carboxylase (see Figure 19.12). The level of phosphorylation is in turn regulated by glucagon and insulin, the former increasing, and the latter decreasing it, although the exact mechanisms are unclear. The AMP-activated protein kinase is also activated by a kinase kinase through phosphorylation. The kinase kinase is in turn activated by nanomolar amounts of fatty acyl-CoA. A protein phosphatase inactivates the AMP-dependent kinase. It is thus clear that both the cholesterol and fatty acid biosynthetic pathways are dependent on cytosolic acetyl-CoA and that both are controlled, at least in part, by the AMP-dependent kinase.

The other system controlling cholesterol biosynthesis involves both the cytosolic HMG-CoA synthase and the ER enzyme HMG-CoA reductase and is based on the cellular levels of respective mRNAs. Increasing free cholesterol decreases both enzyme activities by decreasing the levels of their mRNAs and increasing enzyme degradation processes. The half-life of HMG-CoA reductase may be as short as 1.7 h. Cellular uptake of LDL maintains cholesterol biosynthesis at a relatively low level, and this is achieved through an LDL degradation product-free cholesterol. Some authorities have maintained that hydroxylated

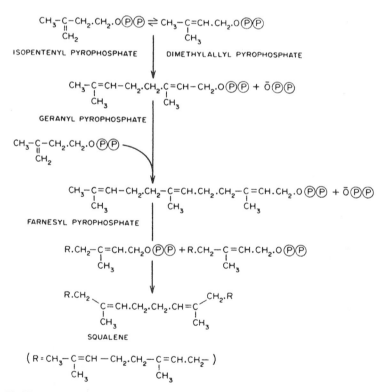

Figure 19.17 Biosynthesis of squalene from mevalonic acid. (Reproduced by permission from Vance DE, Vance JE. Biochemistry of Lipids and Membranes. Menlo Park: Benjamin/ Cummings, 1985, pp. 409–410.)

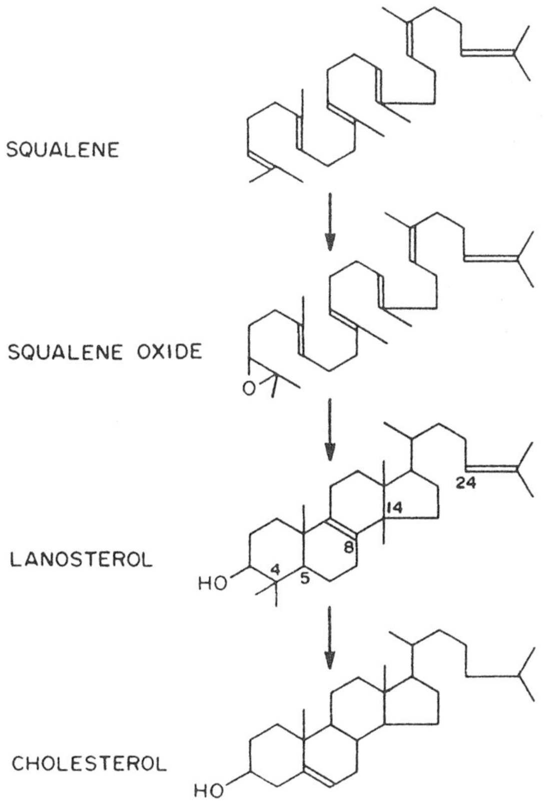

Figure 19.18 Biosynthesis of cholesterol from squalene. (Reproduced by permission from Vance DE, Vance JE. Biochemistry of Lipids and Membranes. Menlo Park: Benjamin/ Cummings, 1985, p. 412.)

cholesterol "metabolites," not free cholesterol, are such inhibitory agents. Some anticholesterol drugs, such as lovastatin, appear to act in the same manner as free cholesterol, as does excess mevalonate. The opposite effect is observed when there is a cellular cholesterol deficiency: mRNAs increase, the quantities of both enzymes increase, and cholesterol biosynthesis is increased. The genes for both enzymes are located on human chromosome 5, although they are separated by a rather large distance. Nevertheless, both enzymes are expressed in a highly coordinated manner.

19.7 SYNOPSIS OF REGULATORY MECHANISMS IN FAT METABOLISM

Situations in which the blood insulin/glucagon ratio is higher than normal lead to fatty acid and cholesterol biosynthesis, whereas low insulin/glucagon ratios are characterized by lipolysis, increased activity of the β-oxidation pathway, and a low level of cholesterol biosynthetic activity. Enzymes that are either activated by insulin or derepressed by low glucagon levels are lipoprotein lipase, which

favors the entry of lipoprotein (chylomicrons and VLDL) triglyceride degradation products into various tissues. Tissue triglyceride biosynthesis is further
favored by the derepression of fatty acyl-CoA glycerol-3-phosphate acyltransferase. Acetyl-CoA carboxylase is derepressed when blood glucagon levels are low,
and increased cellular levels of citrate, which are observed in the fed state,
activate acetyl-CoA carboxylase. Increased cellular levels of malonyl-CoA inhibit
β-oxidation by inhibiting the palmitoyl-CoA–carnitine acyltransferase. Finally,
cellular levels of fatty acid synthetase are increased through the action of insulin
on the translation of this enzyme mRNA. Cholesterol biosynthesis is increased
by the derepression (dephosphorylation) of HMG-CoA reductase.

As blood glucagon levels rise, hormone-sensitive lipase is activated by
phosphorylation, causing fatty acid flow from adipose tissue into the liver. Mean-
while, fatty acyl-CoA glycerol-3-phosphate acyltransferase is inhibited by phosphorylation, thus cutting off triglyceride biosynthesis. Acetyl-CoA carboxylase is
also inhibited by phosphorylation via AMP-dependent protein kinase. Fatty acid
synthetase levels decline as a result of high blood glucagon levels. Low cellular
malonyl-CoA levels cause the derepression of pamitoyl-CoA-carnitine acyltransferase, increasing the activity of the β-oxidative pathway and mitochondrial
acetyl-CoA levels. Ketone body production follows, as well as gluconeogenesis.
Cholesterol biosynthesis ceases because of HMG-CoA reductase phosphorylation. This is the situation typically observed in starvation. Among individual
enzymes that decline in starvation are fatty acid synthetase, acetyl-CoA carboxylase, and HMG-CoA reductase. Starvation is discussed in greater detail in
Chapter 21.

QUESTIONS

Answer Questions 19.1–19.6 by choosing one of the following enzymes, which are involved in regulating various pathways of lipid metabolism.
   a.   Acetyl-CoA carboxylase (malonyl-CoA synthetase)
   b.   Lipoprotein lipase
   c.   Fatty acid synthetase
   d.   Palmitoyl-CoA–carnitine acyltransferase
   e.   Hormone-sensitive lipase

19.1.   Activated by cAMP-dependent protein kinase.
19.2.   Inactivated by an AMP-dependent protein kinase
19.3.   Activated by citrate
19.4.   VLDL is a substrate
19.5.   Controls the rate of the β-oxidation pathway
19.6.   Dehydratase activity
19.7.   A patient has high fasting plasma total cholesterol and triglyceride values. What
        lipoproteins are most likely increased?
            a. Chylomicrons   b. LDL and HDL   c. LDL only
            d. VLDL only   e. LDL and VLDL
19.8.   Several factors control cholesterol biosynthesis either directly or indirectly. Which
        is not a factor?
            a. Insulin   b. Glucagon   c. cAMP
            d. Phosphorylation e. Fatty acyl-CoA

19.9.   Acetyl-CoA is a substrate for all the enzymes *except* which?
     a.   Malic enzyme
     b.   Malonyl-CoA synthetase
     c.   Fatty acid synthetase
     d.   HMG-CoA synthase
     e.   Acetyl-CoA thiolase

19.10.   A high-energy phosphate is *not* required in which reaction?
     a.   Citrate → oxaloacetate + acetyl-CoA
     b.   Fatty acyl-CoA + carnitine → fatty acyl-O-carnitine + CoA
     c.   CDP-choline biosynthesis
     d.   Fatty acid + CoA → fatty acyl-CoA
     e.   Propionyl-CoA + CO_2 → methylmalonyl-CoA

19.11.   2-Monoacylglyceride is a product of which enzyme reaction?
     a.   Fatty acyl-CoA–glycerol-3-phosphate acyltransferase
     b.   Lysolecithinase
     c.   Pancreatic lipase
     d.   Fatty acyl-CoA–glycerol acyltransferase
     e.   Fatty acyl-CoA-acyltransferase

19.12.   Biosynthesis of bile salts involves all of the following, except
     a.   Hydroxylation of cholesterol
     b.   Oxidative shortening of the side chain in the mitochondria
     c.   Cleavage of cholesterol B ring
     d.   Conjugation with taurine
     e.   Reduction of chenodeoxycholate to lithocholate in the small intestine

19.13.   Which is the *least* likely result of prolonged fasting?
     a.   Acidosis
     b.   Increased level of cholesterol biosynthesis
     c.   Excretion in the urine of β-hydroxybutyrate
     d.   Net loss of adipose tissue triglyceride
     e.   Increased cellular levels of NADH

19.14.   Which reaction is promoted by apolipoprotein AI?
     a.   Acyl-CoA + cholesterol → cholesterol ester + CoA
     b.   Triglyceride → glycerol + fatty acids
     c.   Triglyceride + cholesterol → cholesterol ester + lysolecithin
     d.   Phosphatidic acid + acyl-CoA → triglyceride + CoA
     e.   Lecithin + cholesterol → cholesterol ester + lysolecithin

19.15.   An untreated gastrectomized individual most likely excretes in the urine which compound?
     a.   Propionic acid
     b.   Phytanic acid
     c.   Malonic acid
     d.   L-Methylmalonic acid
     e.   Eicosa-5,8,11-trienoic acid

Answer Questions 19.16 and 19.17 on the basis of the following facts: you have 4-*cis*-octenoic acid (/\/̅\COOH) and you are oxidizing it by β oxidation and the Krebs cycle.

19.16.   How many moles of ATP can we produce by oxidizing 1 mol of this acid?
     a.   49
     b.   55
     c.   59
     d.   61
     e.   63

19.17. Which of the following is the least likely intermediate?

a. $CH_3\text{-}(CH_2)_2\text{-}C=C\text{-}C\text{-}S\text{-}CoA$ (with H, H, O substituents)

b. $CH_3\text{-}C(H,OH)\text{-}CH_2\text{-}C\text{-}S\text{-}CoA$ (with O)

c. $CH_3\text{-}(CH_2)_2\text{-}C=C\text{-}C\text{-}S\text{-}CoA$ (with H above, H and O below)

d. $CH_3\text{-}(CH_2)_2\text{-}C(H,OH)\text{-}CH_2\text{-}C\text{-}S\text{-}CoA$ (with O)

e. $CH_3\text{-}(CH_2)_2\text{-}C=C\text{-}C\text{-}CH_2\text{-}C\text{-}S\text{-}CoA$ (with H, H, O, O)

19.18. Which reaction in the following set is rate controlling in lecithin biosynthesis?
a. Choline + ATP → phosphocholine + ADP
b. Phosphocholine + CTP → CDP – Choline + PP_i
c. CDP-choline + diacylglycerol → glycerophosphocholine
d. CDP-choline + glycerol phosphate → glycerophosphocholine
e. Glycerophosphocholine + 2-palmitoyl-CoA → lecithin

19.19. Let us assume that the normal plasma $[HCO_3^-]$ = 25 meq/L and the normal anion gap is 20 meq/L. Suppose your patient, an untreated diabetic, has an anion gap of 30 meq/L. Assuming that pCO_2 remains at 40 mm Hg, what is your patient's plasma pH? pK = 6.1. See also Chapters 3 and 17.
a. 7.5
b. 7.4
c. 7.3
d. 7.2
e. 7.0

19.20. Suppose our patient has a total cholesterol of 250 mg/dL, triglycerides of 200 mg/dL, and HDL cholesterol of 50 mg/dL; what is LDL cholesterol?
a. 200 mg/dL
b. 160 mg/dL
c. 100 mg/dL
d. 50 mg/dL
e. 120 mg/dL

19.21. This compound is an intermediate

$$
\begin{array}{l}
H_2\text{-}C\text{-}O\text{-}\overset{\overset{\displaystyle O}{\|}}{C}\text{-}R_1 \\
R_2\text{-}C\text{-}O\text{-}C\text{-}H \\
\underset{O}{\|}\ \ H_2\text{-}C\text{-}O\text{-}P_i
\end{array}
$$

in the biosynthesis of which compound(s)?
a. Triglyceride
b. Phosphatidylinositol
c. Sphingosine
d. Two of the above
e. All of the above

19.22. cAMP affects the salvage pathway for lecithin biosynthesis. This is accomplished by which of the following?
a. The rate-limiting enzyme is inactivated by phosphorylation.
b. The rate-limiting enzyme must interact with ER to be active; such interaction is inhibited by phosphorylation.
c. The rate-limiting enzyme is activated by phosphorylation.
d. Phosphorylation causes the association of the rate-limiting enzyme with ER, thus inactivating it.

    e. Phosphorylation causes the disassociation of the rate-limiting enzyme from ER, thus activating it in the cytosol.

19.23. NADPH is required for fatty acid biosynthesis. Which reaction or pathway supplies a portion of the required NADPH?

    a. β Oxidation

    b. Cytoplasmic oxaloacetate → malate

    c. Pyruvate → lactate

    d. Dihydroxyacetone phosphate → glycerol-3-phosphate

    e. Malate → pyruvate + CO_2

19.24. All of the following are true about long-chain fatty acid chain elongation except

    a. Performed with the conventional fatty acid synthetase multifunctional enzyme.

    b. Malonyl-CoA utilized

    c. Process takes place in endoplasmic reticulum

    d. Associated with unsaturation reactions in arachidonic acid biosynthesis from linoleic acid

    e. Requires activation of the fatty acid to its CoA form

In Questions 19.25–19.27, mark as follows:

    a. β Oxidation of fatty acids

    b. Fatty acid biosynthesis

    c. Both

    d. Neither

19.25. It is located in peroxisomes.

19.26. The β-hydroxy fatty acyl residue is an intermediate.

19.27. Pantothenic acid is a prosthetic group.

Answers

19.1. (e) Other than hormone-sensitive lipase, only acetyl-CoA carboxylase is affected by phosphorylation, but this event is controlled by an AMP-sensitive kinase.

19.2. (a) Phosphorylation of acetyl-CoA carboxylase results in its *inactivation*.

19.3. (a) Citrate is necessary for acetyl-CoA carboxylase to function.

19.4. (b) Lipoprotein lipase, an extracellular enzyme, causes the hydrolysis of VLDL and chylomicron triglycerides. Hormone-sensitive lipase catalyzes the hydrolysis of intracellular (storage) triglyceride.

19.5. (d) Palmitoyl-CoA–carnitine acyltransferase is rate controlling in fatty acid degradation. Its effector is malonyl-CoA, which inhibits its activity.

19.6. (c) Fatty acid synthetase has all the activities that would be necessary to reverse the β-oxidation pathway. Thus, a cis double bond is generated from β-hydroxy fatty acyl-CoA residues by a dehydration process.

19.7. (e) LDL is a cholesterol carrier, whereas in a fasting serum sample, VLDL is the principal triglyceride carrier.

19.8. (c) HMG-CoA reductase is inhibited by phosphorylation. The phosphorylation is carried out by an AMP-dependent protein kinase, not a cAMP-dependent kinase. Glucagon affects the degree of phosphorylation by an as yet unknown mechanism.

19.9. (a) Malic enzyme converts malate to pyruvate with the generation of NADPH from NADP.

19.10. (b) This reaction is catalyzed by palmitoyl-CoA–carnitine acyltransferase and does not require ATP. The acyl-CoA is sufficiently "activated" to be able to react with carnitine.

19.11. (c) Pancreatic lipase, during the normal digestive process, causes the removal of fatty acyl residues from positions 1 and 3 of triglycerides.

19.12. (c) The cholesterol B ring is opened in the biosynthesis of active vitamin D. This does not occur in bile salt formation.

19.13. (b) Fasting, accompanied by high blood glucagon levels, results in the phosphorylation and inactivation of HMG-CoA reductase. Additionally, the biosynthesis of HMG-CoA synthase and HMG-CoA reductase may be restricted at the transcription level.

19.14. (e) ApoA-I, found in HDL, activates lecithin–cholesterol acyltransferase (LCAT).

19.15. (d) The metabolism of propionyl-CoA requires vitamin B_{12} at the level of methylmalonate metabolism (see Figure 19.6). In an untreated gastrectomized individual, the intrinsic factor would be missing and vitamin B_{12} would not be absorbed.

19.16. (c) The 4-cis-octenoic acid (8 carbons, one double bond) must be activated through the use of 2 ATP equivalents. Three β-oxidation cycles would be necessary (5 ATP each) to generate 4 acetyl-CoA molecules (12 ATP each). Each double bond reduces ATP yield by 2. Total ATP yield: $12(4) + 5(3) - 2 - 2 = 59$.

19.17. (c) See Figure 19.7. To metabolize this compound, one β-oxidation cycle would have to occur with compound e as an intermediate and compound a as a product. Compound a can now be hydrated to the D-β-hydroxy hexanoyl-CoA, and an epimerase would then cause the formation of its L isomer compound. The latter can then be oxidized through two β-oxidation cycles, with compound b as an intermediate.

19.18. (b) See Figure 19.14. The phosphocholine cytidyltransferase is rate controlling.

19.19. (d) There is an excess of "anion gap" anions (ketone bodies) of 10 meq/L. Because the sum of cations and anions must be equal, the 10 meq/L is lost from bicarbonate, giving $[HCO_3^-] = 15$ meq/L. Using the Henderson-Hasselbalch equation, we have pH $= 6.1 + \log 15/(0.03 \times 40) = 6.1 + \log 12.5 = 7.2$.

19.20. (b) LDL cholesterol $= 250 - 50 - (200/5) = 160$ mg/dL.

19.21. (d) The compound shown is phosphatidic acid. It is a precursor of triglycerides (Figure 19.4) and some phosphoglycerides, such as phosphatidylinositol [Equations (19.14) and (19.15)].

19.22. (b) The CDP transferase is activated by dephosphorylation, because this permits it to bind to the ER. It is active only in the ER.

19.23. (e) NADPH is necessary for fatty acid biosynthesis. It is generated by the HMPS and the cytoplasmic malic enzyme.

19.24. (a) Fatty acyl synthetase is used for the de novo biosynthesis of palmitic acid. Elongation of fatty acids occurs by a reversal of β oxidation in the mitochondria and by a set of separate enzymes in the ER.

19.25. (a) β Oxidation occurs largely in the mitochondria but also occurs in the peroxisomes.

19.26. (c) β-Hydroxyl fatty acyl residues are intermediates in both β oxidation (substrate for β-hydroxyacyl-CoA dehydrogenase, Figure 19.5), and in the fatty acid synthetase system (substrate for the dehydratase activity).

19.27. (b) Pantothenic acid is a prosthetic group in fatty acid synthetase. In β oxidation, pantothenic acid participates only as a component of CoA.

PROBLEMS

19.1. Predict what would happen to blood glucose levels if a patient were not able to generate ketone bodies. Which enzyme defect would result in this effect?

19.2. A 25-year-old woman was admitted to a hospital with a mild bleeding disorder reminiscent of chronic aspirin consumption. Her skin bleeding time was 7–9 minutes (normal is 2–5 minutes). Addition of arachidonic acid to her platelet-rich plasma failed to aggregate the platelets, and extracts of her tissue biopsy material failed to inhibit platelet aggregation by ADP. Analysis of platelet extracts by thin-layer chromatography showed normal concentrations of leukotrienes, but not of related compounds. Address the following:
   a. What is indicated by the platelet tests? (Hint: Consult chapter 16.)
   b. Suggest a reason this patient is suffering from a bleeding disorder, giving full biochemical details.
   c. What test(s) should be performed to confirm the diagnosis?
   d. It is known that essential fatty acid deficiencies result in severe cutaneous and neurologic distress. What conclusions can you make from this case regarding the reasons that polyunsaturated fatty acids are essential in human nutrition?

19.3. An 8-year-old male child was suffering from a severe neurologic disorder syndrome, including areflexia, ataxia, and actual nerve degeneration. His total serum bilirubin was 21.6 mg/dL, direct bilirbuin accounting for 14.8 mg/dL (normal is less than 0.4 mg/dL). His blood vitamin E level was less than 1 μg/mL (normal is 3.8–15.5 μg/mL). Fecal fat was 14.5% of the administered dose (normal is less than 5%). Address the following:
   a. Describe the underlying biochemical problem in this child. Be sure to consider the bilirubin data, fecal fat value, and why blood vitamin E level is low.
   b. How would you treat the apparent vitamin E deficiency?
   c. What other causes may be responsible for the type of syndrome seen in this patient?
   d. In another patient, similar neurologic symptoms were observed, however, her bilirubin level was normal and fecal fat excretion was also normal. Her plasma vitamin E level was 4.2 μg/mL, but her total serum lipid was 1630 mg/dL (normal is 320–570 mg/dL). Why the vitamin E-related neurologic symptoms?

19.4. A 6-year-old girl was admitted to a metabolic study unit with extensive skin xanthomas, serum cholesterol of 1100 mg/dL, and triglyceride of 369 mg/dL. Radioactively tagged LDL showed a fractional catabolic rate of 0.12 pools/day (normal is 0.43 pools/day). The girl suffered a heart attack soon thereafter, after which a coronary artery bypass operation was performed. Another was performed 6 weeks thereafter and finally, the patient received a heart and liver transplant. Her cholesterol then fell down to 270 mg/dL and the fractional catabolic rate of administered LDL had increased to 0.31 pools/day. Address the following:
   a. What was the underlying disease in this child? Why was it necessary to transplant both the heart and the liver?
   b. What is the fractional catabolic rate? Why did it not go to normal following the transplants? Why did cholesterol remain slightly elevated?
   c. The patient was shown to synthesize 36 mg ApoB per kg body weight per day before transplant. After the transplant, this was reduced to 16.7 mg. Explain why on the basis of cholesterol homeostasis.
   d. Discuss the rationale of treating this type of disorder by HMG-CoA reductase inhibitors (e.g., lovastatin), ileal bypass surgery, or portocaval shunt surgery.

BIBLIOGRAPHY

Goodridge AG. Regulation of the gene for fatty acid synthase. Fed Proc 45:2399–2405, 1986.

Hardie DG, Carling D, Sim ATR. The AMP-activated protein kinase: a multisubstrate regulator of lipid metabolism. Trends Biochem Sci January 20, 1989.

Kim KH, Lopez-Casillas F, Bai DH, Luo X, Pape ME. Role of reversible phosphorylation of acetyl-CoA carboxylase in long-chain fatty acid synthesis. FASEB J 3:2250–2256, 1989.

Reddy JK, Mannaerts GP. Peroxisomal lipid metabolism. Annu Rev Nutr 14:343–370, 1994.

Schaefer EJ, Levy RI. Pathogenesis and management of lipoprotein disorders. N Engl J Med 312:1300–1310, 1985.

Staff writers. Regulation of cholesterol biosynthesis. Nutr Rev 45:92–94, 1987.

Vance DE, Vance JE. Biochemistry of Lipids and Membranes. Menlo Park: Benjamin/Cummings, 1985.

Zeisel SH, Blusztajn JK. Choline and human nutrition. Annu Rev Nutr 14:269–296, 1994.

20

Protein and Amino Acid Metabolism

After completing this chapter, the student should

1. Be familiar with the reasons why amino acids are required in the diet: the significance of essential amino acids, the concept of nitrogen balance, the meaning of obligatory nitrogen loss, and the nature of protein deficiency diseases.
2. Know the names and modes of action of all proteolytic enzymes and their zymogens, if any, and the hormones that regulate protein digestion; understand the mechanisms of amino acid absorption and their disorders; understand amino acid traffic patterns in the bloodstream, including their changes in the various dietary states and hepatic encephalopathy.
3. Understand the factors that control cellular protein degradation and turnover; be able to solve problems involving protein half-lives and fractional catabolic rates; and understand how whole-body protein turnover may be estimated.
4. Know in detail how amino acids can lose their nitrogen by transamination and deamination reactions and combination of the two; know in detail how nitrogen is disposed of in the organism: the alanine, glutamine, and urea cycles; be able to recite the names of all enzymes, cofactors, and intermediates, and be familiar with their regulatory mechanisms; be able to recognize and draw structures of all intermediates involved in these reactions.
5. Know which amino acids are ketogenic, glucogenic, and both ketogenic and glucogenic; be able to give the degradative pathways of amino acids (however, it is not necessary to memorize the details of tryptophan, tyrosine, histidine, branched-chain amino acid, or lysine catabolism; only the highlights, such as cofactors required, associated pathologies or diagnostic utility, and relationships with other metabolic pathways should be recognized).
6. Know the origin and mode of synthesis of biologically important nitrogenous compounds, such as those listed in Table 20.9.

20.1 NUTRITIONAL ASPECTS OF AMINO ACID AND PROTEIN METABOLISM

20.1.1 Essential Amino Acids

The primary purpose of carbohydrate and fat metabolism is to provide the organism with energy. The third major component of the human diet, the protein, is required primarily for the purpose of replacing tissue protein broken down as part of normal tissue metabolism and to provide the organism with certain required nitrogenous substances. The replacement of tissue protein requires two raw materials that are usually provided by dietary protein: the *essential amino acids*, which are amino acids that cannot be synthesized in the human organism, and nitrogen, which is provided by both the essential and nonessential dietary amino acids. The nitrogen requirement can be supplied by an inorganic nitrogen source, such as ammonium salt.

Essential amino acids are lysine, leucine, isoleucine, valine, methionine, phenylalanine, tryptophan, threonine, and histidine. Their approximate daily requirements are given in Table 20.1. All other amino acids found in the human organism are nonessential; that is, they can be synthesized either from the essential amino acids or from various glycolytic intermeidates and nitrogen. Human proteins are in a constant state of breakdown and biosynthesis, *turnover*. This means that free amino acids are constantly being generated by protein breakdown (*catabolism*) and are then reutilized to rebuild the protein (*anabolism*). Were the reutilization process 100% efficient, very little dietary protein would be required. The recovery of amino acids is not 100% efficient, however; of the approximately 300 g protein degraded per day in a normal human being, 15–30 g is not available for its rebuilding and must be replaced from the outside. This is *obligatory nitrogen loss* and is a result of oxidation of amino acids, loss from the skin, urine, and gastrointestinal tract, and conversion to other nitrogenous substances.

Table 20.1 Essential Amino Acids and Their Daily Requirements (mg/kg Body Weight per Day)

Amino acid	Adults	Infants
Lysine	12	103
Leucine	14	161
Isoleucine	10	70
Valine	10	92
Methionine/cysteine	13	58
Phenylalanine/tyrosine	14	125
Tryptophar	4	17
Threonine	7	87
Histidine	8–12	28

Source: Values taken from Young VR, Bier DM. A kinetic approach to the determination of human amino acid requirements. Nutr Rev 45:289–298, 1987.

Dietary amino acids are a good source of energy in some organs. Thus, almost 50% of oxygen consumed by the liver is used for amino acid oxidation, and in the small intestine it is almost 80%. In the muscle and kidney, however, these figures are only 7 and 12.5%, respectively. Oxidation of amino acids is accomplished by converting them to glycolysis or Krebs cycle intermediates, such as acetyl coenzyme A (acetyl-CoA); α-ketoglutarate, or pyruvate. Because amino acids can be converted to acetyl-CoA, they can also generate storage fat. Amino acid metabolism is thus closely associated with that of carbohydrates and fats. The energy yields of amino acids are provided in Table 20.2.

If adequate amounts of carbohydrate are present in the diet, the amount of dietary protein converted to energy is limited. It is said that carbohydrate has a *sparing* effect on protein. In fasting or starvation, however, protein must be broken down to yield blood glucose and energy. Under such circumstances, more nitrogen will be excreted than taken in, because nitrogen must be removed from amino acids before they can be converted to glucose or glycolysis/Krebs cycle intermediates. The concept of *nitrogen balance* is useful in defining the protein nutritional state of an individual. Normal adults are in zero nitrogen balance; that is, they excrete as much nitrogen as they take in. A positive nitrogen balance exists when less nitrogen is excreted than taken in. This occurs during growth, in pregnancy, or during recovery from a debilitating illness. A negative nitrogen balance is present where more nitrogen is excreted than is taken in, as during starvation or a wasting illness. A normal adult loses some 54 mg nitrogen per kg body weight per day, or an equivalent of 337 mg protein/kg/day. To maintain a zero nitrogen balance, an adult must ingest some 730 mg of an "average" protein per kg body weight per day. A growing child requires 1800–2200 mg protein/kg/day, depending on age.

Not all proteins are equal nutritionally: some may have a good complement of essential amino acids, and others may be deficient in one or more essential

Table 20.2 Net ATP Yields from the Catabolism of Amino Acids

Amino acid	ATP yield (in mol/mol amino acid)
Alanine	16
Arginine	29
Aspartic acid	16
Glutamic acid	25
Histidine	21
Isoleucine	41
Leucine	40
Lysine	35
Methionine	18
Phenylalanine	39
Proline	30
Serine	13
Threonine	21
Tyrosine	42
Valine	20

amino acids. The nutritional value of a protein may be expressed in terms of its biologic value (BV), or net protein utilization (NPU). Both ratings must be determined in a growing rat. BV is defined as the ratio of the protein retained to that absorbed, whereas NPU is the ratio of protein retained to that administered in the diet. NPU, but not BV, depends on the digestibility of the protein, and both depend on its essential amino acid content. For a quick assessment of the nutritional value of a protein, one can compute its chemical score, which depends solely on the content of one of its component essential amino acids (also called the limiting amino acid). Comparison must be made to a reference protein that is considered "ideal," or nearly so. Human milk proteins and egg proteins have been used as such reference substances. Animal proteins usually have high chemical scores, but plant proteins have lower scores. For example, wheat protein is deficient in lysine, corn protein in lysine and tryptophan, and rice protein in lysine and threonine.

In the absence of an adequate protein intake, the subject goes into a negative nitrogen balance, even though calorie intake may be normal. If untreated, a protein deficiency disease called kwashiorkor develops. This is characterized by a failure to grow, skin lesions, edema, and anemia. It is estimated that from 1 to 7% of all preschool children in the developing countries suffer from kwashiorkor, although in the United States it is rare. Kwashiorkor is characterized by low plasma protein levels, as low as 3 g/dl. The main components lost are serum albumin and transferrin, and their levels in plasma may serve as diagnostic tools in suspected protein deficiency. Low plasma protein levels result in the movement of water from extracellular spaces to intracellular compartments, giving rise to the characteristic edematous condition observed in kwashiorkor. It may coexist with a general state of caloric malnutrition called marasmus. Edema is usually not observed in marasmus.

Severe negative nitrogen balance may occasionally have to be corrected by hyperalimentation or total parenteral nutrition (TPN). Intravenous solutions used in TPN contain essential and nonessential amino acids, plus a source of calories in the form of fat and carbohydrate. They "spare" the administered amino acids and allow them to be used for tissue repair. The TPN fluid must also contain all other nutritional factors required for life, including essential fatty acids, vitamins, and minerals. Severe metal and essential fatty acid deficiencies have been observed in situations in which such inclusions had not been made.

20.1.2 Protein Digestion and Absorption

Dietary protein is degraded into free amino acids and small peptides in the stomach and the small intestine. The enzymes involved in this process are *proteinases*, or proteolytic enzymes. *Endopeptidases* are proteinases that catalyze the hydrolysis of peptide linkages anywhere in the protein chain, whereas *exopeptidases* cause the removal of either the N- or the C-terminal amino acids from proteins. Major digestive proteinases are secreted by cells in the form of zymogens, whose activation to the active enzymes occurs via the removal of small peptides. The nature of such cleavage and the sizes of peptides removed from each zymogen are listed in Table 20.3. Both the gastric and pancreatic zymogen secretions are regulated by hormones: gastrins in the stomach and

Table 20.3 Properties of Some Well-Characterized Digestive Proteinases

Enzyme	Zymogen	Source	Size of fragment removed during activation	Means of activation	Specificity
Pepsin	Pepsinogen	Stomach	42 amino acids	HCl and pepsin	Amino group contributed by Tyr, Phe, Leu
Trypsin	Trypsinogen	Pancreas	Hexapeptide	Enterokinase	Carboxyl group contributed by basic amino acids
Rennin	Not known	Stomach	Not known	Not known	Removes glycopeptide from κ-casein
Chymotrypsin	Chymotrypsinogen	Pancreas	Two dipeptides, creating a three-subunit enzyme	Trypsin and chymotrypsin	Carboxyl group contributed by aromatic amino acids
Elastase	Proelastase	Pancreas	Decapeptide (?)	Trypsin	Amino group contributed by small amino acids
Carboxypeptidase A	Procarboxy-peptidase A	Pancreas	Two large fragments, MW 54,000	Trypsin	C-terminal amino acids except basics, Pro and Cys
Carboxypeptidase B	Procarboxy-peptidase B	Pancreas	Uncertain	Trypsin	C-terminal basic amino acids

cholecystokinin in the small intestine. Their mode of action was described in Chapter 16.

The stomach environment is acidic as a result of HCl secretion by the parietal cells. The acidic pH serves to denature many proteins, thus making them susceptible to proteolysis. The chief cells of the stomach produce pepsinogen, which is activated to pepsin by the HCl (see Table 20.3). The optimum pH of peptic activity is around 2, and pepsin is inactivated at neutrality. Another stomach enzyme is rennin or chymosin, which is present in infants but not in adults. It removes a glycopeptide from milk-κ-casein, disrupting the casein micelle and promoting milk protein coagulation and digestion.

The small intestinal tract receives its zymogens from the pancreas via the pancreatic duct. In addition, the pancreas secretes large amounts of bicarbonate, thus neutralizing the stomach contents and creating an environment with pH 7–7.5, the optimum pH of intestinal enzymes. Secretion of bicarbonate is controlled by the hormone secretin (Chapter 16). Pancreatic juice contains the following zymogens: trypsinogen, chymotrypsinogen, proelastase, and procarboxypeptidases A and B. Trypsinogen is activated to the active enzyme trypsin by the intestinal mucosal enzyme enterokinase, and trypsin, in turn, activates the other zymogens: chymotrypsinogen to chymotrypsin, proelastase to elastase, and procarboxypeptidases to carboxypeptidases. These enzymes, in concert with intestinal mucosal enzymes, such as di- and tripeptidases and aminopeptidases, convert peptic protein digests to amino acids or di- and tripeptides, which are then absorbed into the intestinal mucosal cells. Homologies among the various digestive tract enzymes and hormones have been discussed in Chapters 4 and 16.

Free amino acids absorbed into the intestinal mucosal cells are channeled into the portal circulation. Small peptides absorbed are broken down in the intestinal mucosal cells into free amino acids, which are also exported into the portal circulation. There are several amino acid transport systems that serve to bring amino acids across membranes into cells, including the intestinal mucosal cells. Such transport mechanisms exist in intestinal brush borders, kidney tubules, and hepatocytes. The various types of transporters are shown in Table 20.4. Several of these depend on the operation of the Na^+/K^+-ATPase, so that the

Table 20.4 Amino Acid Transport Systems of Eukaryotic Cells

System	Specificity	Dependence on the Na^+/K^+ pump
ASC	Neutral amino acids, especially serine, alanine, and cysteine	Yes
A	Neutral amino acids, especially glycine and alanine	Yes
L	Neutral amino acids, especially branched chain and phenylalanine	No
Gly	Glycine, proline, hydroxyproline	Yes
N	Histidine, asparagine, glutamine	Yes
Anionic	Glutamate, aspartate	Yes
Cationic	Basic amino acids, cystine	No

amino acid is transported into the cells with Na^+. Such systems may thus be classified as active. The L and the cationic amino acid transport systems seem to work via facilitative rather than active processes.

Regulation of amino acid transport is achieved via adaptive processes; that is, the systems respond to specific amino acid levels in their environment. The A and L systems have been studied most thoroughly. The activities of both systems are increased when amino acid levels are low. The V_{max} rises, whereas the K_m remains unchanged. This indicates that the number of transport particles rises but their affinity for amino acids remains the same. For A, all amino acid concentrations must decrease to observe an increase in transport activity. In the L system, the decline of only one amino acid concentration is sufficient. The level of system A activity is regulated at the transcription level (mRNA biosynthesis), whereas that of system L activity is regulated at the translation level (no change in mRNA concentration). In addition to these adaptive effects, the following hormones have been shown to stimulate system A activity: glucagon, glucocorticoids, insulin, growth hormone, and the thyroid hormones.

A number of amino acid transport disorders may be associated with one or several of the systems described in Table 20.4. These are characterized by the excretion of amino acids in the urine but no increase in amino acid levels in the bloodstream. They are usually of hereditary origin. The most common disorder is cystinuria, characterized by the excretion of cystine. Because cystine is only slightly water soluble, cystinuria is often accompanied by the deposition of cystine-containing stones in the genitourinary tract. Cystinuria is apparently caused by a defect in the cationic amino acid transport system. Another disease that affects this system is lysinuric protein intolerance, which is associated with a failure to transport lysine, ornithine, arginine, and citrulline across membranes. Citrulline and ornithine are urea cycle intermediates (see later), and a disruption of their interorgan traffic results in hyperammonemia.

The best known amino acid transport disorder is Hartnup disease, which seems to be the result of a defect in the A system, affecting largely the transport of tryptophan. Intestinal bacteria cleave the unabsorbed tryptophan into indole, among other compounds, which then yield dyes that stain the pediatric patient's diaper blue. Hartnup disease also results in pellagra-like symptoms, because tryptophan is a precursor of NAD^+ in the human organism (see later). Another absorption disorder, iminoglycinuria, is apparently caused by a disorder in the Gly system and results in excessive urinary losses of proline and glycine. The Fanconi syndrome is a disorder, in which a number of amino acids are excreted in the urine along with other compounds. This may be caused by a hereditary kidney tubule defect or, occasionally, kidney damage by toxic substances.

20.2 AMINO ACID POOLS AND PROTEIN TURNOVER

20.2.1 Interorgan Amino Acid Traffic

Portal circulation carries amino acids to the liver, and the general circulation then distributes them throughout the organism. The amino acid content of plasma depends on the dietary state of the individual. After a meal, the free amino acid concentration in plasma increases by about 200–250% compared with that seen in the postabsorptive state, and more than 50% of these amino acids are branched chain. Liver does not extract these amino acids from the portal circulation very efficiently and prefers to retain and metabolize the others, especially the aromatic. The branched-chain amino acids are preferentially extracted from the bloodstream by the muscle. In the postabsorptive state (8 h or more after feeding), the source of plasma amino acids is largely the muscle, not the liver. Muscle releases largely alanine and glutamine, and these then predominate in the bloodstream. Alanine is also contributed by the intestinal mucosal cells and kidney. On the other hand, kidney synthesizes and exports serine, and the intestinal mucosa exports proline.

The brain receives a mixture of amino acids, which must be in balance to allow the brain to function optimally. Such function is disrupted in severe liver disease, and the resulting syndrome is hepatic encephalopathy. The damaged liver does not metabolize sufficient amounts of aromatic amino acids or glucose, causing aromatic amino acid levels in plasma to rise and hyperglycemia. The latter stimulates insulin production, which in turn causes an excessive entry of branched-chain amino acids into muscle, lowering their levels in the bloodstream. The blood aromatic to branched-chain amino acid ratio thus rises, causing an excessive entry of the aromatics into the brain and disrupting its normal neurotransmitter concentrations. The patient may lapse into a coma and can be brought back by administration of valine. The latter apparently competes with the aromatics for entry into the brain, indicating that both types of amino acids may be transported into the brain by the same transport mechanism.

Each tissue, including the bloodstream, has a free amino acid pool. This amounts to a total of about 100 g. By far the largest fraction, 50–80%, is located in muscle. Kidney accounts for about 4%, liver for 10%, and the bloodstream another 4%. Glutamine and glutamate are major components of such pools. Free amino acid pools are in equilibrium with tissue protein. Tissue proteins are in a constant state of turnover, that is, biosynthesis and degradation from and to free amino acids. Only plasma proteins, which are largely synthesized in the liver, are not in equilibrium with the plasma free amino acid pool.

It was stated earlier in this chapter that amino acids may be oxidized to yield energy or that amino acids can give rise to glucose. In doing so, nitrogen must be released and excreted, largely in the urine. Normal amino acid nitrogen excretion forms are urea, ammonium ions, creatinine, and uric acid. Creatinine is formed when the high-energy creatinine phosphate undergoes spontaneous hydrolysis, and the muscle is its principal tissue of origin. Uric acid is a nucleic acid degradation product. Thus, creatinine and uric acid arise from amino acids indirectly compared with urea and ammonium ions, which result from amino acids by more direct routes. The normal nitrogen excretion pattern in human beings is shown in Table 20.5. It has long been recognized that urea and uric acid excretion may rise drastically after a meal, and this phenomenon has been called exogenous nitrogen metabolism. On the other hand, creatinine excretion does not depend on the dietary state of the individual and, for this reason, was deemed to represent an endogenous nitrogen metabolism. From a clinical point of view, the determination of urea and uric acid in the urine is of little value. On the other hand, the determination of fasting serum urea, uric acid, creatinine,

Table 20.5 Excretion of Nitrogenous Substances in a Normal Human Adult Urine in a 24 h Period

Compound	Amount excreted (g)	Total nitrogen excreted (%)
Ammonia	0.7	2.5–4.5
Protein	0–0.1	—
Creatinine	1–1.6	3–4
Creatine	0–0.1	—
Uric acid	0.6–0.7[a]	1–2
Urea	30[a]	80–90
Amino acids	0.6–1.2	1–2

[a]Average diet.
Source: From Varley H. Practical Clinical Biochemistry. New York: Interscience, 1963.

and NH_3/NH_4^+ levels is of great diagnostic significance. These compounds, plus bilirubin and free amino acids, are referred to as serum nonprotein nitrogen (NPN). The interorgan movement of amino acids and their nitrogenous excretion products is summarized in Figure 20.1. Glucose traffic is also indicated for reference purposes.

20.2.2 Protein Degradative Mechanisms

All proteins in the human organism have a finite life span; that is, they are constantly being degraded and resynthesized. This is turnover. Protein turnover was discovered in the 1930s by Schonheimer, Rittenberg, and their coworkers, who found that isotopically labeled dietary amino acids were rapidly incorporated into tissue protein. Protein turnover must therefore have a catabolic and an anabolic arm. When an individual is in a zero nitrogen balance, the two arms are exactly equal. However, one may exceed the other in positive or negative nitrogen balance. Protein anabolism (biosynthesis) was discussed in Chapter 12, and it is clear that a great deal of knowledge exists in regard to this process. Much less is known, however, about the intracellular protein catabolic process.

Protein degradation in tissues is accomplished by lysosomal and nonlysosomal proteinases. Lysosomal proteinases are often termed cathepsins, several of which belong to the serine proteinase homology group. Lysosomal protein degradation is relatively slow and is subject to regulation by hormones: insulin decreases protein degradation, whereas glucagon, glucocorticoids (except in the liver), and thyroxine stimulate it. This apparently occurs via their effects on the gene expression of the lysosomal proteinases. One degradative mechanism involves the recognition of a Lys-Phe-Glu-Arg-Gln (KFERQ) sequence in proteins to be degraded by a specific "binding protein." This binding protein combines with the protein to be degraded (e.g., RNAse), followed by recognition of the complex by a lysosomal membrane receptor. Such proteins are then internalized by the lysosome and degraded.

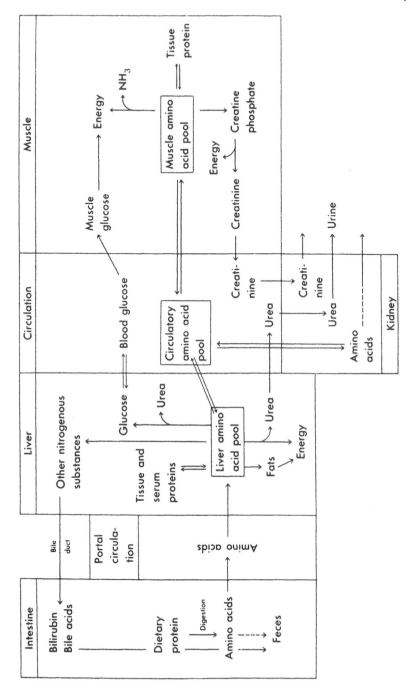

Figure 20.1 Amino acid traffic in the human organism.

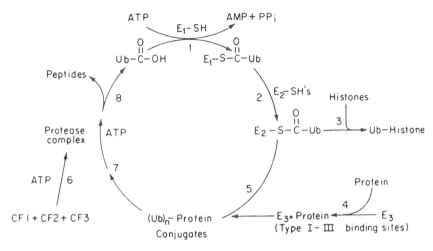

Figure 20.2 Function of ubiquitin in extralysosomal protein degradation. Ub is ubiquitin; E_1, E_2, and E_3 are activating enzymes; CF_1, CF_2, and CF_3 are degradation enzymes. (Reproduced with permission from Hershko A. Ubiquitin-mediated protein degradation. J Biol Chem 263:15237–15240, 1989.)

The nonlysosomal degradation of proteins is rapid and apparently unaffected by hormones. A major system involves a small-molecular-weight protein called ubiquitin, which combines with the protein to be degraded and makes it susceptible to proteolytic attack. This combination involves the carboxyl groups of ubiquitin and the N-terminal groups of proteins. ATP is required for this reaction. Before combining with the protein, ubiquitin must be activated by two enzymes, and this process too requires ATP. Ubiquitin best combines with large and/or denatured proteins. Bulky N-terminal residues, such as tryptophan or leucine, also enhance the reaction with ubiquitin. It is thus the nature of the proteins themselves that determines whether they are degraded by the ubiquitin-mediated system. This process is illustrated in Figure 20.2.

Another nonlysosomal protein degradative system is dependent on calcium ions. They combine with specific protein residues in close proximity to each other: proline, glutamate, serine, and threonine (PEST sequences). It is believed that a calcium-requiring proteinase (a metalloenzyme) recognizes the calcium and combines with it, thus achieving an active status, and then hydrolyzes the protein in the vicinity of the PEST sequence.

20.2.3 Protein Turnover

It was just stated that protein turnover has anabolic and catabolic arms. In a subject in a steady metabolic state, these are exactly equal. It may then be of interest to determine the absolute rates of protein synthesis/degradation. Individual protein turnover rates may be expressed in terms of half-lives ($t_{1/2}$) or fractional catabolic rates or simply in terms of grams protein synthesized and degraded per unit time. The same parameters can be derived for whole-body protein turnover.

Plasma proteins have historically been the easiest to study. Thus, a first-

order catabolic expression describing the disappearance of an injected isotopically labeled plasma protein can be written as

$$\frac{dS_B}{dt} = \frac{-qS_B}{B} \qquad (20.1)$$

where S_B is the specific activity of the protein, B is the total plasma pool of the
protein, and q is a proportionality constant termed the *turnover rate*, or total flux
of the protein per unit time. If we define q/B as k (because q and B are constants),
we can then call k the *fractional catabolic rate*, or the fraction of B turning over per
unit time. If we now replace q/B in Equation (20.1) with k and integrate the
resulting equation, we have

$$\ln S_B = \ln S_B^0 - kt \qquad (20.2)$$

Rearranging this equation, we obtain

$$kt = \ln \frac{S_B^0}{S_B} \qquad (20.3)$$

Now, suppose $S_B = \frac{1}{2} S_B^0$, where S_B^0 is the initial specific activity of protein B at
the time of mixing in vivo; Equation (20.3) gives

$$kt_{1/2} = \ln 2 = 0.69 \qquad (20.4)$$

where $t_{1/2}$ is the *half-life* of the protein, the time it takes for half of the administered radioactivity to disappear or for one-half of the total B to turn over. The
fractional catabolic rate k, on the other hand, indicates the fraction of total B
replaced per unit time. As can be seen from Equation (20.4), one can be calculated from the other.

The half-life of a serum protein may be determined by plotting $\ln S_B$ versus t
in Equation (20.2). Ln S_B^0 is the y intercept, whereas k is the slope of the straight-
line plot. The $t_{1/2}$ can also be read directly from the graph, as shown in Figure
20.3. Human IgG and serum albumin have half-lives of 8–12 and 7–10 days,
respectively, whereas in rats, these figures are about 5 and 3 days. The half-life of
albumin increases when dietary protein decreases, and excess dietary protein
does the opposite. The half-life of IgG does not depend on dietary protein.

The determination of S_B^0 provides a means of estimating B. For instance, if a
rat is injected with 5 mg radioactive serum albumin containing 150,000 dpm/mg
and a subsequent plot of S_B versus time is extrapolated to 1000 dpm/mg on the y
axis, this means that the rat has a total of $5 \times 150,000/1000$, or 750 mg circulating
serum albumin. If the rat weighs 250 g, the rat then has 3 mg albumin per g body
weight. Half-life and pool determinations in circulation can be calculated for any
substance, such as glucose, creatinine, or drugs.

Whole-body protein turnover may be evaluated using the so-called Picou
and Taylor-Roberts model, illustrated in Figure 20.4. In this very simple model,

$$I + C = S + E_T = Q \qquad (20.5)$$

where I is nitrogen (N) entering the total-body metabolic N pool from the diet, C
is that entering from tissue protein, E_T is total N excreted, and Q is total N flux. C
and S are thus representative of total body protein turnover, its catabolic and its
anabolic arms respectively. Experimentally, an isotopically labeled amino acid

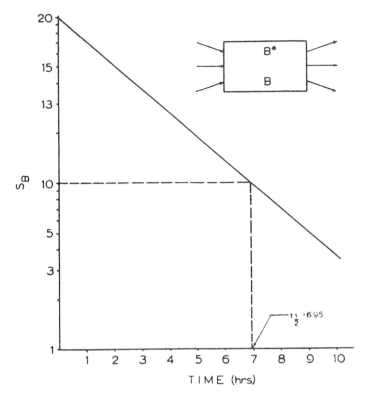

Figure 20.3 First-order disappearance of a radioactive protein B injected into the bloodstream of an animal. Specific activity is on the y axis. The half-life of B is about 7 days. (Reproduced with permission from Zilversmit DB. The design and analysis of isotope experiments. Am J Med 29:832–848, 1960.)

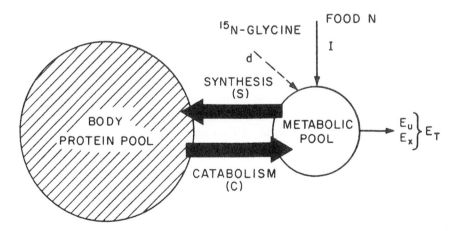

Figure 20.4 The Picou and Taylor-Roberts model for studying whole-body protein turn-over. Nitrogen enters the metabolic pool via I and C, and exits via E_T and S. [^{15}N]-glycine is infused continuously, and represents the label for overall nitrogen entry into the pool. (Reproduced with permission from Steffee WP, Goldsmith RS, Pencharz PB, Scrimshaw NS, Young VR. Dietary protein intake and dynamic aspects of whole body nitrogen metabolism in adult humans. Metabolism 25:281–297, 1976.)

(e.g., [^{15}N]-glycine) is gradually infused into the subject, and ^{15}N excretion is measured. When ^{15}N excretion stabilizes, then the following equation applies:

$$\frac{e_u}{d} = \frac{E_u}{Q} \tag{20.6}$$

Equation (20.6) holds true as long as there is no percholation of [^{15}N]-glycine from the metabolic N pool to tissue protein and back. The [^{15}N]-glycine infused, d, is representative of the sum of I and C, that is, the total N entering the metabolic pool. Isotopic N excreted as urea is indicated by e_u. Because d, e_u, and E_u are measurable, Q can be calculated. Because I is known, C can be calculated by subtracting I from Q. This method yields a C value of 3–4 g protein/kg body weight per day in the human being, or 210–280 g protein synthesized and degraded per day in a 70 kg person. At equilibrium, $S = C$.

20.3 METABOLIC PATHWAYS COMMON TO ALL AMINO ACIDS

20.3.1 Transamination and Decarboxylation

In the preceding sections, attention was focused on amino acid metabolism in the intact animal. We now examine the metabolic pathways of individual amino acids, which take place in the cells of various human tissues. The first reaction in the metabolic pathways of many amino acids is the loss of nitrogen through transamination or deamination. Conversely, the biosynthesis of many non-essential amino acids involves the addition of nitrogen to amino acid precursors: amination and transamination. Decarboxylation, or loss of CO_2, is another reaction shared by many amino acids.

Transamination, often also referred to as aminotransfer, is applied to those enzymatic reactions in which an amino group is exchanged between an amino acid and an α-keto acid. This type of reaction is catalyzed by a group of transferases called transaminases or aminotransferases. They are active in both the cytosol and the mitochondria of most cells. An essential prosthetic group of such enzymes is pyridoxal phosphate, and the reaction is generally of the ping-pong type.

There are numerous transminases, each specific to a given substrate pair. Some may be primarily mitochondrial; others, cytosolic. For example, glutamate-oxaloacetate transminase (GOT), also called aspartate aminotransferase (AST), is primarily a mitochondrial enzyme. AST is extensively used in the diagnosis of heart and liver disorders (see Chapter 5). The AST reaction is represented by Equation (20.7).

$$\text{Glutamate + oxaloacetate} \rightleftarrows \alpha\text{-ketoglutarate + aspartate} \tag{20.7}$$

The most common acceptors of amino groups in transamination reactions are α-ketoglutarate, oxaloacetate, and pyruvate. Transamination reactions are readily reversible. Some amino acids, such as lysine, do not transaminate in the manner indicated in Equation (20.7).

The reason certain amino acids are essential in human diets is because the carbon skeletons cannot be synthesized. It was reasoned formerly that the re-

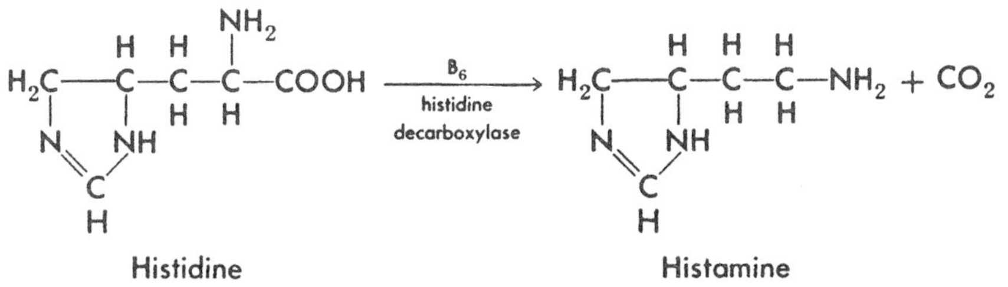

Figure 20.5 Conversion of histidine to histamine by decarboxylation.

quirements for essential amino acids could thus be met by their α-keto analogs and that the respective amino acids could then be generated by transamination with glutamate, aspartate, or alanine. This was indeed found to be the case, especially with glutamate. This discovery has found application in clinical medicine in patients with chronic renal failure. By administering α-keto analogs of essential amino acids, the intake of protein could be minimized and the patients required less dialysis time. Chronic kidney failure patients must undergo frequent hemodialysis to remove nitrogenous waste products, such as urea, from the bloodstream. Any dietary regimen that minimizes nitrogen intake would be extremely beneficial.

Decarboxylation, or loss of the α-carboxyl group as CO_2, is another reaction common to most amino acids. It, too, requires pyridoxal phosphate as a coenzyme. Decarboxylation reactions are irreversible. For example, see Figure 20.5, which shows the decarboxylation of histidine to produce histamine. Table 20.6 lists transamination and decarboxylation products of some representative amino acids.

20.3.2 Deamination Reactions

An amino acid is deaminated when it loses its nitrogen in the form of NH_3 and generates an α-keto acid. It is a redox reaction using NAD^+, FAD, or FMN as cofactors, and it may occur in either the mitochondria or the cytosol. The most potent L amino acid deaminase is glutamate dehydrogenase, which catalyzes the reaction

$$\text{Glutamate} \xrightleftharpoons[\quad]{NAD^+ \quad NADH + H^+} \text{alpha-ketoglutarate} + NH_3 \qquad (20.8)$$

Glutamate dehydrogenase is a zinc-containing allosteric enzyme with a molecular weight of nearly 280,000. It is affected by several modulators, most notably ATP (negative effector) and ADP (positive effector). Thus, when the energy charge is low, glutamate dehydrogenase generates NADH, and the α-ketoglutarate produced may enter the Krebs cycle to amplify this effect.

In addition to glutamate dehydrogenase, cells contain various amino acid deaminases, most often referred to as L-amino acid oxidases. In addition, there is the very active glycine oxidase, which also deaminates D amino acids. The L amino acid oxidases utilize FMN as a cofactor, whereas glycine oxidase utilizes FAD. The $FMNH_2$ generated by L amino acid oxidases, unlike $FADH_2$, cannot enter the oxidative phosphorylation system and, instead, undergoes reoxidation

Table 20.6 Transamination and Decarboxylation Products of Some Amino Acids

Amino acid	Transamination product	Decarboxylation product	Notes
Lysine	Does not transaminate	Cadaverine	Cadaverine is toxic and has odor of rotting flesh
Ornithine	Glutamic-γ-semialdehyde	Putrescine	Putrescine is toxic and has the odor of putrid flesh
Histidine	Imidazole pyruvic acid	Histamine	Histamine is a mediator of the allergic response
Phenylalanine	Phenylpyruvic acid	Phenylethylamine	Phenylpyruvic acid is found in the serum of patients with phenylketonuria
Cysteine	Mercaptopyruvic acid	Cysteamine, taurine[a]	Cysteamine is a component of CoA Taurine is a component of conjugated bile salts
Glutamic acid	α-Ketoglutarate	γ-Aminobutyric acid (GABA)	GABA is a neurotransmitter
Tryptophan	Indolepyruvic acid	Serotonin[b]	Serotonin is a neurotransmitter
Serine	Hydroxypyruvic acid	Ethanolamine	Ethanolamine is a component of phosphatidyletha-nolamines

[a]After oxidation of the –SH group to $-SO_3^-$.
[b]Also called 5-hydroxytryptamine; in addition to being decarboxylated, tryptophan is also hydroxylated to give serotonin.

with oxygen to generate hydrogen peroxide, as shown by Equations (20.9) and (20.10), for example:

$$\text{Leucine} \underset{}{\overset{\text{FMN} \quad \text{FMNH}_2}{\rightleftharpoons}} \alpha\text{-ketoisocaproic acid} + NH_3 \tag{20.9}$$

$$FMNH_2 + O_2 \rightarrow FMN + H_2O_2 \tag{20.10}$$

The hydrogen peroxide formed is degraded through the action of catalase, or, less often, by one of the peroxidases. Serine and threonine lose nitrogen via dehydratases (lyases; see Figures 20.12 and 20.13).

Glycine oxidase converts glycine to glyoxylic acid according to Equation (20.11). Its action on D-amino acids may be fortuitous, but this provides the organism with the means of dealing with them.

$$\text{Glycine} \underset{}{\overset{\text{FAD} \quad \text{FADH}_2}{\rightleftharpoons}} \underset{\text{Glyoxilic acid}}{H-\overset{\overset{\displaystyle O}{\|}}{C}-COOH} + NH_3 \tag{20.11}$$

The FMN-dependent L-amino acid oxidases are relatively sluggish, and a more rapid way of deaminating amino acids other than glutamate and glycine is to combine transamination with α-ketoglutarate, then deaminating the glutamate formed via glutamate dehydrogenase:

$$\text{Alanine} + \alpha\text{-ketoglutarate} \leftrightarrows \text{pyruvate} + \text{glutamate} \tag{20.12}$$

$$\text{Glutamate} + NAD^+ \leftrightarrows \alpha\text{-ketoglutarate} + NH_3 + NADH + H^+ \tag{20.13}$$

Net:

$$\text{Alanine} + NAD^+ \leftrightarrows \text{Pyruvate} + NH_3 + NADH + H^+ \tag{20.14}$$

Reaction (20.12) is catalyzed by glutamate-pyruvate transaminase (GPT), also known as alanine aminotransferase, and Equation (20.13) is catalyzed by glutamate dehydrogenase. Note that these reactions are completely reversible. The reverse of deamination, for example, if one wanted to synthesize alanine from ammonia and pyruvate, is *amination*.

20.4 DISPOSAL OF AMMONIA

20.4.1 The Alanine Cycle

Transmination and deamination-amination reactions play a vital role in the metabolic interrelationships of muscle and liver. It has been observed that blood alanine levels are increased in exercising individuals. The origin of alanine is the muscle, and its destination is the liver. Alanine arises in the muscle by transamination of amino acids (e.g., the branched chain) with pyruvate. Their carbon skeletons then become oxidized to yield energy. The resulting alanine is exported into the bloodstream and extracted from there by the liver. In the liver, alanine loses its nitrogen, most likely by reactions depicted by Equations (20.12) through (20.14), and the resulting pyruvate is then converted to glucose via gluconeogenesis. The glucose is returned to the muscle, completing the *alanine cycle*. The ammonia generated is converted into urea (see later). Alanine thus serves as a nontoxic vehicle for removing ammonia from the muscle and other tissues. The alanine cycle is in many ways similar to the Cori cycle (see Chapters 17 and 18). Both cycles are illustrated in Figure 20.6.

The reason ammonia must be removed from tissues is its toxicity above concentrations of 1 mM. This is largely a result of its effect on the Krebs cycle: as

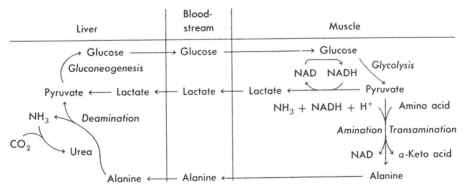

Figure 20.6 The alanine and Cori cycles. Amination of pyruvate or deamination of alanine assumes the participation of glutamate dehydrogenase as shown in Equation (20.13). In the muscle, transamination of pyruvate to alanine predominates over amination.

tissue NH_3 concentrations rise, the glutamate dehydrogenase reaction equilibrium is shifted toward glutamate biosynthesis from α-ketoglutarate. The latter then becomes unavailable for participation in the Krebs cycle. Urea is a relatively nontoxic substance generated from ammonia of whatever source in the liver. Some ammonia may also be excreted directly into the urine (see later).

20.4.2   The Glutamine Cycle

Another major system for removing ammonia from tissues is the glutamine cycle. It is active in the muscle, and in the brain, the astrocyte cells are especially active in glutamine biosynthesis. Glutamine is synthesized from glutamate and NH_3 by glutamine synthetase using ATP as an energy source:

$$\text{Glutamate} + \text{ATP} \rightarrow \gamma\text{-glutamylphosphate} + \text{ADP} \qquad (20.15)$$

$$\gamma\text{-glutamyl phosphate} + NH_3 \rightarrow \text{glutamine} + P_i \qquad (20.16)$$

A similar, although less prevalent reaction catalyzes the conversion of aspartic acid to the corresponding amide, asparagine. The enzyme involved is asparagine synthetase. Glutamine is exported by the tissues in which it is formed into the bloodstream, from which it is extracted by the kidney and intestinal mucosal cells. Both tissues are rich in glutaminase, which causes the hydrolysis of glutamine to glutamate and ammonia. The ammonia may pick up a proton to be converted to the ammonium ion, and, if in the kidney cells, is excreted in the urine. Thus, most, if not all, urinary NH_4^+ is the product of the glutaminase reaction. Excretion of the ammonium ion provides a means for the organism to excrete protons and to spare the sodium and potassium electrolytes.

In kidney cells, the glutamate generated by glutaminase may be metabolized to carbon dioxide and water and the CO_2 returned to the bloodstream in the form of bicarbonate. Some glutamate may be returned to its tissue of origin, completing the glutamine cycle (Figure 20.7). In intestinal mucosal cells, glutamate is used largely for the synthesis of proline, whereas the ammonia is channeled into the liver via the portal circulation. The portal circulation also carries ammonia generated by bacterial action in the intestinal lumen and resorbed into the intestinal muscosal cells. The liver thus receives large amounts of ammonia from both the alanine cycle and the portal circulation in addition to that produced by its own metabolic processes. All the ammonia is processed into urea.

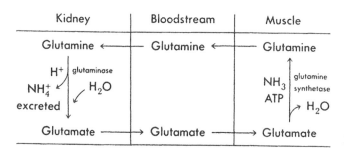

Figure 20.7   The glutamine cycle linking muscle and kidney.

20.4.3 The Urea Cycle

In humans and many other vertebrates, ammonia arising from deamination reactions or other sources is excreted in the form of urea. These animals are called *ureotelic*. Fish excrete nitrogen in the form of ammonium ions and are therefore *ammonotelic*. Animals that need to conserve water excrete their nitrogen in the form of crystalline uric acid. They are *uricotelic*, or purinotelic. One often finds animals that convert uric acid to allantoin via uric acid oxidase (Figure 20.8). Allantoin is more water soluble than uric acid. Uric acid oxidase is absent from primates.

The overall reaction for urea production is

$$2NH_3 + HCO_3^- + H^+ \rightarrow \underset{\text{Urea}}{NH_2-\overset{\overset{\displaystyle O}{\|}}{C}-NH_2} + H_2O \tag{20.17}$$

NH_3 is the actual substrate for the first reaction in the urea cycle. The overall process requires an energy equivalent of four ATP per molecule of urea formed. The first two reactions in the urea cycle (Figure 20.9) take place in the mitochondria, and the rest takes place in the cytosol. Liver is the only organ that contains all the urea cycle enzymes in sufficient quantity to generate substantial quantities of urea. However, other organs may have individual urea cycle enzymes, so there is an extensive traffic of urea cycle intermediates from one organ to another.

The initial urea cycle mitochondrial reaction is catalyzed by carbamoyl (carbamyl) phosphate synthetase I (CPS I). This is an allosteric enzyme, which accounts for as much as 20% of all mitochondrial protein and is inactive without a positive effector, N-acetylglutamate. N-acetylglutamate is synthesized in the cytosol from acetyl-CoA and glutamate via N-acetylglutamate synthase. It is activated by high cellular arginine and glutamate levels. Two ATP equivalents are required in this reaction. An enzyme similar to CPS I, called CPS II, is present in the cytosol and is concerned with the biosynthesis of carbamoylphosphate used in pyrimidine biosynthesis (see Chapter 10). Instead of ammonia, CPS II uses glutamine as a nitrogen source and is not activated by N-acetylglutamate.

The second reaction in the urea cycle is the condensation of carbamoylphosphate with ornithine, a basic amino acid not found in proteins but readily formed from glutamate (see later). The product is another basic amino acid called

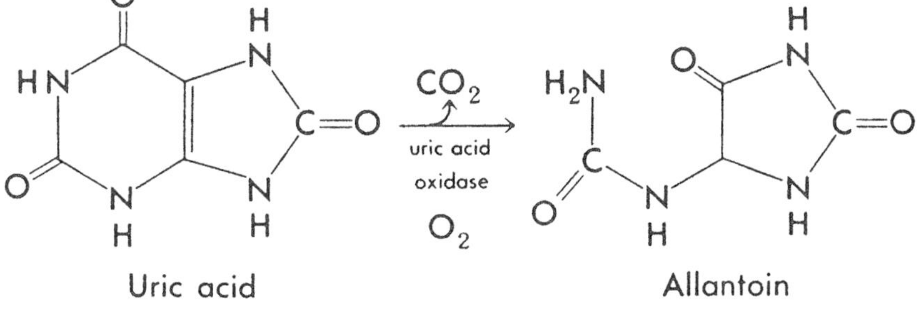

Figure 20.8 Conversion of uric acid to allantoin with uric acid oxidase.

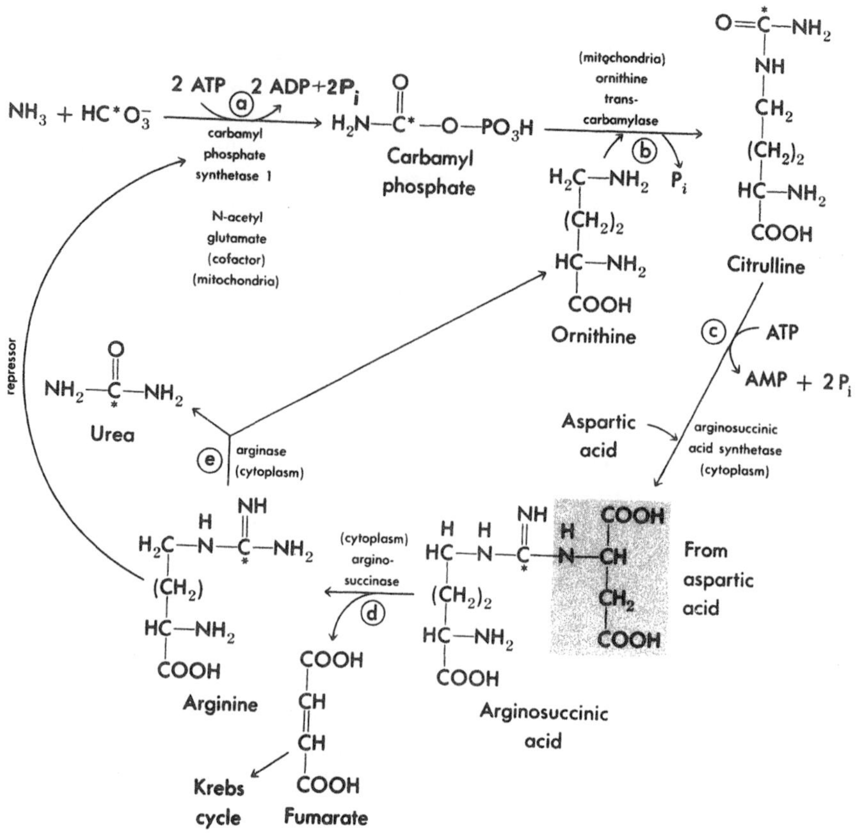

Figure 20.9 The urea cycle. The bicarbonate is marked by an asterisk to facilitate its tracing through the pathway; a, b, c, d, and e indicate urea cycle lesions, hyper-ammonemia I and II, citrullinemia, arginosuccinic aciduria, and argininemia, respectively.

citrulline, which is not found in proteins either. Citrulline is exported from the mitochondria into the cytosol, where it condenses with a molecule of aspartic acid to form arginosuccinate. This is an energy-requiring process. Arginosuc-cinate is then split into arginine and fumarate by arginosuccinase (arginosuc-cinate lyase). The last reaction of the urea cycle involves the degradation of arginine to urea and ornithine. The latter is then transported into the mitochon-drion to complete the cycle. Urea diffuses into the bloodstream, from which it is extracted by the kidneys to be excreted in the urine.

Note that the second nitrogen atom of urea originates from the amino group of aspartate. Cytosolic amino acid nitrogen is the source of aspartate nitrogen, as shown in Equation (20.18) through (20.20):

$$\text{Amino acid + oxaloacetate} \xrightarrow[\text{transamination}]{} \alpha\text{-keto acid + aspartate} \qquad (20.18)$$

$$\text{Aspartate} \xrightarrow[\text{urea cycle}]{} \text{fumarate} \xrightarrow[\text{Krebs cycle}]{} \text{malate} \qquad (20.19)$$

$$\text{Malate} \xrightarrow[\text{Krebs cycle}]{\text{NAD}^+ \quad \text{NADH} + \text{H}^+} \text{oxaloacetate} \tag{20.20}$$

The oxaloacetate produced may now repeat the cycle. Alternatively, the fumarate produced in the urea cycle may enter the Krebs cycle to become metabolized or to yield glucose. Depletion of oxaloacetate, for example under conditions of starvation or fasting or in malonate poisoning of the Krebs cycle, limits the extent of urea formation.

A number of inherited disorders of urea cycle metabolism are known. Hyperammonemia I and II are associated with CPS I and ornithine transcarbamylase deficiencies, respectively. Citrullinemia, arginosuccinic aciduria, and argininemia are associated with low levels of arginosuccinic acid synthetase, arginosuccinase, and arginase, respectively. All such disorders are associated with mental retardation, convulsions, and failure to thrive if not treated. Treatment involves the feeding of low-protein diets or, experimentally, the administration of α-keto analogs of essential amino acids instead of protein.

The function of urea cycle is regulated in part by cellular levels of N-acetylglutamate as stated above, in part by availability of NH_3, and in part by the adjustment of all five urea cycle enzyme levels in the cell. High-protein diets cause an increase in the activity of all five enzymes. Because their mRNAs are also increased, this regulation must occur at the transcriptional level. One may imagine that this effect is brought about by hormones. However, injections of glucagon and corticosteroids do not bring about a concerted response from the five enzymes. At least for CPS I and arginosuccinate synthetase, cAMP is a powerful transcription promoter. Steroids apparently work in the same fashion, although through a different mechanism.

It has been stated that the liver is the principal urea producer, yet several urea cycle intermediates are produced by other organs as well and must be moved to other organs to be processed. Thus, intestinal mucosal cells are able to convert ornithine to citrulline, but citrulline cannot be converted to arginine in that location. Citrulline must be transported to either the kidney or liver, where conversions to arginine and urea are possible. Kidney, on the other hand, cannot convert ornithine to citrulline.

In addition to being the principal NH_3 detoxifier, the urea cycle is also believed to play a crucial role in regulating the acid-base balance of the organism. It has been argued (without consensus) that the organism produces either an excess of protons (acid) or an excess of bicarbonate (base), and proponents of both sides of the issue have invoked the urea cycle as the means by which disaster is averted. What seems to be certain, however, is that amino acid catabolism results in the production of excess acid in the form of sulfuric and hydrochloric acids. The protons produced react with bicarbonate via the carbonic anhydrase reaction to form carbon dioxide, and the latter is then lost through the lungs. The bicarbonate lost is replaced in the kidneys by the metabolism of glutamate, which arises there through operation of the glutamine cycle. A loss of kidney function results in metabolic acidosis, because the kidney cannot replenish the bicarbonate lost through amino acid catabolism. Note also that the operation of the urea cycle diminishes in acidosis. This is because the substrate of CPS I is NH_3. Normally, the NH_4^+/NH_3 ratio is about 40 ($pK = 9$), but in acidosis, this ratio becomes much higher. The availability of ammonia, as opposed to ammonium ion, thus has a profound effect on the operation of the urea cycle. Bicarbonate concentration variations seem to have little effect, because CPS I is saturated with bicarbonate under normal circumstances.

20.5 FATE OF THE CARBON SKELETON OF AMINO ACIDS

20.5.1 General Considerations

In addition to being incorporated into tissue proteins, amino acids, after losing their nitrogen atoms by deamination and/or transamination, may be catabolized to yield energy or to form glucose. Conversely, the nonessential amino acids may be synthesized from carbohydrate metabolism intermediates and ammonia or from essential amino acids. This section is devoted to the mechanisms of such metabolic processes and their interrelationships with carbohydrate and lipid metabolic pathways.

From the point of view of their catabolic fates, amino acids may be divided into three categories: those that can give rise to glucose and glycogen, those that can give rise to acetyl-CoA and acetoacetate and hence ketone bodies, and those that can give rise to both: the *glucogenic, ketogenic* and both *glucogenic and ketogenic*. Table 20.7 lists the amino acids in each category, and Figure 20.10 shows the carbohydrate and fat metabolism intermediates generated by each amino acid. As with acetyl-CoA, ketogenic amino acids are not capable of generating glucose on a net basis. Only the glucogenic and the glucogenic-ketogenic amino acids may do so. All three types of amino acids can give rise to storage fat.

20.5.2 Metabolism of Serine, Glycine, Threonine, and Cysteine

Both serine and glycine are nonessential amino acids. They are also interconvertible. They can be obtained from the diet or, in the case of serine, from the

Table 20.7 Classification of Amino Acids on the Basis of Their Metabolic Fate

Glucogenic	Ketogenic	Glucogenic and ketogenic
Alanine	Leucine	Isoleucine
Glutamic acid	Lysine	Phenylalanine
Aspartic acid		Tyrosine
Methionine		Tryptophan
Cysteine/cystine		
Arginine		
Histidine		
Serine		
Glycine		
Threonine		
Proline/hydroxyproline		
Valine		

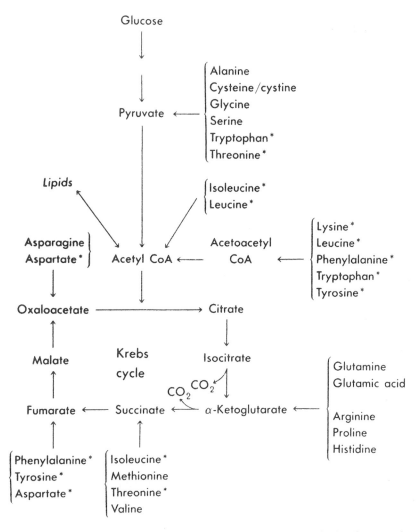

Figure 20.10 Entrance of amino acids into the Krebs cycle and glycolysis pathways. Amino acids that can yield more than one intermediate are marked by an asterisk.

glycolysis intermediate 3-phosphoglyceric acid (Figure 20.11). The major source of glycine besides the diet is serine. The reversible conversion of serine to glycine requires tetrahydrofolate (THF; see Chapter 6), and it is catalyzed by serine hydroxymethyltransferase:

Serine + THF ⇆ glycine + 5,10-methylene THF   (20.21)

This reaction is readily reversible. Another means of metabolizing serine, which accounts for its glucogenic character, as well as that of glycine, is the conversion of serine to pyruvate, as indicated in Figure 20.12. This reaction is catalyzed by serine dehydratase. A similar enzyme, threonine dehydratase, converts threonine to α-ketobutyrate, and the latter is then converted to propionyl-CoA, as indicated in Figure 20.13. Another similar enzyme, cysteine desulfhydrase, con-

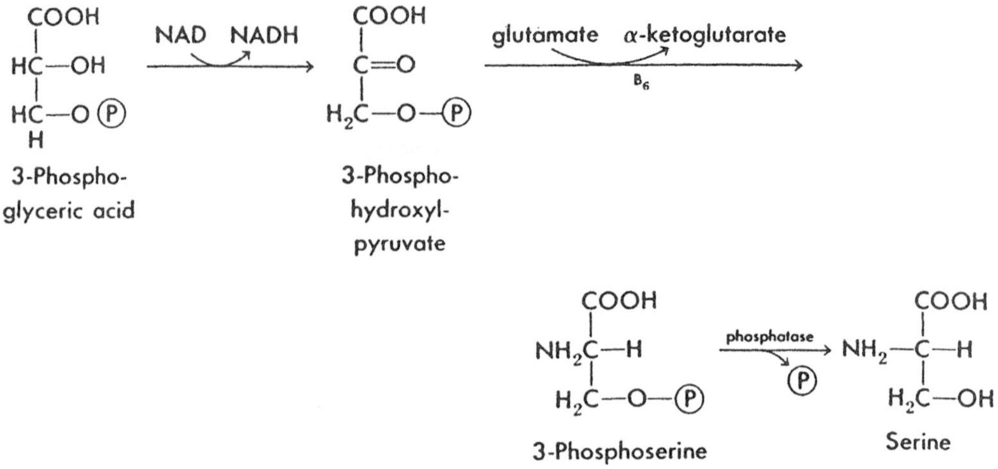

Figure 20.11 Conversion of 3-phosphoglyceric acid to serine. 3-Phosphoglyceric acid originates from dihydroxyacetone phosphate, a glycolysis intermediate.

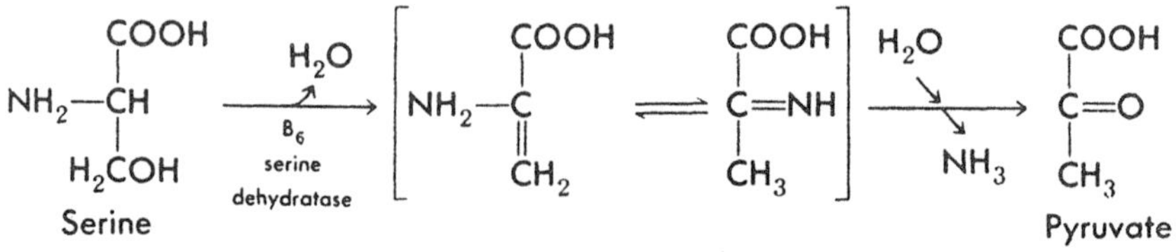

Figure 20.12 Conversion of serine to pyruvate.

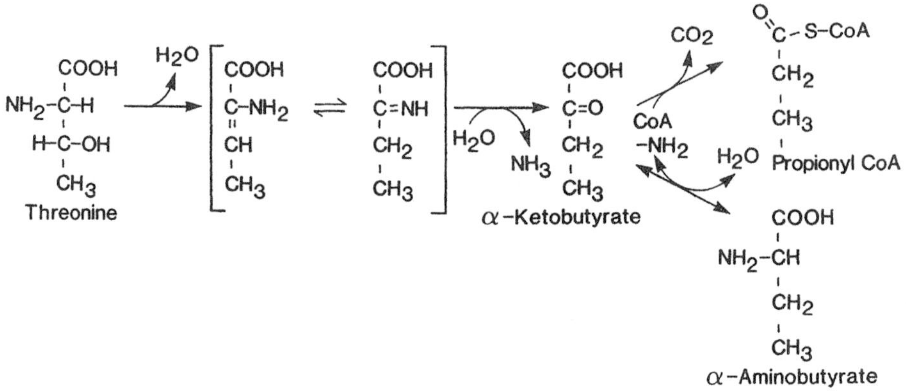

Figure 20.13 Conversion of threonine to α-aminobutyrate and propionyl-CoA.

verts cysteine to pyruvate, as shown in Figure 20.14. Both threonine and cysteine are glucogenic, because propionyl-CoA can be converted to succinate, as shown in Chapter 19. Succinate gives rise to oxaloacetate, a gluconeogenesis intermediate. Pyruvate, too, is converted to glucose via the gluconeogenesis pathway (see Chapter 18). α-Ketobutyrate may be aminated to α-aminobutyrate,

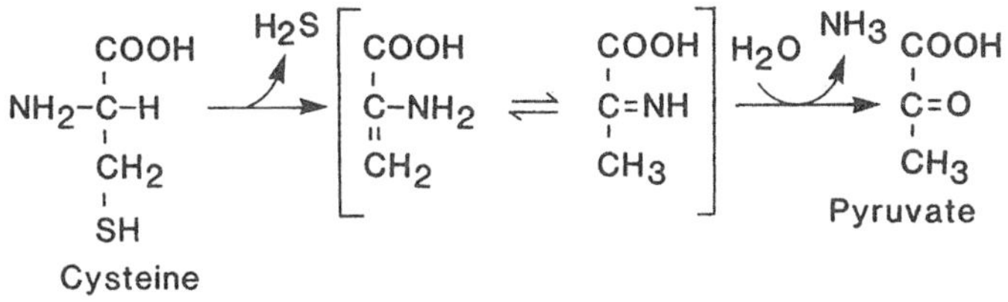

Figure 20.14 Conversion of cysteine to pyruvate. The H_2S is eventually oxidized to SO_4^{2-}.

and the latter is found in both the circulation and various tissues. However, its only fate is to be converted back to α-ketobutyrate and metabolized via propionyl-CoA.

The hydrogen sulfide released by cysteine desulfhydrase (Figure 20.14) is oxidized to sulfate, which is largely excreted in the urine. Some sulfate may become activated by ATP, however, to give active sulfate. This compound participates in various sulfation reactions, such as those associated with connective tissue proteoglycan biosynthesis. The oxidation of H_2S is a stepwise process. An especially interesting enzyme in this pathway is sulfite oxidase, which converts sulfite to sulfate. It is among a handful of mammalian enzymes that contain molybdenum as a prosthetic group. Sulfate is not formed in a genetic disorder characterized by the absence of sulfite oxidase.

Returning now to glycine: it was stated earlier that glycine and serine are interconvertible. The major pathway for glycine catabolism, however, appears to be its degradation to CO_2 and a THF-bound one-carbon unit. This reaction is catalyzed by glycine synthase, also known as the glycine cleavage enzyme:

$$\text{Glycine} + \text{THF} \xrightarrow[]{\text{NAD}^+ \quad \text{NADH} + \text{H}^+} \text{5,10-methylene THF} + CO_2 + NH_3$$

$$(20.22)$$

The one-carbon unit may in turn be converted to carbon dioxide and thus generate 9 mol ATP per mol glycine degraded (see Chapter 6). In an inborn error of glycine metabolism, nonketotic hyperglycinemia, glycine synthase is apparently absent, with the result that glycine levels in the blood are increased and glycine is excreted in the urine. The interrelationships among the serine and glycine metabolic pathways are summarized in Figure 20.15.

A minor pathway of glycine metabolism is its conversion to glyoxalate via glycine oxidase [see Equation (20.11)]. Glyoxylate may in turn be converted to formaldehyde and CO_2, followed by a combination of formaldehyde with THF to form 5,10-methylene THF. Another pathway for glyoxylate is to give rise to oxalate via oxidation with FAD and an oxidase. A third pathway is to combine with α-ketoglutarate to form α-hydroxy-β-ketoadipic acid and CO_2. This reaction is catalyzed by α-ketoglutarate-glyoxylate carboligase. The α-hydroxy-β-ketoadipic acid eventually yields CO_2 and α-ketoglutarate, thus disposing of the glyoxylate as CO_2 (see Figure 20.16). In a genetic disorder called oxaluria I, the α-ketoglutarate-glyoxylate carboligase is apparently absent and much of the glyoxylate is instead channeled into oxalate production. Patients with this disor-

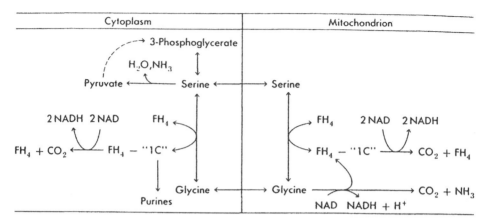

Figure 20.15 Interrelationships between the serine and glycine metabolic pathways. FH$_4$-"C" indicates 5,10-methylenetetrahydrofolate. (Adapted from Yoshida T, Kikuchi G. Comparative study on major pathways of glycine and serine catabolism in vertebrate livers. J Biochem 72:1503–1516, 1972.)

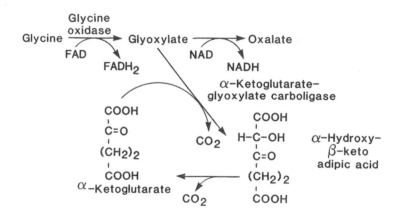

Figure 20.16 Oxidation of glycine to oxalate and CO_2.

der excrete large amounts of oxalic acid in urine and show a high incidence of calcium oxalate stone formation in the genitourinary tract.

Additional reactions of glycine include its ability to become conjugated with bile acids to form conjugated bile salts (see Chapter 19), formation of heme (Chapter 7), formation of purine nucleotides (Chapter 10), formation of creatine (see later), and the formation of hippuric acid from benzoic acid. In the last case, an amide linkage is formed between the carboxyl group of benzoic acid and the amino group of glycine.

20.5.3 Metabolism of Methionine and Biosynthesis of Cysteine

A large proportion of sulfur present in the human organism is derived from dietary methionine and cystine/cysteine. Only methionine is essential, although cystine and cysteine exert potent sparing effects on the methionine requirement. Methionine is thus essential, not because of its sulfur content but because the organism cannot synthesize its carbon chain. The metabolism of methionine begins with its condensation with ATP to form S-adenosylmethionine (SAM; Figure 20.17). The enzyme involved in this reaction is methionine adenosyltransferase. The methyl group becomes "activated" and may be transferred to a number of receptors. Thus, in the biosynthesis of phosphatidylcholine from phosphatidylethanolamine (Chapter 19), ethanolamine acts as the methyl group acceptor:

$$3SAM + \text{phosphatidylethanolamine} \rightarrow \text{phosphatidylcholine} +$$
$$3S\text{-adenosylhomocysteine} \qquad\qquad\qquad\qquad (20.23)$$

Other well-known methyl group acceptors are guanidoacetic acid, the precursor of creatine, norepinephrine, the precursor of epinephrine, lysine, the precursor of carnitine, and many proteins that are modified posttranslationally by methylation. Methyl group transfer using SAM as the donor is often referred to as transmethylation. SAM complements THF-bound one-carbon units as a one-carbon donor in various metabolic pathways. Although the two types of one-carbon units are not exchangeable, they are, nevertheless, interconvertible, as was discussed in Chapter 6 and as is shown in Figure 20.17. It is seen that the methyl group of methionine can be generated from THF-bound methyl groups in the presence of vitamin B_{12} and with homocysteine acting as the methyl group acceptor. Another means of recovering methionine from homocysteine is to use betaine as the methyl donor (Figure 20.18). Additional means of exchanging methionine-derived methyl groups with THF-bound one-carbon units is through the metabolism of choline, as is also shown in Figure 20.18. Note that two of the three methyl groups of choline end up as THF-bound one-carbon units, whereas the third is transferred to homocysteine.

There are two pyridoxal phosphate-requiring enzymes in the homocysteine degradation pathway, which are associated with genetic diseases. In homocystinuria, cystathionine synthase is defective, and large amounts of homocystine are excreted in the urine. Some homocystinurics respond to the administration of large doses of vitamin B_6. In cystathioninuria, cystathionase is either defective or absent. These patients excrete cystathionine in the urine. Cystathionase is often underactive in the newborns with immature livers, and cysteine and cystine become essential amino acids. Human milk protein is especially rich in cysteine, presumably to prepare the newborn for such a contingency.

Methionine is intimately related to lipid metabolism in the liver. Methionine deficiency is one of the causes of the fatty liver syndrome. Lack of methionine prevents the methylation of phosphatidylethanolamine to phosphatidylcholine, resulting in an ability by the liver to build and export very low density lipoprotein. The syndrome can be treated by the administration of choline, and for this reason, choline has often been referred to as the lipotropic factor.

The carbon skeleton of methionine is converted to α-ketobutyrate (Figure 20.17), which is catabolized to propionyl-CoA and then to succinate. The sulfur atom is transferred to serine in the cystathionase reaction to yield cysteine. Cysteine is nonessential, because it can be derived from serine and methionine.

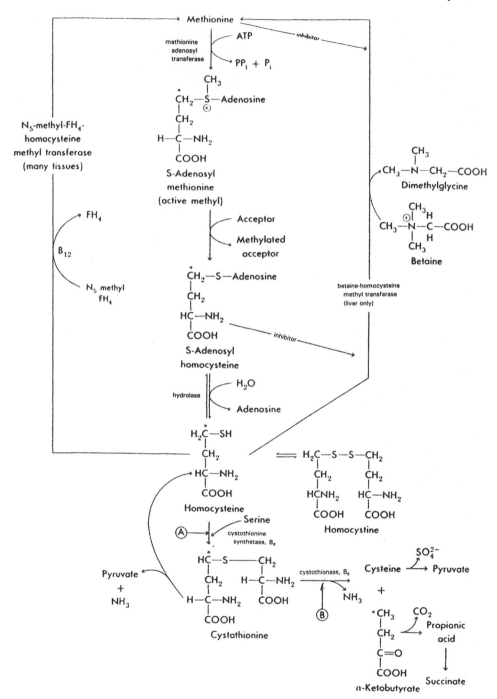

Figure 20.17 Metabolism of methionine. FH_4 indicates tetrahydrofolate. A and B indicate defects in homocystinuria and cystathioninuria, respectively, and the asterisk indicates the fate of the methionine carbon skeleton.

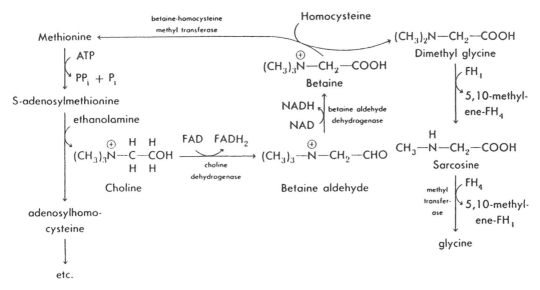

Figure 20.18 Metabolism of choline, indicating the fate of each methyl residue originally derived from SAM. FH_4 is tetrahydrofolate.

As already pointed out, cysteine may be metabolized to pyruvate, or it can be oxidized to cystine. It can also be converted to taurine, $NH_3^+-CH_2-CH_2-SO_3^-$. Taurine is obtained by oxidizing the –SH group of cysteine and losing the carboxyl group of decarboxylation. Taurine is quite abundant in most tissues and is said to be the most abundant "amino acid" of the human organism. One of its functions is to conjugate primary bile acids (Chapter 19).

20.5.4 Metabolism of Alanine, the Acidic Amino Acids, and Imino Acids

Alanine, aspartate, and glutamate are catabolized by being converted to pyruvate, oxaloacetate, and α-ketoglutarate, respectively, by deamination and/or transamination. Conversely, they may be biosynthesized from their respective α-keto analogs. Asparagine and glutamine, whose biosynthesis was discussed earlier in this chapter, are metabolized by being converted to aspartic and glutamic acids by the action of asparaginase and glutaminase, respectively.

Glutamic acid is also the precursor of nonessential amino acids proline, hydroxyproline, and ornithine. Biosynthesis of proline occurs largely in the intestinal mucosal cells and is irreversible. Proline is catabolized back to glutamate by a separate liver and kidney pathway, as shown in Figure 20.19. Hydroxyproline is found almost entirely in collagen, whereas ornithine is a urea cycle intermediate that must be constantly replenished from glutamate because of its participation in the biosynthesis of arginine. Ornithine transaminase (Figure 20.19), which interconverts ornithine and glutamic acid semialdehyde, is apparently defective in gyrate atrophy, a serious retinal disorder. In such patients, blood ornithine levels are elevated. Hydroxyproline may be degraded to

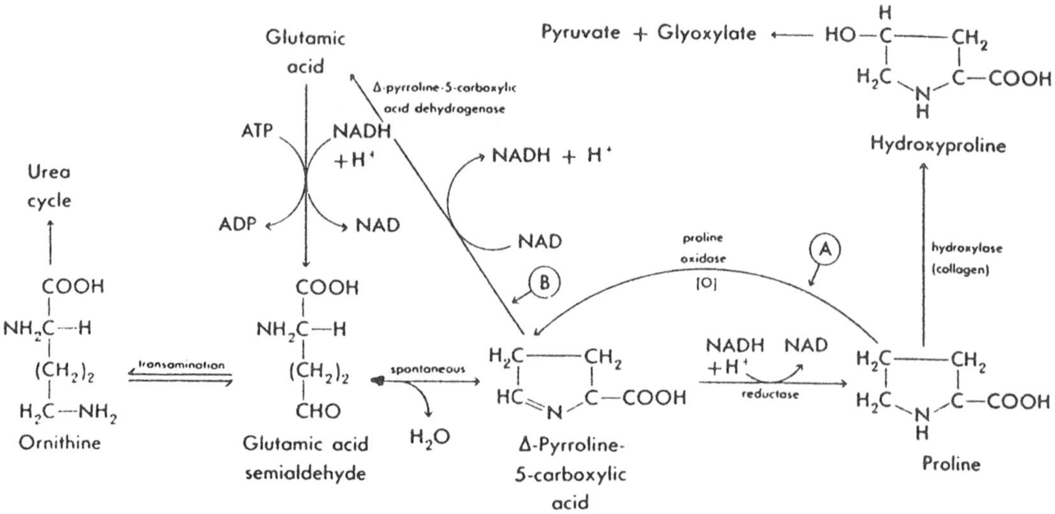

Figure 20.19 Biosynthesis and degradation of proline, hydroxyproline and ornithine. Proline oxidase and δ-pyrroline-5-carboxylic acid dehydrogenase are both mitochondrial enzymes. A and B indicate defects in hyperprolinemia I and II, respectively.

pyruvate and glyoxylate, although much of it is excreted in the urine in the form of small peptides that are breakdown products of collagen.

20.5.5 Metabolism of Branched-Chain Amino Acids

The first two steps in the degradation of leucine, isoleucine, and valine are identical: they are transaminated to their α-keto analogs and then decarboxylated. A common transaminase removes the nitrogen from leucine and isoleucine, whereas the same dehydrogenase decarboxylates all three α-keto analogs. The mechanism of action of this enzyme is very similar to that of pyruvate dehydrogenase. It is absent in the hereditary maple syrup urine disease, which is characterized by the excretion of branched-chain amino acid α-keto analogs in the urine. The latter and their various reaction products give the affected urine its characteristic maple syrup odor.

The degradation of branched-chain amino acids is shown in Figure 20.20. Note that leucine metabolism produces β-hydroxy-β-methylglutaryl (HMG)-CoA as an intermediate, which was encountered in the cholesterol and ketone body biosynthetic pathways (Chapter 19). It is also obvious that valine produces only propionyl-CoA and is therefore glucogenic. Isoleucine produces both acetyl-CoA and propionyl-CoA and thus both ketogenic and glucogenic. Leucine is entirely ketogenic, because it produces only ketone body precursors. The degradation of branched-chain amino acids occurs in the mitochondria.

A minor pathway of valine catabolism is concerned with its conversion to leucine. Because leucine is an essential amino acid, its synthesis from valine is clearly not sufficiently significant to meet the organism's daily demand for leucine. In this reaction, isobutyryl-CoA (see Figure 20.20) is condensed with a molecule of acetyl-CoA to give β-ketoisocaproate, which is then transaminated to give β-*leucine*. A mutase is then used to convert β-leucine to leucine. This mutase

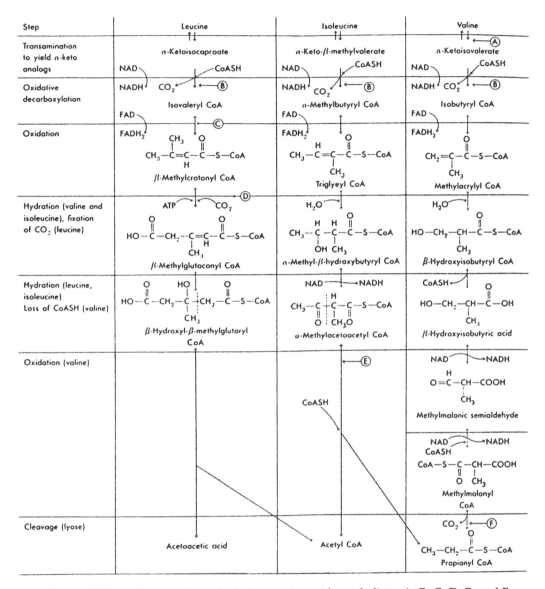

Figure 20.20 Pathways of branched-chain amino acid metabolism. A, B, C, D, E, and F indicate defects in valinemia, maple syrup urine disease, isovaleric acidemia, β-hydroxyisovaleric aciduria, α-methyl-β-hydroxybutyric aciduria, and methylmalonic aciduria, respectively.

reaction requires the vitamin B_{12} coenzyme. In vitamin B_{12} deficiency, β-leucine is excreted in the urine. These reactions are summarized in Equation (20.24):

$$\text{Isobutyryl-CoA} \xrightarrow[\text{Acetyl-CoA}]{} CH_3\text{–}CH\text{–}\underset{\underset{O}{\|}}{C}\text{–}CH_2\text{–}COOH \xrightarrow[-NH_2]{} CH_3\text{–}CH\text{–}\overset{NH_2}{CH}\text{–}CH_2\text{–}COOH$$

Isobutyryl-CoA   Acetyl-CoA   β-ketoisocaproate (CH₃, O)   β-leucine (CH₃)   (20.24)

$$\xrightarrow[\text{B}_{12},\ \text{mutase}]{} \text{leucine}$$

20.5.6 Metabolism of Aromatic Amino Acids

Tryptophan, an essential amino acid, gives rise to glucogenic and ketogenic end products, as well as a number of physiologically important nitrogenous compounds, such as serotonin and NAD$^+$. The fate of tryptophan is summarized in Figure 20.21.

Catabolism of tryptophan can be divided into the serotonin and 3-hydroxyanthranilic acid pathways, the latter being by far the more prevalent. It may lead to the formation of NAD$^+$ or to α-ketoadipic acid. Only about 3% of 3-

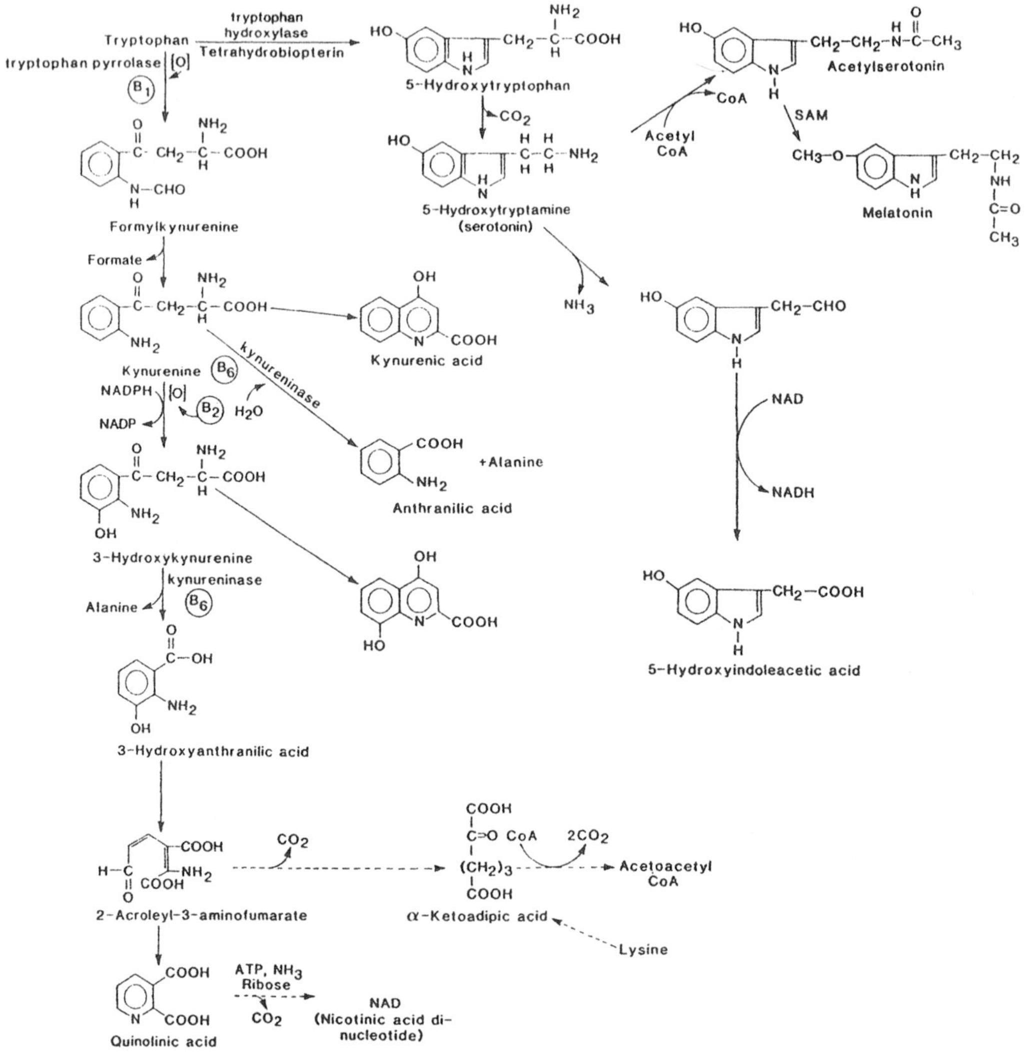

Figure 20.21 Catabolism of tryptophan by the serotonin and 3-hydroxyanthranilate pathways. B_1, B_2, and B_6 indicate the participation of coenzymes derived from the respective vitamins. Notice that tryptophan is glucogenic and ketogenic, because it produces alanine on the one hand, and acetoacetyl-CoA on the other.

hydroxymethylanthranilic acid is converted to NAD^+, and it would be necessary to ingest approximately 60 mg tryptophan per day to satisfy the human niacin requirement. Nevertheless, this pathway is important for supplying at least a part of the niacin (some estimates go as far as 50%). Thus, a vitamin B_6 deficiency stops tryptophan catabolism and elicits pellagra-like symptoms. Conversely, pellagra has been treated with tryptophan. Pellagra-like symptoms are also elicited by vitamin B_1 deficiency and in Hartnup disease (see earlier). NAD^+ exerts a negative feedback effect on tryptophan pyrrolase, the first enzyme of this pathway.

Tryptophan catabolism is also associated with several dead-end pathways, for example the formation of kynurenic and xanthurenic acids. Normal urine contains small amounts of hydroxykynurenine, kynurenine, kynurenic acid, and xanthurenic acid. When large amounts of tryptophan are fed to animals, the excretion of these compounds increases. Xanthurenic acid is excreted in massive quantities in vitamin B_6 deficiency.

Focusing our attention on the serotonin branch of Figure 20.21, it is seen that the initial hydroxylation reaction requires tetrahydrobiopterin, which was introduced in Chapter 16 and is discussed further here. Serotonin per se is a neurotransmitter, and it can give rise to melatonin in the pineal gland. Melatonin is synthesized at night, and is believed to be associated with the phenomenon of circadian rhythms. Serotonin is metabolized to 5-hydroxyindoleacetic acid, which is excreted in the urine. Normal 5-hydroxyindoleacetic acid excretion is about 7 mg/day, whereas in carcinoid tumor patients, this may be as high as 400 mg/day. Carcinoid is an intestinal tumor that may metastasize into the liver.

The metabolic pathways of phenylalanine and tyrosine are identical, because the essential phenylalanine must be converted to tyrosine to become metabolized. Figure 20.22 illustrates this pathway, which is termed the liver pathway to distinguish it from those leading to catecholamine biosynthesis. It is localized in the cytosol, with the exception of tyrosine transaminase, which is also present in the mitochondria.

The first step in the liver pathway is catalyzed by phenylalanine hydroxylase. Tetrahydrobiopterin is a cofactor. This redox cofactor is also required for the hydroxylation of tyrosine to form L-dopa (Chapter 16) and for the hydroxylation of tryptophan to form 5-hydroxytryptophan. The structure of tetrahydrobiopterin is given in Figure 20.23. In the process of phenylalanine hydroxylation, the tetrahydrobiopterin is oxidized to dihydrobiopterin. The reduced form is then recovered via NADH and dihydrobiopterin reductase, as shown in Figure 20.23. Dihydrobiopterin, although similar in structure to folic acid, is synthesized in the human organism from GTP.

A number of genetic disorders are associated with phenylalanine and tyrosine metabolism. The best known is the classic phenylketonuria, discovered in 1934 by Folling. It is characterized by the virtual absence of phenylalanine hydroxylase from the organism. As a result, phenylalanine is converted to a large extent to phenylpyruvate, phenyllactate, and phenylacetate (Figure 20.22). Their levels and that of phenylalanine in the bloodstream are elevated. Hyperphenylalaninemia may also result from the absence of dihydrobiopterin reductase or any enzyme required for dihydrobiopterin biosynthesis from GTP. Although the etiologies of such disorders differ from that of classic phenylke-

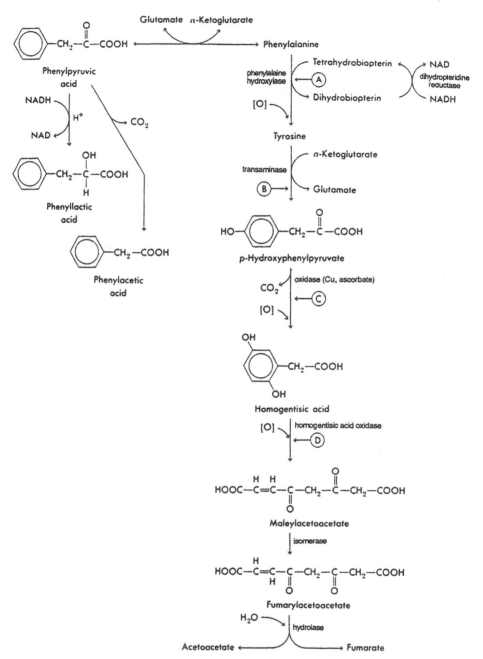

Figure 20.22 Catabolism of phenylalanine and tyrosine. A indicates the lesion in classic phenylketonuria; B indicates a tyrosinemia caused by tyrosine transaminase deficiency; C indicates a tyrosinemia caused by *p*-hydroxyphenylpyruvate oxidase deficiency and the lesion in neonatal tyrosinemia; D indicates alcaptonuria.

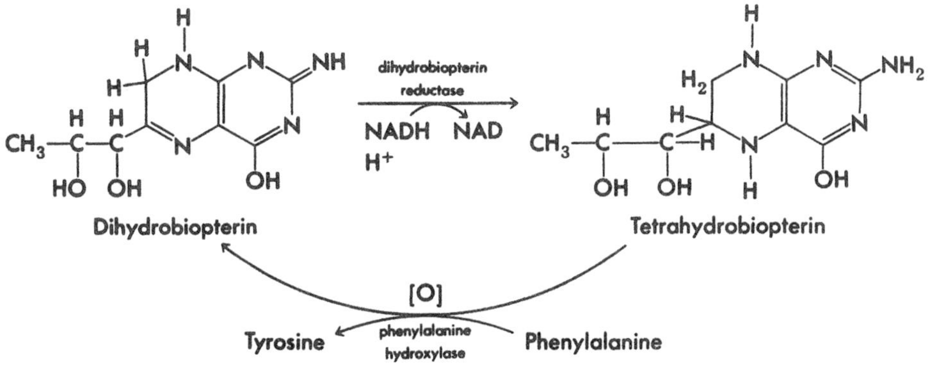

Figure 20.23 Interconversions of dihydro- and tetrahydrobiopterins.

tonuria, their effect is the same: hyperphenylalaninemia. Such nonclassic phenylketonurias may be treated by the administration of those intermediates that cannot be synthesized. Classic phenylketonuria is treated by the dietary restriction of phenylalanine.

Additional errors of phenylalanine and tyrosine metabolism include tyrosinosis, or hereditary tyrosinemia, neonatal tyrosinemia, and alcaptonuria. In the first case, there is a probable defect in p-hydroxyphenylpyruvate oxidase. In neonatal tyrosinemia, the problem is transient and may be solved by the administration of ascorbic acid. Ascorbic acid is apparently a cofactor for p-hydroxyphenylpyruvate oxidase. Alcaptonuria is a benign disorder in which homogentisic acid oxidase is inoperative and homogentisic acid is excreted in the urine. Air oxidizes the homogentisic acid to a pigment, giving urine a black color. This pigment also accumulates in the patient's tissues.

Tyrosine gives rise to a variety of hormones, neurotransmitters, and other nitrogenous substances. The biosynthesis of thyroxine and the catecholamines was described in Chapter 16. In the melanoblasts, tyrosine gives rise to *melanins*, which are pigments of the eyes, skin, and hair:

$$\text{Tyrosine} \xrightarrow{\text{tyrosinase}} \text{L-dopa} \rightarrow \text{Melanins} \tag{20.25}$$

The initial reaction in this pathway is catalyzed by tyrosinase, a copper enzyme. Its absence produces albinism, lack of all pigment. The structure of L-dopa is shown in Figure 16.9.

20.5.7 Metabolism of Basic Amino Acids

In addition to giving rise to urea, arginine is also converted to creatine phosphate. Creatine phosphate is a high-energy substance used to store chemical energy for muscular work. It can transfer its high-energy bond to ADP through the action of creatine kinase (CPK or CK). CPK determinations are extremely important in the diagnosis of myocardial infarcts and skeletal muscle disorders, such as muscular dystrophy (see Chapter 5). Creatinine is the product of the spontaneous loss of the phosphate residue from creatine phosphate without recovery of the high-energy bond. It has no function in the physiology of the organism and is excreted in the urine. Its plasma levels are high in patients with kidney failure: the normal level is 0.6–1.5 mg/dl, whereas in patients with renal disease this may rise to 10–15 mg/dl. Normally, some 2 g creatinine is excreted per day. The metabolic pathway leading to the formation of creatinine and creatine phosphate is shown in Figure 20.24.

Arginine is a precursor of nitric oxide (NO) in the human organism. NO is a powerful vasodilator and a neurotransmitter. It is formed as indicated in Equation (20.26):

$$\text{Arginine} \xrightarrow{\text{[O], NO synthase}} \text{citrulline} + \text{NO} \tag{20.26}$$

NO synthase is activated in response to Ca^{2+}, which is released in the endothelial cells in response to acetylcholine or bradykinin interaction with their respective cell surface receptors. The NO synthesized diffuses into smooth muscle cells of the blood vessels causing them to relax. Nitroglycerin, a drug used to treat angina pectoris patients, causes vasodilation by giving rise to NO.

Histidine, an essential amino acid, is metabolized to glutamate and a tetrahydrofolate-bound one-carbon unit. This pathway is shown in Figure 20.25. Two inborn errors of metabolism are associated with this pathway: histidinemia and formiminoglutamic aciduria. Histidinemia is caused by the absence of histidase and is characterized by high blood and urinary levels of histidine and imidazoleacetic, imidazolepyruvic, and imidazolelactic acids. Formiminoglutamic acid-

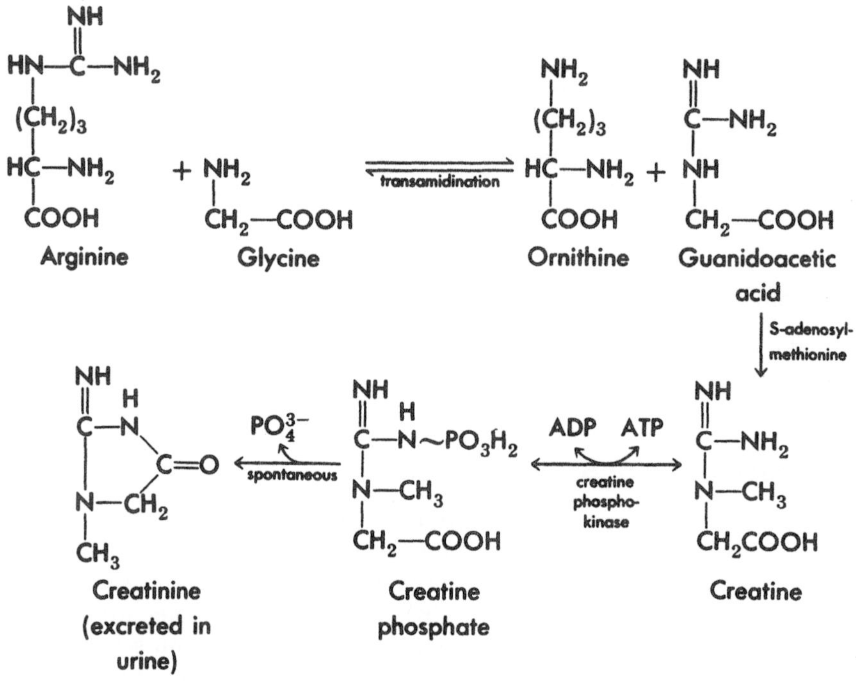

Figure 20.24 Biosynthesis of creatine, creatinine phosphate, and creatine from arginine.

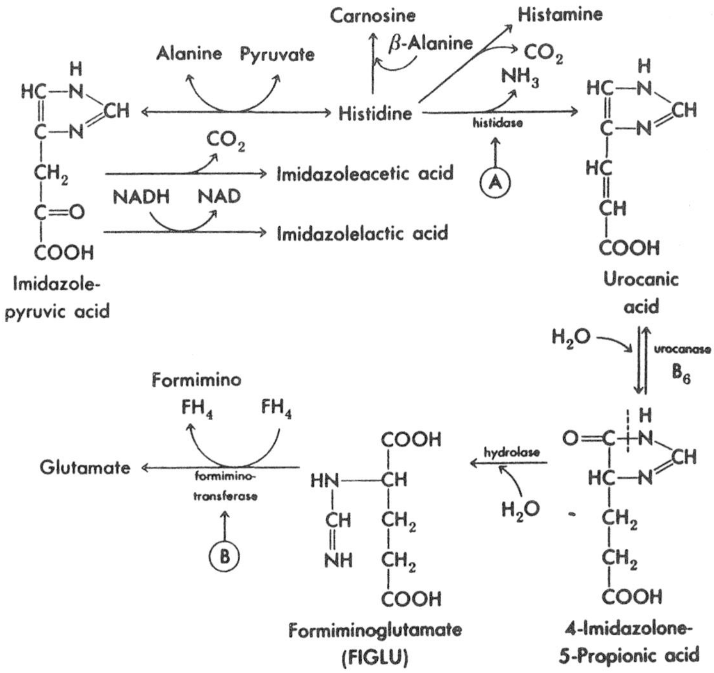

Figure 20.25 Catabolism of histidine. A and B indicate lesions in histidinemia and formiminoglutamic aciduria, respectively.

uria is characterized by the excretion of formiminoglutamic acid in the urine. This is a result of the absence of formiminotransferase.

The catabolism of lysine merges with that of tryptophan at the level of β-ketoadipic acid. Both metabolic pathways are identical from this point on and lead to the formation of acetoacetyl-CoA (Figure 20.21). Lysine is thus ketogenic. It does not transaminate in the classic way. Lysine is a precursor of carnitine: the initial reaction involves the methylation of ϵ-amino groups of protein-bound lysine with SAM. The N-methylated lysine is then released proteolytically and the reaction sequence to carnitine completed. See Equation (19.6) for the structure of carnitine.

20.5.8 Inborn Errors of Amino Acid Metabolism

Throughout this chapter, we have had occasion to refer to genetic diseases associated with amino acid metabolism. Such defects are characterized by amino acidemias and amino acidurias. The former indicate elevated amino acid levels in serum, whereas the latter indicate their excretion in the urine. A patient may have an amino aciduria without an amino acidemia. This is the case with amino acid transport disorders. It is unusual, however, to have an amino acidemia without amino aciduria.

Inborn errors of amino acid metabolism are usually inherited as autosomal recessive traits, which result in the inability to metabolize a specific amino acid.

An amino acid-metabolizing enzyme is absent or defective. The blood level of the offending amino acid or its catabolism intermediate becomes so high that it "spills over" into the urine. Such inborn errors may be successfully treated by restricting the dietary intake of the offending amino acid. If the disorder is not treated soon after birth, irreversible brain damage or even death may result. Untreated phenylketonurics do not develop an IQ (intelligence quotient) beyond 25 ± 15. Table 20.8 lists a number of such disorders. As can be seen, the incidence of each disease is quite rare. Taken together, on the other hand, along with the amino acid transport disorders, these inborn errors occur in about 325 in 1 million births.

Table 20.8 Some Inborn Errors of Amino Acid and Nitrogen Metabolism

Disorder	Incidence per live births	Catabolic pathway involved	Enzyme deficiency
Phenylketonuria	1:12,000 1:8000[a]	Phenylalanine	Phenylalanine hydroxylase
Histidinemia	1:20,000 1:12,000[a]	Histidine	Histidase
Maple syrup urine disease	1:300,000 1:120,000[a]	Branched-chain amino acids	Branched-chain α-ketoacid decarboxylase
Homocystinuria	1:200,000 1:280,000[a]	Methionine	Cystathionine synthase
Cystathioninuria	1:150,000	Methionine	Cystathionase
Tyrosinemia	1:600,000[b]	Tyrosine	p-Hydroxyphenylpyruvate oxidase
Nonketotic hyperglycinemia	1:150,000	Glycine	Glycine cleavage enzyme
Hyperlysinemia and hypersaccharopinuria	1:300,000	Lysine	First two lysine degradation enzymes
Alcaptonuria	1:200,000	Tyrosine	Homogentisic acid oxidase
Arginosuccinic aciduria	1:150,000	Urea cycle	Arginosuccinase
Hyperammonemia I	Unclear	Urea cycle	Carbamoylphosphate synthetase
Hyperammonemia II	Unclear	Urea cycle	Ornithine transcarbamylase
Citrullinemia	Unclear	Urea cycle	Arginosuccinate synthetase
Argininemia	Unclear	Urea cycle	Arginase
Gyrate atrophy	Unclear	Ornithine	Ornithine transaminase
Formiminoglutamic aciduria	Unclear	Histidine	Formiminotransferase
Oxaluria	Unclear	Glycine	α-Ketoglutarate-glyoxylate carboligase
Hyperprolinemia I	Unclear	Proline	Proline oxidase
Hyperprolinemia II	Unclear	Proline	δ-Pyrroline-5-carboxylate dehydrogenase

[a]In Belgium, Denmark, France, Germany, Great Britain, Ireland, the Netherlands, and Switzerland. (Data from collective results of mass screening for inborn errors in eight European countries. Acta Paediatr Scand 62:413–416, 1973.)
[b]May be as high as 3:10,000 in French Canadians in Quebec.

Table 20.9 Amino Acids as Precursors of Various Nitrogenous Substances

Amino acid	Nitrogenous substance	Function
Glycine	Purines	Component of nucleic acids
	Creatine	Forms creatine phosphate with ATP
	Creatinine	Diagnostic importance in nephrology
	Porphyrins	Components of hemoglobins
	Glutathione	Biologic reducing agent
	Hippuric acid	Detoxication of benzoic acid
Arginine	Urea	Excretion product for nitrogen
	Creatine	See glycine
	NO	Vasodilator and neurotransmitter
Aspartate	Purines and pyrimidines	Components of nucleic acids
Glutamate	γ-Aminobutyric acid	Neurotransmitter
Tyrosine	Melanins	Biologic pigments
	Epinephrine	Adrenal medulla hormone
	Norepinephrine	Neurotransmitter
	Thyroxine	Thyroid hormone
Tryptophan	Serotonin	Neurotransmitter
	Melatonin	Mediator of circadian rhythms
	Nicotinic acid	Forms NAD and NADP
Serine	Ethanolamine and choline	Components of phosphoglycerides
Histidine	Histamine	Mediator of allergic response
	Carnosine	Possible olfactory function
Cysteine	Taurine	Conjugates bile acids
	Cysteamine	Component of CoA
	Glutathione	See glycine
Lysine	Carnitine	Fatty acid catabolism

20.5.9 Amino Acids as Precursors of Biologically Active Substances

Amino acids serve as precursors for a number of important nitrogenous compounds. Many of these have been discussed in this and previous chapters. Table 20.9 lists some of the more important biologically active nitrogenous compounds that originate from amino acids.

QUESTIONS

20.1. Anaplerotic reactions replace substances present in catalytic amounts, which are indispensable for the operation of biochemical cycles. Which is an anaplerotic reaction?
   a. Phenylalanine → tyrosine
   b. 3Methionine + ethanolamine → choline + 3homocysteine
   c. Glutamic semialdehyde + alanine → pyruvate + ornithine
   d. Alanine + oxaloacetate → pyruvate + aspartate
   e. Glutamine → ammonia + glutamate
20.2. The degradation of proteins in cells may involve all of the following, except
   a. Melatonin
   b. Cathepsins
   c. Calcium ions

d. ATP
e. Ubiquitin

20.3. Symptoms of pellagra may appear with the deficiency of which amino acid?
a. Tyrosine
b. Tryptophan
c. Methionine
d. Lysine
e. Asparagine

20.4. In the following table, which is incorrect?

Biochemical reaction	*One-carbon unit involved*
a. Formiminoglutamate → glutamate + 1C	THF, formate level
b. Homocysteine + 1C → methionine	SAM
c. Guanidoacetic acid + 1C → creatine	SAM
d. Glycine → ammonia + CO_2 + 1C	THF, formaldehyde level
e. Sarcosine → glycine + 1C	THF, methyl level

20.5. Tetrahydrobiopterin is associated with all of the following, except
a. Hydroxylation of tyrosine to form melanins
b. Biosynthesis of serotonin
c. Biosynthesis of tyrosine
d. Metabolism of catecholamines
e. Metabolism of GTP

20.6. The metabolism of which amino acid cannot produce propionyl-CoA?
a. Tryptophan
b. Threonine
c. Methionine
d. Valine
e. Isoleucine

20.7. Deamination of aspartate to oxaloacetate and ammonia best occurs via which reaction(s)?
a. Aspartate dehydrogenase using FMN as a redox cofactor
b. Combination of AST and glutamate dehydrogenase
c. Combination of glycine oxidase and asparaginase
d. Combination of asparaginase and glutaminase
e. Asparaginase using THF and NAD^+ as cofactors

20.8. The two tissues that best extract glutamine from the bloodstream are
a. Intestine and kidney
b. Liver and muscle
c. Brain and kidney
d. Liver and kidney
e. Muscle and kidney

20.9. Which reaction is responsible for the most if not all urinary NH_4^+/NH_3?
a. Glutamate → α-ketoglutarate + ammonia
b. Aspartate → fumarate + ammonia
c. Glutamine → glutamate + ammonia
d. Glycine → $2CO_2$ + ammonia
e. Asparagine → aspartate + ammonia

20.10. Which is not a substrate for a urea cycle enzyme?
a. Carbamoylphosphate
b. Ornithine
c. Citrulline
d. NH_4^+
e. Arginine

20.11. The enzyme that initiates the activation of all major pancreatic zymogens in the small intestine is
   a. Chymotrypsin
   b. Pepsin
   c. Enterokinase
   d. Carboxypeptidase A
   e. Trypsinogen
20.12. In the Picou and Taylor-Roberts protein turnover model, which is correct?
   a. Total flux $Q = I + C$
   b. $C = S + E_T$
   c. $F = E_T - Q$
   d. $C + S = I + E_T$
   e. $Q - E_T = S$
20.13. Which equation is not able to give you the correct fractional catabolic rate, assuming that all other necessary data are available? See text for abbreviations.
   a. $dS_B/dt = -qS_B/B$
   b. $k = S_B^{0}/S_B \ (\ln t_{1/2})$
   c. $\ln S_B = \ln S_B^{0} - kt$
   d. $k = 0.69/t_{1/2}$
   e. $dS_B/dt = k\hat{S}_B$

The curve shown in Figure 20.26 represents the turnover of rat serum albumin when radioactive albumin is injected into the animals (curve B). Determine the required parameters from this curve in Questions 20.14 and 20.15:

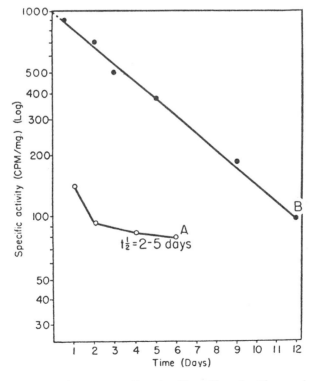

Figure 20.26 Turnover of rat serum albumin. (Reproduced with permission from Jeffay H, Winzler RJ. J Biol Chem 1958; 231:101–116.)

20.14.   The half-life of rat serum albumin is about
a.   9 days
b.   12 days
c.   4.5 days
d.   6 days
e.   3.4 days

20.15.   What is the total serum albumin pool in the rat if 5 mg labeled serum albumin is injected, specific activity 134,000 dpm/mg?
a.   134 mg
b.   500 mg
c.   670 mg
d.   1.2 g
e.   2.1 g

20.16   Assume you are treating your uremic patient with α-keto analogs of essential amino acids and are thus giving the patient no nitrogen. Which α-keto analog would be inappropriate?
a.   Phenylalanine
b.   Isoleucine
c.   Histidine
d.   Tryptophan
e.   Lysine

In Questions 20.17–20.24, use the following key:
a.   1, 2, and 3 are correct.
b.   1 and 3 are correct.
c.   2 and 4 are correct.
d.   Only 4 is correct.
e.   All are correct.

20.17   Pyrroline-5-carboxylic acid:
1.   Is in equilibrium with its open form, α-glutamic semialdehyde
2.   May be reduced to proline
3.   Can be converted to ornithine
4.   Can be converted to glutamic acid

20.18.   The alanine cycle involves
1.   The movement of alanine from liver to muscle for energy production
2.   Conversion of alanine to glucose and ammonia in the liver
3.   Removal of nitrogen from the peripheral tissue to kidneys
4.   Conversion of pyruvate to alanine in peripheral tissue

20.19.   Phenylalaninemia may result from
1.   An inability of tyrosine to be converted to phenylalanine
2.   Failure to hydroxylate phenylalanine
3.   Failure to deaminate phenylalanine
4.   Inability to form tetrahydrobiopterin from dihydrobiopterin

20.20.   The urea cycle operates at less than normal capacity when
1.   The patient suffers from ketosis.
2.   Dihydrobiopterin levels in the cell are below normal.
3. N-acetylglutamate levels in the cell are below normal.
4.   The amino acid pool is larger than normal.

20.21.   Valine
1.   Metabolism compromised in maple syrup urine disease
2.   May give rise to leucine in mammals
3.   Is an essential amino acid
4.   Is both ketogenic and glucogenic

20.22. In hepatic encephalopathy,
   1. Excessive amounts of branched-chain amino acids enter the brain.
   2. The liver produces excessive amounts of aromatic amino acids.
   3. Liver tryptophan pyrrolase does not function, inducing excess conversion of tryptophan to serotonin.
   4. Blood aromatic amino acid to branched-chain amino acid ratios are increased.

20.23 A patient with cystine in the urine (cystinuria)
   1. Cannot synthesize cysteine from methionine
   2. Has a defective cationic amino acid transport system
   3. Has a high blood cystine level
   4. May have genitourinary stones

20.24 Urea cycle:
   1. Its enzyme are located both in the mitochondria and cytosol
   2. Utilizes four ATP equivalents to synthesize one urea molecule
   3. Produces fumarate
   4. Activity regulated in part by tissue amino acid pools

In a–e are listed a number of disease entities. Answer Questions 20.25–20.28 on the basis of these diseases:
   a. Hepatic encephalopathy
   b. Gyrate atrophy
   c. Chronic kidney failure
   d. Homocystinuria
   e. Carcinoid tumor

20.25. Brought about by vitamin B_{12} deficiency.
20.26. Associated with ornithine transaminase deficiency
20.27. Associated with excessive amounts of indoleacetic acid in urine
20.28. Associated with excessive amounts of creatinine in the bloodstream

Answers

20.1. (c) Ornithine is required to maintain the urea cycle. Conversion of glutamate to ornithine via glutamate semialdehyde is therefore an anaplerotic reaction.

20.2. (a) Melatonin is a compound synthesized from serotonin. It has a function in the circadian rhythm activity and has nothing to do with intracellular protein degradation.

20.3. (b) Tryptophan provides some of the human daily niacin requirements. Hence niacin deficiency with pellagra-like symptoms develops if the diet contains insufficient amounts of tryptophan.

20.4. (b) The conversion of homocysteine to methionine requires 5-methyl-THF and the vitamin B_{12} coenzyme.

20.5. (a) Hydroxylation of tyrosine to L-dopa in the pigment cells involves tyrosinase, a copper enzyme and requires no tetrahydrobiopterin.

20.6. (a) Tryptophan metabolism does not produce any propionyl-CoA precursors, such as α-ketobutyrate. The other four amino acids do.

20.7. (b) Deamination of all amino acids other than that of glutamate and glycine occurs fastest by combining transamination with α-ketoglutarate, followed by deamination of the glutamate formed by glutamate dehydrogenase.

20.8. (a) Intestinal cells convert glutamate into proline for export, whereas the kidney uses glutamate to make bicarbonate. Both tissues may also return glutamate to the bloodstream and its tissue of origin to complete the glutamine cycle.

20.9. (c) Glutamine is subject to glutaminase action in the kidneys. One product, ammonia, is excreted as ammonium ion in the urine.

20.10. (d) The actual substrate for carbamoylphosphate synthetase is ammonia (NH_3).

20.11. (c) Enterokinase activates trypsinogen to trypsin, and the latter activates all the other zymogens.

20.12. (a) Total flux is equal to either total nitrogen input or output; that $Q = I + C = E_T + S$.

20.13. (b) This equation is nonsensical. The other four are derived from the basic equation in a.

20.14. (e) One can read the half-life from the curve, where specific activity is 500 (one-half of the extrapolated initial specific activity of 1000). Alternatively, one can calculate the half-life from k, the fractional catabolic rate; $-k$ is equal to the slope of the curve: $\ln 1000 - \ln 100/0 - 12 = -0.19 = -k$. k is therefore 0.19, and the half-life is $0.69/0.19 = 3.6$ days.

20.15. (c) Total dpm injected is $134,000 \times 5 = 670,000$; because the extrapolated *in vivo* specific activity is 1000 dpm/mg, the total pool B is $670,000/1000 = 670$ mg.

20.16. (e) Lysine α-keto analog is not able to transaminate to give the essential amino acid lysine.

20.17. (e) All are correct; glutamate semialdehyde forms an internal Schiff base to give pyrroline-5-carboxylic acid, and the reaction is reversible.

20.18. (c) Alanine cycle carries nitrogen from peripheral tissue to liver, where alanine loses the N and the pyruvate formed is used in the gluconeogenesis process.

20.19. (c) Failure to hydroxylate phenylalanine may be caused by classic phenylketonuria (absence of phenylalanine hydroxylase) or the absence of a cofactor, such as tetrahydrobiopterin.

20.20. (b) The urea cycle is retarded in ketosis because of the concurrent acidosis. This raises the cellular level of the ammonium ion and lowers ammonia, the natural substrate for the urea cycle. N-acetylglutamate is a positive effector for carbamoylphosphate synthetase.

20.21. (a) Valine, an essential amino acid, is glucogenic, but it can give rise to some leucine via a vitamin B_{12}-requiring reaction. It is not metabolized in maple syrup urine disease.

20.22. (d) In hepatic encephalopathy, serum branched-chain amino acids are low, and the aromatic are high. This is a result of the inability of the liver to process aromatic amino acids and an excessive entry of branched-chain amino acids into the muscle.

20.23. (c) In cystinuria, there is cystine excretion in the urine, but no cystinemia. Cystine stones may deposit in the genitourinary tract because of the low solubility of cystine in water.

20.24. (e) All are true for the urea cycle.

20.25. (d) Conversion of the THF-bound one-carbon unit to methyl groups in methionine results in a decline in vitamin B_{12} deficiency, because this vitamin is required to methylate homocysteine.

20.26. (b) Gyrate atrophy is associated with ornithinemia.

20.27. (e) Indoleacetic acid is a degradation product of serotonin, and carcinoid tumor patients excrete large amounts of this degradation product in the urine.

20.28. (c) In chronic renal disease, creatinine is not cleared by the kidneys and accumulates in the bloodstream.

PROBLEMS

20.1. A newborn child was found to be lethargic and jaundiced and, at 6 days of age, showed elevated blood phenylalanine levels. He was placed on a low-phenylalanine diet with the result that blood phenylalanine levels declined yet remained much higher than those of classic phenylketonuria patients. During the next 4 years, his physical and mental capabilities developed much more slowly than those of normal or classic phenylketonuric patients on the same diet. At the age of 2.5 years, his urinary 5-hydroxyindoleacetic acid and vanillylmandelic acid levels were found to be lower than normal. In addition, oral challenge with phenylalanine in normal and classic phenylketonuric patients results in about a 10-fold increase in serum "biopterin" levels. This patient failed to show this response.

Provide a diagnosis for this patient, and explain all the chemical data provided on the basis of your diagnosis. How would you treat this patient? What scientific conclusion can you make regarding the normal relationship between blood phenylalanine and "biopterin" levels?

20.2. An adolescent went into delirium after eating a high-protein meal. He had an extremely high blood ammonia level and excreted orotic acid and uracil in the urine. His blood also contained increased glutamine and lysine levels. Despite heroic symptomatic treatment, the patient expired after 2 weeks. His liver tissue showed normal urea cycle enzyme levels, except that for ornithine transcarbamylase (OTC), whose activity was only 10% that of normal liver. The K_m of OTC was normal. Liver carabmylphosphate levels were about 10 times normal. Theoretical computer simulations indicated that urea can be produced at normal rates when liver OTC levels are higher than 0.3% of normal.

What do you think was wrong with this patient? Why were blood ammonia levels so high? Why was the patient excreting orotic acid and uracil?

20.3. An adolescent developed a persistent scaly and dirty-looking rash and severe neurologic symptoms, such as difficulty in walking and maintaining balance. He was in and out of the hospital for several years with no relief. His laboratory data showed increased levels of serum bicarbonate (31 meq/L), normal urinary porphyrins and porphobilinogen, and a massive excretion of amino acids, indican, and indoxyl sulfate.

What is the problem with this patient? What do the rash and neurologic symptoms mean? Why were porphyrins and porphobilinogen determined? Why is serum bicarbonate high? What is the meaning of amino acid and indole derivative excretion? How would you treat this patient?

BIBLIOGRAPHY

Bender DA. Amino Acid Metabolism, 2d ed. New York: John Wiley, 1985.

Bernardini P, Fischer JE. Amino acid imbalance and hepatic encephalopathy. Annu Rev Nutr 2:419–454, 1982.

Fuller MF, Garlick PJ. Human amino acid requirements: can the controversy be resolved? Annu Rev Nutr 14:217–241, 1994.

Halperin ML, Jungas RL, Cheema-Dhadlim S, Brosnan JT. Disposal of the daily acid load: an integrated function of the liver, lungs and kidneys. Trends Biochem Sci May:197–199, 1987.

Jungas RL, Halperin ML, Brosnan JT. Quantitative analysis of amino acid oxidation and related gluconeogenesis in humans. Physiol Rev 72:419–448, 1992.

Kilberg MS. Amino acid transport in isolated hepatocytes. J Membr Biol 69:1–12, 1982.

Wellner D, Meister A. A survey of inborn errors of amino acid metabolism and transport in man. Annu Rev Biochem 50:911–968, 1981.

21

Integration of Metabolism

After completing this chapter, the student should

1. Be able to give the effects of insulin, glucagon, epinephrine, and the glucocorticoids on individual metabolic processes, and explain how these pathways change and interact if such hormone levels should change.
2. Be able to give the metabolic processes that normally take place in the fed state, the three fasting-starvation states, and in insulin-dependent diabetes.
3. Be able to convert the volumes of O_2 utilized or CO_2 produced into daily energy requirements, and determine which types of foods are being oxidized from these data; know the meaning of RQ and be able to use it in caloric requirement calculations.
4. Understand the meaning of BMR, and calculate this for individuals on the basis of weight and surface area; be able to estimate energy requirements for people leading different lifestyles.

21.1 INTRODUCTION

In previous chapters we learned about the nature of hormones, metabolic pathways, and the effects of such hormones as insulin, glucagon, epinephrine, and the glucocorticoids on individual metabolic reactions and enzymes. The objective of this chapter is to look at the overall picture of hormonal control of intermediary metabolism, that is, to integrate the metabolisms of the three major sources of energy: carbohydrates, lipids, and proteins. To illustrate these interrelationships, we examine three metabolic states: the fed state, the fasting state, and the diabetic state. Last, we should remember that normal metabolism takes place in an oxygen atmosphere and that CO_2 is the end product of metabolic activity. Surprisingly, large amounts of information on metabolic activity can be garnered from data on O_2 consumption and CO_2 production in human beings. Such measurements serve as a basis for calculating minimal human energy requirements, and sample calculations are presented at the end of this chapter.

21.2 EFFECT OF HORMONES ON INDIVIDUAL METABOLIC PATHWAYS

Let us now consider the effects of insulin, glucagon, epinephrine, and the glucocorticoids on individual metabolic pathways learned in Chapters 18 through 20. We begin with insulin, an anabolic hormone. In such situations as the fed state, when blood glucose and therefore insulin levels are high and glucagon levels low (high insulin/glucagon ratio), glycogen is synthesized in the muscle and liver from glucose entering cells. Glycolysis is also stimulated in the liver, producing pyruvate and acetyl coenzyme A (acetyl-CoA). The latter gives rise to lipids in the adipose and other tissues. Cholesterol biosynthesis also increases in activity. Protein synthesis is stimulated in part because insulin stimulates amino acid entry into cells; protein synthesis can hardly proceed in the absence of insulin. On the other hand, gluconeogenesis, lipolysis, and glycogenolysis are shut down. Events taking place in the fed state are summarized in Figure 21.1.

When blood insulin levels decline in response to low glucose levels, glucagon levels rise and shut down glycolysis, fat biosynthesis (lipogenesis), and cholesterol biosynthesis. Glycogen degradation is turned on and its biosynthesis shut off. Lipid degradation (lipolysis) is switched on, resulting in an increase of β-oxidation activity and possibly increased ketone body formation. Protein synthesis declines, but protein and amino acid degradation continues for the purpose of energy production and glucose biosynthesis. Thus, with a low insulin/glucagon ratio, gluconeogenesis in liver proceeds to maintain blood glucose at nearly normal levels, and fatty acids and ketone bodies provide the bulk

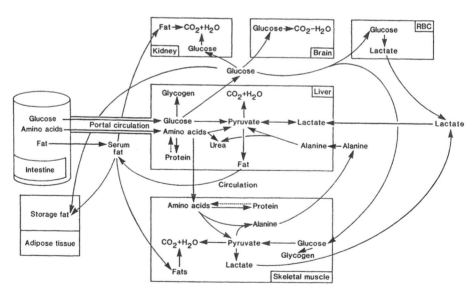

Figure 21.1 Metabolite and fuel movements in the fed state (high insulin/glucagon). Arrows indicate net movement of metabolites. There is a net synthesis of glycogen and fat in the liver. Glucose is converted to pyruvate and lactate during muscular activity. Both the Cori and alanine cycles are shown.

of the organism's energy requirement. Epinephrine has the same effects as glucagon in most tissues, a notable exception being the skeletal muscle.

The glucocorticoids are secreted in increased amounts in stress situations; this may also accompany a low insulin/glucagon ratio. Increases in blood glucocorticoid levels have been associated with a decreased protein content in all tissues except the liver. Apparently this is caused by a decrease of amino acid transport into these tissues and possibly an increased catabolic activity. Liver proteins, on the other hand, increase under the influence of glucocorticoids, most likely because these hormones stimulate amino acid entry into the liver. Testosterone, a steroid male hormone, is *anabolic*: its effect on protein metabolism is to stimulate protein accumulation in all tissues, especially the muscle. Glucocorticoids act in concert with glucagon to increase the rate of gluconeogenesis, in part because of their action to increase amino acid entry into the liver. In addition, as with glucagon and epinephrine, glucocorticoids serve to increase the activity of hormone-sensitive lipase and thus lipolysis. The action of glucocorticoids is slower than that of insulin, epinephrine, and glucagon.

There are no glucagon receptors in the skeletal muscle, and glucagon therefore has no effect on muscle metabolism. Epinephrine then becomes a major factor in regulating muscle metabolism. Gluconeogenesis does not take place in the muscle because it lacks glucose-6-phosphatase. Therefore, glucose-6-phosphate generated from muscle glycogen by the action of epinephrine, as well as exogenous glucose, is channeled into glycolysis. Muscle glycolysis enzymes, unlike those from the liver, are insensitive to cAMP regulation. In fact, increases in cAMP have a mild stimulatory effect on muscle phosphofructokinase I. In the muscle, therefore, epinephrine stimulates glycolysis.

During exercise, when blood epinephrine levels rise, muscle glycogen is converted to lactate via glycolysis. Lactate is removed from the muscle and channeled into the liver, where it is reconverted to glucose via gluconeogenesis and the glucose is returned to muscle. This is the Cori cycle. When muscle glycogen is depleted after prolonged exercise or by fasting, the muscle switches to fatty acids as its principal fuel. In the resting state, the principal fuel for muscle metabolism are the fatty acids. Table 21.1 summarizes the effects of hormones on the various metabolic pathways, and Table 21.2 shows hormone effects on the regulatory enzymes of the pathways.

21.3 FASTING AND STARVATION

Our knowledge of what happens to intermediary metabolism during fasting and starvation has been worked out by a number of investigators, especially by G. F. Cahill and his associates. Fasting has been divided into three broad stages: the initial (early) stage (0–2 days of low calorie intake), the intermediate stage (2–24 days), and the prolonged stage (more than 24 days). These three stages differ from each other with regard to their metabolic pathways. All three stages are, of course, characterized by relatively high blood glucagon and epinephrine levels and low insulin levels. Insulin/glucagon ratios are thus lower than normal. In addition, blood glucocorticoid levels may be higher than normal.

Figure 21.2 represents the flux of various metabolites in the human organism in the initial state of fasting. Note that no foodstuffs enter the metabolic

Table 21.1 Hormone Effects on Intermediary Metabolic Pathways

Pathway	Hormone			
	Insulin	Glucagon[a]	Epinephrine	Glucocorticoids
Gluconeogenesis	↓	↑	↑	↑
Glycolysis				
Liver	↑	↓	↓	↓ [b]
Muscle			↑	
Glycogenolysis	↓	↑	↑	
Glycogenesis	↑	↓	↓	
Lipolysis	↓	↑	↑	↑
Lipogenesis	↑	↓	↓	
Cholesterol biosynthesis	↑	↓	↓	
Protein biosynthesis	↑	↓	↓	↑ [c]
Protein degradation				
Liver	↓	↑	↑	↓
Muscle	↓		↑	↑

[a]Does not affect skeletal muscle.
[b]Indirect effect; interferes with glucose utilization (entry) by cells.
[c]In liver only; includes plasma proteins. In other tissues, glucocorticoids favor protein degradation.

Table 21.2 Hormone Direct or Indirect Effects on Some Regulatory Enzymes

Enzyme[a]	Hormone			
	Insulin	Glucagon	Epinephrine	Glucocorticoids
Carbohydrate metabolism				
Glycogen synthase	↑	↓	↓	
Phosphorylase system	↓	↑	↑	
Glucokinase	↑	—	—	
PFK I	↑	↓	↑	
Pyruvate kinase	↑	↓		
Pyruvate dehydrogenase	↑	(↓)	(↓)	
Pyruvate carboxylase	↓	↑	↑	
PEP carboxykinase	↓	↑	↑	↑
Fructose-1,6-diphosphatase	↓	↑	↑	↑
Glucose-6-phosphatase	↓	↑	↑	↑
Lipid metabolism				
Acetyl-CoA carboxylase	↑			
Lipoprotein lipase	↑			
Hormone-sensitive lipase	↓	↑	↑	↑
Fatty acid synthetase	↑	↓	↓	
Fatty acyl-CoA–glycerol-3-phosphate acyltransferase	↑	↓	↓	
HMG-CoA reductase	↑	↓	↓	
Amino acid metabolism: transaminases				↑

[a]PEP, phosphoenolpyruvate; HMG, β-hydroxy-β-methylglutaryl.

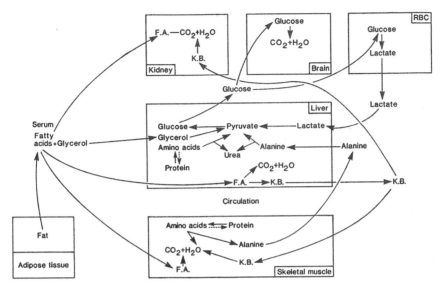

Figure 21.2 Metabolite movements in the organism during the early stage of starvation (low insulin/glucagon). FA indicates fatty acids. There is a *net* loss of protein and storage fat, and amino acids and lactate are converted to glucose. In the fasting state, there is no glycogen, and the intestinal tract does not contribute anything. Note that the red blood cells (RBC) are absolute glucose utilizers. The white blood cells, retina, adrenal medulla, and intestinal mucosal cells belong to the same category. In the fasting state, the kidney and muscle utilize practically no glucose. In prolonged starvation, muscle ceases to use ketone bodies (KB).

network from the outside. Glycogen is being broken down to glucose in the liver, and glucose for export is also made from lactate, amino acids, and glycerol by the process of gluconeogenesis. Fatty acids, derived from the degradation of storage fat, provide fuel for muscle (including the heart) and kidney, as do ketone bodies. Nerve tissue (e.g., brain) and other tissues, such as the red and white blood cells, the retina, and adrenal medulla, remain glucose utilizers. Lactic acid is returned by these tissues (except the nerve tissue) to the liver for gluconeogenesis. Quantitative data on the early stages of fasting are listed in Table 21.3.

As the fasting state continues, we reach the intermediary stage. This is characterized by the depletion of glycogen, which no longer serves as a source of blood glucose, leaving only gluconeogenesis to perform this task. Protein biosynthesis is limited and protein and amino acid degradation begin to decline. Fatty acids continue to provide fuel for the metabolism of muscle and the kidneys. Ketone bodies, in addition to providing fuel for the muscle, heart, and kidneys, begin to be utilized by the nerve tissue as the availability of glucose declines.

In the advanced stages of fasting, ketone bodies cease to provide substantial metabolic fuel for skeletal and heart muscle and kidneys. They are used almost exclusively by the brain, which also continues to use glucose, albeit in drastically lowered amounts. Muscle, heart, and kidneys depend exclusively on fatty acids for their subsistence. Glucose continues to be used exclusively by the

Table 21.3 Daily Flux of Metabolites at Two Stages of Fasting (grams)[a]

Pathway	24 h Fast	Adapted (prolonged) fast (5–6 weeks)
Protein degradation to amino acids for gluconeogenesis	0.75	20
Glycerol production by adipose tissue	16	15
Fatty acid production by adipose tissue	160	150
Fatty acid utilization by muscle, heart, kidney	120	112
Ketone body production by the liver	60	57
Glucose export by liver	180[a]	80[b]
Glucose utilization by nerve tissue	144	44
Glucose utilization by other tissues[c]	36	36
Ketone body utilization by nerve tissue	0	47
Ketone body utilization by heart, muscle, kidney	60	0
Ketone body excretion	0	10
Lactate + pyruvate returned to liver	36[d]	50[e]

[a]From glycogen and gluconeogenesis.
[b]From gluconeogenesis only.
[c]Glucose-requiring tissues, such as red blood cells.
[d]From tissue in note c.
[e]From glucose-requiring tissues, including brain.
Source: Data from Cahill GF. Starvation in man. N Engl J Med 282:668–675, 1970.

red and white blood cells, retina, and renal medulla. Protein and amino acid degradation is only a third or less of what it was during the early fasting stage. Thus, the limited utilization of glucose by the organism and the extensive use of fatty acids and ketone bodies serve to conserve precious protein and may allow a starving subject to remain alive for a long time. Quantitative data on the prolonged stage of fasting are listed in Table 21.3.

Several carbohydrate metabolism enzymes show a net decline or rise as a result of starvation. Among the specific enzymes, whose activities decline, are glycogensynthase, phosphofructokinase I (PFK I), pyruvate kinase, pyruvate dehydrogenase, and glucose-6-phosphate dehydrogenase. Pyruvate carboxylase, phosphoenolpyruvate carboxykinase, fructose-1-6-diphosphatase, and glucose-6-phosphatase are increased. The result is that in prolonged starvation, gluconeogenesis is the only carbohydrate metabolic pathway of the liver that shows a highly elevated activity.

When glucose is given to an animal after prolonged fasting, glycogen is apparently not synthesized immediately. Instead, most of the glucose (up to 85%) is first transformed into lactate, and then reconverted to glucose and glycogen via gluconeogenesis. If gluconeogenesis is artificially inhibited under such conditions (e.g., by inhibiting PEPCK with 3-mercaptopicolinate), very little glycogen deposition takes place. The conversion of glucose to lactate under these circumstances apparently occurs at nonhepatic sites, and lactate is then transported to the liver via the Cori cycle. The inability of the organism to synthesize glycogen immediately may be explained by the need to recover the needed enzyme machinery, which was dismantled during prolonged fasting.

It is interesting that patients undergoing β-blocker therapy (usually for hypertension) may simulate the starvation state. This is because the β blocker prevents the combination of epinephrine with the β-adrenergic receptors. The result may be hypoglycemia, because in the absence of epinephrine effects, gluconeogenesis declines in activity.

21.4 DIABETES MELLITUS

Diabetes mellitus is the best known disorder involving lack of insulin. The term "diabetes," however, is used in a broader sense to indicate polyuria, including diabetes insipidus. Even diabetes mellitus, which signifies increased levels of blood glucose, may or may not be associated with the underproduction of insulin. Thus, in insulin-dependent diabetes, there is an outright loss of insulin, usually as a result of degeneration of the β cells. These patients must receive exogenous insulin. An example of this disease is juvenile-onset diabetes. In non–insulin-dependent diabetes, the bloodstream contains plenty of insulin, but it does not act on tissues. This may be caused by a decline in the number of insulin receptors in peripheral tissues, as often happens in obese individuals, or the reaction of insulin with its tissue receptors may be blocked. Patients with untreated diabetes have hyperglycemia (high blood glucose), which when in excess of about 160 mg/dL spills over into the urine, resulting in glucosuria. The 160 mg/dL figure is the *renal threshold* for glucose. Along with the glucose, large quantities of water are excreted (polyuria).

Diagnosis of diabetes mellitus may be achieved by first looking at the fasting blood sugar level, which normally amounts to 70–105 mg/dL. Diabetes mellitus of one form or another is suspected if blood glucose exceeds this range, at which time a glucose tolerance test may be performed. The patient is given an oral dose of glucose, and then blood glucose levels are measured for a period of up to 3 h. Figure 21.3 shows normal and pathologic glucose tolerance curves. Other diagnostic strategies also exist. For instance, a fasting blood glucose of 140

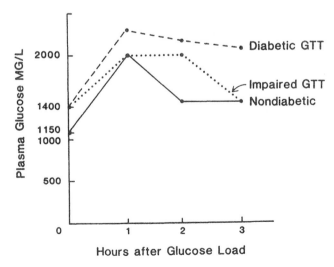

Figure 21.3 Glucose tolerance curves in the normal and diabetic patient. GTT indicates "glucose tolerance test." (Reproduced by permission from Skillman T. Diabetes mellitus. In Kaplan LA, Pesce AJ, eds. Clinical Chemistry. St. Louis: CV Mosby, 1984, p. 545.)

mg/dL or above, or a level of 200 mg/dL 2 h following a meal, is considered diagnostic of diabetes mellitus. Last, glycosylated hemoglobin (see Chapter 7) is an important tool in recognizing diabetes mellitus as well as a means of following therapy. Total glycosylated hemoglobin is given as 5–8% in normal individuals (6.5% mean); in untreated diabetics this may rise to as high as 20%.

Treatment of insulin-dependent diabetes involves the administration of insulin. In less severe cases of this diabetic form or in patients with adult-onset diabetes who have retained some β cell function, it is possible to "squeeze" the pancreas with such drugs as tolbutamide (orinase), tolazamide, or chlorpropamide, which act directly on the pancreas to increase insulin production. In most non–insulin-dependent diabetes situations, the dietary restriction of carbohydrate and fat is sufficient to control the disease.

Metabolically, insulin-dependent diabetes resembles starvation. However, such metabolic consequences are exaggerated in diabetes, which if untreated (unlike starvation) does not become stabilized and may lead to the rapid demise of the patient. Table 21.4 lists some metabolites in normal, fasting, and diabetic individuals. All metabolic effects exhibited in a diabetic are largely caused by an absolute or relative excess of glucagon and an absolute or relative dearth of insulin. The insulin/glucagon ratio in a diabetic is substantially lower than that of the normal individual. There is a high concentration of blood glucose and excretion of glucose in the urine. Only scant amounts of glucose can then enter the cells.

Because insulin normally inhibits lipolysis, a diabetic has an extensive lipolytic activity in the adipose tissue. As is seen in Table 21.4, plasma fatty acid concentrations become remarkably high. β-Oxidation activity in the liver increases: because of a low insulin/glucagon ratio, acetyl-CoA carboxylase is relatively inactive and acyl-CoA–carnitine acyltransferase is derepressed. β-Oxidation produces acetyl-CoA which in turn generates ketone bodies. Ketosis is perhaps the most prominent feature of diabetes mellitus. Table 21.5 compares ketone body production and utilization in fasting and in diabetic individuals. It may be seen that, whereas in the fasting state ketone body production is roughly equal to excretion plus utilization, in diabetes this is not so. Ketone bodies therefore accumulate in diabetic blood.

Table 21.4 Arterial Concentrations of Metabolites in Normal, Fasting, and Untreated Diabetics (mM)

Metabolite	Fed state		Fasted		Diabetic (untreated)
	Resting	Exercise	Overnight	24 Days	
Ketone bodies	0.075	0.072	0.29	6.8	11.0
Glucose	4.33	4.90	5.42	3.53	22.2
Lactate	1.06	2.84	0.625	0.553	1.98
Pyruvate	0.062	0.138	0.064	0.050	0.13
Free fatty acids	0.694	0.833	0.511	0.841	1.51
Glycerol	0.043	0.143	—	—	0.17
Alanine	0.253	0.435	0.3	0.1	0.15

Source: Data from Fenselau, A. Ketone body metabolism in normal and diabetic man. In Brownlee M, ed. Diabetes mellitus, Vol. III. New York: Garland STPM Press, 1981, p. 145.

Table 21.5 Ketone Body Production and Utilization in Fasting and Diabetes Mellitus (g/24 h)

Process	State		
	Short-term fast	Long-term fast	Untreated diabetic
Total production	115 ± 23	130 ± 20	131
Urinary excretion	2.5	14	24
Utilization			
Total	110	110	50–70
Brain	20	40	30–40
Kidney	—	31	20
Heart	3–5	3–5	3–5
Skeletal muscle	34	14	5

Source: Data from Fenselau, A. Ketone body metabolism in normal and diabetic man. In Brownlee M, ed. Diabetes mellitus, Vol. III. New York: Garland STM Press, 1981, p. 193.

Another observable difference between the diabetic and the fasting state is the high concentration of very low density lipoprotein (VLDL) and chylomicrons in the diabetic and their lowering in the prolonged fasting state. Insulin-dependent lipoprotein lipase is nonfunctional in the diabetic, resulting in an incomplete lipid clearance from the bloodstream. In addition, the liver may not be able to handle the enormous fatty acid influx in the diabetic, converting the excess to VLDL.

Protein degradation and amino acid metabolism are highly elevated in the diabetic, because the stimulatory effect of insulin on protein synthesis is nonexistent and the relative excess of glucagon and glucocorticoids causes protein breakdown to continue. Indeed, muscle wasting is a cardinal symptom of the untreated diabetic. Insulin also inhibits amino acid release into the bloodstream, and this may be a reason a moderate rise in plasma amino acid levels is observed in the diabetic. Such increased amino acids are largely of the branched-chain type, and alanine levels are in fact lower than normal. Nevertheless, alanine uptake by the liver is twice that of the normal individual, and it continues to be a major actor in the gluconeogenesis process.

The low insulin/glucagon ratio favors gluconeogenesis in the diabetic. It is twice as active in the diabetic as in the normal individual. Glucose is synthesized from alanine and lactate and exacerbates an already excessively high blood glucose level.

21.5 METABOLIC INFORMATION DERIVED FROM O_2 CONSUMPTION AND CO_2 PRODUCTION MEASUREMENTS

21.5.1 Type of Foodstuff Utilized in Metabolism

The generation of ATP by the passage of electrons from reduced redox cofactors to O_2 is not 100% efficient. Only about 40% of calories contained within carbohydrates, proteins, and lipids oxidized can be harnessed in the form of chemical energy—ATP. The rest appears in the environment as heat. In addition, the energy contained within ATP and related substances also eventually appears in the environment as heat. Thus, it is possible to determine the amounts of food-stuffs being metabolized by an animal by measuring its heat output. Although heat output may be measured directly in whole-body calorimeters, it is more convenient to calculate it by measuring O_2 utilized and CO_2 produced by an animal.

The simplest parameter to express the relationships between O_2 utilized and CO_2 produced is via the respiratory quotient (RQ). This is defined as the ratio of number of moles of CO_2 produced to moles O_2 consumed. For the combustion of glucose,

$$C_6H_{12}O_6 + 6O_2 \rightarrow 6H_2O + 6CO_2 \tag{21.1}$$

The RQ is 6/6 = 1, which is assumed to be the case for all carbohydrates. On the other hand, for the metabolism of palmitic acid (a lipid),

$$C_{16}H_{32}O_2 + 23O_2 \rightarrow 16CO_2 + 16H_2O \tag{21.2}$$

The RQ is 16/23 = 0.71, which is assumed to be the case for all fats. For proteins, which are the sums of their component amino acids, the RQ is generally taken as 0.8. Thus, if a person were metabolizing only fat, RQ would be 0.71. Normally the RQ is around 0.82, however, it is possible to observe more extreme values. In a marathon runner, for example, the initial RQ is indeed close to 1, indicating that carbohydrate is largely being metabolized. At the end of the run, blood sugar is down by some 40% and the RQ is 0.77, indicating that most of the calories toward the end derive from fat metabolism.

The energy produced by the combustion of foodstuffs is measured in calories or J (see Chapter 2). An excellent approximation of how many calories of energy a person is generating in an hour is provided by multiplying O_2 consumption by the factor 4.82, which represents the average kilocalorie yield per L O_2 consumed. A person consuming 20 L O_2 per hour is generating 20 L/h × 4.82 kcal/L = 96 kcal/h. This multiplies to 2304 kcal per day. A more accurate estimate of this, as well as a breakdown of foodstuffs oxidized, is provided by the following sample calculation: a person excretes 0.5 g N/h (in urea, for example), consumes 20 L O_2/h, and exhales 16 L CO_2/h. We proceed as follows:

1. Amount of protein oxidized per hour = 0.5 g N × 1 g protein/0.16 g N = 3.12 g protein. Here we note that the average N content of proteins is 16%. We then use Table 21.6 to determine how many L O_2 are consumed per gram protein oxidized. This is 3.12 × 0.95 = 2.96 L, and CO_2 produced is 3.12 × 0.76 = 2.37 L.

Table 21.6 O_2, CO_2, and Calorie Relationship Among the Most Common Foods

	RQ	O_2 consumed (L/g)	CO_2 exhaled (L/g)	Yield (kcal/L O_2)
Carbohydrate	1.0	0.74	0.74	5.1
Fat	0.71	2.0	1.42	4.7
Protein	0.80	0.95	0.76	4.2

2. We can now calculate nonprotein O_2 consumed and CO_2 produced by subtracting 2.96 L from 20 L and 2.37 L from 16 to give 17.04 L O_2 and 13.63 L CO_2. The non-protein RQ = 13.63/17.04 = 0.80.

3. If we now consult Table 21.7, we find that an RQ of 0.80 corresponds to the yield of 4.80 kcal/LO_2/h, giving a total nonprotein energy yield of 17.04 × 4.80 = 81.8 kcal/h. Table 21.7 also indicates that 33.4% of the energy, or (81.8 × 33.4)/100 = 27.3 kcal come from carbohydrate metabolism and 66.6% or (81.8 × 66.6)/100 = 54.5 kcal come from fat metabolism. Protein metabolism produces 2.96 L × 4.2 kcal/L = 12.4 kcal (See Table 21.6).

4. To determine the weight of fat and carbohydrate being utilized, we may refer again to Table 21.7, where it was stated that carbohydrate in this particular example consumes 31.7% of the nonprotein O_2, and fat consumes 68.3%. This translates to 17.04 × 0.317 = 5.40 L O_2 for carbohydrate and 17.04 × 0.683 = 11.6 L O_2 for fat. Because, per Table 21.6, carbohydrate consumes 0.74 L O_2 per gram and fat consumes 2.0 L/g, total carbohydrate being used per hour is 5.40/0.74 = 7.3 g, and total fat used is 11.6/2.0 = 5.8 g.

5. The subject is oxidizing 3.12 g protein, 7.3 g carbohydrate, and 7.3 g fat per hour. Total energy production is 27.3 + 54.5 + 12.4 = 94.2 kcal, which is fairly close to the approximate value just calculated from the total amount of O_2 used.

Note also that the information given in Table 21.6 can provide us with more accurate values for the calorie value per gram of each foodstuff: for carbohydrates, 5.1 × 0.74 = 3.8 kcal/g; for fats, 4.7 × 2 = 9.4 kcal/g; and for proteins, 4.2 × 0.95 = 4.0 Kcal/g. Compare this with the approximate values provided in Chapter 2.

In the preceding example, the subject was generating about 2261 kcal per day. This most likely represents an average daily energy output. It is higher during active phases of the day and lower when the subject is asleep. The energy output while the subject is at a complete rest is the *basal metabolic rate* (BMR). It is usually measured after some 12 h of fasting in the postabsorptive state to avoid the so-called specific dynamic action, an unexplained surge of heat production

Table 21.7 Energy Yields Obtained from Different Fat and Carbohydrate Mixtures

| RQ | % Total O_2 consumed by | | % Heat produced by | | Kilocalories per liter O_2 |
	Carbohydrate	Fat	Carbohydrate	Fat	
0.71	0	100	0	100	4.69
0.75	14.7	85.3	15.6	84.4	4.74
0.80	31.7	68.3	33.4	66.6	4.80
0.82	38.6	61.4	40.3	59.7	4.83
0.85	48.8	51.2	50.8	49.3	4.86
0.90	65.9	34.1	67.5	32.5	4.92
0.95	82.9	17.1	84.0	16.0	4.99
1.00	100	0	100	0	5.05

after eating. Specific dynamic action is especially high after a meal high in protein. BMR is considered the amount of energy that is absolutely necessary to sustain life. Its average value for all human beings is 1500 kcal/day or 1 kcal/kg/h, although rather wide variations are observed from individual to individual. To be more precise, that is, to take into account individual size and weight variations, BMR is generally calculated on the basis of the person's *surface area*, which is estimated using the DuBois equation:

$$\log A = 0.425 \log W + 0.725 \log H + 1.8564 \qquad (21.3)$$

where A is the subject's surface area in m^2, W is the weight, and H is the height in cm. A 75 kg person who is 1.8 m (5.91 feet) tall has a surface area of about 1.94 m^2. In all mammals, the BMR expressed in this fashion is approximately the same, about 1100 kcal/m^2/day. Large variations are observed if the weight is used, however. For instance, BMR in the human is about 32 kcal/kg/day, whereas in a mouse it is 212 kcal/kg/day.

BMR was used in the past as an aid to clinical diagnosis. It is increased in hyperthyroidism, Addison's disease, and shock. It also decreases with age: in males at 1 year of age, BMR is 53 kcal/m^2/h, at age 20 it is 38.6 kcal/m^2/h, and at 80 it is 33 kcal/m^2/h. It is also somewhat larger in males than females. A large proportion of the BMR is ascribable to the need to turn over proteins. During a typical day, a subject turns over 400 g protein. This represents about 4 mol peptide bonds, and each peptide bond requires an equivalent of about 5 ATP molecules for biosynthesis. This is 20 mol ATP per day. At 8 kcal per mole of ATP, this translates to about 400 kcal/day. Because ATP biosynthesis is only about 40% efficient in terms of harnessing the energy of combusted foodstuffs, the total energy required to generate those 20 mol ATP is close to 1000 kcal, or two-thirds of the total BMR (1500 kcal). BMR also accounts for such processes as glycoside bond biosynthesis and the maintenance of cation differences across membranes.

21.5.2 Estimating Human Energy Requirements

Our daily activities require a certain number of calories in the form of food. If our food supply exceeds substantially our energy needs, obesity develops. This condition is a serious problem in the United States. Tables are available that indicate energy requirements for the various activities of our daily lives, and these can be used to estimate our energy needs. Table 21.8 indicates some such values, plus the daily activity of an average U.S. soldier after basic training. From this we can then calculate the daily energy requirement for a typical U.S. trooper.

Table 21.8 shows that the various daily activities in an 80 kg U.S. soldier account for 874 kcal. The BMR may be calculated from the approximation just given (1 kcal/kg/h) by $1 \times 80 \times 24 = 1920$ kcal. Adding the two numbers, 1920 and 874, we get a total of 2794. A 10% surcharge is usually added to take into account the specific dynamic action. This amounts to about 279 kcal to give a grand total calorie requirement of $279 + 2794 = 3073$ kcal/day. A more accurate assessment of energy needs in a soldier would have to take into account his or her sex and average height. For an 80 kg male soldier about 1.8 m in height and about 20 years of age, the BMR would amount to 38.6 kcal/m^2/h, his surface area would be 2 m^2, and his total BMR would then be 38.6 kcal/m^2/h $\times$ 24 h $\times$ 2

Table 21.8 Daily Activities and Energy Requirements in U.S. Soldiers (Not Including the BMR[a])

Activity	Calorie value (kcal/kg/h)[b]	Hours engaged in activity per day	Calorie requirement (kcal/day)
Sitting	0.4	8.2	262.4
Lying down	0.1	4.0	32.0
Standing	0.5	1.0	40.0
Walking	2.0	0.9	144.0
Personal activity	0.7	0.8	44.8
Light activity	1.3	0.6	62.4
Physical training	7.0	0.5	280.0
Miscellaneous	1.0	0.1	8.0
Total		16.1	873.6

[a]Sleeping not included: it is part of the BMR.
[b]Assume an 80 kg soldier.
Source: Adapted from Consolazio CF, and Johnson HL. Measurement of energy cost in humans. Fed Proc 30:1444–1453, 1971.

$m^2 = 1853$ kcal, which is somewhat less than the result of the approximation shown earlier.

QUESTIONS

21.1. Which would *not* be expected to take place in the fed state?
   a. Blood fatty acid levels are increased.
   b. Blood VLDL is increased.
   c. Lipid is synthesized in the adipose tissue.
   d. Glucose in the liver is converted to acetyl-CoA.
   e. Two of the above.

21.2. Injection of epinephrine into an animal causes
   a. Increase in the activity of the Cori cycle
   b. Increase in blood glucose levels
   c. Increase in blood lactate levels
   d. All of the above
   e. None of the above

21.3. The basal metabolic rate
   a. Can be approximated by 5 kcal/L O_2/h
   b. Varies greatly from one species to another if expressed on the basis of surface area
   c. Is much greater in a 200-pound lumberjack than in a 200-pound medical student of the same age and sex
   d. Is increased in an individual with hyperthyroidism
   e. Is usually calculated from the respiratory quotient

21.4. A marathon runner with a respiratory quotient of 0.95 is
   a. Nearing the end of his journey
   b. Metabolizes largely carbohydrate
   c. Metabolizes largely fat
   d. Metabolizes largely ketone bodies
   e. Metabolizes equal amounts of carbohydrate and fat

21.5.   The O_2 consumption in an individual is 21.6 L/h. Approximately how many calories does she consume per day?

        a. 1500   b. 2000   c. 2500   d. 3000

        e. Impossible to calculate from information given

21.6.   Which is the most dramatic difference between metabolic states observed in the early and prolonged starvation stages?

    a. Blood glucagon levels in prolonged starvation are much higher than in early starvation.

    b. In prolonged starvation, protein degradation is much lower than that of early starvation.

    c. Use of ketone bodies is greatly diminished in prolonged starvation than early starvation.

    d. The use of fatty acids as a fuel is much higher in prolonged starvation than in early starvation.

    e. Amino acid degradation in prolonged starvation is much higher than that of early starvation.

21.7.   In prolonged starvation, which tissue remains primarily a glucose metabolizer?

        a. Skeletal muscle   b. Brain

        c. Red blood cells   d. Kidney   e. Liver

21.8.   Which is seen in untreated diabetes mellitus but not in starvation?

    a. Increased blood fatty acid levels

    b. Increased blood VLDL levels

    c. Increased levels of gluconeogenesis

    d. Increased levels of ketone bodies in blood

    e. Net catabolism of tissue protein

21.9.   Which is not a consequence of increased blood glucocorticoid levels?

    a. Net protein degradation in the muscle

    b. Net protein degradation in the liver

    c. Increased gluconeogenesis

    d. Increased lipolysis

    e. Increased movement of amino acids into the liver

21.10.   To utilize ketone bodies, a tissue must have a functioning

    a. Krebs cycle

    b. Gluconeogenesis pathway

    c. Glycolysis pathway

    d. Cholesterol biosynthesis pathway

    e. Hexose monophosphate shunt pathway

21.11.   In prolonged starvation, the major source of blood glucose is

    a. Glycogen

    b. Lactate and glycerol

    c. Ketone bodies

    d. Fatty acids

    e. Amino acids and lactate

21.12.   Which does *not* occur in the fed state?

    a. Increased cholesterol biosynthesis

    b. Net biosynthesis of glycogen in the muscle and liver

    c. Increased activity of pyruvate dehydrogenase in adipose tissue

    d. Increased secretion of glucocorticoids

    e. Increased rate of protein synthesis.

21.13.   Prolonged starvation differs from early starvation in that

    a. Nerve tissue switches from a primarily glucose utilization to ketone body utilization.

b. Muscle and kidney, in contrast to early starvation, do not utilize ketone bodies in prolonged starvation.

c. Glycerol utilization increases in prolonged starvation.

d. Fatty acid production from storage fat in adipose tissue increases in prolonged starvation.

e. Two of the above.

Answers

21.1. (a) Fatty acids increase in the bloodstream in a lipolysis environment, when blood glucagon levels are increased.

21.2. (d) Epinephrine increases muscle glycolysis, and therefore blood lactic acid production and an amplified Cori cycle. In the liver, epinephrine stimulates gluconeogenesis and blood glucose will therefore rise.

21.3. (d) BMR is increased in thyrotoxicosis cases. It is roughly the same in the two persons and is about the same in all species when calculated on the basis of surface area as opposed to weight. Total calorie consumption, not BMR, is calculated on the basis of the 5 kcal/L O_2/h.

21.4. (b) An RQ of 0.95 is closest to 1, which is characteristic of carbohydrate metabolism. In a marathon runner, this is observed at the beginning of the race.

21.5. (c) Using the approximation of 4.82 kcal/L O_2, we have $21.6 \times 4.82 = 104$ kcal/hour and $104 \times 24 = 2496$ kcal/day.

21.6. (b) Protein degradation rate is lowered drastically as the organism adapts to starvation. Glucagon levels remain about the same, as do ketone body and fatty acid utilization (see Figure 21.2).

21.7. (c) Most tissues switch to either fatty acid or ketone body utilization except the red and white blood cells, retina, and adrenal medulla. Even brain utilizes largely ketone bodies.

21.8. (b) Increased lipoprotein levels are seen in diabetes mellitus but not in starvation.

21.9. (b) Glucocorticoids have a protein catabolic activity in all tissues except liver. There, glucocorticoids stimulate protein synthesis.

21.10. (a) Ketone bodies are converted to acetyl-CoA, which must be metabolized via the Krebs cycle.

21.11. (e) Lactate and amino acids provide the largest glucose source (see Table 21.3). Glycerol is a minor, although an important glucose precursor as well.

21.12. (d) Blood glucocorticoid levels are up in stressful situations and in starvation. They are depressed, if anything, in the fed state.

21.13. (e) The correct answers are a and b (see Table 21.3). Glycerol and fatty acid production remain the same in early and prolonged starvation.

PROBLEMS

21.1. A 38-year-old woman weighing 213 kg had a fasting blood glucose level of 155 mg/dL and an insulin level of 28 μU/mL (normal is 6–24 μU/mL). She was given a glucose tolerance test, and after 90 minutes her blood glucose was 250 mg/dL, where it stayed for another 180 minutes. Her blood insulin level rose to 100 μg/dL during that period. Her lymphocytes bound between 1.1 and 1.4% of administered insulin per 56×10^6 cells. Following a weight reduction regimen, she lost 13 kg and her lymphocytes were able to bind 3.2% of administered insulin per 56×10^6 cells. This value is near normal.

Discuss the biochemical basis for this patient's disorder. What would her glucose tolerance curve be following the weight reduction program? What would her fasting blood glucose level be? Why was her blood insulin elevated before the weight reduction regimen, and what should it be following the weight loss?

21.2. A 29-year-old male was admitted to the hospital in a "confused" state. His blood glucose level was 650 mg/dL, glycosylated hemoglobin was 11% of total (normal is 4–6%), and serum "anion gap" was 27 meq/L (normal is 10–18 meq/L, with a mean of 16 meq/L). He was breathing rapidly in the Kussmaul style.

   Provide a biochemical explanation for this person's disorder. What is the difference between this patient and that in Problem 21.1? What is the significance of "Kussamaul" breathing? What is the significance of the elevated "anion gap" and glycosylated hemoglobin? Can you estimate this patient's blood pH and some electrolytes? How would you treat him?

BIBLIOGRAPHY

Brownlee M. Handbook of Diabetes Mellitus, Vol. 3. Intermediary Metabolism and Its Regulation. New York: Garland STPM Press, 1981.

Cahill GF, Jr. Starvation in man. N Engl J Med 282:668–675, 1971.

Consolazio CF, Johnson HL. Measurement of energy cost in humans. Fed Proc 30:1444–1453, 1971.

APPENDIXES

Appendix A: Common Biochemical Abbreviations

A	Adenine or adenosine
AA	Arachidonic acid
ACAT	Acyl CoA—cholesterol acyl transferase
ACP	Acyl carrier protein
ACTH	Adrenocorticotrophic hormone
ADH	Antidiuretic hormone (vasopressin)
ADP	Adenosine diphosphate
Ala	Alanine
ALA	δ-Aminolevulinate
AMP	Adenosine monophosphate
cAMP	Cyclic AMP
Arg	Arginine
Asn	Asparagine
AST	Aspartate aminotransferase (Glutamate-oxaloacetate transaminase)
ATP	Adenosine triphosphate
ATPase	Adenosine triphosphatase
BMR	Basal metabolic rate
BV	Biological value
C	Cytosine or cytidine
CAP	Catabolite activator protein
CDP	Cytidine diphosphate
CMP	Cytidine monophosphate
CoA	Coenzyme A
CoQ	Coenzyme Q (ubiquinone)
COMT	Catecholamine-O-Methyl Transferase
CPK (or CK)	Creatine phosphokinase
cpm	Counts (disintegrations) per minute
CPS	Carbamoyl phosphate synthetase
CT	Calcitonin
CTP	Cytidine triphosphate
Cyclic AMP (cAMP)	Adenosine 3′,5′-cyclic monophosphate
Cyclic GMP (cGMP)	Guanosine 3′,5′-cyclic monophosphate
Cys	Cysteine
Cyt	Cytochrome

DCCD	Dicyclohexylcarbodiimide
DHAP	Dihydroxyacetone phosphate
DNA	Deoxyribonucleic acid
cDNA	Complementary DNA
DNase	Deoxyribonuclease
DNP	Dinitrophenol
DOPA	L-Dihydroxyphenylalanine
2,3-DPG	2,3-Diphosphoglycerate
EDTA	Ethylenediaminetetraacetic acid
EPA	Eicosapentaenoic acid
ER	Endoplasmic reticulum
FA	Fatty acid
FAD	Flavin adenine dinucleotide (oxidized form)
FADH$_2$	Flavin adenine dinucleotide (reduced form)
FDP	Fructose 1,6-diphosphate
FFA	Free fatty acid
FH$_4$	Tetrahydrofolic acid
fMet	N-Formylmethionine
FMN	Flavin mononucleotide (oxidized form)
FMNH$_2$	Flavin mononucleotide (reduced form)
Fru	D-fructose
FSH	Follicle stimulating hormone
Fuc	Fucose
G	Guanine or guanosine, or ganglioside (depending on context)
$\Delta G_0'$	Standard free energy change
ΔG	Free energy change
GABA	γ-Aminobutyric acid
Gal	D-Galactose
Gal NAc	N-Acetyl-D-galactosamine
GDP	Guanosine diphosphate
GH	Growth hormone (somatotropin)
Glc	D-Glucose
Glc NAc	N-Acetyl-D-glucosamine
GlcUA	Glucuronic acid
Gln	Glutamine
Glu	Glutamate
Gly	Glycine
GMP	Guanosine monophosphate
GOT	Glutamate–oxaloacetate transaminase (aspartate aminotransferase)
GSH	Glutathione (reduced)
GSSG	Glutathione (oxidized)
GTP	Guanosine triphosphate
GTPase	Guanosine triphosphatase
Hb	Hemoglobin
HbC	Carbon monoxide hemoglobin
HbO$_2$	Oxyhemoglobin
HDL	High-density lipoprotein
His	Histidine
HMG CoA	β-Hydroxy-β-methylglutaryl CoA
HMPS	Hexose monophosphate shunt
Hp	Haptoglobin

HVA	Homovanillic acid
ICSH	Interstitial cell stimulating hormone
IDL	Intermediate density lipoprotein
IdUA	L-Iduronic acid
IgG	Immunoglobulin G
Ile	Isoleucine
IMP	Inosine monophosphate
IP_3	Inositol-1,4,5-triphosphate
pI	Isoelectric point
ITP	Inosine triphosphate
K_a	Association constant
KB	Kilobases (DNA or RNA)
Kcal	Kilocalories
K_d	Disassociation constant
K_i	Inhibition constant
K_m	Michaelis–Menten constant
L	Liter
dL	Deciliter
LCAT	Lecithin–Cholesterol Acyl Transferase
LDH	Lactate dehydrogenase
LDL	Low-density lipoprotein
Leu	Leucine
LH	Luteinizing hormone
Lys	Lysine
Man	Mannose
MAO	Monoamine oxidase
Mb	Myoglobin
MDH	Malate dehydrogenase
meq	Milliequivalent
Met	Methionine
Met Hb	Methemoglobin
MHPG	3-Methoxy-4-hydroxyphenylglycol
MSH	Melanocyte stimulating hormone
MW	Molecular weight
NAD^+, NAD	Nicotinamide adenine dinucleotide (oxidized form)
NADH	Nicotinamide adenine dinucleotide (reduced form)
$NADP^+$, NADP	Nicotinamide adenine dinucleotide phosphate (oxidized form)
NADPH	Nicotinamide adenine dinucleotide phosphate (reduced form)
Neu NAc	N-Acetylneuraminic acid (sialic acid)
NPN	Nonprotein nitrogen
NPU	Net protein utilization
PBG	Porphobilinogen
PC	Phosphatidylcholine or pyruvate carboxylase (depending on context)
PE	Phosphatidylethanolamine
PEP	Phosphoenolpyruvate
PEPCK	Phosphoenolpyruvate carboxykinase
PFK	Phosphofructokinase
PG	Prostaglandin
Phe	Phenylalanine
P_i	Inorganic orthophosphate
PI	Phospatidyl inositol

PLP	Pyridoxal phosphate
PP$_i$	Inorganic pyrophosphate
PRL	Prolactin
PRPP	5-Phosphoribosyl-1-pyrophosphate, phos-phoribosylpyrophosphate
PS	Phosphatidylserine
PTH	Parathyroid hormone
RDS	Respiratory distress syndrome
RE	Reticuloendothelial system
RNA	Ribonucleic acid
hnRNA	Heterogenous nuclear RNA
mRNA	Messenger RNA
rRNA	Ribosomol RNA
tRNA	Transfer RNA
RNase	Ribonuclease
RQ	Respiratory quotient
S	Svedberg unit
SAM	*S*-Adenosylmethionine
Ser	Serine
SM	Sphingomyelin
T	Thymine or thymidine
$t_{1/2}$	Half-life
T$_3$	Triiodothyronine
T$_4$	Thyroxine
TBG	Thyroxine-binding globulin
THF	Tetrahydrofolate
Thr	Threonine
TI	Total plasma iron
TIBC	Total iron-binding capacity
TPN	Total parenteral nutrition
TPP	Thiamine pyrophosphate
Trp	Tryptophan
TSH	Thyroid stimulating hormone
TTP	Thiamine triphosphate
TSH	Thyroid stimulating hormone
TX	Thromboxane
U	Uracil or uridine
UDP	Uridine diphosphate
UDP gal	Uridine diphosphate galactose
UDP glc	Uridine diphosphate glucose
UMP	Uridine monophosphate
UTP	Uridine triphosphate
V	Volts
mV	Millivolts
Val	Valine
VLDL	Very low density lipoprotein
VMA	Vanillylmandelic acid
V_{max}	Maximum velocity
Xyl	Xylose

Appendix B: Atomic Numbers and Weights of Biologically Important Elements

Element	Symbol	Atomic number	Atomic weight
Calcium	Ca	20	40.1
Carbon	C	6	12.0
Chlorine	Cl	17	35.5
Chromium	Cr	24	52.0
Cobalt	Co	27	58.9
Copper	Cu	29	63.6
Fluorine	F	9	19.0
Hydrogen	H	1	1.00
Iodine	I	53	127
Iron	Fe	26	55.8
Lead	Pb	82	207
Lithium	Li	3	6.94
Magnesium	Mg	12	24.3
Manganese	Mn	25	54.9
Molybdenum	Mo	42	96.0
Nitrogen	N	7	14.0
Oxygen	O	8	16.0
Phosphorus	P	15	31.0
Potassium	K	19	39.1
Selenium	Se	34	79.0
Sodium	Na	11	23.0
Sulfur	S	16	32.1
Zinc	Zn	30	65.4

Appendix C: Selected Normal Clinical Biochemistry Analytes

Electrolytes and gases

Anion gap (meq/L)	7–14 (mean 12)
Bicarbonate (meq/L)	
Arterial blood	18–23
Arterial plasma	21–28
Venous plasma	22–29
Calcium (mg/dL)	
Total	8.4–10.2
Ionized	2.25–2.60
Carbon dioxide (pCO_2, whole blood, mm Hg)	35–48 (M), 32–45 (F)
Chloride (meq/L)	98–106
Osmolality (mOsmol/kg)	275–295
Oxygen (pO_2, arterial blood, mm Hg)	83–108
pH (arterial blood)	7.35–7.45
Phosphorus (inorganic, mg/dL)	2.7–4.5
Potassium (meq/L)	3.5–5.1
Sodium (meq/L)	136–146
Total CO_2 (arterial blood, meq/L)	19–24

Nitrogenous substances

Amino acid nitrogen (mg/dL)	4.0–6.0
δ-Aminolevulinic acid (urine, mg/day)	1.7–7.0
Ammonia (ug N/dL)	15–49
Bilirubin (mg/dL)	
Total	0.2–1.0
Conjugated (direct)	0–0.2
Coproporphyrin (urine, ug/day)	34–234
Creatinine (mg/dL)	0.5–1.2
Non-protein nitrogen (NPN, mg/dL)	
Blood	<50
Serum	<35
Urea nitrogen (BUN, mg/dL)	7–18
Uric acid (mg/dL)	4.5–8.2 (M), 3.0–6.5 (F)
Urobilinogen (fecal, mg/day)	40–280

Lipid metabolism indicators

Cholesterol (mg/dL)	
Total	140–310

HDL cholesterol	30–70 (M), 30–80 (F)
LDL cholesterol, age 40–49	90–205 (M), 80–190 (F)
Fat (fecal, g/day)	<7
Ketone bodies	Undetectable
Triglycerides (mg/dL), age 40–49	56–298 (M), 44–186 (F)

Hormones and their derivatives

C-peptide (ng/mL)	1.5–5.0 (M), 1.4–5.5 (F)
Glucagon (pg/dL)	
Normal	30–210 (mean 75)
Hyperglycemic diabetes	1525 ± 578
Homovanillic acid (HVA, urine, mg/day)	<15
Insulin (fasting, μU/mL)	6–24
Thyroxine (total, μg/dL)	5–10 (M), 5.5–10.5 (F)
Triiodothyronine (total, ng/dL)	115–190
Vanillylmandelic acid (VMA, urine, mg/day)	2–7

Metals (also see *Electrolytes*)

Copper (μg/dL)	70–140
Iron (TI, μg/dL)	50–160 (M), 40–150 (F)
Iron-binding capacity (TIBC, μg/dL)	250–400
Lead (whole blood, μg/dL)	<30 (child), <40 (adult)
Magnesium (meq/L)	1.3–2.1
Zinc (μg/dL)	70–150

Blood proteins

α_1-Antitrypsin (M-phenotype, mg/dL)	220 ± 20
Ceruloplasmin (mg/dL)	30± 12.4
Ferritin (ng/mL)	15–200 (M), 12–150 (F)
Fibrinogen (plasma, mg/dL)	200–400
Haptoglobin (mg/dL)	83–267 (mean 175)
Hemoglobin (whole blood, g/dL)	13.5–17.5 (M), 12.0–16.0 (F)
IgA (mg/dL)	90–450 (mean 210)
IgG (mg/dL)	565–1765 (mean 1047)
IgM (mg/dL)	60–250 (mean 125)
Serum protein panel (g/dL)	
Albumin	3.5–5.0 (mean 4.2)
α_1-globulin	0.1–0.3 (mean 0.2)
α_2-globulin	0.6–1.0 (mean 0.8)
β-globulin	0.7–1.1 (mean 0.9)
γ-globulin	0.8–1.6 (mean 1.2)
Total protein (g/dL)	6.4–8.3
Transferrin (mg/dL)	200–400 (mean 295)

Enzymes

Acid phosphatase (total, U/L)	2.5–11.7 (M), 0.3–9.2 (F)
Alanine aminotransferase (ALT, SGPT, U/L)	8–20
Aldolase (U/L)	3.1–7.5 (M), 2.7–5.3 (F)
Alkaline phosphatase (ALP, SMA 12, U/L)	30–90 (M), 20–80 (F)
Amylase (U/L)	25–125
Aspartate aminotransferase (AST, SGOT, U/L)	8–20
Creatine phosphokinase (CPK, CK, U/L)	38–174 (M), 96–140 (F)
γ-glutamyl transferase (U/L)	22.1 ± 11.7 (M), 15.4 ± 6.58 (F)
Lactate dehydrogenase (LDH, U/L)	210–420
Lipase (U/L)	<200

Miscellaneous substances

Galactose (mg/dL)	5
Glucose (fasting, mg/dL)	70–105
Lactate (venous blood, mg/dL)	4.5–19.8
Pyruvate (mg/dL)	0.3–0.9

Note: Normal values are for adult serum or plasma, unless otherwise noted.

Abbreviations: dL, deciliter; F, female; g, gram(s); kg, kilogram(s); L, liter; M, male; meq, milliequivalents; mg, milligram(s); mL, milliliter(s); mm, millimeter(s); m0smol, milliosmole(s); ng, nanogram(s); pg, picogram(s); U, international unit, defined as 16.7×10^{-9} moles of substrate transformed by an enzyme per second; μg, microgram(s)

Source: Tietz, NW. 1983. *Clinical Guide to Laboratory Tests.* Philadelphia: WB Saunders.

Index

T - #0130 - 160425 - C0 - 254/178/34 - PB - 9780824797362 - Gloss Lamination